SIDE EFFECTS OF DRUGS
ANNUAL 14 (1990)

Complementary to this volume:

SIDE EFFECTS OF DRUGS ANNUALS 1 – 13 (1977 – 1989)
Edited by M.N.G. Dukes

MEYLER'S SIDE EFFECTS OF DRUGS, 11th EDITION (1988)
Edited by M.N.G. Dukes

SEDBASE – The Side Effects of Drugs Database

DRUG-INDUCED DISORDERS
Edited by M.N.G. Dukes

Vol. 1 Drug-Induced Hepatic Injury (1985)
B.H.Ch. Stricker and P. Spoelstra

Vol. 2 Drug-Induced Diseases in the Elderly (1986)
F.I. Caird and P.J.W. Scott

Vol. 3 Treatment-Induced Respiratory Disorders (1989)
G.M. Akoun and J.P. White

Vol. 4 Drug-induced Immune Disease (1990)
J. Descotes

UNWANTED EFFECTS OF COSMETICS AND DRUGS USED IN DERMATOLOGY, 2nd EDITION (1985)
J.P. Nater and A.C. de Groot

IMMUNOTOXICOLOGY OF DRUGS AND CHEMICALS, 2nd EDITION (1986)
J. Descotes

DRUGS AND HUMAN LACTATION (1988)
P.N. Bennett and the WHO Working Group

DRUG SAFETY IN PREGNANCY (1990)
P.I. Folb

RESPONSIBILITY FOR DRUG-INDUCED INJURY (1988)
M.N.G. Dukes and B. Swartz

SIDE EFFECTS OF DRUGS ANNUAL 14

A worldwide yearly survey of new data and trends

EDITORS

M.N.G. DUKES M.D., M.A., LL.M.

Professor of Drug Policy Science
University of Groningen, The Netherlands

L. BEELEY M.A., F.R.C.P.

Drug and Therapeutics Unit, The Queen Elizabeth Hospital
Birmingham, United Kingdom

1990
ELSEVIER, Amsterdam – New York – Oxford

ISBN 0 444 81346 2
ISSN 0378-6080

This book is printed on acid-free paper.

Published by:
Elsevier Science Publishers B.V. (Biomedical Division)
P.O. Box 211
1000 AE Amsterdam
The Netherlands

Sole distributors for the U.S.A. and Canada:
Elsevier Science Publishing Co. Inc.
655 Avenue of the Americas
New York, NY 10010
U.S.A.

Printed in The Netherlands

Contributors

G. AGNELLI, M.D.
Istituto di Semeiotica Medica, University of Perugia, Via Enrico dal Pozzo, 06100 Perugia, Italy

S. AGOSTON, M.D.
Research Group of the Institutes of Experimental Anesthesiology and Clinical Pharmacology, University of Groningen, Oostersingel 59, 9713 EZ Groningen, The Netherlands

G. ANSELL, M.D., F.R.C.P., F.R.C.R.
101 Childwall Park Avenue, Liverpool L16 0JF, U.K.

K.M. ARANKO, M.D.
Department of Clinical Pharmacology, University of Helsinki, Paasikivenkatu 4, SF-00250 Helsinki, Finland

J.K. ARONSON, M.A., D.Phil., M.B., F.R.C.P.
MRC Unit and University Department of Clinical Pharmacology, Radcliffe Infirmary, Woodstock Road, Oxford OX2 6HE, U.K.

A.V. ASTAKHOVA, M.D.
All-Union Center for Study on Side Effects of Drugs, Ministry of Health, Per. Rachmanovsky 3, Moscow 1-51, U.S.S.R.

N. BAILEY, M.R.C.P.
West Midlands Clinical Trials Unit, Clinical Research Block, Queen Elizabeth Hospital, Edgbaston, Birmingham B15 2TH, U.K.

A.G.C. BAUER, M.D.
Havenziekenhuis, Haringvliet 2, 3011 TD Rotterdam, The Netherlands

G. BLACKLEDGE, M.D., PH. D., F.R.C.P.
West Midlands Clinical Trials Unit, Queen Elizabeth Hospital, Edgbaston, Birmingham B15 2TH, U.K.

R. BOUILLON, M.D.
Laboratory for Experimental Medicine and Endocrinology (LEGENDO), Catholic University of Leuven, Gasthuisberg, Herestraat 49, 3000 Leuven, Belgium

D. CAPELLÀ, M.D.
Unitat de Farmacologia Clìnica, Universitat Autònoma de Barcelona, Spanish Centre for Drug Monitoring in the WHO International Programme, Ciutat Sanitaria de la Vall d'Hebron, 08035 Barcelona, Spain

N.H. CHOULIS, M.D.
Department of Pharmacy, University of Athens, 104 Solonos Street, 106 80 Athens, Greece

A.C. DE GROOT, M.D., PH.D.
Department of Dermatology, Carolus Hospital, P.O. Box 1101, 5200 BD 's Hertogenbosch, The Netherlands

A. DEL FAVERO, M.D.
University of Perugia, Institute of Clinical Medicine, Policlinico Monteluce, 06 100 Perugia, Italy

J. DESCOTES, M.D., PH.D., Pharm.D.
Lyons Poison Control Center and Laboratory of Fundamental and Clinical Immunotoxicology, INSERM U80 – CNRS UA1177-UCBL, Alexis Carrel Faculty of Medicine, 69008, Lyons, France

P.A.G.M. DE SMET, PH.D.
Drug Information Center, Royal Dutch Association for the Advancement of Pharmacy, Alexanderstraat 11, 2514 JL The Hague, The Netherlands

S. DITTMANN, M.D., D.SC.MED.
Central Institute of Hygiene, Microbiology and Epidemiology, Britzer Strasse 1-3, 1190 Berlin, F.R.G.

M.N.G. DUKES, M.D., M.A., LL.M.
Drug Policy and Management Division, World Health Organization, 8, Scherfigsvej, 2100 Copenhagen Ø, Denmark

C.J. ELLIS, M.D., F.R.C.P.
Department of Communicable and Tropical Diseases, East Birmingham Hospital, Bordsley Green East, Birmingham B9 5ST, U.K.

S. ERILL, M.D.
Esteve Foundation, Llobet i Vall-Llosera 2, 08032 Barcelona, Spain

J.-C. EVREUX, M.D.
Post-Marketing Drug Surveillance, Regional Center, Edouard Herriot Hospital, 69003 Lyons, France

P.I. FOLB, M.D., F.R.C.P.
Department of Pharmacology, University of Cape Town Medical School, Groote Schuur Hospital, Observatory 7925, South Africa

B. GHODSE, M.A., M.B., M.R.C.P.
42 Alwyne Road, London, SW19 7AE, U.K.

A.H. GHODSE, M.D., PH.D., F.R.C.Psych.
Department of Psychiatry, St. George's Hospital Medical School, Jenner Wing, Cranmer Terrace, London SW17 ORE, U.K.

A.I. GREEN, M.D.
Department of Psychiatry, Harvard Medical School, Massachusetts Mental Health Center, 74 Fenwood Road, Boston, MA 02115, U.S.A.

E. HELSING, PH.D.
Nutrition Programme, World Health Organization, 8 Scherfigsvej, 2100 Copenhagen Ø, Denmark

J.E. IDÄNPÄÄN-HEIKKILÄ, M.D.
The National Board of Health, Siltasaarenkatu 18A, PB 223, 00530 Helsinki 53, Finland

I.A. JAFFE, M.D.
Department of Medicine, College of Physicians and Surgeons of Columbia University, 630 West 168th Street, New York, NY 10032, U.S.A.

T.C. JERRAM, M.B., M.R.C.Psych.
High Royds Hospital, Menston, Ilkley LS29 6AQ, West Yorkshire, U.K.

H.M.J. KRANS, M.D.
Department of Endocrinology and Metabolic Diseases, University Hospital, Building 1, C4-R, Rijnsburgerweg 10, 2333 RC Leiden, The Netherlands

W. LAMMERS, M.D.
Dean's Office, College of Medicine, P.O. Box 22979, Bahrain

J.-R. LAPORTE, M.D.
Unitat de Farmacologia Clìnica, Universitat Autònoma de Barcelona, Spanish Centre for Drug Monitoring in the WHO International Programme, Ciutat Sanitaria de la Vall d'Hebron, 08035 Barcelona, Spain

C. LAROUSSE, M.D.
Pharmacologie Clinique et Centre de Pharmacovigilance, Hôtel-Dieu, B.P. 1005, 44035 Nantes Cédex 01, France

Y. LE NORMAND, M.D.
Centre de Pharmacovigilance, Hôtel-Dieu, B.P. 1005, 44035 Nantes Cédex 01, France

V.K. LEPAKHIN, M.D.
Pharmacological Committee, Ministry of Health, Kropotkinsky Pereulok 25/9, Moscow, U.S.S.R.

I. LUNDE, M. Pharm.
Pharmaceuticals, World Health Organization, Regional Office for Europe, 8, Scherfigsvej, 2100 Copenhagen Ø, Denmark

M. MALINGE, M.D.
Département d'Anesthésie, Hôtel-Dieu, 11, rue Gaston Veil, 44035 Nantes Cédex 01, France

G.T. McINNES, M.B., F.R.C.P.
University of Glasgow, Department of Medicine and Therapeutics, Gardiner Institute, Western Infirmary, Glasgow G11 6NT, U.K.

R.H.B. MEYBOOM, M.D.
Netherlands Centre for Monitoring of Adverse Reactions to Drugs, P.O. Box 5406, 2280 HK Rijswijk, The Netherlands

T. MIDTVEDT, M.D.
Department of Medical Microbial Ecology, Karolinska Institutet, Box 60 400, 104 01 Stockholm, Sweden

J.C. MUCKLOW, M.D., F.R.C.P.
Department of Clinical Pharmacology, North Staffordshire Hospital Centre, Newcastle Road, Stoke-on-Trent ST4 6QG, U.K.

J.P. NATER, M.D.
Department of Dermatology, University of Groningen, Oostersingel 59, 9713 EZ Groningen, The Netherlands

F.A. NELEMANS, M.D., PH.D.
Foundation for Therapeutic Evaluation of Medicine, Saturnus 109, 1115 TJ Duivendrecht, The Netherlands

I. NIR, M.D., PH.D
Department of Pharmacology and Experimental Therapeutics, Hebrew University, Hadassah Medical School, P.O. Box 12065, 91010 Jerusalem, Israel

O.R. ØDEGAARD, M.D.
Department of Clinical Chemistry, Aker Hospital, Trondhjemsveien 235, 0514 Oslo 5, Norway

B.C.P. POLAK, M.D.
Department of Ophthalmology, Erasmus University, Eye Hospital, Schiedamse Vest 180, 3011 BH Rotterdam, The Netherlands

H.D. REUTER, PH.D.
Department of Medicine I, University Hospital, Joseph-Stelzmann-Strasse 9, 5000 Cologne 41, F.R.G.

G. REYBROUCK, M.D.
Public Health Laboratory, School of Public Health, Catholic University of Leuven, Kapucijnenvoer 33, 3000 Leuven, Belgium

F.J. RICHARDSON, M.D.
Research Group of the Institutes of Experimental Anesthesiology and Clinical Pharmacology, University of Groningen, Oostersingel 59, 9713 EZ Groningen, The Netherlands

C. SALZMAN, M.D.
Department of Psychiatry, Harvard Medical School, Massachusetts Mental Health Center, 74 Fenwood Road, Boston, MA 02115, U.S.A.

M. SCHOU, M.D.
Psychiatric Hospital, 2 Skovagervej, 8240 Risskov, Denmark

R.P. SEQUEIRA, PH.D.
Department of Pharmacology and Clinical Pharmacology, College of Medicine and Medical Sciences, Arabian Gulf University, P.O. Box 22979, Manama, Bahrain

J.A. STEINER, M.B., D. Phil., F.R.A.C.P., M.B.A.
Gensia Europe Ltd., Wolfelands, High Street, Westerham, Kent TN16 1RQ, U.K.

F.A. VAN ASSCHE, M.D.
Department of Gynecology, Catholic University of Leuven, Gasthuisberg, Herestraat 49, 3000 Leuven, Belgium

PH. VANHOVE, M.D.
Center for Thrombosis and Vascular Research, Department of Medical Research, Catholic University of Leuven, Gasthuisberg, Herestraat 49, 3000 Leuven, Belgium

P.L.C.M. VAN RIEL, M.D.
Department of Rheumatology, University Hospital, Postbus 9101, 6500 HB Nijmegen, The Netherlands

R. VERHAEGHE, M.D.
Center for Thrombosis and Vascular Research, Department of Medical Research, Catholic University of Leuven, Gasthuisberg, Herestraat 49, 3000 Leuven, Belgium

J. VERMYLEN, M.D.
Center for Thrombosis and Vascular Research, Department of Medical Research, Catholic University of Leuven, Gasthuisberg, Herestraat 49, 3000 Leuven, Belgium

M. VERSTRAETE, M.D.
Center for Thrombosis and Vascular Research, Department of Medical Research, Catholic University of Leuven, Gasthuisberg, Herestraat 49, 3000 Leuven, Belgium

K.-W. VON EICKSTEDT, M.D.
Neue Landstrasse 15A, 3000 Hannover 51, F.R.G.

Contents

Special reviews

How to use this book

THE SCOPE OF THE 'ANNUAL'

The Side Effects of Drugs Annual has been published each year since 1977. It is designed to provide a critical and up-to-date account of new information relating to adverse drug reactions and interactions from the clinician's point of view. The *Annual* can be used independently or as a supplement to the standard encyclopedic work in this field, *Meyler's Side Effects of Drugs*, the eleventh edition of which was published in November, 1988.

℞ *SPECIAL REVIEWS*

As new data appear, older findings may be discredited and existing concepts may require revision. Twenty 'special reviews' deal critically with such topics, interpreting conflicting evidence and providing the reader with clear guidance. Special reviews are identified by the traditional prescription symbol and are printed in italic type. Older papers cited in these reviews are either listed by name or via cross-references to previous Annuals or past editions of Meyler's Side Effects of Drugs, which can be found in most medical libraries.

SELECTION OF MATERIAL

In compiling the *Side Effects of Drugs Annual* particular attention is devoted to those publications which provide essentially new information or throw a new light on problems already recognized. In addition, some authoritative new reviews are listed. Publications which do not meet these criteria are omitted. Readers anxious to trace all references on a particular topic, including those which duplicate earlier work, are advised to consult *Adverse Reactions Titles*, a monthly bibliography of titles from approximately 3400 biomedical journals published throughout the world, compiled by the Excerpta Medica International Abstracting Service.

PERIOD COVERED

The present *Annual* reviews all reports presenting significant new information on adverse reactions to drugs from July 1st 1988 to February 1990. During the production of this *Annual*, more recent papers have been included.

CLASSIFICATION

Drugs are classified according to their main field of application or the properties for which they are most generally recognized. In borderline cases, however, some supplementary discussion has been included in other chapters relating to secondary fields of application. Fixed combinations of drugs are dealt with according to their most characteristic component.

DRUG NAMES

Drug products are in general dealt with in the text under their most usual non-proprietary names; where these are not available, chemical names have been used; fixed combinations usually have no proprietary connotation and here trade names have been used as necessary.

SYSTEM OF REFERENCES

References in the text are coded as follows:

R: In the original paper, the point is *reviewed* in some detail with reference to other literature.

r: The original paper *refers* only briefly to the point, on the basis of evidence adduced by other writers.

C: The original paper presents *detailed original clinical evidence* on this point.

c: The original paper provides *clinical evidence*, but only *briefly*.

The code has not been applied to animal pharmacological papers.

The various Editions of *Meyler's Side Effects of Drugs* are cited in the text as SED-9, SED-10 etc.; *SED Annuals 1–13* are cited as SEDA-1, SEDA-2 etc.

INDEXES

Index of Drugs: This index provides a complete listing of all references to a drug in this volume.

Index of Side Effects: This index is necessarily selective, since a particular side effect may be caused by very large numbers of compounds; the index is therefore mainly directed to those side effects which are particularly serious or frequent, or are discussed in special detail. Before assuming that a given drug does not have a particular side effect, one should consult the relevant chapters.

To help the clinical reader, side effects are classified according to the system or phenomenon involved. All adverse reactions involving the skin will for example be found together, listed under both general and specific headings; in looking for drugs causing 'erythema' or 'pruritus', one will thus also be able to check rapidly whether these drugs also affect the skin or hair in other ways.

For *interactions,* the reader should refer to the *Index of Drugs* where all interactions are listed under the drugs concerned, irrespective of the chapter in which they appear.

It should be borne in mind that American spelling has been used throughout, e.g. anemia, estrogen etc. (instead of anaemia, oestrogen etc.).

The indexes have been compiled by Dr. H. Kettner, Middelburg, The Netherlands.

The great cholesterol carrousel

Graham Dukes and Elisabet Helsing

Of all the delicious absurdities to which human creativity in its more puckish moments has given birth, the great steam carrousel — the roundabout to end all roundabouts — must rank as one of the most delectable. Somewhere, surely, there must be one of them left to warm the heart? Mark well, it must be a *genuine* steam carrousel, and not an anemic mummy turning tamely on electricity and compressed air in some fairground museum. Out in the hustle of a country summer wakes it must be, with stalls and sideshows and hawkers noising all around, and everything of its own self pounding away to feed the eyes, the ears, the nose and the very soul with thrills; there must be swarthy men shovelling coke into the engine grate, furious steam to feed the organ, gasps of smoke going up into the dusk ... and there must be horses in white and gold and decked in glittering things, prancing proudly and unendingly to the music, forever and magnificently going nowhere.

The serious things in life (which include many but not all of the medicines with which ingenious industry has blessed us) are not supposed to be like that at all. By the light of day we are deemed to consecrate our resources to progress, our minds to considering our current course and the way ahead, and to make our choices dispassionately and with a proper sense of our responsibilities to one another and ourselves. The idea is quite noble. The practice is sometimes rather more akin to the carrousel; we go around in circles, and choose to be excited by it, losing the while sight of the horizon.

Alliteration apart, we would surely never have set the name of cholesterol alongside that of the carrousel of yore had we not alighted one day, while rummaging through some medical journals of 30 years ago, on an advertisement dated 1961 for a lipid-lowering medicine. It was, the reader of the time was given to understand, a breakthrough; a group of right-minded physicians had voted it the most substantial medical advance of the previous year. Having through much effort gained a better understanding of the molecular biology concerned, science had now created an instrument wherewith to control some part of it; a neat adjustment to the body's metabolic processes was within the reach of the prescribing pad. The cholesterol problem had been solved.

When looking back on some of the promises, the genuine hopes and the explanations of 30 years ago, one sometimes gets a feeling which we can only term *déjà vu* in reverse; we have heard much the same things said since — not once only, but on a fair number of occasions. That would not matter if society had been proceeding in a fairly straight line, or at least a progressive spiral, slowly edging towards a better world. In some fields of drug research, that is the way things have gone; the goal — be it the non-surgical cure of peptic ulcer or the non-soporific relief of hay fever — has been a well-defined and necessary one, and we have moved towards its attainment. On both counts, the lipid-lowering story is less exemplary. For the largest part of the target population, views differ as to what we want to achieve and whether we should be trying to achieve what-

*The Side Effects of Drugs Essay is written each year by an external contributor. Dr. Elisabet Helsing is head of the Nutritional Programme, World Health Organization, Scherfigsvej 8, 2100 Copenhagen Ø, Denmark.

Side Effects of Drugs Annual 14 M.N.G. Dukes and L. Beeley, editors ever it may be with drugs. But quite apart from that, we have in this field anything but a clean record on safety. Neither of us as individuals is particularly prone to undue worry, least of all about the need to measure and meddle with our own blood cholesterol. But if we set alongside one another the history of drug treatment in this field and the sometimes ill-defined objectives which such treatment has been supposed to serve, we look ahead into the 1990s with concern, for society does not seem to have learnt sufficiently from experience. If that makes us gloomy Cassandras, then so be it.

THE DRUGS

The drug which we encountered in our yellowed journal of 1961 was triparanol — Mer-29 — of unhallowed memory. It is not the most typical story with which to begin, but it is the earliest.

The tale is untypical in that the problems which the drug induced arose relatively early in its career, rather than after a long period of treatment; in that particular case there was also a very clear failure on the part of the manufacturer to do what he could have done to predict the drug's ill effects, and to detect and report them when they did occur. There is, however, another familiar element in the story: the injury which triparanol caused was attributable not to any direct toxicity of the drug itself but to the very metabolic interference which it was both claimed and designed to produce, namely a blockage in the last phase of endogenous formation of cholesterol. As a result its precursor desmosterol rapidly accumulated in the system, resulting in a range of serious effects varying from hair loss to cataract and worse. The drug itself was hastily withdrawn. Injured patients hurried to court to sue the manufacturer, and the entire history of triparanol was chronicled as one of the drug disasters of the age. The more general lesson which could and should however have been learnt is surely that whosoever interferes chemically and incautiously with lipid metabolism does so at his peril. Even with a less unsubtle form of interference than that offered by triparanol one might be expected to upset a complex system of checks and balances, inviting consequences which it may be difficult to predict or overview.

In the case of ICI's clofibrate, the first major clinical reports on which dated from the late 1960s, there is no need to raise the question of serious fault on the part of the drug's originators; by all accounts it had been respectably studied in both animals and man; after marketing, too, the company went along willingly with a project coordinated by the World Health Organization to examine its long-term effects in 3 European centers (1). The interpretation of certain findings from that study has not gone entirely unquestioned, but it did show a disproportionate mortality among treated males as compared to controls, attributable primarily to a greater incidence of gastrointestinal tumors and in part to problems with gallstones. The direct result of that study was an almost universal restriction of the indication for clofibrate; a product which had come into very widespread use for a dozen different lipid disorders was henceforth to be used only for those relatively few patients with severe familial hyperlipidemias in whom, because of the poor prognosis of the condition itself, one could accept some degree of alternative risk.

This time, the primary lesson was essentially that some of the risks of lipid interference might emerge only after a very long period of treatment in human subjects. The average period of observation in the clofibrate trial was 13.2 years — 5.3 years in the trial itself and 7.9 years of follow-up — and the very fact that the interpretation of it all is disputed points to the fact that with any other drug used for such a purpose trials are needed which are even larger and longer-lasting. The emergence of the specter of late risk created the need for very conscientious long-term safety monitoring of such drugs in the future, but it also demanded a great deal of caution in marketing. From that time onwards there could surely be no reason to release or sell any new drug immediately for the treatment of lipid disorders as a whole; the starting point would necessarily be the small population at grave risk.

The WHO findings of the mid-1970s left at least one important question unanswered. Were the risks which had become manifest with clofibrate a reflection of the drug's own properties? Or were they — as had been the case with triparanol — an unforeseen consequence of the very effect which the drug had been designed to achieve? The answer has emerged only slowly, and has come primarily from the epidemiologists. The 1986 Multiple Risk Factor Intervention Study (2,3) like earlier work from the group headed by McMichael (4) showed that low cholesterol levels in middle-aged men were correlated with a higher incidence of cancer, particularly colorectal tumors, and the general impression today (although even that is disputed) is that the low cholesterol was the cause rather than the consequence of the cancers (5). Such evidence has sometimes been interpreted to mean that an all too drastic reduction in lipids, induced with drugs or by other means, is the cause of the sort of problems which clofibrate encountered. Again, however, the truth is elusive, and we shall look at some of the complexities in a moment. At this point let us merely record the now widely-held view that one can easily go too far in lowering cholesterol; any measure designed to lower cholesterol levels in the population should be cautious and selective so that it does not further reduce these levels in individuals in whom it is already low enough; to do so could be to increase further their existing risk of tumors and probably (cholesterol being such an essential part of physiology) to invite other problems as well.

The lessons presented by gemfibrozil and probucol are rather different from those which one learned with clofibrate. Both arrived on the tables of regulatory agencies in the late 1970s, and with the experience of clofibrate fresh in mind several such agencies boldly set out to demand that before they could be marketed the manufacturers should provide some proof that their products did indeed help to prevent coronary heart disease or improve its prognosis, as well as demonstrating the drug's long-term safety. The result of such demands was sometimes deadlock, sometimes outrage, but also some useful discussion as to what evidence society reasonably can and should demand before it exposes itself to new drugs the expressed aim of which is to confer a very long-term benefit. Patents and returns on research investment being what they are, it is unrealistic to call for 10 years of clinical study before a new drug is sold at all, yet that in fact is what medical logic would demand. For neither drug could one extrapolate from its effects on the lipid spectrum either to its likely effects on coronary disease or to its possible late adverse effects, as the lipid effects of each were different from those of the drugs which had gone before; whereas clofibrate, for example, acted mainly by inhibiting the synthesis and promoting the breakdown of very-low-density lipoproteins, gemfibrozil primarily raised triglycerides and high-density lipoprotein (HDL)-associated cholesterol, the effect on low-density lipoprotein (LDL) being variable; probucol reduced both HDL- and LDL-cholesterol. Despite several studies in the decade since gemfibrozil and probucol first emerged, there is persisting uncertainty as to how useful and safe those effects will be in the long term as compared with others. And let us be clear what we mean by 'the long term'; we shall not really be able to conclude that we know enough about any such a drug until it has been prescribed in early middle age to a great many carefully monitored patients, and until these have been followed for the rest of their lives. By that time, will gemfibrozil, probucol or most of their contemporaries still be around?

Several of the other drugs which have come (and sometimes also gone) deserve only brief mention; a fair number of such horses prance exotically on the cholesterol carrousel in the course of a decade, chasing one another to the accompaniment of much noise, yet largely leaving us where we were before. Sometimes no one really seems to care how useful and safe they really are. Do you remember dextrothyroxine, that curious and unsuccessful effort to dissociate the lipid effects of thyroid completely from the endocrine? And what is one to think of the various congeners of clofibrate, not one of which has been subjected to the sort of painstaking long-term study which clofibrate enjoyed? Some of them are as close as no matter to clofibrate itself, others deviate sufficiently in their lipid effects to merit quite separate study; in either case one gets worried from time to time to see the promoters of some such products veering across the thin red line which distinguishes enterprise from recklessness.

In the meantime some old products, carthorses rather than carrousel horses, have plodded unspectacularly along, each contributing in some measure to the field. It is good that they have been there. Niacin and neomycin have done something for those who tolerate them. The ion-exchange resins still feature at the top of the U.S. Cholesterol Education Program's list of top hits and deserve to do; their troublesome interactions (and their dreadful impalatability) apart, they probably represent the safest drug-based approach imaginable, for they do not get into the bodily system al all.

It was towards the end of the 1980s that all these products first threatened to be upstaged by something which promised to be both new and spectacular. The inhibitors of hydroxymethylglutaryl coenzyme A (HMG-CoA) reductase — lovastatin, simvastatin and their siblings — were not merely placed upon the market; they arrived with fanfares of trumpets worthy of an army of Liberaces. The HMG-CoA reductase inhibitors were both different from and similar to what had gone before (6). Essentially, they competitively inhibit the rate-limiting enzyme in cholesterol biosynthesis, reducing LDL-cholesterol by some 25–45%. With some years of clinical research to hand one is told that the effect is maintained so long as treatment continues. As to adverse effects: over this same period of time one seems to have no great trouble. The transaminases may rise; there may be rhabdomyolysis when lovastatin is part of a multi-drug regimen; suggestions that one might with these drugs induce cataract have been rejected with some explanation. What one will see after 10 or 20 years is in the lap of the gods. That is all one can say with certainty.

There are some drugs the very chemistry of which gives one the creeps; there are others where the toxicology and the early human studies forbode doom. The HMG-CoA reductase inhibitors are not like that; one can deliver an honest speech about them and leave the audience jubilant. Nor can one be too sombre about selective enzyme inhibitions as such; the trick was pulled off nicely with carbidopa 20 years ago with no apparent ill consequences. Why, then, does one have something of a sinking feeling in the stomach at the HMG-CoA reductase phenomenon? The best answer is that the community seems to be rushing headlong into the mist. It is precisely the phenomenology which is worrying. In this particular field, suggestions of hepatic effects and cataract are not unfamiliar from past experience, but we talk them away; when one early member of the series causes lymphomas in dogs, we are assured that this is irrelevant to the safety of its congeners; we deal in the same way with any suggestion that one should not meddle lightly with cholesterol synthesis; the cries of 'breakthrough' have been heard many times before, yet once again they seduce us into long-term use of something which has been tested only relatively briefly and modestly, as compared with the scale on which it is now to be used. One must hope fervently that all the assurances which we are given will prove truly justified; for the HMG-CoA reductase inhibitors are riding the crest of a mighty wave of fashion and fear with respect to high cholesterol levels and have become subtly intermingled with it, to the point where one no longer knows where honest epidemiology ends and salesmanship begins. Too many of the experts who are urging the doctor to measure cholesterol, the medical correspondents who are seizing the public's attention and the armed guards who pounce upon the critics of the cholesterol-lowering mania prove to have been processed or pampered by those who stand to benefit commercially from what is happening. The horses are prancing much faster and the steam organ blowing far more vigorously than ever before; and woe betide the critic who dares suggest that we may be taking risks or at best going nowhere exotically.

THE TARGET AND THE MEANS

At this point one must come down to earth and see what, in the present state of knowledge, we would essentially want *any* therapy in this field to do for us. It is quite beyond dispute that one should do something about the high cholesterol levels — e.g. 7.5 mmol/l or above (7) — in order to reduce the risk of coronary heart disease (8); the more moderate the elevation, the more modest the measures which one can justify to deal with it. Bearing in mind both the demonstrated and theoretical problems which could arise if cholesterol levels fall too far, the view is also widely held that a cholesterol level of some 5.2 mmol/l is a sensible objective and that one should not aim any lower. Beyond that, there is controversy; in particular we still do not really know the relative merits in the long run of primarily lowering LDL-cholesterol, raising HDL-cholesterol (or one of its fractions) or doing both in variable degrees; and it would be surprising if such details did not prove to matter.

How attainable, then, is the current objective without having to resort to drugs at all? The purely physiological answer is that one will very often come a long way with healthy living alone, notably by some adjustments to diet and a sensible approach to tobacco, alcohol, body weight and exercise. Ever since the work of Keys, Grande and others in the 1950s some basic effects of changing fatty acid intake on cholesterol have been known (9). Precisely what nutritionists or dieticians call for is in addition likely to depend on the national dietary tradition within which they work; however, even modest shifts in eating habits can, provided they are maintained, have a drastic effect on coronary heart disease. In Britain, the 1984 Committee on Medical Aspects of Food Policy suggested no more than cutting total fat intake from 40% to 35% of the diet, mainly by replacing some saturated fats with energy from unrefined carbohydrate (10), and in Western countries the manufacturers of foods have done a great deal in two decades to ensure that, as WHO likes to put it, healthy choices become easy choices. Some of the basic points in the dietary outline recommended by America's National Cholesterol Education Program (11) are simple to learn and apply. Diet very often works, provided it is given a chance; it will reduce not only cholesterol but also body weight and blood pressure, and in all 3 ways improve the prognosis as regards coronary disease; drugs may be avoided completely, or used as modest supplements where diet alone is not entirely successful.

The nutritional answer is hence reasonably clear, and yet there are several adders under the grass.

The first is that one could even conceive of a prescribed diet producing unwanted effects. Since, for example, there are suspected links between fat and carcinogenesis, one will need to be cautious about faddism; as Diane Birt has pointed out, 'the essential fatty acids in the fat, the degree of their unsaturation, and the location of their unsaturation are all important in determining the influence of a dietary fat source on carcinogenesis' (12).

The other adders have been put there by non-nutritionists. A cholesterol-lowering diet is not complicated, difficult or unpleasant, but it can easily be made to look so, by comparison with the simple taking of a tablet. Prescribing is quick and tempting for the doctor, as compared with the giving of advice on diets and lifestyles. Health systems are much more prone to cover the costs of prescriptions, however much they may complain about them, than to invest in making adequately qualified dietary advisors available everywhere; even those systems which are by now gravely concerned about the escalating costs of using the HMG-CoA reductase inhibitors are doing nothing to correct that structural imbalance. And while no one will knock daily at the doctor's door to stress the merits of diet, there are plenty already at his door to talk about the virtues and simplicity of drugs.

CONCLUSIONS

Any reviewer in any field whose principal conclusion is that knowledge is still inadequate and that more research is called for deserves to be summarily executed; it is a time-wasting truism, for most decisions in medicine and life are and have to be taken on the basis of incomplete knowledge. We do in fact at the present day know sufficient to tackle the principal risks of lipid derangement without creating new ones. Dietary adjustment within tolerable limits and a firm prohibition on smoking are in very many cases quite sufficient to take an individual who so wishes out of the risk zone. Drugs will be called for in the minority with severe familial lipid disorders, and in those who clearly are not responding to diet; as a measure of last resort they may be tried in the high-risk yet obdurate individual who continues to smoke and over-indulge and who conceivably may prove more compliant with drugs than with diet. In the meantime the supplementary research which we do need should complement our meagre knowledge of these matters in women and in the elderly (4,7); and it must ensure the very long-term monitoring of patients on whatever drugs society sees fit to accept.

That big business has found itself much attracted to the lipid-lowering field is hardly surprising; something like a fifth of the population of a well-to-do industrialized country may be in need of some advice and intervention where their blood lipids are concerned (13) and it is incredibly lucrative to offer them a bubble-pack solution. Fortunately, big business means foods as well as drugs, so that even in that quarter some potential counterbalance is to hand. What one continues to hope is that the community will take a more sensible path before the next drug-induced disaster forces it to do so. Perhaps the hope is in vain; the expectation of finding health in a bottle is as ancient and eternal as the ecstasy of the fairground, and indeed it was among the lights of the fair that the patient medicine man of old sold his wares most successfully. We are up on the carrousel once more, carried entirely away by the hues, the motion, the glorious cacophony of it all, and quite believing for some brief moment that this is life.

REFERENCES

1. Report of the Committee of Principal Investigators (1984) WHO Cooperative Trial on Primary Prevention of Ischaemic Heart Disease with Clofibrate to lower serum cholesterol: final mortality follow-up. *Lancet, 2,* 600.
2. Martin HJ, Hulley SB, Browner WS et al (1986) Serum cholesterol, blood pressure and mortality; implications from a cohort of 361,662 men. *Lancet, 2,* 933.
3. Sherwin RW, Wentworth DN, Cutler JA et al (1987) Serum cholesterol levels and cancer mortality in 361,662 men screened for the multiple risk factor intervention trial. *J. Am. Med. Assoc., 257,* 943.
4. McMichael AJ, Jensen OM, Parkin DM et al (1984) Dietary and endogenous cholesterol and human cancer. *Epidemiol. Rev., 6,* 192.
5. Editorial (1989) Low cholesterol and increased risk. *Lancet, 1,* 1423.
6. Verschoor L (1990) Behandeling van hypercholesterolemie met cholesterolsyntheseremmers. *Geneesmiddelenbulletin, 24,* 13.
7. Hjermann I, Velve Byre K, Leren P (1981) Effect of diet and smoking intervention on the incidence of coronary heart disease. *Lancet, 2,* 1303.
8. Westlund K (1990) Epidemiological aspects: quantitative assessment of the preventive potential in nutrition. Paper presented at: First European Conference on Food and Nutrition Policy, Budapest, 1–5 October.
9. Keys A, Anderson JT, Grande F (1965) Serum cholesterol response to changes in the diet. III. Differences among individuals. *Metabolism, 14,* 766.
10. Committee on Medical Aspects of Food Policy (1984) *Diet and Cardiovascular Disease.* H.M. Stationery Office, London.
11. National Cholesterol Education Program (1988) Report of the Expert Panel on detection, evaluation and treatment of High Blood Cholesterol in Adults. NIH Publications, Bethesda Md.
12. Birt, DF (1990) The influence of dietary fat on carcinogenesis: lessons from experimental models. *Nutr. Rev., 48,* 1.
13. Sempios C, Fulwood R, Haines C et al (1989) The prevalence of high blood cholesterol levels among adults in the United States. *J. Am. Med. Assoc., 262,* 45.

R.P. Sequeira and W. Lammers

1 Central nervous system stimulants and anorectic agents

CENTRAL NERVOUS SYSTEM STIMULANTS

XANTHINE DERIVATIVES AND OTHER RESPIRATORY STIMULANTS *(SED-11, 1; SEDA-12, 2; SEDA-13, 1)*

Caffeine *(SED-11, 1; SEDA-12, 2; SEDA-13, 1)*

Excessive caffeine intake and fertility Considerable interest has been generated by the reports suggesting a relationship between caffeine intake and reduced fertility (1[R], 2[r]). Wilcox et al (1[R]) suggest that women who consume the caffeine equivalent of more than 1 cup of brewed coffee per day are less likely to become pregnant than those whose intake is lower. Failure to conceive within 12 months was nearly 5 times as great among higher caffeine users (1[R]). These epidemiological studies require further verification. It is interesting to note a hypothesis proposed by Casas et al (3[r]) to explain the effects of caffeine on fertility; methylxanthines modulate the dopaminergic control of prolactin release and caffeine has been shown to decrease plasma levels of prolactin. There is a known association between hypoprolactinemia and infertility.

A recent study showed that the semen of men who drank more than 4 cups of coffee per day and smoked in excess of 20 cigarettes per day had fewer motile spermatozoa and more dead cells than the semen of men who never drank coffee or smoked. The authors emphasise that they have not shown, however, any alteration in the fertility of men who consumed coffee and smoked cigarettes (4[C]).

Side Effects of Drugs Annual 14
M.N.G. Dukes and L. Beeley, editors

Caffeine and fetal arrhythmia Three cases of fetal arrhythmia resulting from excessive intake of caffeine by the mother during pregnancy have been reported (5[C]). In all 3 cases echocardiography of the fetal heart did not show any abnormalities. Following delivery in one of the cases the baby's urine was tested and found to contain caffeine. These cases show the importance of considering maternal caffeine abuse as a possible cause of fetal arrhythmia.

Caffeine overdosage A case of acute caffeine overdosage associated with rhabdomyolysis and resultant acute renal failure has been reported (6[C]).

A previously healthy 21-year-old man ingested approximately 3.75 g of caffeine in a suicide attempt. Approximately 4 h later he developed restlessness, nausea, vomiting, muscle twitching and palpitations. The patient was initially discharged without treatment. However, he continued to experience symptoms and sought medical attention 3 days later when he received 25 mg promethazine intramuscularly and was again discharged. On the 5th day after ingestion he presented with continued symptoms and a decrease in urine output with a creatinine clearance of 6.2 ml/min; serum creatinine of 16 mg/dl and creatine phosphokinase of 1134 U/l. He recovered after intravenous volume expansion with 5–6 l normal saline over 24 h, and 72 h of peritoneal dialysis.

A further case of caffeine overdosage was reported by Leson et al (7[C]).

A 16-year-old male ingested 30–35 'pink hearts' each containing 200–225 mg of caffeine (Estimated total dose 6–8 g caffeine). He developed vomiting and complained of left-sided chest pain. ECG revealed tachycardia and occasional bigeminy. Blood analysis showed hypokalemia, hyperglycemia and respiratory alkalosis. Respiratory rate, blood pressure and temperature were normal. The patient was found to have an unusually long elimination half-life (16 h) for caffeine. He recovered within 2 days of the ingestion.

THEOPHYLLINE AND RELATED SUBSTANCES *(SED-11, 3; SEDA-12, 2; SEDA-13, 1)*

Theophylline *(SED-11, 3; SEDA-12, 2; SEDA-13, 1)*

Drug-drug interaction Ranitidine, unlike cimetidine, is thought not to interact with theophylline. However 2 recent reports suggest that this may not be true. Simultaneous administration of theophylline and *ranitidine* to 3 patients resulted in reduction of theophylline clearance rate causing severe nausea and vomiting with subsequent development of abdominal pain (8[C]). These findings were later challenged (9[C]) on the basis of deficiencies in the case-reports. Skinner et al (10[c]) describe 2 patients in whom ranitidine produced an alteration in steady-state serum theophylline concentration. An earlier in vitro study (11[r]) with human hepatic microsomes showed that ranitidine had about 1/5 the inhibitory effect of cimetidine on normal enzymes. However, the inhibitory effect was nearly equal to that of cimetidine on induced enzymes and it is possible that phenytoin, an inducer of cytochrome P-450 enzymes, could have played a role in the case of one of the 2 patients.

It seems unlikely that ranitidine will interact with theophylline in the majority of patients, but it may be prudent to use caution when ranitidine is given to patients receiving theophylline.

Erythromycin is well known to inhibit the metabolism of theophylline (SEDA-12, 4). A case of a 16-year-old asthmatic female who developed theophylline toxicity while receiving erythromycin for her eczema is described (12[C]). These authors question the wisdom of decreasing theophylline dosage by 25% to prevent toxicity during erythromycin therapy because in addition to the effect of erythromycin in causing theophylline toxicity, theophylline can decrease the bioavailability of erythromycin (13[C]).

An interaction between mexiletine and theophylline causing a 30–35% reduction in theophylline clearance aggravating ventricular arrhythmia has been described (14[C]). This finding has to be viewed with caution because the patient had a history of 2 acute myocardial infarctions, coronary artery bypass surgery and left ventricular aneurysmectomy earlier. Nevertheless, this report supports the suggestion of an interaction in earlier report (15[C]).

Theophylline overdosage management and associated complications Hypermagnesemia complicating the treatment of theophylline toxicity is described in 2 patients (16[C]). These patients were treated with oral charcoal and magnesium citrate. They developed hypermagnesemia which resulted in either respiratory failure or prolongation of ventilatory support. Neither patient had renal disease. In one case diminished bowel function due to tricyclic antidepressant overdosage may have contributed to magnesium toxicity. These authors recommend that sorbitol be considered the cathartic agent of choice in the treatment of theophylline toxicity with oral charcoal.

Theophylline and pyridoxine metabolism A placebo-controlled, double-blind clinical trial on normal volunteers showed that theophylline treatment decreases the circulating pyridoxal-5′-phosphate (PLP) levels (17[C]). A daily supplement of 10 mg pyridoxine restored the circulating levels of PLP to normal. This can be explained by the following observations: (a) In vitro, theophylline acts as a non-competitive inhibitor of pyridoxal kinase. (b) Levels of pyridoxal kinase in the body are such that concentrations of theophylline used for therapeutic purposes can produce only partial inhibition of the enzyme. These authors, however, speculate that with increased plasma concentration (as in the case of theophylline overdosage), inhibition of pyridoxal kinase may be sufficient to cause a decrease in PLP which may play a role in theophylline-induced seizures.

Theophylline and cognitive functions A double-blind, cross-over study with theophylline and placebo investigated the potential side effects of theophylline on behavior, attention, memory and fine motor function in children with asthma (18[C]). A neuropsychological battery of tests to assess cognitive performance was used.

The subjects, parents and teachers filled out questionnaires concerning the behavior and attention. While on theophylline, these children experienced more 'stomach-aches' and 'shaking hands'. However, contrary to some earlier reports, no behavioral side effects of theophylline were found. The authors rightly point out that the small number of subjects studied ($n = 17$), the wide variation in plasma theophylline levels and the fact that behavior was assessed for only $3\frac{1}{2}$ days limit the validity of their negative findings.

Aminophylline *(SED-11, 4; SEDA-12, 4; SEDA-13, 2)*

Aminophylline-induced allergy A delayed-type hypersensitivity reaction has been reported in an 83-year-old woman with a long-standing history of obstructive lung disease. The reaction was attributed to the 'ethylene diamine' component of aminophylline (19[C]), a finding supported by another study (20[C]).

Aminophylline and beta-agonists In a prospective study Laaban et al (21[C]) have evaluated the occurrence of cardiac arrhythmias during combined therapy with aminophylline and terbutaline in 29 patients with status asthmaticus. The serum concentration of aminophylline was 12.1 $\pm$ 3.8 μg/ml. Five patients exhibited severe ventricular arrhythmias and another 14 developed rare unifocal premature ventricular contractions. These arrhythmias were clinically well tolerated and resolved spontaneously.

STIMULANT AND ANORECTIC AGENTS *(SED-11, 10; SEDA-13, 3)*

AMPHETAMINES AND RELATED AGENTS *(SED-11, 12; SEDA-12, 2; SEDA-13, 3)*

Amphetamines *(SED-11, 12; SEDA-12, 2; SEDA-13, 3)*

In a retrospective study (22[R]) of all cases of amphetamine toxicity in a metropolitan university emergency department during a 6-month period in 1987–1988, 127 patients who were amphetamine-positive by toxicological analysis were identified. The most commonly reported symptoms were altered mental status including mental agitation, hallucination, suicidal ideation, delusions and confusion. Other symptoms included chest pain, palpitations, headaches, seizures and abdominal pains. Laboratory analysis revealed that 37% patients had ingested methamphetamine or amphetamine alone, and 26% both drugs. The remaining 37% of patients used amphetamines in addition to drugs such as alcohol, benzodiazepines, aspirin and cocaine.

Most patients received no specific treatment and were managed conservatively. Those requiring treatment for agitation responded either to diazepam or to haloperidol. Admission may be required to exclude myocardial infarction, angina, stroke or sepsis in few cases.

3,4-Methylenedioxymethamphetamine; MDMA; 'Ecstasy'

'Ecstasy' has been increasingly abused as a recreational drug. The effects of MDMA are usually euphoric, causing a heightened sense of self-awareness and insightfulness and an increased sense of closeness to others. However, 3 cases have been described in whom dysphoric episodes were produced by the drug (23[c]). These subjects experienced panic attacks in response to recreational use of MDMA.

MDMA and its congeners cause damage to nerve endings concerned with serotoninergic transmission in animal species (24[r], 25[r]). Whether such changes are reversible or not is unclear. It has been aptly said: 'the price of ecstasy shall be damage to the capacity to feel pleasure' (26[r]).

Methylphenidate *(SED-11, 16; SEDA-12, 2; SEDA-13, 3)*

It has been claimed that methylphenidate can cause dramatic dysphoria when used as an infusion in patients with borderline disorders and schizophrenia (27[c]). Others, however, have not found any evidence to support this claim (28[c]). Instead, individual borderline patients may experience dysphoria as a part of their pre-infusion psychopathology. Apart from the fact that some schizophrenic patients exhibited characteristic psychotogenic effects, their affective responses to methylphenidate varied in a similar way to those of non-psychiatric subjects.

A case of methylphenidate-induced *delusional disorder* in a child with attention deficit disorder (ADD) with hyperactivity has been reported (29[C]).

Although the manufacturer of methylphenidate discourages the use of this drug (Ritalin) in children with ADD and seizure, a previous study (30[C]) and a more recent study (31) suggested that it produces no significant changes in epileptiform features or background activity on EEG. It did not alter the plasma concentration of antiepileptic drugs (carbamazepine, phenytoin, phenobarbital and valproic acid). It is argued that methylphenidate is safe and effective treatment for certain children with seizure and concurrent ADD.

Phenylpropanolamine (norephedrine, PPA) *(SED-11, 21; SEDA-13, 3)*

PPA is widely used and freely available as an over-the-counter (OTC) drug. A 150 mg dose (less than contained in 2 diet aids), or 75 mg PPA with 400 mg caffeine resulted in a significant increase in blood pressure into the hypertensive range in 6 subjects investigated (32[C]). Since 1982, at least 19 North American cases of intracranial hemorrhage have been associated with the ingestion of OTC products containing phenylpropanolamine (33[C]). Overdose in a suicide attempt accounted for only 4 of the cases, whereas most of the rest occurred after dosages of PPA (sometimes with caffeine) that were equal to or less than that contained in two diet aid capsules (150 mg). The cause of stroke in these cases was attributed to an acute, transient increase in blood pressure induced by PPA.

In contrast to these case-reports, 2 retrospective record reviews indicate only mild adverse reactions to PPA (34[R], 35[R]).

In the United States, PPA is currently contained in 116 drug products, 65 available over the counter and 51 obtained by prescription; 106 of these are decongestants and/or cough/cold remedies. The remainder are dietary aids usually containing 75 mg of sustained-release PPA. Lake et al (33[C]) have evaluated, by a double-blind, randomized, cross-over trial on 16 normotensive subjects, the effect of 2 doses of PPA (75 and 150 mg), and a 400 mg dose of caffeine alone and in combination with 75 mg PPA. The study also included a placebo-treated group. Their results indicate that 150 mg PPA substantially increases blood pressure. They recommend that physicians inform patients who may consume PPA (i.e. those with allergies, those with eating disorders, overweight persons) and patients at risk for stroke (the elderly and hypertensive patient) of the risks of taking more than the recommended amounts of PPA and of combining caffeine with PPA.

Lake et al (36[R]) have reviewed 37 cases (published in North America and Europe since 1960) that received a diagnosis of acute mania, paranoid schizophrenia and organic psychosis attributed to PPA ingestion. They found that more cases followed the ingestion of (a) combination products than PPA alone, (b) OTC products than those obtained by prescription, and (c) recommended dose than overdoses. Groups at particular risk appear to be those with a past or family psychiatric history, children under 6 years and post-partum women.

Phencyclidine *(SED-11, 86; SEDA-12, 38; SEDA-13, 29)*

The pharmacokinetics of phencyclidine after massive overdose have been described. (37[C]).

On admission to hospital the patient was diagnosed as having a 'toxic-metabolic-encephalopathy' with elevated serum creatine and serum aspartate amino-transferase. While in the medical intensive care unit, he had protracted seizures, which were controlled by barbiturate and tubocurarine, and he developed rhabdomyolsis. On hospital day 11 (13 days after ingestion), he passed 2 plastic bags containing phencyclidine through his rectum. One bag was ruptured. Starting on day 12 he made a rapid neurological recovery and was discharged the next day.

Analysis of pharmacokinetic data have revealed that phencyclidine shows first-order kinetics over a wide range of plasma concentrations with a terminal half-life of 12.5 h. The low renal clearance, large volume of distribution (6.2 l/kg) and metabolic consequences of severe phencyclidine intoxication argue against the widely used practice of acidification of urine as an adjunct to the treatment of phencyclidine intoxication.

Cocaine *(SED-11, 11; SEDA-12, 35; SEDA-13, 25) (see also Chapter 4)*

Cocaine-induced rhabdomyolysis Pogue and Nurse (38[C]) have reported 4 adults with rhabdomyolysis following the use of cocaine. Although a direct causal relationship was not proved, the clinical association suggested that cocaine was responsible for the development of rhabdomyolysis. All patients had used cocaine within 24 h of presentation and this was confirmed by toxicological screening.

A case of rhabdomyolysis produced by intravenous cocaine in a 25-year-old woman with AIDS, chronic herpes simplex and hepatitis B infection has been reported (39[C]). These and other reports (40[C]–42[C]) suggest that cocaine-induced rhabdomyolysis is being increasingly recognized.

Thorough clinical evaluation is necessary before diagnosing rhabdomyolysis due to cocaine to exclude other causes of an increase in creatine kinase, especially of myocardial infarction. Knowlton (43[C]) warns against attributing every increase in creatine kinase among users of cocaine to rhabdomyolysis in the absence of cinical evidence.

The pathophysiology of cocaine-induced rhabdomyolysis is unknown, but several known effects of the drug could be responsible. These include vasoconstriction, hyperthermia and seizures. Increased muscle activity associated with seizures is a common cause of rhabdomyolysis (44[R]).

Free-base cocaine and airway complications The increasing popularity of illicit cocaine use has been accompanied by a proliferation of techniques for getting the drug into the body; these include intranasal snorting, intravenous injection, and smoking 'free based' cocaine ('crack'). In the latter technique the usual street cocaine, in the form of the hydrochloride salt, is combined with an alkaline substance such as sodium bicarbonate, and the resultant mixture is dissolved in ether. The upper layer then contains relatively pure cocaine crystals, which are smoked in a water pipe or cigarette. They can also be used for intravenous injection.

Gordon (45[C]) reports a case of a 19-year-old female who developed marked respiratory distress and pleuritic chest pain following free-base cocaine smoking. A ventilation-perfusion scan revealed reactive airways disease of the large airways and concomitant mucous plugging of small airways. This was thought to be caused by the free-base cocaine, the impurities of the free-basing process or both. The patient made a full recovery with bronchodilators and corticosteroid therapy. An unusual complication of 'crack' smoking is severe thermal injury to the airways due to either inhalational injury or intratracheal ignition of the ether vehicle used in free-basing cocaine (46[C]). The resulting severe airways disease and tracheal stenosis required reconstructive surgery.

Recurrent massive hemoptysis and pulmonary hemorrhage temporally related to smoking free-base cocaine is described in a 20-year-old woman (47[C]).

Bronchoscopy revealed localized brisk hemorrhage to the anterior segment of right upper lobe. Following lobectomy the patient made uneventful recovery. Lung biopsy revealed intrapulmonary hemorrhage with hemosiderin-laden macrophages, and small zones of granulation tissues. Three weeks after discharge, the patient had a massive hemoptysis after smoking free-base cocaine, which resolved spontaneously.

A similar case has been previously described (48[C]). It is suggested that cocaine-induced intense vasoconstriction was the probable cause of the pulmonary hemorrhage.

'Crack' has been reported to cause pneumomediastinum. A review of the literature revealed 9 cases of cocaine-mediated pneumomediastinum, each with an uncomplicated clinical course (49[C], 50[CR], 51[C]). The cause of pneumomediastinum is probably the inhalation technique rather than the drug itself.

Attention is drawn to the use of free-base cocaine as an increasingly frequent cause of chest pain among adolescents (52[C], 53[Cr], 54[C]). The cause of chest pain in such cases may be forceful repetitive coughing or the development of pneumomediastinum when the hot cocaine-saturated vapors are sucked deeply into the respiratory tract followed by a sustained Valsalva maneuver. Free-base cocaine can also cause chest pain by inducing cardiac arrhythmias, by precipitating myocardial infarction, or by inducing coronary vasospasm.

Cocaine and cardiovascular complications Myocardial infarction is now a well-recognized complication of cocaine abuse (for review, see Ref. 55[R]). A case has now been reported of in a 38-year-old man who died following simultaneous acute thromboses of 2 major epicardial coronary arteries shortly after intravenous cocaine use. The finding of layers of mural thrombus of varying age, from acute to 2–3 days, in both coronary arteries has not been previously reported in cocaine-associated deaths (56[C]).

The cardiotoxic effects of cocaine have been described in 2 other papers (57[C], 58[CR]). The extent to which cocaine produces arrhythmias is uncertain; acute myocardial infarction is a demonstrated risk even in subjects without preexisting coronary disease.

In a review of records of 3712 drug abusers, 13 patients were identified with neurological deficits attributable to the use of of cocaine. Ischemic manifestations were the most frequent, occurring in 7 patients; 3 had subarachnoid hemorrhage and another 3 had intracerebral hemorrhage. Of the 6 patients with computed tomographic findings of cerebral infarction, 5 had subcortical infarcts. Two of the 4 patients who presented with subarachnoid hemorrhage had a congenital intracranial aneurysm; one of the patients with cerebral hemorrhage had an arteriovenous malformation. It is probable that cocaine-induced hypertension might be responsible for some of these events (59[Ct]).

A case of acute ischemia of the upper limb due to an accidental intra-arterial injection is reported in a young female drug addict who presented with a very painful distal upper limb (60[C]). The patient was managed with brachial plexus anesthesia and intravenous infusion of heparin, followed by aspirin and dipyridamole. She made a good recovery.

Cocaine use and nasal complications A questionnaire on cocaine use patterns and associated adverse effects on the nasal passages given to 464 adolescents revealed that cocaine users had frequent symptoms such as sniffing, sinus problems and diminished olfaction. Those who had snorted cocaine at least 25 times (but less than daily) had nasal membrane irritation with nasal crusts and scabs, recurrent nose bleeds, or both. It is suggested that an astute otolaryngologist should consider cocaine abuse as a cause of puzzling or recalcitrant rhinitis (61[C]).

A new complex of symptoms has been described in association with cocaine snorting in 2 patients and cocaine packing of the nostrils in another. Each patient, in varying degrees, had nasal bridge collapse, a perforated nasal deformity secondary to the collapse, nasal bleeding secondary to the perforated nasal septum and voice changes with pharyngeal ulcerations secondary to palatal retraction (62[C]).

Botulism associated with maxillary sinusitis following intranasal cocaine abuse has been reported in 2 cases (63[Cr], 64[C]). The history of intranasal cocaine use 10 days before the development of the illness is similar to the recognized 4–14 days incubation period seen in patients with wound botulism.

Cocaine-induced panic attacks Louie et al (6[C]) have described panic attacks developing after cocaine use in 10 patients. Compared to the primary panic disorder, these patients showed atypical trends with regard to the following: (a) more had psychosensory symptoms, fewer had agoraphobia and none had school-phobia; (b) all were extremely sensitive to the anxiogenic effect of caffeine and a few developed panic attack or visual illusions; (c) more had lack of sensitivity to the anxiogenic effect of marijuana; (d) there was a worsening of their clinical condition with tricyclic antidepressants and substantial improvement after taking clonazepam or carbamazepine. The timing of the onset of symptoms, i.e. after 1–6 years of cocaine use, and the fact that only one among these patients had a first-degree relative with panic disorder were more suggestive of 'acquired' than 'primary' panic disorder. Typically, these acute attacks included tachycardia, hyperventilation, paresthesias, tremor, diaphoresis, hot and cold flushes, vomiting and fear of going insane. They soon began to occur independently of cocaine use and persisted despite several months of abstinence from cocaine. The authors say that the atypical symptoms and response to benzodiazepine medication are suggestive of limbic neuronal hyperexcitability induced by cocaine through a kindling mechanism or through behavioral sensitization. Interestingly, an epidemiological study based on 5896 subjects has revealed that the risk of panic attacks was highest in cocaine users who reported no marijuana use during the follow-up interval (66[R]).

Cocaine and venous thrombosis In a retrospective study carried out at the University of Texas Medical Branch, 12 cases of upper-extremity deep vein thrombosis (UEDVT) were documented between 1987 and 1988. Among them, 5 cases were associated with intravenous cocaine abuse. Although superficial thrombophlebitis has been well known as a complication of intravenous drug abuse, deep vein thrombosis is unusual. Thus the occurrence of UEDVT in a young subject should alert the clinician to the possibility of intravenous cocaine abuse (67[cR]).

Cocaine use during pregnancy and associated complications Several studies have been carried out during the past 2 years and the risks of cocaine abuse to the mother, the fetus and the newborn are becoming clearer. A retrospective matched cohort study (68[R]) of 55 women who admitted to the use of cocaine ('crack') during pregnancy and 55 non-drug-using women who delivered during the same period showed that the drug users had an increased incidence of: (a) delivery at 37 weeks or earlier, (b) intrauterine growth retardation (IUGR), and (c) premature rupture of the membranes. Abnormal neurobehavioral symptoms such as tremulousness, irritability and muscular rigidity which were mild and self-limiting were noticed in the newborns of the drug users.

In another cohort study, pregnancy outcome and health status of infants born to 53 cocaine abusers were compared with those of another group of 100 unexposed women and their infants (69[R]). The findings were similar to those of Cherukuri et al (68[R]) discussed above. In addition, in this study the authors also noted a higher incidence of cardiac anomalies among infants born to mothers who abused cocaine. In both these studies the authors rightly point out the possibility that many of the observed adverse effects may be related to life-style rather than the pharmacological effect of the drug itself. However, it is possible that the increased incidence of IUGR was a consequence of chronic hypoxia and that the reduced gestational period was related to altered myometrial response to catecholamines.

A large population of pregnant women was tested for drug use at the time of their admission to hospital for delivery in Chicago (70[R]). During the study period 138 of 1776 patients (8%) who were delivered of infants were found to have cocaine in their urine. The perinatal outcome of these 138 patients was compared with that of 88 control patients. The findings are comparable to those of Cherukuri et al (68[R]) and Little et al (69[R]). Also, when compared to the control infants, infants of mothers who used cocaine had more neonatal morbidity and longer hospitalization, thus making more demand on health care resources (70).

Yet another study examines the prevalence of drug abuse among women during pregnancy. A prospective study (71) has been carried out on 1226 mothers recruited from a general prenatal clinic in Boston. On the basis of either interviews or urine assays conducted prenatally or postpartum, 27% of the subjects had used marijuana and 18% had used cocaine. When only positive urine samples were considered, the corresponding values were 16 and 9%, respectively. The percentage of women found positive by urine analysis is comparable to the other study reported earlier (70[R]). Lower birth weight, shorter length and small head circumference were suggestive of impaired fetal growth.

The recent addition of 3 more cases to those reported earlier makes a total of 9 cases of placental abruption that have been temporally related to cocaine abuse (72[Cr], 73[C], 74[R]). The known hypertensive and vasoconstrictor effects of cocaine provide a mechanism for abruption.

A case of fetal death in utero followed by spontaneous abortion has been reported. Toxic levels of cocaine were found in the fetus at postmortem (75[C]).

The first reported case of cocaine-associated maternal intracerebral hemorrhage occurred in the postpartum period in a 25-year-old woman (76[C]).

The patient admitted using 'crack' before the seizure episode. A CT scan revealed a small intracerebral hemorrhage in the left frontoparietal area. Aneurysms and vascular malformations were ruled out by carotid angiography and EEG was normal. The patient was discharged on phenytoin with no neurological sequelae.

It is especially interesting to note that in this patient the seizure and hypertension were associated with cocaine use, although her physician initially believed that she had postpartum eclampsia.

Components of fetal behavioral state organization reflect the successful integration of the CNS, have a specific developmental time table and can be studied with fetal ultrasonographic technique. A study was performed on 20 fetuses and newborns exposed in utero to cocaine to determine the effect on CNS maturation and state organization (77[C]). Abnormal or delayed-state behavior was identified in 13 of 20 fetuses. State organization was evaluated as suspect or abnormal for 16 of the 20 exposed newborns. A disorganized behavioral state in the fetus successfully predicted abnormal newborn behavior. These findings support the concept that cocaine exposure disrupts development and fetal assessment of state is predictive of neonatal outcome.

Fulroth et al (78[R]) have described a study performed on 86 infants who were born to women with a history of cocaine and/or heroin use during pregnancy.

The newborns were observed for a 5-day period in hospital using a standardized abstinence scoring system and urine drug measurements in both mother and infant. Mild withdrawal occurred in 26% of the cocaine group, and another 6% had withdrawal which needed treatment.

The authors recommend that these infants be followed up closely after discharge from the nursery, as growth retardation, microcephaly and abnormal behavior may all be suggestive of potential long-term neurological or developmental problems.

Infants prenatally exposed to cocaine have a high incidence of cardiorespiratory abnormalities and an increased risk of sudden infant death syndrome. The prospective evaluation of 32 cocaine-exposed and 18 methadone-exposed infants revealed 13 infants with an abnormal cardiorespiratory pattern. Theophylline treatment resulted in normalization of the respiratory pattern and there were no further problems (79[C]).

Maternal use of cocaine during pregnancy causing neonatal ventricular tachycardia has been reported (80[C]). The woman admitted using intranasal cocaine once every 7–10 days during the 2 initial and 3 final months of gestation. There was no placental abruption or meconium staining of the amniotic fluid. These authors recommend screening for cocaine metabolites in neonates with ventricular tachycardia.

Reports describing the effects of maternal cocaine use on the fetus and infant have addressed mainly those effects produced by maternal or placental pathology and to the direct transplacental effects of cocaine itself. What happens after birth to infants who continue to be exposed to free-base cocaine is described in a study by Bateman and Heagarty (81[C]).

They report 4 infants or toddlers (age 3 months to 3 years 11 months), all residents of Harlem, New York, whose urine contained cocaine and its principal metabolite methyl ecgonine, presumably as a result of passive inhalation of crack vapors used by adult care-takers. Two had transient neurological symptoms such as drowsiness and unsteady gait and 2 had seizures whose cause could not be determined by laboratory investigations. Cocaine and its metabolites were found in the urine of these children and the authors suggest that passive cocaine inhalation may have contributed to their symptoms. They also point out the potential environmental effects of cocaine smoking.

REFERENCES

1. Wilcox A, Weinberg C, Band D (1988) Caffeinated beverages and decreased fertility. *Lancet, 2,* 1453.
2. Christianson RE, Oechsli FW, Van den Berg, BJ (1989) Caffeinated beverages and decreased fertility. *Lancet, 1,* 378.
3. Casas M, Ferrer S, Calaf J et al (1989) Dopaminergic mechanism for caffeine induced decrease in fertility. *Lancet, 1,* 731.
4. Marshburn PB, Sloan CS, Hammond MG (1989) Semen quality and association with coffee drinking, cigarette smoking and ethanol consumption. *Fertil. Steril., 52,* 162.
5. Oei SG, Vosters RPL, Van der Hagen NLJ (1989) Fetal arrhythmia caused by excessive intake of caffeine by pregnant women. *Br. Med. J., 298,* 568.
6. Wrenn KD, Oschner I (1989) Rhabdomyolysis induced by a caffeine overdose. *Ann. Emerg. Med., 18,* 155.
7. Leson CL, McGuigan MA, Bryson SM (1988) Caffeine overdose in an adolescent male. *Clin. Toxicol., 26,* 407.
8. Roy AK, Cuda MP, Levine KA (1988) Induction of theophylline toxicity and inhibition of clearance rates by ranitidine. *Am. J. Med., 85,* 525.
9. Muir JG, Powell JR, Bauman JH (1989) Induction of theophylline toxicity and inhibition of clearance rates by ranitidine. *Am. J. Med., 86,* 513.

10. Skinner MH, Leslie L, Blaschke TF (1989) Theophylline toxicity subsequent to ranitidine administration: a possible drug – drug interaction. *Am. J. Med.*, *86*, 129.
11. Hoensoh HP, Hutzel H, Kirch W et al (1985) Isolation of human hepatic microsomes and their inhibition by cimetidine and ranitidine. *Eur. J. Clin. Pharmacol.*, *29*, 199.
12. Tenenbein M (1989) Theophylline toxicity due to drug interaction. *J. Emerg. Med.*, *7*, 249.
13. Paulsen O, Hoglund P, Nilsson LG et al (1987) The interaction of erythromycin with theophylline. *Eur. J. Clin. Pharmacol.*, *32*, 493.
14. Kessler KM, Interian Jr, A, Cox AM et al (1989) Proarrhythmia related to a kinetic and dynamic interaction of mexiletine and theophylline. *Am. Heart J.*, *117*, 964.
15. Katz A, Buskila D, Sukenik S (1987) Oral mexiletine theophylline interaction. *Int. J. Cardiol.*, *17*, 227.
16. Weber CA, Santiago RM (1989) Hypermagnesemia: a potential complication during treatment of theophylline intoxication with oral charcoal and magnesium containing cathartics. *Chest*, *95*, 56.
17. Ubbink JB, Delport R, Becker PJ, Bissbort S (1989) Evidence of a theophylline induced vitamin B_6 deficiency caused by noncompetitive inhibition of pyridoxal kinase. *J. Lab. Clin. Med.*, *113*, 15.
18. Rappaport L, Coffman H, Guare R et al (1989) Effect of theophylline on behaviour and learning in children with asthma. *Am. J. Dis. Child.*, *143*, 368.
19. Saaven A, Lippman ML (1987) Aminophylline allergy. *Am. J. Med.*, *82*, 1002.
20. Patruno C, De Simone D, Monaco G (1988) Attualita in tema di sensibilizzazione da etilindiamina. *Quad. Med. Chir.*, *4*, 21.
21. Laaban JP, Iung B, Chauvet JP et al (1988) Cardiac arrhythmias during the combined use of intravenous aminophylline and terbutaline. *Chest*, *94*, 496.
22. Derlet RW, Rice P, Horowitz BZ, Lord RV (1989) Amphetamine toxicity: experience with 127 cases. *J. Emerg. Med.*, *7*, 157.
23. Whitaker-Azmitia PM, Aronson TA (1989) 'Ecstasy' (MDMA)-induced panic. *Am. J. Psychiatry 146*, 119.
24. Finnegan KT, Ricuarte GA, Ritchie LD (1988) Orally administered MDMA causes a long term depletion of serotonin in rat brain. *Brain Res.*, *447*, 141.
25. Battaglia G, Yeh SY, De Souza B (1988) MDMA induced neurotoxicity: parameters of degeneration and recovery of brain serotonin neurons. *Pharmacol. Biochem. Behav.*, *29*, 269.
26. Edwards G (1989) Blasted with ennui: dangers in another drug fashion. *Br. Med. J.*, *298*, 136.
27. Lucas PB, Gardner DL, Wolkowitz OM et al (1987) Dysphoria associated with methylphenidate infusions in borderline personality disorder. *Am. J. Psychiatry*, *144*, 1577.
28. Robinson AS, Bailine S. Lieberman J (1988) Dysphoria associated with methylphenidate infusion. *Am. J. Psychiatry*, *145*, 9.
29. Bloom AS, Russell LJ, Weiskopf B et al (1988) Methylphenidate induced delusional disorder in a child with attention deficit disorder with hyperactivity. *J. Am. Acad. Child Adolesc. Psychiatry*, *27*, 88.
30. McBride MC, Wang D, Torres CF (1986) Methylphenidate in therapeutic doses does not lower seizure threshold. *Ann. Neurol.*, *20*, 428.
31. Feldman H, Crumrine P, Handen BL et al (1989) Methylphenidate in children with seizures and attention-deficit disorder. *Am. J. Dis. Child.*, *143*, 1081.
32. Lake CR, Zaloga G, Clymen R et al (1988) A double dose of phenylpropanolamine causes transient hypertension. *Am. J. Med.*, *85*, 339.
33. Lake CR, Zaloga G, Bray J et al (1989) Transient hypertension after two phenylpropanolamine diet aids and the effects of caffeine: a placebo controlled follow up study. *Am. J. Med.*, *86*, 427.
34. Elkins BR, Spoerke DG (1983) An estimation of non-prescription diet aids from seventy exposure cases. *Vet. Hum. Toxicol.*, *25*, 81.
35. Aselton P, Jick H, Hunter JR (1985) Phenylpropanolamine exposure and subsequent hospitalization. *J. Am. Med. Assoc.*, *253*, 977.
36. Lake CR, Masson EB, Quirk RS (1988) Psychiatric side effects attributed to phenylpropanolamine. *Pharmacopsychiatry*, *21*, 171.
37. Jackson JE (1989) Phencyclidine pharmacokinetics after a massive overdose. *Ann. Intern. Med.*, *111*, 613.
38. Pogue VA, Nurse HM (1989) Cocaine associated acute myoglobinuric renal failure. *Am. J. Med.*, *86*, 183.
39. Reinhart WH, Slowman-Kovacs, Leapman SB (1988) Rhabdomyolysis after intravenous cocaine. *Am. J. Med.*, *85*, 579.
40. Krohn KD, Slowman-Kovacs, Leapman SB (1988) Cocaine and rhabdomyolysis. *Ann. Intern. Med.*, *108*, 639.
41. Roth D, Alarcon FJ, Fernandez JA et al (1988) Acute rhabdomyolysis associated with cocaine intoxication. *N. Engl. J. Med.*, *319*, 673.
42. Zamora-Quezada JC, Dinerman H, Stadecker MJ et al (1988) Muscle and skin infarction after free-basing cocaine (Crack). *Ann. Intern. Med.*, *108*, 564.
43. Knowlton AA (1989) Acute rhabdomyolysis associated with cocaine intoxication. *N. Engl. J. Med.*, *320*, 667.
44. Curry SC, Chang D, Connor D (1989) Drug and toxin induced rhabdomyolysis. *Ann. Emerg. Med.*, *18*, 1068.
45. Gordon III, K (1989) Case report: free based cocaine smoking and reactive airway disease. *J. Emerg. Med.*, *7*, 145.

46. Taylor RF, Bernard GR (1989) Airway complications from free basing cocaine. *Chest, 95,* 476.
47. Godwin JE, Harley RA, Miller KS, Hefner JE (1989) Cocaine, pulmonary hemorrhage and hemoptysis. *Ann. Intern. Med., 110,* 843.
48. Murray RJ, Albin RJ, Mergner W et al (1988) Diffuse alveolar hemorrhage temporally related to cocaine smoking. *Chest, 93,* 427.
49. Palat D, Denson M, Sherman M et al (1988) Pneumomediastinum induced by inhalation of alkaloidal cocaine. *NY State J. Med., 88,* 438.
50. Hunter JG, Loy HC, Markovitz L et al (1986) Spontaneous pneumomediastinum following inhalation of alkaloidal cocaine and emesis case report and review. *Mt. Sinai J. Med. (NY), 53,* 491.
51. Mir J, Galvete J, Plaza M et al (1986) Spontaneous pneumomediastinum after cocaine inhalation. *Respiration, 50,* 230.
52. Schwartz RH (1989) Chest pain in an adolescent: think of cocaine. *Pediatrics, 83,* 639.
53. Woodward GA, Selbst SM (1987) Chest pain secondary to cocaine use. *Pediat. Emerg. Care, 3,* 153.
54. Wiener MD, Putnam CE (1987) Pain in the chest in a user of cocaine. *J. Am. Med. Assoc., 258,* 2087.
55. Frishman WH, Karpenos A, Molloy TJ (1989) Cocaine induced coronary artery disease. *Med. Clin. North Am., 73,* 475.
56. Stenberg RG, Winniford MD, Hillis LD et al (1989) Simultaneous acute thrombosis of two major coronary arteries following intravenous cocaine use. *Arch. Pathol. Lab. Med., 113,* 521.
57. Isner J, Estes M, Thomson P et al (1986) Acute cardiac events temporarily related to cocaine. *N. Engl. J. Med., 315,* 1438.
58. Mathias D (1986) Cocaine-associated myocardial ischemias: a review of clinical and angiographic findings. *Am. J. Med., 81,* 675.
59. Jacobs IG, Roszler MH, Kelly JK et al (1989) Cocaine abuse: neurovascular complications. *Radiology, 170,* 223.
60. Berger JL, Nmier M, Desmonts JM (1988) Continuous axillary plexus block in the treatment of accidental intra-arterial injection of cocaine. *N. Engl. J. Med., 318,* 930.
61. Schwartz RH, Estroff T, Fairbanks DNF, Hoffmann NG (1989) Nasal symptoms associated with cocaine abuse during adolescence. *Arch. Otolaryngol. Head Neck Surg., 115,* 63.
62. Deutsch HL, Millard Jr, JV (1989) A new cocaine abuse complex: involvement of nose, septum, palate and pharynx. *Arch. Otolaryngol. Head Neck Surg., 115,* 235.
63. Kudrow DB, Haake DA, Mathisen GE (1988) Botulism associated with *Clostridium botulinum* sinusitis after intranasal cocaine abuse. *Ann. Intern. Med., 109,* 984.
64. McDonald KL, Rutherford GW, Friedman SM et al (1985) Botulism and botulism-like illness in chronic drug abusers. *Ann. Intern. Med., 102,* 616.
65. Loie AK, Lannon RA, Ketter TA (1989) Treatment of cocaine induced panic disorder. *Am. J. Psychiatry, 146,* 40.
66. Anthony JC, Tien AY, Petronis KR (1989) Epidemiology evidence on cocaine use and panic attacks. *Am. J. Epidemiol., 129,* 543.
67. Lisse JR, Davis CP, Thurmond-Anderle ME (1989) Upper extremity deep vein thrombosis increased prevalence due to cocaine abuse. *Am. J. Med., 87,* 457.
68. Cherukuri R, Minkoff H, Feldman J et al (1988) A cohort study of alkaloidal cocaine ('Crack') in pregnancy. *Obstet. Gynecol., 72,* 147.
69. Little BB, Snell LM, Klein VR, Gilstrap LC (1989) Cocaine abuse during pregnancy: maternal and fetal complications. *Obstet. Gynecol., 73,* 157.
70. Neerhoff MG, MacGregor SN, Retzky SS, Sullivan TP (1989) Cocaine abuse during pregnancy: peripartum prevalence and perinatal outcome. *Am. J. Obstet. Gynecol., 161,* 633.
71. Zuckerman B, Frank DA, Hingson R et al (1989) Effects of maternal marijuana and cocaine use on fetal growth. *N. Engl. J. Med., 320,* 763.
72. Townsend RR, Laing FC, Jeffrey Jr, BB (1988) Placental abruption associated with cocaine. *Am. J. Radiol., 150,* 1339.
73. Acker D, Sachs BP, Tracey KJ et al (1983) Abruptio placentae associated with cocaine use. *Am. J. Obstet. Gynecol., 143,* 146.
74. Chasnoff IJ, Burns WJ, Schnoll SH et al (1985) Cocaine use in pregnancy. *N. Engl J. Med., 313,* 666.
75. Critchley H, Woods SM, Barson AJ et al (1988) Fetal death in utero and cocaine abuse: case report. *Br. J. Obstet. Gynaecol., 95,* 195.
76. Mercado A, Johnson Jr, G, Calver D, Sokol RJ (1989) Cocaine, pregnancy and postpartum intracerebral hemorrhage. *Obstet. Gynecol., 73,* 467.
77. Hume RF, O'Donnell KJ, Stanger CL et al (1989) In utero cocaine exposure: observation of fetal behavioural state may predict neonatal outcome. *Am. J. Obstet. Gynecol., 161,* 685.
78. Fulroth R, Phillipa B, Durand DJ (1989) Perinatal outcome of infants exposed to cocaine and/or heroin in utero. *Am. J. Dis. Child., 143,* 905.
79. Chasnoff IJ, Hunt CE, Kletter R, Kaplan D (1989) Prenatal cocaine exposure is associated with respiratory pattern abnormalities. *Am. J. Dis. Child., 143,* 583.
80. Geggel RL, McInery J, Estes III, NAM (1989) Transient neonatal ventricular tachycardia associated with maternal cocaine use. *Am. J. Cardiol., 63,* 383.
81. Bateman DA, Heagarty MC (1989) Passive freebase cocaine ('Crack') inhalation by infants and toddlers. *Am. J. Dis. Child., 143,* 25.

M.N.G. Dukes

2 Antidepressant drugs

MONOAMINE OXIDASE (MAO) INHIBITORS *(SED-11, 31; SEDA-12, 8; SEDA-13, 6)*

Iproniazid

Overdose The long-term eclipse of the MAO inhibitors, largely because of their interaction problems, has sometimes caused physicians to lose sight of one of their relative advantages over the tricyclic antidepressants, namely their safety in overdosage. Fatalities and even severe short-term consequences are rare. Jourdan et al (1^C) reported a case where the dose of iproniazid taken by a young woman – apparently 3 g – was sufficient to put her into coma for 4 days. Although during this period she exhibited some abnormalities, notably hypoglycemia, a slight increase in ALT and pulmonary congestion, her circulatory system remained stable and the autonomic nervous system was normal; after recovery she experienced a month of 'melancholia' but had no residual injury. The only reservation one needs to make is the unreliability of the information sometimes given by potential suicides as to what their drug intake actually has been.

Selegiline

Selegiline (L-deprenyl) is a propinylamine derivative and a type B MAO inhibitor which has come into use only recently.

Interactions The interaction of earlier MAO inhibitors with tyramine-containing foods (and the known difficulty in avoiding it in daily life) is sufficiently serious to engender caution when newer members of the group are used; nevertheless, physicians continue to be taken by surprise.

A man of 34 with a long history of chronic and cyclic depression was included in a clinical trial of selegiline, receiving a dose of 20 mg daily and being instructed on the use of a low-tyramine diet. After 3 weeks of treatment he nevertheless experienced a severe hypertensive episode with throbbing headache, starting half an hour after taking a meal rich in tyramine and lasting for 90 min. With further instruction on his diet he continued therapy for a total of 11 weeks, showing good tolerance despite an increase in the prescribed dose to 40 mg daily (2^C).

The reader may be reminded that a useful table of tyramine-rich foods was provided in SEDA-13 (p. 7).

Much less familiar is the possibility of a severe interaction between a MAO inhibitor and endogenous catecholamines. An unusual case which appears to fall into this category was described by Menza and Golbe in 1988:

A woman of 41 with idiopathic Parkinson's disease had been treated for a long period with levodopa/carbidopa, latterly supplemented (because of difficulty in dose adjustment) with selegiline and bromocriptine. Because of her problems she underwent implantation of autologous adrenal medulla tissue into the left caudate in the hope of improving her condition; both selegiline and bromocriptine were discontinued before the operation. Following surgery the patient experienced visual hallucinations for some days but thereafter improved and her Parkinson symptoms were well-controlled for the next 2–3 weeks on reduced doses of levodopa/carbidopa. A month after surgery there was a clear need for supplementary treatment and selegiline was restarted in a dose of 5 mg/b.d. Within 2 days she experienced anorexia, euphoria and insomnia; she was unusually talkative and irritable. The patient discontinued selegiline 6 days after the onset of these symptoms and within 2 days her behavior normalized (3^C).

It is not at all clear whether one is dealing with a direct adverse effect of selegiline, i.e. in-

(Biomedical Division)
Side Effects of Drugs Annual 14
M.N.G. Dukes and L. Beeley, editors

duction of something resembling hypomania (which is not a recognized effect of MAO inhibitors) or, as the authors themselves suggest, the combination of the drug and the adrenal implant. If the latter is the case, it is tempting to draw the analogy to the interaction with exogenous catecholamines.

Tranylcypromine

Cardiovascular Reports of *hypertensive episodes* with tranylcypromine and other MAO inhibitors continue to appear (4[c], 5[c]), but on most instances there is doubt as to whether one is dealing with a true adverse effect or with an interaction with tyramine, alcohol or some other nutrient which has been ingested but gone unrecorded.

Nervous system Pande and Max have described the occurrence of *dystonia* in a woman of 65 who had been receiving tranylcypromine 10 mg twice daily for 3 days in an attempt to control major long-term depression which had failed to respond to other agents. The condition receded 48 h after drug withdrawal but returned on rechallenge with the original dose. Although this patient had been receiving a series of other drugs, notably for a cardiac disorder, and also seems to have shown a dystonic reaction to propranolol, the positive rechallenge left little doubt that tranylcypromine was responsible (6[C]).

Withdrawal reactions It is clear that in some patients the withdrawal of a MAO inhibitor will induce either a fortified recurrence of the original condition or new symptoms, which may include anxiety, perceptual disturbances and psychosis. One cannot thus entirely share the surprise expressed by Absher and Black when they describe '... the first report of a withdrawal delirium caused by the discontinuation of tranylcypromine', though earlier cases have indeed involved other members of the class.

A woman of 62 had been stable on treatment with tranylcypromine (90 mg/d) for a year but recurrent depressant symptoms led to her admission to hospital, where the dose was increased to 110 mg/d and lithium was added. Because of an episode of orthostatic hypotension, both the tranylcypromine and a thiazide diuretic (which she had been receiving for hypertension) were withdrawn but the next day she became delirious; the delirium became more pronounced over a period of 3 days, with disorientation, agitation and paranoia. She was ultimately controlled on lithium only (7[C]).

There are, all the same, elements of doubt as to what actually happened in this case, notably because during her hospital stay there had also been and interruption of the oral antidiabetic therapy which she had been receiving for a long period, and her recovery from the delirium in fact coincided with the resumption of her glibenclamide.

TRICYCLIC ANTIDEPRESSANT DRUGS AND CONGENERS *(SED-11, 36; SEDA-13, 8)*

Amitriptyline

Nervous system *Hypomanic reactions* to tricyclic antidepressants are not unknown (SED-11, 40) though they are rarely severe. A severe case in a man with AIDS was described by Holmes et al in 1989; although there were other aggravating factors in the history and nortriptyline was clearly better tolerated the temporal association with amitriptyline is undeniable, and there was both a positive rechallenge and evidence of a dose–effect relationship (8[c]).

Endocrine, metabolic Earlier studies have on various occasions looked specifically for any influence which tricyclic antidepressants may have on carbohydrate metabolism and appear to have excluded any consistent effect. A case reported in 1988 does however seem to show that a diabetic patient who takes a tricyclic drug may be rendered unaware of impending symptoms of hypoglycemia. In that case a woman of 24 with unstable diabetes who normally recognized an oncoming hypoglycemic episode by the appearance of adrenergic symptoms was prescribed 25 mg/d amitriptyline for depression. Over the next 2 weeks she experienced several hypoglycemic episodes marked by violent derangement of her behavior but without the usual adrenergic warning signs. As soon as the drug was discontinued the phenomenon vanished (9[c]). A warning to diabetic patients that this *masking of hypoglycemia* can occur thus seems appropriate.

Amoxapine *(SED-11, 49; SEDA-12, 15)*

Nervous system The neuroleptic malignant syndrome ('malignant hyperthermia') has been reported with a range of drug products, the neuroleptics being the most prominent, but there is no known association with the typical tricyclic antidepressants. Amoxapine is however not a typical tricyclic agent, having structural links to the neuroleptics. It would therefore not be surprising if it were to precipitate the syndrome. Whether a fatal case published by Washington et al in 1989 proves the association is dubious, since it relates to a patient who had received a series of drugs, though he was taking amoxapine when the syndrome occurred. After a month of treatment of 200 mg daily (and 5 days after increasing this to 300 mg) a typical malignant hyperthermia appeared and rapidly proved fatal. Drugs taken in the recent past had comprised thiothixene, imipramine, alprazolam and diphenhydramine (10[c]).

Desipramine (and imipramine)

Sexual function As pointed out when discussing fluoxetine (below), derangement of sexual function by the tricyclic antidepressants has often been discussed. Desipramine may be added to the list following a recent report on a woman of 38 who lost her ability to attain orgasm on masturbation so long as she was treated with desipramine (rising doses to 150 mg/d). Although there was no follow-up or rechallenge, the case is interesting in that an effect on the reaction to masturbation is perhaps less likely to be confused by other factors (e.g. emotional changes during depression) than is the ability to attain orgasm during normal coitus (11[c]).

Hypersensitivity Morrow et al have described 2 fatal cases of hypersensitivity myocarditis and hepatitis, in middle-aged men; in one desipramine had been prescribed in rising doses (up to 200 mg/d) and in the other imipramine had been given in a dose of 50 mg/d. Taking the 2 cases together the authors suggest that hypersensitivity reactions to imipramine may be mediated through its primary metabolite, i.e. desipramine (12[c]).

Interactions The still emergent picture of *fluoxetine* interactions is discussed later in the present chapter. One fairly clear risk is that fluoxetine may raise blood levels of desipramine if the two drugs are given concurrently. Two recent cases in adults 33 and 75 years of age with blood level measurements seem to provide clear evidence of this interaction and have led to a firm warning from the authors concerned that fluoxetine and desipramine must not be used together in the customary doses (13[c], 14[c]).

'SECOND GENERATION' ANTIDEPRESSANT DRUGS *(SED-11, 50; SEDA-13, 11)*

Amfebutamone (bupropion, mefebutamone) *(SED-11, 55)*

Nervous system For several antidepressants developed in the past (e.g. maprotiline) doubt as to the frequency in which they precipitated *seizures* has persisted for a long time, though the existence of the effect was beyond doubt. Davidson, in 1989, provided a useful review of the issue as regards amfebutamone. Of 4097 patients treated during clinical studies, 37 developed seizures. The frequency was 0.35–0.44% when using a dose of 450 mg/d or less, and 2.19% when using higher doses. Fourteen of the patients concerned had predisposing factors, including cerebral palsy, brain tumors or head trauma, while 25 were receiving other medication (15[R]). Naturally, these same risk factors are present in a proportion of any population eligible for antidepressant therapy.

Fluoxetine *(SED-11, 55; SEDA-12, 17; SEDA-13, 12)*

The massive introduction of fluoxetine, particularly in the United States, followed by an overwhelming public relations campaign has produced a phenomenon not unfamiliar in the adverse reactions world; many patients appear to have been transferred without any clear reason from other drugs on which they were well-maintained, and some of these have experienced distressing effects with the new agent; the switch from trazodone to fluoxetine and back again is becoming a particularly familiar one.

Nervous system There is now evidence from various directions that fluoxetine may precipitate an *extrapyramidal disorder*, though probably only where there are strongly predisposing factors. One recent report describes a woman of 38 who had been treated successfully in the past with trazodone for her depression. When she was admitted to hospital for other reasons she was given haloperidol for a concurrent myoclonic disorder and the trazodone was withdrawn; the depression recurred and she was now given fluoxetine in a dose of 20 mg/d. She developed generalized muscle stiffness of extrapyramidal type which became progressively more severe over the next 4 days. Once fluoxetine was replaced by trazodone the muscular symptoms waned over a 12-day period (16[C]). Although the physician concluded that extrapyramidal effects might be induced by fluoxetine alone or its combination with a neuroleptic (see also 'interactions' below), one is dealing here with an unusual case; bearing in mind the propensity of neuroleptics alone to induce extrapyramidal effects and the fact that the patient was suffering from cerebral palsy, one would again hesitate to conclude that fluoxetine itself will induce parkinson-like symptoms in a normal patient.

The same reservation applies to 2 cases reported by Bouchard et al where fluoxetine indeed seems to have aggravated pre-existing parkinsonism in 2 women with an existing history of parkinsonian disorders (17[c]).

The fact that fluoxetine might occasionally induce *seizures* in normal doses and would certainly be capable of doing so in severe overdosage emerged during the clinical trials of this compound (SED-11, 55), and a number of case reports since then confirm this as a problem. Reports include one on a woman of 35 with a seizure-free history who developed major motor convulsions within 3 days of starting fluoxetine 20 mg/d with no other evident cause (18[C]) and another on an elderly woman on multiple drug therapy who went into seizures (with confusion and incontinence) 5 days after starting on a normal dose of fluoxetine to replace amoxapine (19[c]).

Manic and hypomanic reactions have been described earlier with fluoxetine and in 1989 Saran et al described what may have been precipitation of a *panic attack*.

A man of 41 with a history of obsessive compulsive disorder and panic attacks had been treated with trazodone but had tended to experience sedation; it was therefore replaced by fluoxetine 20 mg/d. He became anxious within 2 days and was admitted to hospital on the sixth day with a panic attack. He was successfully returned to trazodone and alprazolam (20[C]).

Endocrine, metabolic Hwang et al described a man of 70 in whom mineral derangement with hyponatremia followed replacement of trazodone by fluoxetine in normal doses. The reduced sodium and chloride levels were detected after 10 days, and after 2 weeks reduced serum and urine osmolarity were consistent with the picture of *inappropriate secretion of antidiuretic hormone*. The picture normalized within 10 days of drug withdrawal, and trazodone was reinstated (21).

Sexual function The tricyclic antidepressants have produced in the past a long series of case reports pointing to derangement of sexual function (SED-11, 42) and although the effect is assumed to be anticholinergic there is often a problem in distinguishing drug effects from those due to the depression itself. Much the same problem has arisen with the 'second-generation' products; 2 recent cases – one male and one female – of *anorgasmia* temporarily associated with prescribing and withdrawal of fluoxetine (one with positive rechallenge) serve as a reminder that the same type of effect can be encountered in some individuals with this drug (22[c]). Although similar cases in both sexes have been described by others, together with some evidence that it is a dose-dependent effect (23[c]), there is no reason to think that the problem will be any more frequent than it is with the tricyclic agents.

Overdose Overdosage data are only secondary to the field covered by these volumes, but where antidepressant drugs are concerned the risk of attempted suicide is evident. One may therefore note that a woman of 31 described by Finnegan and Gabiola survived with no major problems a dose believed to be 1400 mg, taken alongside a small dose of clonazepam. Gastric lavage was performed only 4 hours later, but her symptoms remained relatively mild; she was drowsy but arousable, and could be discharged after 4 days (24[c]). The finding is encouraging, though it is not clear why a patient with a history of multiple suicide attempts should have been given access to some 8–10 weeks' supply of any antidepressant drug.

Interactions With newer antidepressant drugs it remains difficult to analyze the unexpected reactions which may occur when they are only part of a complex of antidepressant measures (e.g. including lithium, tricyclic agents, MAO inhibitors or tryptophan) as is not uncommonly the case. In the case of fluoxetine and other drugs raising the availability of serotonin in the central nervous system there may be drug interactions with this process which have not yet been identified. A fatality reported by Kine et al illustrates the assessment problem:

A woman of 45 who had been treated with 40 mg doses of fluoxetine was hospitalized beause of the severity of her depression and tranylcypromine (20 mg, rising to 30 mg/d) was added; 2 days later the treatment was extended to include tryptophan 500 mg and thioridazine 50 mg. Two hours after the last drug had been added to the regimen she complained of headache, muscle cramps and insomnia; her gait became unsteady and she developed fever. She was moved to intensive care where she experienced a seizure, lost consciousness and exhibited hypotension, ventricular tachycardia and raised AST and ALT. She died after 44 hours. While considering the possibility of a neuroleptic malignant syndrome, the authors tend to attribute her death to the combined effects of fluoxetine, tranylcypromine and tryptophan on serotonin (25[C]).

That fluoxetine could cause a serious 'serotonin syndrome' when given alongside MAO inhibitors has of course been known for some years (SEDA-9, 22 and subsequent volumes) and as pointed out in the previous Annual the manufacturer stressed from June 1988 onwards that this particular combination should be avoided. Slightly less florid was the combination received by a 53-year-old woman described by Noveske et al:

The patient had for a period been receiving fluoxetine 20 mg/d and lorazepam but experienced inadequate relief and was therefore given lithium 900 mg/d in addition. Within 2 days she developed ataxia, confusion and involuntary movements of the limbs. There was pyrexia, jerky breathing and a reduced leukocyte count. The drugs were withdrawn, resulting in irregular improvement and she was later maintained without problems on lithium and nortriptyline only. The authors considered that the case represented a toxic encephalopathy due to fluoxetine with lithium (26[C]).

It would seem, firstly, that one must be cautious when using fluoxetine (and perhaps other serotonin-raising drugs?) as part of any psychopharmacological multi-drug regimen, and secondly that if problems suggesting an interaction do occur it may be well to replace it with a tricyclic agent.

Mianserin *(SED-11, 52; SEDA-12, 19; SEDA-13, 13)*

Nervous system '*Restless legs*' is a poorly understood syndrome which occasionally comes suddenly to the fore in association with a particular disorder or a particular drug. Pak et al have described three women in their forties, all of whom were treated with mianserin in doses rising from 30 mg/d to 60 or 90 mg/d over a period of a week. Within 12 days all patients had developed unpleasant sensations in their legs, and in 2 of them there were involuntary leg movements at night. In 2 patients the symptoms disappeared following drug withdrawal, while in the third reduction of the dose for 30 mg/d was sufficient to relieve the symptoms. In 1 patient a rechallenge was attempted and proved positive. None of the patients had previously experienced neurological disorders (27).

Dyskinesias have been described with most antidepressant drugs in incidental cases. There is a questionable report of induction of oral dyskinesias in a woman of 30 treated with mianserin 30 mg daily; the dyskinesia became evident within 2 weeks of starting treatment, which continued for 8 weeks until the depression had passed: the drug was then withdrawn and the oral dyskinesia disappeared within 3 days. However, choreoathetoid movements then appeared, apparently precipitated by the drug withdrawal, and persisted for 8 weeks. One should add that this was a case of mental retardation and the authors themselves suggest that recent treatment with amitriptyline may have played a role in the oral dyskinesias (28[C]).

Endocrine, metabolic In a woman of 77 a severe *edematous reaction* to mianserin has been described, involving the face, tongue and buccal mucosa, with partial obstruction of the pharynx. The woman had some days before been admitted to hospital for severe dehydration with hyponatremia and essential hypertension, and it was after supportive treatment for this primary condition that mianserin was prescribed for her depression, together with diazepam and atenolol. The edematous reaction appeared within 2 days and regressed rapidly after the antidepressant was withdrawn (29[C]).

Maprotiline *(SED-11, 51; SEDA-12, 18; SEDA-13, 13)*

Liver National Centres for Adverse Reaction Monitoring have in the course of the years received various reports of hepatic reactions to maprotiline, but one would not consider it a proven association. Weinstein et al described in 1988 a case in which a woman of 63 who had been switched from trazodone (which had proven ineffective) to maprotiline 150 mg/d showed biochemical evidence of a liver disorder; there were elevations in AST, alkaline phosphatase and γ-glutamyl transferase, but there were no clinical changes and the total bilirubin was normal. All measures began to normalize once the drug was withdrawn and recovery was complete. In the absence of rechallenge and with little relevant evidence of hepatic effects in the literature it remains doubtful whether there is here a cause-and-effect relationship (30[c]).

Trazodone *(SED-11, 50; SEDA-12, 20; SEDA-13, 14)*

An unusual approach to determining the *safety of a drug in the elderly* was followed by Spivak et al, who discussed 8 case reports on patients aged 60–76 years suffering from a range of conditions which are relatively common in this age group. They sought on this basis to determine how trazodone, which they regarded as a relatively safe antidepressant drug, might be expected to affect this particular population. The absence of serious cardiovascular and anticholinergic effects as compared with the tricyclic compounds was in part counterbalanced by a series of unwanted effects, of themselves mild, which could nevertheless prove problematical in this age group. They included urinary retention in a man with prostatic hypertrophy; orthostatic hypotension with syncope in cases of angina pectoris; paroxysmal supraventricular tachycardia or hypertension which could affect any elderly patient adversely; drowsiness, nausea and vomiting in a case of chronic atrial fibrillation or premature ventricular contractions; and drowsiness with loss of balance which was sufficiently severe to lead to withdrawal of the product in 4 of the 8 patients (31[C]).

ACKNOWLEDGEMENTS

The author would like to acknowledge the support which he received in the preparation of this Chapter from a specialized section of the Working Group on Human Toxicological Assessment at the University of Copenhagen.

REFERENCES

1. Jourdan Ch, Artu F, Lamy et al (1988) Acute MAOI intoxication: a case with coma for four days. *J. Toxicol. Clin. Exp. 8*, 395.
2. McGrath PJ, Stewart JW, Quitkin FM (1989) A possible L-deprenyl induced hypertension reaction. *J. Psychopharmacol., 9*, 310.
3. Menza MA, Golbe LI (1988) Hypomania in a patient receiving deprenyl (selegiline) after adrenal–striatal implantation for Parkinson's disease. *Clin. Neuropharmacol., 11*, 549.
4. Kraus R (1989) Hypertensive episodes with tranylcypromine treatment. *J. Clin. Psychopharmacol., 9*, 232.
5. Keck P, Pope HG, Nierenberg AA (1989) Autoinduction of hypertensive reactions by tranylcypromine? *J. Clin. Psychopharmacol., 9*, 48.
6. Pande AC, Max PA (1989) A dystonic reaction occurring during treatment with tranylcypromine. *J. Clin. Psychopharmacol., 9*, 229.
7. Absher JR, Black DW (1988) Tranylcypromine

withdrawal delirium. *J. Clin. Psychopharmacol., 8*, 379.
8. Holmes VF, Fricchione GL (1989) Hypomania in an AIDS patient receiving amitriptyline for neuropathic pain. *Neurology, 30*, 305.
9. Sherman KE, Bornemann M (1988) Amitriptyline and asymptomatic hypoglycemia. *Ann. Intern. Med., 109*, 683.
10. Washington C, Haines KA, Tam CW (1989) Amoxapine-induced neuroleptic malignant syndrome. *DICP (Ann. Pharmacother.), 23*, 713.
11. Yeragani VK (1988) Anorgasmia associated with desipramine. *Can. J. Psychiatry, 33*, 76.
12. Morrow PL, Hardin NJ, Bonadies J (1989) Hypersensitivity myocarditis and hepatitis associated with imipramine and its metabolite, desipramine. *J. Forensic Sci., 34*, 1016.
13. Goodluck PJ (1989) Influence of fluoxetine on plasma levels of desipramine. *Am. J. Psychiatry, 146*, 552.
14. Bell IR, Cole JO (1988) Fluoxetine induces elevation of desipramine level and exacerbation of geriatric nonpsychotic depression. *J. Clin. Psychopharmacol., 8*, 447.
15. Davidson J (1989) Seizures and bupropion: a review. *J. Clin. Psychiatry, 50*, 256.
16. Brod TM (1989) Fluoxetine and extrapyramidal side effects. *Am. J. Psychiatry, 146*, 1352.
17. Bouchard RH, Purcher E, Vincent P (1989) Fluoxetine and extrapyramidal side effects. *Am. J. Psychiatry, 146*, 1352.
18. Ware MR, Stewart RB (1989) Seizures associated with fluoxetine therapy. *DICP (Ann. Pharmacother.), 23*, 428.
19. Weber JJ (1989) Seizure activity associated with fluoxetine therapy. *Clin. Pharm., 8*, 296.
20. Saran A, Halaris A (1989) Panic attack precipitated by fluoxetine. *J. Neuropsychiatry Clin Neurosci., 1*, 219.
21. Hwang AS, Magraw RM (1989) Syndrome of inappropriate secretion of antidiuretic hormone due to fluoxetine. *Am. J. Psychiatry, 146*, 399.
22. Lydiard RN, George MS (1989) Fluoxetine-related anorgasmy. *South. Med. J., 82*, 933.
23. Kine MD (1989) Fluoxetine and anorgasmia. *Am. J. Psychiatry, 146*, 804.
24. Finnegan KT, Gabiola JM (1988) Fluoxetine overdose. *Am. J. Psychiatry, 145*, 1604.
25. Kine SS, Mauro LS, Scala-Barnett DM et al (1989) Serotonin syndrome versus neuroleptic malignant syndrome as a cause of death. *Clin. Pharm., 8*, 510.
26. Noveske FG, Hahn KR, Flynn RJ (1989) Possible toxicity of combined fluoxetine and lithium. *Am. J. Psychiatry, 146*, 1515.
27. Paik I-H, Lee C, Choi B-M et al (1989) Mianserin-induced restless legs syndrome. *Br. J. Psychiatry, 155*, 415.
28. Otani K, Kaneko S, Fukushima Y et al (1988) Involuntary movements associated with mianserin treatment: a case report. *Br. J. Psychiatry, 154*, 113.
29. Leibovitch G, Maaravi Y, Shalev O (1989) Severe facial oedema and glossitis associated with mianserin. *Lancet, 2*, 871.
30. Weinstein RP, Gosselin JY (1988) Case report of hepatotoxicity associated with maprotiline. *Can. J. Psychiatry, 33*, 233.
31. Spivak B, Radvan M, Meltzer M (1989) Side effects of trazodone in a geriatric population. *J. Clin. Psychopharmacol., 9*, 62.

Mogens Schou

3 Lithium

LITHIUM *(SED-11, 71; SEDA-12, 26; SEDA-13, 17)*

℞ *Lithium treatment and the kidneys*

Observation in the 1970s of morphological changes in the kidneys of lithium-treated patients caused serious concern among psychiatrists. Many asked themselves whether perhaps the patients' mental health was being bought at the expense of their kidney function, and whether patients given lithium treatment for many years would eventually develop renal failure and die. The number of patients started on lithium dropped drastically, ongoing treatments were interrupted, relapses developed, and suicides are known to have occurred. Some patients objected violently to being deprived of the treatment that had changed their lives radically, but protests were overruled, and the patients were left in a miserable state (1).

Other psychiatrists were less panicked. Those who had been using lithium for a long time argued that if the treatment had been apt to produce deterioration of the glomerular filtration rate (GFR), they would have seen at least some instances of renal failure among the many patients given lithium for many years. To them the main concern was that a widespread but unfounded 'kidney scare' might deprive seriously ill patients of a treatment which offered vital help (2).

A number of centers decided to subject the matter to systematic scrutiny, and few actions of psychotropic drugs have been as extensively examined as the effects of lithium administration on the kidneys. The matter was the subject of a 'Special Review' in SEDA-4 (p. 22) and has been referred to in all later volumes of SEDA. More than a decade has now passed since the appearance of the first frightening kidney report (3[C]), and the time seemed ripe for a new, critical examination of the laboratory and clinical evidence. One was published in 1988 (4[R]) and should be consulted for detailed data, arguments and references. Its main findings are analyzed here.

Both cross-sectional and longitudinal studies of lithium effects of the kidney have been carried out. In the former studies, values obtained from lithium-treated patients were compared with generally used reference ranges, with values from healthy subjects, or with values from patients not on lithium. According to 26 papers more than 2700 patients have been subjected to such examinations. In the longitudinal studies, kidney function was examined repeatedly in the same patients during lithium treatment. In some of the studies the patients were examined both before and during the treatment; in other studies the patients were examined during lithium treatment and again after its discontinuation. According to 15 papers more than 800 patients have been subjected to such examinations, some of the patients having been on lithium treatment for up to 18 years.

Cross-sectional studies *Cross-sectional studies without a control group are of little informative value as far as averages are concerned, for there is nothing to compare with. In several of the studies a number of individual patients showed GFR values lower than the lowest limit of the reference range, but it is impossible to know whether this had to do with the lithium treatment or with characteristics of the patient group not related to lithium. No patient developed renal failure.*

Cross-sectional studies using control groups of healthy subjects or of patients not given lithium provide more relevant information. Five of the studies contain GFR data (5[C]–9[C]). None of them showed a significant difference between the glomerular filtration rate of the lithium-treated patients and of the controls. No patient developed renal failure.

Side Effects of Drugs Annual 14
M.N.G. Dukes and L. Beeley, editors

Data from the cross-sectional studies have been analyzed for possible correlations between the GFR and time on lithium. None of the studies revealed a strong correlation. One study (10[C]) showed a weak negative correlation, but there were only a few GFR values lower than 50% of the reference mean, and the scatter of the data was pronounced.

Longitudinal studies Information bearing directly on the effect on GFR of treatment duration as well as of start and stop of the treatment comes from the longitudinal studies. In 6 studies the GFR was determined before and during lithium treatment (11[C]-16[C]). None of them showed a significant fall in GFR. No patient developed renal failure.

In 4 studies the GFR was determined repeatedly in the same patients during lithium treatment (7[C],16[C]–18[C]). None of them showed a statistically significant correlation between the GFR and the number of years on lithium. No patient developed renal failure.

Of the two studies with determinations of the GFR during lithium treatment and again after its discontinuation, one (7[C]) showed no significant change in GFR. The other (19[C]) showed a rise in ^{51}Cr-EDTA clearance. It should be noted, however, that the patients selected for discontinuation of lithium included those who during lithium treatment had had ^{51}Cr-EDTA values that were lower than the mean value minus 2 standard deviations. It need not be a sign of altered GFR when patients thus selected show a rise in ^{51}Cr-EDTA clearance on re-examination. The creatinine clearance did not change.

A recent cohort study revealed that among 234 patients given lithium treatment for up to 8 years and with a total lithium exposure time of 624 years, only two showed a falling creatinine clearance, and a causal relation to the lithium treatment was questionable (20[C]).

After psychiatric lithium usage for more than 35 years and treatment of very large numbers of patients, not a single case of renal failure has occurred which can be ascribed with reasonable certainty to the lithium treatment. A case of supposedly lithium-induced uremia was reported in 1979 (21[C]), but the causal role of lithium was highly questionable (22[C]). It was not until 1–3 months after discontinuation of lithium that the patient developed severe renal deterioration, and there was evidence of independent kidney disease: renal arteriosclerosis, hypertension, proteinuria, anemia, and a elevated sedimentation rate.

On the basis of the total evidence available today one must conclude that lithium treatment, even when given for many years, does not lead to any change in the GFR.

Serum creatinine concentration Serum creatinine values have been recorded in many studies in an attempt to disclose deterioration of the GFR and threatening renal failure. This might have been appropriate if filtration rates had fallen by 50% or more during lithium treatment. But they did not, and the serum creatinine values accordingly do not provide information of relevance for the GFR.

Nephrotic syndrome There have been occasional reports about development of a nephrotic syndrome with proteinuria and edema formation during lithium treatment or during treatment with lithium in combination with other psychotropic drugs (for references, see Ref. 4[R]). The frequency is so low that one might consider coincidence the most likely explanation; even if the proteinuria disappeared after discontinuation of lithium, this could have been due to spontaneous recovery.

However, in some instances the proteinuria reappeared when lithium treatment was resumed, and such observations clearly inculpate lithium, either as sole cause or as precipitating agent (23[C]–25[C]). Proteinuria developing during lithium administration has, on the other hand, been seen to disappear in spite of continued treatment (26[C]).

Even if lithium treatment did induce or precipitate a nephrotic syndrome in these patients, such conditions are rare and reversible. In a cohort of patients followed systematically during lithium treatment for up to 7 years and with a total lithium exposure time of more than 500 years, not a single patient developed a nephrotic syndrome (16[C]).

Urine volume and renal concentrating ability In the cross-sectional and longitudinal studies, urine volumes and renal concentrating abilities were also measured, primarily on the assumption that changes in these variables might predict later, functionally more ominous, changes in the GFR. As pointed out above, there were no such *changes to portend, and the main outcome of the examinations was a confirmation of what had been known for a long time, namely that lithium treatment may affect renal water handling.*

Morphological changes *It was the morphological kidney changes that made such an impression in the 1970s, because they were felt to reflect severe kidney damage and a serious prognosis. The picture is different today (27[C], 28[C]). Structural changes in the glomeruli of lithium-treated patients may occur, but they are non-specific and can be found also in the kidneys of patients about to start, but not yet having started, lithium treatment. Those morphological changes that are specifically associated with lithium treatment are confined to the distal tubules and collecting ducts; they are reversible; and they do not signify risk of falling GFR or renal failure.*

Conclusions *Lithium treatment, even when given for many years, does not lead to change in the GFR, let alone renal failure. It is time that misleading and anxiety-inducing references to 'the nephrotoxic effect of lithium' come to an end.*

One sometimes wonders how 'the kidney scare' could attain such dimensions and lead to such dire consequences. Even today many psychiatrists are diffusely uneasy about lithium and hesitate to start or continue treatment with this valuable drug. The development of this situation presumably had to do with overlapping responsibilities among specialists not very well acquainted with each others' problems and obligations. Nephrologists regarded lowered renal concentrating ability as a sign of serious kidney disease, and they felt it their duty to guard patients against the—apparently deleterious—effects of a drug they knew little about. And psychiatrists, concerned about not doing harm with their treatment, tended to trust the warnings of pathologists and nephrologists rather than the reassuring experiences of their own profession from more than 25 years of lithium treatment.

Use of terms such as 'lithium-induced nephropathy' or 'chronic lithium-induced renal insufficiency' without specification of whether this meant progressive deterioration of GFR, morphological changes in a kidney biopsy, or moderate lowering of the ability to concentrate the urine, has undoubtedly scared many psychiatrists into forgetting to weigh the factual risk of relapse and suicide with a discontinuation of lithium treatment against the hypothetical risk of renal failure with its continuation. We know now that the latter risk is non-existent, and psychiatrists can confidently use lithium prophylaxis for the protection of their manic-depressive patients.

GENERAL

The proceedings of The Second British Lithium Conference (29) contain many papers and reviews about side effects of and interactions with lithium (30[C]–43[C]).

Systematic enquiry among patients on maintenance lithium treatment (44[C]) revealed that whereas *thirst*, *increased urination* and *dry mouth* were the most common side effects, the patients perceived *cognitive changes* and *weight gain* as more troublesome and more likely to provoke non-compliance and interruption of treatment.

Animal studies have suggested that intake of additional potassium may counteract lithium-induced side effects (45–47). A clinical study showed that addition of 16 mmol of potassium per day in slow-release capsules ameliorated lithium-induced *hand tremor* and *ankle edema*; the side effects reappeared on discontinutation of potassium and abated on its resumption (48[C]).

EFFECTS ON ORGANS AND SYSTEMS

Neuromuscular system *Downbeat nystagmus* is usually secondary to cerebellar or cervico-medullary dysfunction (49[C], 50[C]) and may be seen as a sequel of lithium intoxication (50[C]–52[C]), perhaps even in non-toxic patients who are given additional drugs (50[C], 53[C]).

Akathisia can develop during lithium monotherapy but is a rare side effect (54[C]), possibly a dose-independent idiosyncratic reaction. It may abate during treatment with lorazepam (55[C]).

There have been case-reports about *writer's cramp* (56[C]) and *alexithymia* (inadequacy of experiencing and expressing emotions) (57[C]) associated with lithium therapy.

Lithium is occasionally used to treat painful dystonia seen after withdrawal of levodopa treatment of Parkinson's disease. In one case development of *neuroleptic malignant-like syndrome* was ascribed to lithium (58[C]), but it could also have been caused by the levodopa withdrawal itself.

A special review has been devoted to lithium effects on the *cerebellum* (59[R]).

Lithium-induced *tremor* has been treated with the relatively selective β_1-adrenoceptor blocker, atenolol, which may offer advantages over other beta-blockers (60[C]).

Mind *Memory impairment* during long-term lithium treatment may or may not be caused by the therapy, and there can be discrepancy between objective and subjective evaluation of cognitive functions (61[C]). In a systematic study, 18 bipolar patients were tested initially and after 6 years of lithium treatment. The mean memory test scores remained remarkably stable with only one of the 10 subtests showing a statistically, but not clinically, significant decrease, possibly caused by the age gain (62[C]). The patients' subjective complaints of impaired memory functioning correlated with the level of depression at the time of testing.

A patient developed *paranoid ideas* and *visual and auditory hallucinations* during lithium treatment, which disappeared when lithium was discontinued (63[C]); no rechallenging was attempted. A case of *mania* induced by lithium augmentation of antidepressant treatment has been reported (64[C]).

Lithium-treated unipolar ($n = 50$) and bipolar ($n = 50$) patients in remission were scored for *life satisfaction* and *social adjustment*. They did not differ significantly from healthy controls ($n = 50$); during remission the patients showed no residual impairment (65[C]). No significant group differences were found when *cognitive functioning* was compared in healthy controls, medication-free, carbamazepine-treated, and lithium-treated manic-depressive patients (66[C]).

Thyroid Figures for the frequency with which thyroxine-requiring *hypothyroidism* develops during lithium treatment (e.g. 'eight of 42 patients' (67[C])) are difficult to assess when the total lithium exposure time is not given. Only two studies, a Swedish (68[C]) and a Danish (69[C]), have provided such values. They both found an incidence of 2 cases per 100 years of lithium exposure, but we need corresponding incidence values from other geographical regions.

Antithyroid antibodies may increase the risk of developing lithium-induced hypothyroidism, but apparently their presence is neither a sufficient nor a necessary condition. Among 60 lithium-treated patients 7 had antithyroid antibodies and were euthyroid, 10 were hypothyroid without antithyroid antibodies, and 6 presented both antithyroid antibodies and hypothyroidism (70[C], 71[C]).

Cases of lithium-induced hypothyroidism presenting as carpal tunnel syndrome (pain and numbness in arms and hands) and responding to thyroxine remind us of the many guises that hypothyroidism can take (72[C], 73[C]).

Metabolic A useful review of *weight gain* with antidepressants and lithium (74[R]) quoted rather old observations concerning the latter drug. They were updated in a Letter to the Editor (75[C]), which pointed out that weight gain during lithium treatment has been found to be positively correlated with a diagnosis of bipolar illness, with coadministration of antidepressant drugs, and with the patients' body weight before lithium treatment started (76[C]). It may be prudent to give specific instructions about exercise and the avoidance of calorie-rich food and drinks to obese patients who start lithium treatment, particularly obese bipolar patients who may be less physically active when they are no longer manic. Supplementary treatment with antidepressants should be avoided.

Gastrointestinal After a few days of lithium carbonate treatment a patient developed *nausea* and vomited bright red blood. Gastroscopy revealed a *Mallory-Weiss tear* at the posterior wall, a syndrome sometimes produced by substances that can produce severe retching (77[C]). Three patients in well tolerated lithium treatment developed nausea within 2 hours after addition of 5 mg of the anticholinergic drug trihexyphenidyl, which does not by itself induce nausea (78[C]).

Complaints of *dry mouth* occur but are are not among the more frequent of lithium's side effects. A study with use of objective salivation tests nevertheless showed *hyposalivation* in 10 out of 14 lithium-treated patients (79[C]); the paper did not state whether these patients suffered subjectively from dry mouth.

Urinary system Evidence relating to this issue and published before the summer of 1988 has been reviewed in detail (4[R]) and is analyzed in the introductory 'Special Review'. Later publications on lithium and the urinary system have consolidated the conclusions, notably that lithium treatment of even many years' duration does not affect the *glomerular filtration rate* significantly even though urine flow may be increased and concentrating ability decreased (80[C]–86[C]). A single study (87[C]) showed a statistically significant moderate fall in creatinine clearance in men (not in women), but the sample size at 3 years of treatment duration was only 8. In a study on 50 patients maintained at a mean serum lithium level of 0.54 mmol/l none of the kidney variables changed significantly (88[C]). One lithium-treated patient had reduced glomerular filtration rate which was secondary to hypothyroidism and which normalized during treatment with thyroxine (89[C]).

Lowered renal concentrating ability is more pronounced when lithium has been given concurrently with neuroleptics or antidepressants for more than 2 years than when lithium has been given alone or concurrently with these drugs for less than 2 years (90[C]).

Urinary excretion of albumin and retinol-binding protein may be increased (91[C]), but this has not been shown to be of clinical relevance. There have been two more reports of lithium-induced *nephrotic syndrome with proteinuria* which resolved when lithium was discontinued (92[C], 93[C]). One of the patients also suffered from diabetes.

Skin and appendages Cutaneous side effects of lithium include *psoriasis* with *psoriatic arthritis* (94[C]–97[C]), *nail dystrophy* (98[C]), *alopecia areata* (99[C], 100[C]), and *subcorneal pustular dermatosis (Sneddon-Wilkinson disease)* (101[C]).

Second-generation effects A woman taking lithium throughout pregnancy had a *stillbirth* (102[C]). *Ebstein's anomaly* is found with increased frequency among children born of mothers on lithium treatment (103[C]), but studies of series of children with this malformation indicate that lithium is a rare cause (104[C], 105[C]). A mother given lithium during pregnancy gave birth to a baby with a port-wine stain (106[C]).

Intoxication The appearance of occasional reports of lithium intoxication developing with 'therapeutic lithium doses' may have left the impression that poisoning with lithium can occur capriciously even when treatment guidelines are followed. Systematic inquiry does not support this notion.

A study was carried out on the frequency and circumstances of lithium intoxications developing in a population of 372 000 over a 9-year period (20[C]). The point prevalence of lithium usage was 1.5 er 1000 persons in the population, and the total lithium exposure was accordingly about 5000 patient-years. There were 24 intoxications; none of the patients died, one developed permanent cerebellar damage. Fifteen of the intoxications were caused by deliberate self-poisoning with suicidal intent. Among the 9 remaining intoxications, 4 developed because lithium treatment was continued with unaltered dosage during somatic illness with fever and one during lowered intake of food and fluid in a depressive relapse. One patient was given too high lithium doses by his physician; one, with senile confusion, took more lithium than prescribed; and two patients took too high doses because they felt good on lithium and thought they would feel better on more lithium.

Rather than of capriciousness these observations speak of a high degree of predictability as far as lithium toxicity is concerned. Unintended lithium intoxications can be avoided by adherence to treatment guidelines and precautions.

Acute cases of lithium intoxication usually have milder symptoms than those with a more protracted course (107[C]). Lithium intoxication may present a transitory *Creutzfeldt-Jakob-like syndrome* with myoclonus and EEG showing periodic sharp waves, triphasic waves and diffuse slowing (108[C]–110[C]), in one case after combined treatment with lithium and levodopa (111[C]). Elderly patients, possibly with pre-existing brain pathology, may be especially sensitive to the cerebral effects of lithium (112[C]). A case of severe *generalized polyneuropathy* during lithium intoxication has been described (113[C]).

Lithium intoxication may result in death or permanent *cerebellar sequelae* (32[C], 114[C]–117[C]), but this is infrequent (20[C], 117[C]–119[C]). Treatments of intoxication have included hemodialysis, hemofiltration, peritoneal dialysis, and correction of electrolyte and fluid disturbances (107[C], 115[C]–116[C], 118[C]–123[C]). Administration of dopamine, which increases renal blood flow and increases sodium excretion, was tried with good results in one case (124[C]).

Interaction Interaction continues to be reported with *neuroleptics*, for example *droperidol* (125[C]), *haloperidol, chlorpromazine, perazine* (126[C]), *tiotixene* (*thiothixene*), *fluphenazine* (127[C]), and *thioridazine* (128[C]). High doses of neuroleptics are more dangerous than low (41[C], 129[C]). Interactions with *antidepressants* occur, e.g. development of lithium intoxication after combination with *fluoxetine* (130[C]), of malignant hyperpyrexia after combination with *tryptophan* and *phenelzine* (131[C]), and of myoclonus after combination with *nortriptyline* (132[C]). Combination of lithium and *carbamazepine* is usually safe (133[C]), but when used in brain-damaged adolescents it induced neurotoxic symptoms (134[C]).

Opinion and experience continue to be divided about interaction with *electroconvulsive treatment* (30[C], 135[C]–137[C]).

Case-reports indicate that in patients with pre-existing renal disease the combination of lithium and *angiotensin converting-enzyme inhibitors* such as *enalapril* and *captopril* may lead to aggravation (138[C]–145[C]).

Interaction with *tetracycline* has never been fully established, and a recent study with healthy volunteers showed a decrease, rather than an increase, of serum lithium during tetracycline intake (146[C]). Previously reported evidence of interaction with *diltiazem* (147[C]) has been questioned (148[C]). *Non-steroidal anti-inflammatory drugs*, e.g. *mefenamic acid* (149[C]), continue to attract interest. An editorial on the issue concluded: 'Toxic clinical interactions between lithium and NSAIDs are rare, and probably only occur in a small minority of the instances when the two drugs are used together. They seem to occur in only two situations, first in association with the more potent NSAIDs such as piroxicam, indomethacin and phenylbutazone, which are also very potent PG synthetase inhibitors and, secondly, among medically ill patients who may already have malfunctioning kidneys and who are often subjected to polypharmacy' (150[C]).

Miscellaneous Does *abuse of lithium* ever occur? A patient with a long history of bipolar disorder and alcohol abuse was out of funds for buying alcohol but found that if he combined 2400 mg of lithium carbonate (rather than the prescribed 1800 mg) with about 3 cups of coffee he felt relaxed, light-headed, and giddy. He developed incipient intoxication with a serum lithium level of 3.0 mmol/l and thereafter had no desire to overmedicate with lithium (151[C]).

REFERENCES

1. Kassirer JP (1983) Adding insult to injury. *N. Engl. J. Med., 308*, 898.
2. Schou M, Vestergaard P (1981) Lithium and the kidney scare (Editorial). *Psychosomatics, 22*, 92.
3. Hestbech J, Hansen HE, Amdisen A et al (1977) Chronic renal lesions following long-term treatment with lithium salts. *Kidney Int., 12*, 205.
4. Schou M (1988) Effects of long-term lithium treatment on kidney function: an overview. *J. Psychiatr. Res., 22*, 287.
5. Hullin RP, Coley VP, Birch NJ et al (1979) Renal function after long-term treatment with lithium. *Br. Med. J., 2*, 1457.
6. Coppen A, Bishop ME, Bailey JE et al (1980) Renal function in lithium and non-lithium treated patients with affective disorders. *Acta Psychiatr. Scand., 62*, 343.
7. Vestergaard P, Amdisen A (1981) Lithium treatment and kidney function: a follow-up study of 237 patients in long-term treatment. *Acta Psychiatr. Scand., 63*, 333.
8. Walker RG, Davies BM, Holwill BJ et al (1982) A clinicopathological study of lithium nephrotoxicity. *J. Chronic Dis.,, 35*, 685.
9. Khandelwal SK, Chugh KS, Sakhuja V et al (1983) Renal function in long-term lithium prophylaxis. *Indian J. Med. Res., 77*, 107.
10. Løkkegaard H, Andersen NF, Henriksen E et al (1985) Renal function in 153 manic-depressive patients treated with lithium for more than five years. *Acta Psychiatr. Scand., 71*, 347.
11. Grof P, MacGrimmon D, Saxena B et al (1980) Long-term lithium treatment and the kidney: clinical viewpoint. In: Grof P, Saxena B (Eds.), *Recent Advances in Canadian Neuropsychopharmacology*, p. 153. Karger, Basel.
12. Jensen SB, Rickers H (1984) Glomerular filtration rate during lithium therapy: a longitudinal

study. *Acta Psychiatr. Scand., 70*, 235.

13. Smigan L, Bucht G, Von Knorrig L et al (1984) Long-term lithium treatment and renal function: a prospective study. *Neuropsychobiology, 11*, 33.
14. Amsterdam, JS, Jorkasky D, Potter L et al (1985) A prospective study of lithium-induced nephropathy: preliminary results. *Psychopharmacol. Bull., 21*, 81.
15. Vaamonde CA, Millian NE, Magrinat GS et al (1986) Longitudinal evaluation of glomerular filtration rate during long-term lithium therapy. *Am. J. Kidney Dis., 7*, 213.
16. Schou M, Vestergaard P (1988) Prospective studies on a lithium cohort. 2. Renal function: water and electrolyte metabolism. *Acta Psychiatr. Scand., 78*, 427.
17. Johnson GFS, Hunt GE, Duggin GG et al (1984) Renal function and lithium treatment: initial and follow-up tests in manic-depressive patients. *J. Affect. Disord., 6*, 249.
18. DePaulo JR, Correa EI, Sapir DG (1986) Renal function and lithium: a longitudinal study. *Am. J. Psychiatry, 143*, 892.
19. Bendz H (1985) Kidney function in a selected lithium population: a prospective, controlled, lithium-withdrawal study. *Acta Psychiatr. Scand., 72*, 451.
20. Schou M, Hansen HE, Thomsen K et al (1989) Lithium treatment in Aarhus. 2. Risk of renal failure and of intoxication. *Pharmacopsychiatry, 22*, 101.
21. Hestbech J, Aurell M (1979) Lithium-induced uraemia. *Lancet, 1*, 212.
22. Vestergaard P (1979) Lithium-induced uraemia. *Lancet, 1*, 491.
23. Richman AV, Masco HL, Rifkin SI et al (1980) Minimal-change disease and the nephrotic syndrome associated with lithium therapy. *Ann. Intern. Med., 92*, 70.
24. Alexander F, Martin J (1981) Nephrotic syndrome associated with lithium therapy. *Clin. Nephrol., 15*, 267.
25. Depner TA (1982) Nephrotic syndrome secondary to lithium therapy. *Nephron, 30*, 286.
26. Singer L, Imbs J-L, Singer P et al (1979) Evolution favorable d'un syndrome néphrotiqué malgré la poursuite d'un traitement par le lithium. *Ann. Méd.-psychol., 137*, 584.
27. Walker RG, Dowling JP, Alcorn D et al (1983) Renal pathology associated with lithium therapy. *Pathology, 15*, 403.
28. Walker RG, Kincaid-Smith P (1987) Kidneys and the fluid regulatory system. In: Johnson FN (Ed.), *Depression and Mania: Modern Lithium Therapy*, p. 206. IRL Press, Oxford.
29. Birch NJ (Ed.) (1988) *Lithium: Inorganic Pharmacology and Psychiatric Usage*, 346 pp. IRL Press, Oxford.
30. Ahmed SK, Stein GS (1988) Is there a negative interaction between ECT and lithium? In: Birch NJ (Ed.), *Lithium: Inorganic Pharmacology and Psychiatric Usage*, p. 69. IRL Press, Oxford.
31. Albrecht G (1988) Cutaneous side effects in patients on long-term lithium therapy. In: Birch NJ (Ed.), *Lithium: Inorganic Pharmacology and Psychiatric Usage*, p. 79. IRL Press, Oxford.
32. Balasubramanian K (1988) Cerebellar damage following lithium toxicity. In: Birch NJ (Ed.), *Lithium: Inorganic Pharmacology and Psychiatric Usage*, p. 67. IRL Press, Oxford.
33. Curzon MEJ (1988) Lithium and dental caries. In: Birch NJ (Ed.), *Lithium: Inorganic Pharmacology and Psychiatric Usage*, p. 73. IRL Press, Oxford.
34. Friedlander AH (1988) Lithium/bipolar disorder: their effects on salivary flow, dental caries and periodontal disease. In: Birch NJ (Ed.), *Lithium: Inorganic Pharmacology and Psychiatric Usage*, p. 77. IRL Press, Oxford.
35. Imbs JL, Danion JM, Schmidt M et al (1988) Interaction between lithium and non-steroidal anti-inflammatory drugs. In: Birch NJ (Ed.), *Lithium: Inorganic Pharmacology and Psychiatric Usage*, p. 245. IRL Press, Oxford.
36. Jefferson JW, Greist JH, Carroll JA (1988) Lithium interactions with other drugs. In: Birch NJ (Ed.), *Lithium: Inorganic Pharmacology and Psychiatric Usage*, p. 45. IRL Press, Oxford.
37. King JR (1988) Review of significant side effects. In: Birch NJ (Ed.), *Lithium: Inorganic Pharmacology and Psychiatric Usage*, p. 15. IRL Press, Oxford.
38. Kocsis JH, Shaw ED, Hatterer J et al (1988) Motor and cognitive performance on lithium: relationship to thyroid function. In: Birch NJ (Ed.), *Lithium: Inorganic Pharmacology and Psychiatric Usage*, p. 263. IRL Press, Oxford.
39. Simhandl C, Thau K, Spiel C et al (1988) Side effects (self rating and objective rating) in 265 patients under lithium long term therapy. In: Birch NJ (Ed.), *Lithium: Inorganic Pharmacology and Psychiatric Usage*, p. 157. IRL Press, Oxford.
40. Simhandl C, Kircher S, Denk E et al (1988) Evaluation of renal lesions of lithium patients by non-invasive methods. In: Birch NJ (Ed.), *Lithium: Inorganic Pharmacology and Psychiatric Usage*, p. 249. IRL Press, Oxford.
41. Spring GK (1988) Problems of combined lithium neuroleptic toxicity. In: Birch NJ (Ed.), *Lithium: Inorganic Pharmacology and Psychiatric Usage*, p. 55. IRL Press, Oxford.
42. Srinivasan DP, Hullin RP (1988) Morbidity and mortality of lithium patients. In: Birch NJ (Ed.), *Lithium: Inorganic Pharmacology and Psychiatric Usage*, p. 19. IRL Press, Oxford.
43. Wancata J, Simhandl C, Denk E et al (1988) Reliability of lithium related side effects. In: Birch NJ (Ed.), *Lithium: Inorganic Pharmacology and Psychiatric Usage*, p. 159. IRL Press, Oxford.

44. Gitlin MJ, Cochran SD, Jamison KR (1989) Maintenance lithium treatment: side effects and compliance. *J. Clin. Psychiatry, 50*, 127.
45. Olesen OV, Jensen J, Thomsen K (1975) Effect of potassium on lithium-induced growth retardation and polynuria in rats. *Acta Pharmacol. Toxicol., 36*, 161.
46. Olesen OV, Hestbech J, Thomsen K (1980) Potassium reduction of lithium-induced histological changes of the rat kidney. *Toxicol. Appl. Pharmacol., 55*, 79.
47. Klemfuss H, Kripke DF (1987) Potassium reduces lithium toxicity: circadian rhythm actions are maintained. *Life Sci., 40*, 2531.
48. Cummings MA, Cummings KL, Haviland MG (1989) Use of potassium to treat lithium's side effects. *Am. J. Psychiatry, 145*, 895.
49. Halmagyi GM, Rudge P, Gresty MA et al (1983) Downbeating nystagmus: a review of 62 cases. *Arch. Neurol., 40*, 777.
50. Corbett JJ, Jacobson DM, Thompson HS et al (1989) Downbeating nystagmus and other ocular motor defects caused by lithium toxicity. *Neurology, 39*, 481.
51. Engelhardt A, Neundörfer B (1988) Downbeat-Nystagmus bei Lithiummedikation. *Nervenarzt, 59*, 624.
52. Yoshimoto Y (1987) A case of lithium intoxication with downbeat vertical nystagmus. *Auris, Nasus, Larynx (Tokyo), 14*, 71.
53. Williams DP, Troost BT, Rogers J (1988) Lithium-induced downbeat nystagmus. *Arch. Neurol., 45*, 1022.
54. Patterson JF (1988) Lithium-induced akathisia. *J. Clin. Psychopharmacol., 8*, 445.
55. Yassa R, Groulx B (1989) Lorazepam in the treatment of lithium-induced akathisia. *J. Clin. Psychopharmacol., 9*, 70.
56. Srikanth S, Khanna S, Channabasavanna SM (1988) Writer's cramp associated with lithium. *Clin. Neuropharmacol., 11*, 189.
57. Rybakowski JK, Dyson WL, Amsterdam JD (1988) Alexithymia and somatic conditions in patients with affective illnesses during lithium prophylaxis. *Psychother. Psychosom., 49*, 1.
58. Koehler PJ, Mirandolle JF (1988) Neuroleptic malignant-like syndrome and lithium. *Lancet, 2*, 1499.
59. Johnson FN (1988) The effects of lithium on the cerebellum. *Med. Sci. Res., 16*, 1097.
60. Davé M (1989) Treatment of lithium induced tremor with atenolol. *Can. J. Psychiatry, 34*, 132.
61. Sharma I, Singh P (1988) Cognitive functions in patients of primary affective disorder on prophylactic lithium treatment. *Indian J. Med. Res., 88*, 246.
62. Engelsmann F, Katz J, Ghadirian AM et al (1988) Lithium and memory: a long-term follow-up study. *J. Clin. Psychopharmacol., 8*, 207.
63. Kamlana SH (1989) Lithium-induced paranoid hallucinatory state. *Br. J. Psychiatry, 154*, 273.
64. Yuvarajan R, Yousufzai NM (1988) Mania induced by lithium augmentation: a case report. *Br. J. Psychiatry, 153*, 828.
65. Lepkifker E, Horesh N, Floru S (1988) Life satisfaction and adjustment in lithium-treated affective patients in remission. *Acta Psychiatr. Scand., 78*, 391.
66. Joffe RT, MacDonald C, Kutcher SP (1988) Lack of differential cognitive effects of lithium and carbamazepine in bipolar affective disorder. *J. Clin. Psychopharmacol., 8*, 425.
67. Joffe RT, Kutcher S, MacDonald C (1988) Thyroid function and bipolar affective disorder. *Psychiatry Res., 25*, 117.
68. Smigan L, Wahlin A, Jacobsson L et al (1984) Lithium therapy and thyroid function tests: a prospective study. *Neuropsychobiology, 11*, 39.
69. Maarbjerg K, Vestergaard P, Schou M (1987) Changes in serum thyroxine (T4) and serum thyroid stimulating hormone (TSH) during prolonged lithium treatment. *Acta Psychiatr. Scand., 75*, 217.
70. Leroy M-C, Villeneuve A, Lajeunesse C (1988) Lithium, thyroid function and antithyroid antibodies. *Prog. Neuro-Psychopharmacol. Biol. Psychiatry, 12*, 483.
71. Leroy M-C, Villeneuve A, Lajeunesse C (1988) Lithium and antithyroid antibodies. *Am. J. Psychiatry, 145*, 534.
72. Wood KA, Jacoby RJ (1986) Lithium induced hypothyroidism presenting with carpal tunnel syndrome. *Br. J. Psychiatry, 149*, 386.
73. Deahl MP (1988) Lithium-induced carpal tunnel syndrome. *Br. J. Psychiatry, 153*, 250.
74. Garland EJ, Remick RA, Zis AP (1988) Weight gain with antidepressants and lithium. *J. Clin. Psychopharmacol., 8*, 323.
75. Vestergaard P, Schou M (1989) Weight gain with lithium. *J. Clin. Psychopharmacol., 9*, 227.
76. Vestergaard P, Poulstrup I, Schou M (1988) Prospective studies on a lithium cohort. 3. Tremor, weight gain, diarrhea, psychological complaints. *Acta Psychiatr. Scand., 78*, 434.
77. Ananth J, Savodnik I, Yang H (1988) Lithium-associated Mallory-Weiss syndrome. *J. Clin. Psychiatry, 49*, 412.
78. Swartz CM, Breen KJ (1988) Nausea from taking both lithium and trihexyphenidyl. *Am. J. Psychiatry, 145*, 767.
79. Markitziu A, Shani J, Avni J (1988) Salivary gland function in patients on chronic lithium treatment. *Oral Surg. Oral Med. Oral Pathol., 66*, 551.
80. Dhar NK, Bhatia MS, Agarwal P et al (1987) Renal status in patients on long term lithium therapy. *Ann. Nat. Acad. Med. Sci. India, 23*, 223.
81. Bismuth C, Baud FJ, Godin M (1988) Renal function in lithium treatment. *Arch. Toxicol., 62, (Suppl. 12)*, 179.

82. Bismuth C, Baud FJ, Godin M et al (1988) Fonction rénale lors du traitement par lithium: à propos de 50 cas personnels. *Thérapie, 43*, 419.
83. Conte G, Vazzola A, Sacchetti E (1988) Renal function and long-term lithium therapy. *Med. Sci. Res., 16*, 1137.
84. Hetmar O (1988) The impact of long-term lithium treatment on renal function and structure. *Acta Psychiatr. Scand., 78, Suppl. 345*, 85.
85. Waller DG, Edwards JG, Papasthatis-Papayanni S (1988) A longitudinal assessment of renal function during treatment with lithium. *Q. J. Med. N. Ser., 68*, 553.
86. Welsch M, Danion JM, Singer L et al (1988) Effets indésirables rénaux des sels de lithium. *Thérapie, 43*, 423.
87. Jorkasky DK, Amsterdam JD, Oler J et al (1988) Lithium-induced renal disease: a prospective study. *Clin. Nephrol., 30*, 293.
88. Conte G, Vazzola A, Sacchetti E (1989) Renal function in chronic lithium-treated patients. *Acta Psychiatr. Scand., 79*, 503.
89. Balldin J, Berggren U, Svennerholm L et al (1988) Reduced glomerular filtration rate in a lithium-treated bipolar patient with hypothyroidism: reversal by levothyroxine. *Clin. Nephrol., 29*, 160.
90. Åberg-Wistedt A, Elwin CE, Norée LO et al (1988) Lithium and renal function in relation to concomitant therapy. *Int. Clin. Psychopharmacol., 3*, 277.
91. Jensen HV, Holm J, Hemmingsen L et al (1988) Urinary excretion of albumin and retinol-binding protein in lithium-treated patients. *Acta Psychiatr. Scand., 78*, 375.
92. Wood IK, Parmelee DX, Foreman JW (1989) Lithium-induced nephrotic syndrome. *Am. J. Psychiatry, 146*, 84.
93. Pawel BR, Kaye WA, Khan MY et al (1989) Aggravation of diabetic nephropathy by lithium: a case report and review of the literature. *J. Clin. Psychiatry, 50*, 101.
94. Hóly B, Nejdková A (1986) Psoriasis and lithium. *Acta Univ. Carol. Med. (Praha), 32*, 217.
95. Skerritt PW (1987) Psoriatic arthritis during lithium therapy. *Austr. NZ J. Psychiatry, 21*, 601.
96. Kaur I, Tripathi BM, Kaur S et al (1988) Cutaneous eruptions and lithium. *Indian J. Dermatol. Venerol. Leprosy, 53*, 278.
97. Zirilli G, Di Pompeo MD, Zirilli F (1988) Litio e psoriasi: revisione critica e contributo clinico. *Minerva Psichiatr., 29*, 43.
98. Don PC, Silverman RA (1988) Nail dystrophy induced by lithium carbonate. *Cutis, 41*, 19.
99. Beri A, Murdoch JK (1988) Lithium-associated alopecia. *Can. J. Hosp. Pharm., 41*, 211.
100. Silvestri A, Santonastaso P, Paggiarin D (1988) Alopecia areata during lithium therapy. *Gen. Hosp. Psychiatry, 10*, 46.
101. Sterling GB, Depietro WP (1988) Subcorneal pustular dermatosis (Sneddon-Wilkinson disease) associated with lithium carbonate treatment. *Cutis, 41*, 165.
102. Khandewal SK, Sagar RS, Saxena S (1989) Lithium in pregnancy and still birth: a case report. *Br. J. Psychiatry, 154*, 114.
103. Schou M, Weinstein MR (1980) Problems of lithium maintenance treatment during pregnancy, delivery and lactation. *Agressologie, 21A*, 7.
104. Warkany J (1988) Teratogen update: lithium. *Teratology, 38*, 593.
105. Källen B (1988) Comments on 'Teratogen update: lithium'. *Teratology, 38*, 597.
106. Leung AKC (1987) Port-wine stain associated with maternal use of lithium carbonate. *J. Nat. Med. Assoc., 79*, 877.
107. Gadallah MF, Feinstein EI, Massry SG (1988) Lithium intoxication: clinical course and therapeutic considerations. *Miner. Electrolyte Metabol., 14*, 146.
108. Primavera A, Brusa G, Poeta MG (1989) A Creutzfeldt-Jakob like syndrome due to lithium toxicity. *J. Neurol. Neurosurg. Psychiatry, 52*, 423.
109. Kemperman CJF, Van Gent EM, Rooij JAM et al (1988) Neurotoxiciteit van lithium bij een normale lithiumspiegel. *Ned. Tijdschr. Geneedskd., 132*, 2066.
110. Kemperman CJF, Notermans SLH (1989) Creutzfeld-Jacob like syndrome due to lithium toxicity. *J. Neurol. Neurosurg. Psychiatry, 52*, 291.
111. Brousolle E, Setiey A, Moene Y et al (1989) Reversible Creutzfeldt-Jakob like syndrome induced by lithium plus levodopa treatment. *J. Neurol. Neurosurg. Psychiatry, 52*, 686.
112. Kemperman CJF, Gerdes JH, De Rooij J et al (1989) Reversible lithium neurotoxicity at normal serum level may refer to intracranial pathology. *J. Neurol. Neurosurg. Psychiatry, 52*, 679.
113. Chang Y-C, Yip P-K, Chiu Y-N et al (1988) Severe generalized polyneuropathy in lithium intoxication. *Eur. Neurol., 28*, 39.
114. Nagaraj D, Taly AB (1987) Haemodialysis in lithium poisoning. *J. Assoc. Physicians India, 35*, 247.
115. Rose SR, Klein-Schwartz W, Oderda GM et al (1988) Lithium intoxication with acute renal failure and death. *Drug Intell. Clinical Pharm., 22*, 691.
116. Saxena S, Mallikarjuna P (1988) Severe memory impairment with acute overdose lithium toxicity: a case report. *Br. J. Psychiatry, 152*, 853.
117. Adityanjee (1989) The syndrome of irreversible lithium-effectuated neurotoxicity (SILENT). *Pharmacopsychiatry, 22*, 81.
118. Tunkel AR, D'Antonio J, Engel-Kominsky S et al (1988) Predicting the clinical course in intentional drug overdose. *Arch. Intern. Med., 148*, 253.
119. Simard M, Gumbiner B, Lee A et al (1989) Lithium carbonate intoxication: a case report and review of the literature. *Arch. Intern. Med., 149*, 36.

120. Josephs W, Schilken P, Wiechmann HW et al (1988) Erfolgreiche Detoxikation einer potentiell letalen Lithiumvergiftung mittels Hämofiltration. *Intensivmed. Notfallmed.*, *25*, 241.
121. Karki SD, Holden JMC (1988) Treatment of lithium intoxication. *Psychiatric Annals*, *18*, 708.
122. Gallardo MB, Ortega JMR, Torana MA (1988) Tratamiento con hemodiálisis en las intoxicaciones por litio. *Rev. Clin. Esp.*, *183*, 156.
123. Genser AS, Smith P, Honcharuk L et al (1988) Lithium overdose, when to dialize? A report of 28 consecutive cases. *Vet. Hum. Toxicol.*, *30*, 355.
124. MacDonald TM, Cotton M, Prescott LF (1988) Low dose dopamine in lithium poisoning. *Br. J. Clin. Pharm.*, *26*, 195.
125. Bamrah JS (1988) Neuroleptic-induced pyrexia: a benign variant. *J. Nerv. Ment. Dis.*, *176*, 741.
126. Kiejna A, Krakiewicz A (1988) Neurologic complications in patients treated with lithium. *Psychiatr. J. Univ. Ottawa*, *13*, 164.
127. Addonizio G, Roth SD, Stokes PE et al (1988) Increased extrapyramidal symptoms with addition of lithium to neuroleptics. *J. Nerv. Ment. Dis.*, *176*, 682.
128. Van den Broek WW, Van Hulst AM, Klompenhouwer JL et al (1988) Blijvende neurologische schade bij therapeutische lithium-concentraties in het plasma. *Ned. Tijdschr. Geneeskd.*, *132*, 2063.
129. Kane JM (1988) The role of neuroleptics in manic-depressive illness. *J. Clin. Psychiatry*, *49, Suppl.*, 12.
130. Salama AA, Shafey M (1989) A case of severe lithium toxicity induced by combined fluoxetine and lithium carbonate. *Am. J. Psychiatry*, *146*, 278.
131. Staufenberg EF, Tantam D (1989) Malignant hyperpyrexia syndrome in combined treatment. *Br. J. Psychiatry*, *154*, 577.
132. Devanand DP, Sackeim HA, Brown RP (1988) Myoclonus during combined tricyclic antidepressant and lithium treatment. *J. Clin. Psychopharmacol.*, *8*, 446.
133. Post RM, Kramlinger KG, Uhde TW (1988) Carbamazepine–lithium combination: clinical efficacy and side effects. *Int. Drug Ther. Newslett.*, *22*, 5.
134. Parmelee DX, O'Shanick GJ (1988) Carbamazepine–lithium toxicity in brain-damaged adolescents. *Brain Injury*, *2*, 305.
135. Milstein V, Small JG (1988) Problems with lithium combined with ECT. *Am. J. Psychiatry*, *145*, 1178.
136. Pearlman C (1988) Lithium–ECT interaction. *Convuls. Ther.*, *4*, 182.
137. Rudorfer MV, Potter WZ (1988) Lithium–ECT interaction: a reply to Pearlman. *Convuls. Ther.*, *4*, 183.
138. Douste-Blazy P, Rostin M, Livarek B et al (1986) Angiotensin converting enzyme inhibitors and lithium treatment. *Lancet*, *2*, 1448.
139. Santella RN, Rimmer JM, MacPherson BR (1988) Focal segmental glomerulosclerosis in patients receiving lithium carbonate. *Am. J. Med.*, *84*, 951.
140. Simon G (1988) Combination angiotensin converting enzyme inhibitor/lithium therapy contraindicated in renal disease. *Am. J. Med.*, *85*, 893.
141. Rimmer JM, Santella RN (1988) Combination angiotension converting enzyme inhibitor/lithium therapy contraindicated in renal disease: reply to Simon. *Am. J. Med.*, *85*, 894.
142. Mahieu M, Houvenagel L, Leduc JJ et al (1988) Lithium–inhibiteurs de l'enzyme de conversion: une association à éviter? *Presse Méd.*, *17*, 281.
143. Pulik M, Lida H (1988) Interaction lithium–inhibiteurs de l'enzyme de conversion. *Presse Méd.*, *17*, 755.
144. Rostin M, Douste-Blazy P, Galinier M et al (1988) Lithium et inhibiteur de l'enzyme de conversion: une association dangereuse. *Presse Méd.*, *17*, 1218.
145. Navis GJ, De Jong PE, De Zeeuw D (1989) Volume homeostasis, angiotensin converting enzyme inhibition, and lithium therapy. *Am. J. Med.*, *86*, 621.
146. Frankhauser MP, Lindon JL, Connolly B et al (1988) Evaluation of lithium–tetracycline interaction. *Clin. Pharm.*, *7*, 314.
147. Valdiserri EV (1985) A possible interaction between lithium and diltiazem: case report. *J. Clin. Psychiatry*, *46*, 540.
148. Flicker MR, Quigley MA, Caldwell EG (1988) Diltiazem–lithium interaction: an opposing viewpoint. *J. Clin. Psychiatry*, *49*, 325.
149. MacDonald J, Neale TJ (1988) Toxic interaction of lithium carbonate and mefenamic acid. *Br. Med. J.*, *297*, 1339.
150. Stein G, Robertson M, Nadarajah J (1988) Toxic interaction betwen lithium and non-steroidal anti-inflammatory drugs. *Psychol. Med.*, *18*, 535.
151. O'Boyle M, Emory E (1988) A case of lithium carbonate abuse. *Am. J. Psychiatry*, *145*, 1036.

Alan I. Green and Carl Salzman

4 Drugs of abuse

Cocaine *(SED-11; SEDA-12, 35; SEDA-13, 25) (see also Chapter 1)*

Less than 10 years ago, a major psychiatric textbook described cocaine as a relatively safe agent (1[R]). Many considered that cocaine, the 'champagne of drugs', was not a serious drug abuse problem. The fact that there had been a number of previous cocaine epidemics in the United States and elsewhere was discounted. Today, cocaine use is again at epidemic proportions. A recent review suggested that 36% of senior medical students in the United States had used cocaine (2[C]), 6% of them in the past month (2[C]). Although these data are lower than the national average, they indicate an alarming figure in a group with access to up-to-date information about cocaine's dangers. Since the lay media and the medical literature are filled with new reports of the detrimental effects of this drug, we have decided to devote this year's entire chapter to a review of cocaine and a discussion of the information that is rapidly pouring out of laboratories and clinics throughout the world. We do not imply that toxicity of other drugs of abuse is not important. Rather, the available literature over the past year is so overwhelmingly focussing on cocaine that for us to not do so did not seem appropriate.

Cocaine is a stimulant with a half-life of approximately 90 min. Some users may limit their use and never become heavy users. However, perhaps because the duration of the euphoric effect is less than the half-life, others gradually change to compulsive 'binge' use, in which cocaine is taken every 10–20 min for hours or even days. Controlled use may shift to compulsive use when more drug is available or when it is used intravenously or through smoking—both of which allow for very rapid effects.

Cocaine hydrochloride can be sniffed (snorted, tooted) or injected. Cocaine base (produced either through an organic solvent extraction process or through alkaline precipitation) is not inactivated by heat and, therefore, can be smoked. An inexpensive form of cocaine base (made through alkaline precipitation) known as 'crack' is widely available throughout the major urban areas of the United States. The easy availability and relative low price of crack have been in part responsible for the epidemic of cocaine use now occurring. Although the tendency of smoked cocaine to be rapidly addicting has been an important factor in the morbidity related to cocaine use, even intranasal cocaine administration can result in eventual binge abuse (3[R]).

Cardiovascular effects In the past few years, many reports have appeared, both in the scientific literature and the lay press, of the apparent cardiovascular effects of cocaine. It appears that *cardiotoxicity* may contribute to the lethality of the drug (4[R]). However, since many authors have noted that some of the presumed association of cocaine with cardiovascular effects is inferential, further study would seem appropriate (5[C]).

In a recent review of autopsy results of 40 cocaine-associated deaths, an increased incidence of *myocarditis* was noted as compared to data from 27 victims of sudden trauma (5[C]). The cause of the myocarditis in these patients was not clear; histologic examination revealed mononuclear infiltrates but failed to detect presence of bacteria, fungi or viral inclusions (5[C]). The investigators and others have speculated upon the role of focal ischemia (5[C], 6[R]). A second group has reported the presence of myocardial contraction bands in over 50% of patients following sudden death from cocaine use as compared to 10% of the controls (6[R]). They suggest that contraction band necrosis may contribute to the development of arrhythmias even without pre-existing coronary artery disease (6[R]).

Side Effects of Drugs Annual 14
M.N.G. Dukes and L. Beeley, editors

Cocaine use has also been associated with *myocardial infarction*. About 20 case-reports have appeared in recent years (4[R]). In at least 5 of the cases, no significant pre-existing coronary artery disease was present (4[R], 7[R]). Although the pathogenesis is uncertain, speculation about these cases has centered on a cocaine-induced acute coronary spasm (4[R], 7[R], 8[R]). In the majority of reported cases, however, cocaine-associated myocardial infarction has been noted in patients with pre-existing coronary disease. In such patients, cocaine may precipitate the acute event in a susceptible individual by increasing myocardial oxygen demand and producing coronary vasospasm (4[R]).

Whether cocaine frequently produces clinically significant *cardiac arrhythmias* in man appears to be uncertain (4[R]). Ventricular arrhythmias described in cocaine intoxication syndromes may be related to metabolic acidosis secondary to seizures (4[R]) or to a hypersympathetic state. Although cocaine's 'arrhythmogenic potential' may be modest (4[R]), the hypersympathetic state from cocaine may well be important. A recent report noted an aortic rupture following cocaine use in a 45-year-old man, an effect thought related to the *hypersympathetic* condition (4[R], 9[R]).

Two recent articles, one reporting 3 cases, the other providing a review, have discussed cocaine-associated *stroke* (10[R], 11[C]). None of the 3 cases described had any stroke risk factors (11[C]). In all cases, the stroke occurred shortly after smoking alkaloidal cocaine or crack (11[C]). While the mechanism for this effect is speculative, theories involve direct sympathetic stimulation by cocaine or vasoconstriction secondary to cocaine's ability to increase synaptic levels of serotonin (10[R], 11[C]).

Lastly, a recent study of the effects of cocaine in humans suggests that acute tolerance does not develop to the tachycardia and hypertensive effects of cocaine during a 4-hour controlled infusion (12[R]). Data such as these may begin to explain the profound cardiovascular effects associated with cocaine use in man. Clearly, more research is required.

Cocaine-associated deaths Deaths associated with cocaine use have been linked to hyperthermia, seizures, respiratory arrest, or cardiovascular events (3[R]). At times, the quantity of drug ingested is enormous, such as in the 7 cases of 'mini-packer' syndrome recently described (13[C]). In these cases, death occurred when small-time drug dealers ('mini-packers') swallowed cocaine-filled rubber containers to elude law enforcement detection (13[C]). Subsequent rupturing of the containers led to overdose and death. Other times, seemingly benign amounts of cocaine (by any route, including intravenous, snorting, smoking, oral, anal or vaginal) can lead to death (13[C]–15[C]). One investigator has speculated that some individuals may be particularly prone to toxic cocaine effects, due to reduced levels of pseudocholinesterase, an enzyme involved in cocaine metabolism and inactivation (16[C]). At present, sufficient data are not available to support such an hypothesis.

In a retrospective analysis of death cases brought to the Chief Medical Examiner of New York City over an 11-month period, 15% were noted to be cocaine-related (with detectable levels of cocaine in their blood) (17[R]). Of these cocaine-related cases, more than one-third were homicide victims and 16 were in children age 10 or under. The authors expressed concern about the role of cocaine in violence, and in deaths otherwise described as 'sudden infant death syndrome' (17[R]).

Cocaine use during pregnancy Cocaine use among women appears to have increased over recent years (18[C]). Even among pregnant women, the prevalence rate is high; a recent study of inner-city women measured it at 17% (19[C]). A number of preliminary studies have reported that cocaine use during pregnancy may be associated with spontaneous abortion and placental abruption, as well as reduced birth weight in the neonate (18[C], 20[C]). Over the past year, a number of reports have been published which extend and elaborate upon the previous findings.

One important question concerns the effect of cocaine use by women who discontinue such use upon learning that they have become pregnant. One study has suggested that 'social users' who stop cocaine use in the first trimester do not have babies with abnormalities of birth weight, gestation, or neonatal development (21[R]). A second confirmed the data on birth weight, but indicated that abruptio placentae in the mother and neurobehavioral deficiencies in infants may occur even following cocaine use confined to the first trimester (22[C]).

Studies of women who use cocaine throughout pregnancy have reported abruptio placentae (23[C], 24[R]) as well as low birth weight and early gestational age in their infants (25[C]). The infants appear to have smaller length and head circumference than would ordinarily be expected (18[C]). An ultrasound study utilizing multiple evaluations throughout the pregnancy has also demonstrated abnormal growth patterns (26[C]). One study has reported on genitourinary tract malformations in the infants following birth (27[C]).

Other studies have demonstrated transient EEG abnormalities (28[C]) and auditory system deficits (29[C]) in infants of cocaine-using women. The long-term effect of the auditory system problem is unknown (29[C]). Further studies have reported on birth complications (meconium and tachycardia) (30[C], 31[C]), transient cardiorespiratory pattern abnormalities (32[C]), fetal death (20[C]), and possibly an excess of congenital cardiac abnormalities (30[C]) in these infants. One recent study of women who used 'crack' (and who were presumably therefore in a low socioeconomic group) and had little prenatal care, showed abnormalities in birth weight and gestational age even when compared to a carefully matched control group (33[C]).

The need to carefully control these studies for detrimental effects of prenatal factors other than cocaine use is obviously important. As noted above, cocaine-using women may have poor prenatal care, which by itself may predispose to problems (33[C]). The issue of increased incidence of sudden infant death syndrome (SIDS) in infants born to cocaine-abusing women is a case in point. One study reported such an increased incidence in women who abused cocaine (32[C]). Another review discussed the likelihood that this occurs (34[r]). However, a third report noted that among women who receive prenatal care, the use of cocaine during pregnancy does not increase the risk of SIDS among their infants (35[C]).

Lastly, pregnant women or women in the post-partum period may be at risk for hypertension secondary to eclampsia. A recent report describes a 25-year-old cocaine-using woman who developed a seizure and a frontoparietal intracerebral hemorrhage 4 days after giving birth (36[C]).

Cocaine toxicity in infants Infants born to cocaine-abusing mothers may be at risk for cocaine intoxication via breast feeding (37[C]). This risk may be increased by the fact that plasma cholinesterase, which metabolizes cocaine, is thought to be lower in infants than adults (38[R]). A recent report described an unusual situation in which cocaine-induced seizures occurred in an infant whose mother had applied a topical anesthetic containing cocaine to her nipples to relieve breast- feeding-induced soreness (37[C]). At other times, the source of cocaine in cases of cocaine toxicity of infants is unknown (39[C]). There has been speculation that passive inhalation of freebase cocaine may occur in infants whose mothers are 'crack' smokers (40[C]).

A recent report comments on what may be an indirect form of cocaine toxicity in infants. Crack use may be associated with an increase in violence in the community; children may be accidental victims (41[r]). Fatal child abuse from battery has been described in families where the parents have been using cocaine (41[r]). The extent of this 'toxic effect' of cocaine use in children is unknown.

Hyperthermia Cocaine use can cause significant hyperthermia, which may be associated with a fatal outcome (42[R], 43[C], 44[C]). One case has been described in a young man who was known on the basis of a muscle biopsy to have malignant hyperthermia (44[C]). However, hyperthermia from cocaine intoxication in the absence of a known history of malignant hyperthermia has also been described (43[C]). One group has speculated that the hyperthermia secondary to cocaine intoxication may be a variant of the neuroleptic malignant syndrome (a sometimes fatal complication of antipsychotic drug therapy) that occurs with a significant disruption of dopaminergic function (42[R]). The authors propose that chlorpromazine, which is often suggested as a treatment for cocaine intoxication, may actually worsen the hyperthermia; they suggest the use of bromocriptine (a dopamine agonist) as a treatment for persistent hyperthermia following cocaine intoxication (42[R]).

Neurological effects Cocaine abuse has been associated with a number of neurological effects, including *stroke*, *seizure*, *subarachnoid* *hemorrhage*, *vasculitis*, *respiratory depression* (45[c]), *acute dystonic reaction* (46[C]), and *white matter disease* (45[c]). The dystonic reaction can be transient but reproducible with subsequent cocaine use (46[C]). Two interesting cases of new-onset *migraine* have been described in cocaine users. In both cases, migraine appeared to develop about $1^1/_2$ hours after the cocaine and was partially relieved by further use (47[C]). The authors suggest that cocaine's ability to block the re-uptake of serotonin may be of etiologic importance. They postulate that the migraine develops during cocaine 'withdrawal' accompanied by a lowering of serotonin concentration (47[C]).

Cocaine's ability to stimulate seizure activity produced an unusual manifestation in a 20-year-old woman who was a chronic cocaine abuser. This woman had several seizures over a 3-week period and then presented to the hospital because of psychosis and disturbed behavior over a 2-week period. Diagnosed initially as having a cocaine-induced psychosis, she was subsequently found to have partial complex status epilepticus responsive to anticonvulsant medication (48[C]).

Psychiatric effects Psychostimulants such as cocaine are known to have important psychiatric effects. Cocaine use produces euphoria, which is described as a rush followed by a high. At higher doses, disinhibition, grandiosity, impulsiveness, hypersexuality, psychomotor agitation, hypervigilance and stereotyped behavior can occur; severe panic or frank paranoid psychosis can also develop (3[R]). A recent study in volunteer addicts demonstrated that even a constant 4-hour infusion of cocaine can produce suspiciousness or frank *paranoid behavior* during the time course of the infusion (49[R], 50[R]). Interestingly, the study showed the ability of haloperidol to lessen the cocaine high, but not the initial cocaine rush. The haloperidol effect suggests the importance of dopaminergic action (reuptake blockade) in some of the acute psychiatric symptoms produced by cocaine (49[R], 50[R]).

Studies over a number of years have demonstrated the overrepresentation of mood disorders in patients in treatment programs for cocaine abuse (3[R]). Self-medication with cocaine may be one factor involved in the use of the drug (51[R]). In that regard, 2 patients were recently described whose cocaine use appeared to parallel the dysphoric (winter) periods of apparent seasonal affective disorders (51[C]).

Preliminary studies have suggested that desipramine, a tricyclic antidepressant, may decrease the cocaine craving which can occur during abstinence (3[R]). Some investigators have suggested that this effect of desipramine may be due to its ability to downregulate supersensitive catecholamine receptors (3[R]). In some abstinent patients, the first few desipramine doses may cause a jitteriness which can place patients at risk of relapse to cocaine use (52[C]). Clinical caution, with frequent monitoring, is advised (52[C]).

Renal effects *Acute rhabdomyolysis* has been reported to occur following the use of a number of drugs. Barbiturates, alcohol, methadone, heroin, amphetamine, phenylpropanolamine, phencyclidine, mescaline, and even gasoline (sniffing) have been implicated (53[R], 54[C]). Recently a number of reports have suggested that cocaine deserves an important place on that list (53[R], 55[C], 56[C], 57[R], 58[C], 59[c]).

A recent retrospective study evaluated the association of cocaine use and acute rhabdomyolysis over a 7-year period (57[R]). Of note, most of the 39 cases of renal complications of cocaine-induced rhabdomyolysis were detected quite recently. Routes of administration of cocaine included smoking ($n=11$); snorting ($n=5$); intravenous ($n=11$); and oral ($n=3$). Rhabdomyolysis was defined as myalgia and muscle tenderness and/or a CPK level of over 10 times normal (57[R]).

In this study, acute renal failure occurred in 13 of the 39 patients, and was associated with a more malignant course. Seven of the patients with renal failure developed disseminated intravascular coagulation; 6 of them died. The patients who died also had severe hepatic dysfunction. While only 7 of the 13 patients with acute renal failure (ARF) survived, all 26 patients without ARF did so (57[R]).

Seven prospective case-reports of the development of rhabdomyolysis following cocaine use have been described in the recent literature by 4 groups of investigators (53[R], 55[C], 56[C], 58[C], 59[c]). In 6 of the cases, acute renal failure developed. Other symptoms included myalgia, muscle soreness, discoloration of the urine, myoglobinuria, and elevation of the CPK level

(53[R]). All of the patients recovered with adequate therapy. Adequate hydration may help prevent acute renal failure (53[R]), but hemodialysis may be necessary if it develops (53[R]).

The pathophysiology of the rhabdomyolysis associated with cocaine use remains unclear (57[R], 60[r]). Muscle injury due to traumatic events may be causative in some cases (55[C], 58[C]); however, not all patients show any sign of this or give an appropriate history (57[R], 61[r]). Malignant hyperthermia (see above), which can occur with severe cocaine intoxication, is known to cause rhabdomyolysis (57[R]). The marked sympathomimetic activity of cocaine may facilitate hyperthermia as well as muscle damage (56[C]).

Respiratory effects A number of adverse respiratory effects have been associated with cocaine use. Snorting (tooting) cocaine can result in *nasal symptoms* (including septal perforations) as well as substantial *necrosis* of tissues (midline granuloma) of the upper respiratory tract (62[C]). A recent questionnaire sent to adolescents determined that 47% of daily cocaine snorters complained of nasal irritations, including nosebleeds (63[R]). Two cases of cocaine-related midline granuloma were recently reported (62[C]). The findings, including progressive alterations of the upper respiratory tract, can mimic other forms of midline granuloma. Adequate diagnosis of the cocaine etiology is important as appropriate therapy with antibiotics is effective (62[C]). Another report described a 43-year-old man who developed osteolytic sinusitis and secondary bilateral optic nerve involvement following a 15-year history of daily intranasal cocaine use (64[C]). The optic nerve damage appeared to be due to ischemic necrosis of mucosal and bony structures in close proximity (64[C]).

Inhalation of alkaloidal cocaine (crack) has been associated with *pneumomediastinum* and *pneumothorax* (65[C]). A recent case of pneumomediastinum occurred in a young man who employed vigorous Valsalva maneuvers while smoking cocaine (66[C]). Despite the striking radiographic appearance and physical findings, the course was benign (66[C]). Similarly, *pulmonary hemorrhage* and significant *hemoptysis* secondary to cocaine smoking (perhaps due to cocaine-related vasoconstriction) is also thought to have a generally benign course (67[C]). A recent report described a case of recurrent transient *pulmonary infiltrates*, associated with fever, bronchospasm and eosinophilia (65[C]) in a young female cocaine smoker (65[C]). The syndrome, thought to be a hypersensitivity reaction to the cocaine, occurred on 3 separate occasions, each time following cocaine smoking (65[C]). Fortunately, resolution on each occasion was uneventful. Lastly, cocaine smoking may also cause *necrotizing thermal injury* of the oropharynx (68[c]). The authors of this report speculated that drug-induced decreased sensorium combined with the high temperature of the smoke combined to produce the considerable damage (68[c]).

Miscellaneous Three other reports of cocaine toxicity deserve mention. One was of a 20-year-old woman who developed skin rash, myalgias, and muscle weakness 12 hours after smoking cocaine. Biopsy showed widespread *skin and muscle infarctions* leading to necrosis (69[C]). It was not clear whether an impurity might have been present in the cocaine, but the intravenous route of administration had not been used (69[C]). The second report suggests that severe *hepatotoxicity* can occur with cocaine use (70[C],71[C]). The clinical significance of this, however, for the broad range of users is not known. The third report describes a 38-year-old woman who developed a *central retinal artery occlusion* that appeared to be related to the intravenous injection of a large quantity of cocaine (72[C]). The authors postulate arteriospasm secondary to cocaine as a possible cause (72[C]).

REFERENCES

1. Grinspoon L, Bakalar JB (1980) Drug dependence: nonnarcotic agents. In: Kaplan HI, Freedman AM, Sadock BJ (Eds.), *Comprehensive Textbook of Psychiatry/III, Vol. 2*, p. 1614. Williams and Wilkins, Baltimore.
2. Conard S, Hughes P, Baldwin Jr. DC et al (1989) Cocaine use by senior medical students. *Am. J. Psychiatry, 146*, 382.
3. Gawin FH, Ellinwood Jr. EH (1988) Cocaine and other stimulants: actions, abuse, and treatment. *N. Engl. J. Med., 318*, 1173.
4. Gradman AH (1988) Cardiac effects of cocaine:

a review. *Yale J. Biol. Med., 61*, 137.
5. Virmani R, Robinowitz M, Smialek JE, Smyth DF (1988) Cardiovascular effects of cocaine: an autopsy study of 40 patients. *Am. Heart J., 115*, 1068.
6. Karch SB, Billingham ME (1988) The pathology and etiology of cocaine-induced heart disease. *Arch. Pathol. Lab. Med., 112*, 225.
7. Wang T, Hadidi F, Triana F, Bargout M (1988) Morning report at Charity Hospital: myocardial infarction associated with the use of cocaine. *Am. J. Med. Sci., 295*, 569.
8. Waller BF (1988) Cocaine and the heart. *Indiana Med., 81*, 956.
9 Inoue H, Zipes DP (1988) Cocaine-induced supersensitivity and arrhythmogenesis. *J. Am. Coll. Cardiol., 11*, 867.
10 Levine SR, Welch KMA (1987) Cocaine and stroke. *Curr. Concepts Cerebrovasc. Dis. Stroke, 19*, 779.
11. Levine SR, Washington JM, Jefferson MF et al (1987) 'Crack' cocaine-associated stroke. *Neurology, 37*, 1849.
12. Kumor K, Sherer M, Thompson L et al (1988) Lack of cardiovascular tolerance during intravenous cocaine infusions in human volunteers. *Life Sci., 42*, 2063.
13. Introna F, Smialek JE (1989) The 'mini-packer' syndrome: fatal ingestion of drug containers in Baltimore, Maryland. *Am. J. Forensic Med. Pathol., 10*, 21.
14. Doss PL, Gowitt GT (1988) Investigation of a death caused by rectal insertion of cocaine. *Am. J. Forensic Med. Pathol., 9*, 336.
15. Ettinger TB, Stine RJ (1989) Sudden death temporally related to vaginal cocaine abuse (Letter to Editor). *Am. J. Emerg. Med., 7*, 129.
16. Devenyi P (1989) Cocaine complications and pseudocholinesterase (Letter to Editor). *Ann., Intern. Med., 110*, 167.
17. Tardiff K, Gross E, Wu J et al (1989) Analysis of cocaine-positive fatalities. *J. Forensic Sci., 34*, 53.
18. Zuckerman BS, Frank DA, Hingson R et al (1989) Effects of maternal marijuana and cocaine use on fetal growth. *N. Engl. J. Med., 320*, 762.
19. Frank DA, Zuckerman BS, Amaro H et al (1988) Cocaine use during pregnancy: prevalence and correlates. *Pediatrics, 82*, 888.
20. Critchley HOD, Woods SM, Barson AJ et al (1988) Fetal death in utero and cocaine abuse: case report. *Br. J. Obestet. Gynaecol., 95*, 195.
21. Graham K, Dimitrakoudis D, Pellegrini E, Koren G (1989) Pregnancy outcome following first trimester exposure to cocaine in social users in Toronto, Canada. *Vet. Hum. Toxicol., 31*, 143.
22. Chasnoff IJ, Griffith DR, MacGregor S et al (1989) Temporal patterns of cocaine use in pregnancy: perinatal outcome. *J. Am. Med. Assoc., 261*, 1741.
23. Townsend RR, Laing FC, Jeffrey Jr RB (1988) Placental abruption associated with cocaine abuse. *Am. J. Radiol., 150*, 1339.
24. Collins E, Hardwick RJ, Jeffery H (1989) Perinatal cocaine intoxication. *Med. J. Austr., 150*, 331.
25. Chouteau M, Namerow PB, Leppert P (1988) The effect of cocaine abuse on birth weight and gestational age. *Obstet. Gynecol., 72*, 351.
26. Mitchell M, Sabbagha RE, Keith L et al (1988) Ultrasonic growth parameters in fetuses of mothers with primary addiction to cocaine. *Am. J. Obstet. Gynecol., 159*, 1104.
27. Chasnoff IJ, Chisum GM, Kaplan WE (1988) Maternal cocaine use and genitourinary tract malformations. *Teratology, 37*, 201.
28. Doberczak TM, Shanzer S, Senie RT, Kandall SR (1988) Neonatal neurologic and electronencephalographic effects of intrauterine cocaine exposure. *J. Pediatr., 113*, 354.
29. Shih L, Cone-Wesson B, Reddix B (1988) Effects of maternal cocaine abuse on the neonatal auditory system. *Int. J. Pediatr. Otorhinolaryngol., 15*, 245.
30. Little BB, Snell LM, Klein VR, Gilstrap III LC (1989) Cocaine abuse during pregnancy: maternal and fetal implications. *Obstet. Gynecol., 73*, 157.
31. Geggel RL, McInerny J, Estes III M (1989) Transient neonatal ventricular tachycardia associated with maternal cocaine use. *Am. J. Cardiol., 63*, 383.
32. Chasnoff IJ, Hunt CE, Kletter R, Kaplan D (1989) Prenatal cocaine exposure is associated with respiratory pattern abnormalities. *Am. J. Dis. Child. 143*, 583.
33. Cherukuri R, Minkoff H, Feldman J et al (1988) A cohort study of alkaloidal cocaine ('crack') in pregnancy. *Obstet. Gynecol., 72*, 147.
34. Tudehope DI (1989) Perinatal cocaine intoxication: a precaution. *Med. J. Austr., 150*, 290.
35. Bauchner H, Zuckerman B, McClain M et al (1988) Risk of sudden infant death syndrome among infants with in utero exposure to cocaine. *J. Pediatr., 113*, 831.
36. Mercado A, Johnson Jr G, Calver D, Sokol RJ (1989) Cocaine, pregnancy and postpartum intracerebral hemorrhage. *Obstet. Gynecol., 73*, 467.
37. Chaney NE, Franke J, Wadlington WB (1988) Cocaine convulsions in a breast-feeding baby. *J. Pediatr., 112*, 134.
38. Bingol N, Fuchs M, Daaz V et al (1987) Teratogenicity of cocaine in humans. *J. Pediatr., 110*, 93.
39. Cravey RH (1988) Cocaine deaths in infants. *J. Analyt. Toxicol., 12*, 354.
40. Bateman DA, Heagarty MC (1989) Passive freebase cocaine ('crack') inhalation by infants and toddlers. *Am. J. Dis. Child., 143*, 25.
41. Press S (1988) Crack and fatal child abuse (Letter to Editor). *J. Am. Med. Assoc., 260*, 3132.
42. Kosten TR, Kleber HD (1988) Rapid death during cocaine abuse: a variant of the neuroleptic

malignant syndrome? *Am. J. Drug Alcohol Abuse, 14*, 335.
43. Campbell BG (1988) Cocaine abuse with hyperthermia, seizures and fatal complications. *Med. J. Austr., 149*, 387.
44. Britt BA (1988) Combined anesthetic- and stress-induced malignant hyperthermia in two offspring of malignant hyperthermic-susceptible parents. *Anesth. Analg., 67*, 393.
45. Weingarten K (1988) Cerebral vasculitis associated with cocaine abuse or subarachnoid hemorrhage? (Letter to Editor). *J. Am. Med. Assoc., 259*, 1648.
46. Merab J (1988) Acute dystonic reaction to cocaine (Letter to Editor). *Am. J. Med., 84*, 564.
47. Satel SL, Gawin FH (1989) Migrainelike headache and cocaine use. *J. Am. Med. Assoc., 261*, 2995.
48. Merriam AE, Medalia A, Levine B (1988) Partial complex status epilepticus associated with cocaine abuse. *Biol. Psychiatry, 23*, 515.
49. Sherer MA, Kumor KM, Cone EJ, Jaffe JH (1988) Suspiciousness induced by four-hour intravenous infusions of cocaine. *Arch. Gen. Psychiatry, 45*, 673.
50. Sherer MA (1988) Intravenous cocaine: psychiatric effects, biological mechanisms. *Biol. Psychiatry, 24*, 865.
51. Satel SL, Gawin FH (1989) Seasonal cocaine abuse. *Am. J. Psychiatry, 146*, 534.
52. Weiss RD (1988) Relapse to cocaine abuse after initiating desipramine treatment. *J. Am. Med. Assoc., 260*, 2545.
53. Skluth HA, Clark JE, Ehringer GL (1988) Rhabdomyolysis associated with cocaine intoxication. *Drug Intell. Clin. Pharm., 22*, 778.
54. Krohn KD, Slowman-Kovacs S, Leapman SB (1988) Cocaine and rhabdomyolysis (Letter to Editor). *Ann. Intern. Med., 108*, 639.
55. Lombard J, Wong B, Young JH (1988) Acute renal failure due to rhabdomyolysis associated with cocaine toxicity. *West. J. Med., 148*, 466.
56. Herzlich BC, Arsura EL, Pagala M, Grob D (1988) Rhabdomyolysis related to cocaine abuse. *Ann. Intern. Med., 109*, 335.
57. Roth D, Alarcon FJ, Fernandes JA et al (1988) Acute rhabdomyolysis associated with cocaine intoxication. *N. Engl. J. Med., 319*, 673.
58. Singhal P, Horowitz B, Quinones MC et al (1989) Acute renal failure following cocaine abuse. *Nephron, 52*, 76.
59. Reinhart WH, Stricker H (1988) Rhabdomyolysis after intravenous cocaine. *Am. J. Med., 85*, 579.
60. Herzlich B, Arsura E, Pagala M, Grob D (1989) Cocaine and rhabdomyolysis (Letter to Editor). *Ann. Intern. Med., 110*, 91.
61. Herzlich B, Arsura E, Pagala M, Grob D (1989) Acute rhabdomyolysis associated with cocaine intoxication (Letter to Editor). *N. Engl. J. Med., 320*, 667.
62. Becker GD, Hill S (1988) Midline granuloma due to illicit cocaine use. *Arch. Otolaryngol Head Neck Surg., 114*, 90.
63. Schwartz RH, Estroff T, Fairbanks DNF, Hoffmann NG (1989) Nasal symptoms associated with cocaine abuse during adolescence. *Arch. Otolaryngol Head Neck Surg., 115*, 63.
64. Newman NM, DiLoreto DA, Ho JT et al (1988) Bilateral optic neuropathy and osteolytic sinusitis. *J. Am. Med. Assoc., 259*, 72.
65. Kissner DG, Lawrence WD, Selis JE, Flint A (1987) Crack lung: pulmonary disease caused by cocaine abuse. *Am. Rev. Respir. Dis., 136*, 1250.
66. Palat D, Denson M, Sherman M, Matz R (1988) Pneumomediastinum induced by inhalation of alkaloidal cocaine. *NY State J. Med., 88*, 438.
67. Godwin JE, Harley RA, Miller KS, Hefner JE (1989) Cocaine, pulmonary hemorrhage, and hemoptysis (Letter to Editor). *Ann. Intern. Med., 110*, 843.
68. Bezmalinovic Z, Gonzalez M, Farr C (1988) Oropharyngeal injury possibly due to free-base cocaine (Letter to Editor). *N. Engl. J. Med., 319*, 1420.
69. Zamora-Quezada JC, Dinerman H, Stadecker MJ, Kelly JJ (1988) Muscle and skin infarction after free-basing cocaine (crack). *Ann. Intern. Med., 108*, 564.
70. Perino LE, Warren GH, Levine JS (1987) Cocaine-induced hepatotoxicity in humans. *Gastroenterology, 93*, 176.
71. Porter JM, Sussman MS, Rosen GM (1988) Cocaine-induced hepatoxicity (Abstract and Comments). *Hepatology, 8*, 1713.
72. Devenyi P, Schneiderman JF, Devenyi RG, Lawby L (1988) Cocaine-induced central retinal artery occlusion. *Can. Med. Assoc. J., 138*, 129.

T.C. Jerram

5 Hypnotics and sedatives

BENZODIAZEPINES *(SED-11, 90; SEDA-12, 40; SEDA-13, 33)*

The general problems arising from the use of benzodiazepines are mainly in the area of dependence and withdrawal, but some more specific features such as the effects upon psychological functioning and driving are also worthy of note.

Dependence and withdrawal Increasingly, the indications for benzodiazepine use are being revised, but as they tend to be used for common symptom patterns which are not necessarily associated with specific disease entities, there is inevitably considerable variation in their use. In this connection an important study by Tyrer et al (1[C]) may be helpful. They studied 210 psychiatric out-patients, referred to an ordinary catchment area service. The patients were then randomly allocated to a variety of treatments, including diazepam, an antidepressant, two forms of psychological management, or a placebo. Diazepam was less effective than the 3 active programs and indeed its comparative efficacy became progressively less towards the end of the study period. Given this sort of finding and the known problems with dependence, it is therefore not surprising that there is considerable interest in reducing the use of benzodiazepines overall by methods ranging from government intervention through to anxiety management and avoidance of stimulants such as caffeine.

The reason why dependence occurs is still unclear. Lader and File (2[R]) review this topic in detail and suggest that tolerance, rebound and withdrawal symptoms all reflect a common underlying mechanism which applies to both short-term and long-term treatments, regardless of the dose level used. On the other hand, Kraupl Taylor (3[R]) argues on a more philosophical basis that there are two forms of benzodiazepine dependence. The first one, which he defined as 'therapeutic' dependence, occurs in patients with long-standing and fluctuating disorders in whom benzodiazepines remain effective over lengthy periods; a 'morbid' dependence results in increasing doses and has unpleasant abstinence symptoms. In relation to this the main argument revolves around the question of whether dependence and withdrawal are almost inevitable accompaniments of long-term benzodiazepine usage or whether they occur only in specific patients, e.g., perhaps those with an underlying disturbance of personality. The arguments have been summarized in two parallel papers (4[R], 5[R]). This is an important debate, particularly as in one view benzodiazepines continue to have a useful, if limited, place in treatment, and in the other there is no place for them at all; but it seems unlikely that it will be resolved as it is now no longer possible for satisfactory assessments to be carried out before and after a long enough period of treatment. A further difficulty is the question of whether there are any differences between individual benzodiazepines in their ability to cause dependence. For instance, Feely and Haigh (6[r]) emphasize that there are important pharmacodynamic differences between benzodiazepines and Oswald (7[r]) has repeatedly emphasized that triazolam in its ability to cause day-time anxiety may be specifically associated with the development of rebound anxiety and therefore dependence.

As to management of the benzodiazepine withdrawal syndrome, a consensus is gradually developing that social and psychological treatments form an important part, although there are still occasional reports that some of the symptoms at least may be reduced by adjuvant medication such as propranolol (8[c]). The success of such programs does vary and usually a significant number of subjects refuse to take part in the program or withdraw from it. For instance, Crouch et al (9[c]) assessed 91 patients

Side Effects of Drugs Annual 14
M.N.G. Dukes and L. Beeley, editors

at a tranquillizer withdrawal clinic, but only 44 of these entered their program. Of this a small subgroup of 12 patients entered an experimental group using anxiety management, but only 50% of these were able to discontinue their benzodiazepines. The management of withdrawal in general practice or primary care has been reviewed by Onyett (10[R]) and on an out-patient basis by Petrillo et al (11[R]).

Other effects Further reports have been published describing the study of benzodiazepines upon driving performance and their possible contribution to injuries and accidents. Brookhuis and Borgman (12[c]) compared clorazepate, oxazepam and lorazepam, using an experimental vehicle in normal traffic and found that lorazepam 0.5 mg t.i.d. had the most severe effect. A comparison was also made between those who had been prescribed anxiolytics in the recent past and healthy volunteers. There was a trend for the patients to be slightly less impaired by anxiolytics, but this did not reach statistical significance and the authors were unable to find any support for the statement that patients may be less impaired by the drug than by the underlying anxiety. Girre et al (13[c]) studied just over 2000 subjects who had been involved in an accident of some form or another and measured the concentration of benzodiazepine in their blood. They found benzodiazepines in just under 10% of the cases and a third of these had significant blood alcohol levels. Unfortunately the subjects were a mixed group whose accidents had occurred both while driving and in a variety of other situations and the authors did not compare them to any control group. It is difficult to be sure of the exact significance of the findings, but they are comparable to previous smaller series (SEDA-7, 46).

Dietch and Jennings (14[R]) reported a useful review of what they describe as *aggressive dyscontrol* in patients treated with benzodiazepines which is usually attributed to some form of disinhibition. They reviewed individual case-reports, controlled studies of the effect of benzodiazepines on measures of hostility and data derived from larger-scale studies of the clinical efficacy of benzodiazepines. They found it very difficult to characterize the syndrome precisely but found that it occurred very rarely (in less than 1% of patients treated with these drugs). They found some evidence that clonazepam may be more likely to induce such problems, and that oxazepam is least likely to. There were no consistent predictors as to which patients might develop such symptoms, but overt physical assaults were rare. A brief survey of the effect of psychotropic drugs upon *female orgasm* and whether they inhibited it was reported by Segraves (15[r]). He noted that diazepam and alprazolam had both been reported as inhibiting orgasm.

Finally, Cerqueira et al (16[c]) reported an unusual incident in which five pregnant women ingested 10 g of benzodiazepine. No serious problems occurred in 4 of the women but the 5th had *respiratory depression* and required assisted ventilation for 2 days. She gradually recovered over the next 5 days, but the fetus showed a significant decrease of variability in heart rate which lasted a few hours. Fortunately, all the babies had normal Apgar scores at birth and appeared normal at 6 months.

Benzodiazepines and brain damage

Despite their acknowledged safety as regards most organ-systems, there is still concern that the benzodiazepines might, especially when used for long periods, cause psychological impairment with or without signs of structural brain damage.

The assessment of both of these is difficult, but as regards brain damage Poser et al (17[c]) commented very briefly on their experiences with computed tomographic (CT) scans. They studied 28 patients, comparing them with patients with headache and normal physical and EEG findings and with a group of alcoholic patients: they found that the benzodiazepine group did not differ from controls but were different from alcoholic patients and from those who had mixed alcohol and benzodiazepine use. In contrast to this Lader et al (18[c]) reported briefly on 20 patients who had been taking benzodiazepines for between 2.5 and 20 years. They underwent CT and after routine reporting the films were re-analyzed blindly by taking measurements which reflected loss of cortical tissue and the ventricular area was calculated. These measurements were then compared to similar ones reported in a previous study comparing alcoholic patients and 'normal' controls (19[c]). In the initial reporting 3 of the benzodiazepine group were considered to have abnormal scans: in the further analysis the alcoholic patients had significantly different ventricular/brain ratios (VBR) while the benzodiazepine users were intermediate between them and the controls: those benzodiazepine users with higher scores on the measures of cortical density were older and were more likely to be male. This study was clearly a preliminary one and recognized the potentially confounding effects of alcohol. Rickels, too, reported briefly on a series of 35 long-term benzodiazepine users compared to 26 control patients (20[c]). He found possible changes of mild atrophy in 9 of them and noted that this was very similar to the incidence in Lader et al's control group.

Unfortunately, all these reports were preliminary or brief: there were shortcomings in the provision of control groups and some inconsistencies in the actual measurements used to define cerebral atrophy. At least some of these were overcome in a study by Schmauss and Krieg (21[c]). They investigated 17 in-patients, specifically excluding alcohol abuse and compared them to 22 in-patients suffering from anxiety disorders or with abnormal personalities. Measurements of CSF were made blind in real time: VBRs were calculated from counting of CSF dense pixels and a series of other measurements taken (frontal index, Evans index, etc.). Although there was a trend for these last measures to differ from the controls, this did not reach statistical significance. The main significant finding was of an increase in the VBR in the benzodiazepine group: further there appeared to be a dose effect in that those patients on high doses had significantly higher VBRs than those on low doses. This appears to have been a careful study and suggests that some degree of atrophy may appear subsequent to the use of benzodiazepines and seems to be dose-dependent. It is to be hoped that further studies will confirm or disprove this finding and also add information on any reversibility: it may also be that more sophisticated techniques such as magnetic resonance imaging may help to clarify the issue.

In contrast to the small number of studies of morphological changes, there is a very large literature on possible impairment of psychological functioning. Although this has generated a large number of findings, relatively few of them are of very much relevance to the clinician. He/she is not so concerned with the short-term effects of single or short-term doses on a battery of psychological tests but rather wishes to know whether any specific cognitive impairment, other than that due to sedation, occurs, what effect this has on the patient in behavioral terms and, most importantly, whether it is reversible.

Short-term studies in normal subjects showed clearly that benzodiazepines cause impairment on a variety of psychomotor tasks such as the Digit-Symbol Substitution Test and Copying and Letter Cancellation Tests (22[R], 23[R]). In addition, the critical flicker frequency threshold (CFF) has been widely used as it has been shown to be sensitive to the effects of such drugs, only involves a limited motor activity and is very reliable (24[r]), although it is less clear what its actual significance is (25[R]). An early study of 55 patients suggested that subtle cognitive deficits, especially of memory and verbal learning, may occur, but many of these patients had been abusing their drugs (26[c]). Another report suggested that benzodiazepines may have similar effects to those of narcotic substances (27[c]).

Two recent studies have looked more specifically at patients who have taken benzodiazepines for longer periods. Lucki et al (25[CR]) investigated 43 patients who had been taking benzodiazepines for a mean of 5 years using the tests mentioned above and comparing them to a matched group of anxious, but drug-free, out-patients. Although there was a trend for the benzodiazepine group to perform worse than controls overall, this only reached statistical significance with the CFF. A subgroup of the sample was then assessed before and after taking their usual dose of medication where the most interesting results concerned tests of verbal recall—immediate recall not being affected, but recall at 20 min being significantly impaired. Seventeen of the patients then discontinued their medication, but assessments then showed little difference from their earlier scores except again on the CFF. However, in retrospect, it seems likely that as the tests were conducted within a week or so of abrupt discontinuation, the subjects may well have been experiencing withdrawal symptoms at the time. Golombok et al (28[CR]) carried out a detailed study, using many tests, on 50 chronic benzodiazepine users, a smaller group of patients previously withdrawn from drugs and a control group who were either drug-naive or had taken drugs for a short period in the past. A large amount of data was generated, but the authors postulate that the impairments found could be *attributed to changes in two areas of functioning, namely visual-spatial ability and the ability to sustain attention on a repetitive task under time pressure. On an optimistic note they could find no impairment in global tests of memory, flexibility and reaction time and emphasize that there appears to be a major difference between acute and long-term effects of the drugs.*

These observations on memory function are interesting and contrast with commonly held ideas. Koeppen (29[R]) summarized benzodiazepine effects on memory in both animal and human experiments. The amnesia appears to relate to the consolidation phase of memory in that they do not prevent the acquisition of new material or retrieval of pre-existing material (which may even be improved): there is doubt as to exactly how dose-dependent it is and some tolerance may occur to this effect (30[r]). It has further been argued that different benzodiazepines may have different effects. Scharf et al (31[c]), for instance, compared the effects of triazolam and temazepam. Triazolam caused more amnesia than temazepam and it is possible that this may be explained by their relative affinity for the benzodiazepine receptor.

INDIVIDUAL BENZODIAZEPINES

Alprazolam *(SED-11, 96; SEDA-12, 43; SEDA-13, 35)*

Alprazolam continues to be the subject of investigation, particularly in the United States where its indications appear to be broadening. For instance, Hoehn-Saric and colleagues compared alprazolam with imipramine in generalized anxiety disorder in 60 patients (32[C]). Unfortunately there was no placebo group, but it was found that alprazolam was effective in the early stages of treatment and had more effect upon somatic symptoms, whereas imipramine had more effect upon mood and depressive thinking. The only side effect that occurred significantly with alprazolam was *drowsiness*. Beitman et al (33[c]) reported an open study of 10 patients from a cardiology clinic on the grounds that many such patients with chest pain but no evidence of coronary artery disease are in reality suffering from panic disorder. Again, *sedation* was relatively common and 2 patients receiving higher doses than the others reported *ataxia*, *confusion* and *excessive sedation*. It is also clear that alprazolam shares many, if not all, of the problems of the other benzodiazepines. Juergens and Morse (34[C]) describe in detail 7 patients who had been taking alprazolam for 6 months to 3 years and who developed clear evidence of dependence with tolerance, withdrawal symptoms, and social impairment secondary to drug use. Significantly, 6 of the patients abused other drugs or alcohol either previously or concurrently with the alprazolam. A further case has been reported in which alprazolam may cause the so called 'paradoxical' reaction (35[c]). The patient had been taking alprazolam and tryptophan for some weeks, but after taking her normal dose of alcohol (3 ozs of 80-proof whisky) broke into a neighbor's house destroying property and sustaining lacerations to her wrists. Subsequently she had relatively little recollection of the event but after withdrawal of the alprazolam remained well for the follow-up period of 4 months.

Diazepam *(SED-11, 96; SEDA-12, 44)*

The question of rebound insomnia was investigated in an 18-night sleep laboratory study in Pennsylvania (36[C]), the subjects taking diazepam for 7 of these nights. During this period there was little evidence that tolerance developed and there was the expected degree of daytime sedation. When diazepam was terminated abruptly, there was sleep disturbance on the 6th night after withdrawal, but the total wake time was not then significantly greater than at base line. The authors point out that this pattern is different from that found with the short-acting benzodiazepines where tolerance develops more rapidly and greater sleep disturbance follows withdrawal of the drug. This study also serves as a warning that withdrawal symptoms and rebound insomnia may not be seen unless observations are continued for a prolonged period following withdrawal.

As regards *interactions* with diazepam, Nuotto and Saarialho-Kere investigated whether indometacin potentiated the impairment of psychomotor function caused by diazepam and vice versa (37[c]); there was no evidence that indometacin made the impairment any greater.

Lorazepam

This particular benzodiazepine continues to be a controversial drug in that it remains widely prescribed but is ill-regarded by a number of authorities. Ancill and colleagues had previously noted that lorazepam was the 3rd most commonly prescribed psychotropic drug in a series of 100 elderly patients and questioned whether it was the drug of choice in the elderly. They reviewed in detail a further 20 consecutive elderly patients admitted to hospital in whom lorazepam was the only psychotropic medication (38[C]). All the patients had previously been in long-term care facilities and the use of lorazepam prior to admission had been at a mean dose of 3.8 mg/d for 18 weeks. Nearly all the patients appeared *oversedated* and had an *amnesic syndrome* while a significant number appeared to be *depressed* and *ataxic*. These symptoms all responded well to gradual withdrawal of the drug and the authors were particularly concerned with the presence of a 'pseudo-dementia'. They argue, therefore, that there may be no reason to choose lorazepam over any other drug in this age group but do recognize that it is easier to determine which drugs are to be avoided rather than those to be used. At the other extreme of life a possible new indication for lorazepam was reported in a series of 10 children by Yager and Sheshia (39[C]), whose patients (aged 1–17 yr) suffered from serial seizures—defined as a series of seizures in which consciousness was regained between successive episodes. The patients all had fairly intractable epilepsy as shown by the mixture of other anticonvulsants that they were taking, but even so the majority of them seemed to respond to sublingual doses (1–2 mg) of lorazepam administered by their parents. Side effects were very few and were difficult to disentangle from the effects of the convulsions and of other anticonvulsants.

There have also been several individual case-reports of problems that have occurred with the use of lorazepam. These are often difficult to evaluate as lorazepam is such a widely used drug that a certain number of rare conditions will occur by chance; it is often not possible for practical and ethical reasons to re-challenge with lorazepam, and other causes for the effect cannot be completely excluded. For instance, Engel and Grau (40[c]) reported on a 81-year-old woman who had been taking lorazepam 1 mg/d (duration not stated) and who developed the typical picture of *inappropriate secretion of antidiuretic hormone*. The usual causes for this were excluded as far as was possible and in this instance it was possible to re-challenge and repeat a water-load test. This appeared to confirm that lorazepam did cause the inappropriate secretion. Another brief report was on 2 male patients who developed complete loss of libido when lorazepam was prescribed (41[c]), El-Sayed and Symonds (42[c]) reported on a 47-year-old woman who received radiotherapy for an adenocarcinoma of the uterus. She developed pancytopenia but was able to complete the course of radiotherapy treatment, her blood count returning to normal after the lorazepam was discontinued.

Midazolam *(SED-11, 212; SEDA-12, 203; SEDA-13,35)*

This benzodiazepine is used increasingly by anesthetists mainly as a premedication/inducing agent where its various advantages and disadvantages have been reviewed by White (43[R]). It is also used in intensive care units for sedation where patients are being ventilated and, more controversially, in the technique of 'sedoanalgesia' in which midazolam is combined with some form of local anesthetic for short procedures such as endoscopy. In the intensive care unit Kong et al (44[C]) compared isoflurane with midazolam on the grounds that the latter was the standard agent. They noted that one of the problems with midazolam is that patients often became confused and disruptive and required higher doses which then resulted in oversedation. Two warnings have been sounded about the use of midazolam (45[R], 46[R]). Both have been concerned with the increasing use of midazolam coupled with the use of the benzodiazepine antagonist, flumazenil. It is argued that midazolam does have side effects which may be dangerous and that excessive doses may be used under the mistaken impression that any problems can then be resolved by the use of the antagonist. Further problems may then arise attributable to the flumazenil, which is also a very expensive preparation. These views have been challenged in correspondence (47[r], 48[r]) with particular contributions from clinicians who have very wide experience of using the drug but who have not themselves met with any difficulties (49[c]).

The *anterograde amnesia* that nearly always occurs with midazolam is usually seen as an advantage in such circumstances, but an instance was reported in which the amnesia was prolonged excessively and may have had serious consequences (50[c]). The patient underwent extraction of several teeth and appeared fully conscious, but then swallowed a gauze pack. This proved to be harmless but the patient on subsequent questioning had no recollection of the event. The author suggests that verbal instructions should be reinforced by written advice. *Hypotension* is a well-recognized complication of the use of midazolam which has not previously been recorded following intramuscular usage, but this has now been described (51[c]). A slight decrease in blood pressure was noted in 3 of 14 patients who were treated with intramuscular midazolam for repeated epileptic seizures (52[c]).

Temazepam

An unusual skin reaction to temazepam was reported (53[C]). The patient was an elderly lady who was also taking other drugs including, atenolol, ranitidine and phenytoin. The rash developed very rapidly on several occasions and it eventually transpired that she may have taken temazepam briefly beforehand. The rash was typical of a widespread fixed drug reaction on the trunk and lower limbs. It has also been noted that temazepam, particularly in the 20 mg capsule formulation, is attractive to drug abusers who warm the gel and collect it in a syringe before injecting it (54[c]).

Triazolam *(SED-11, 96; SEDA-13, 36)*

Oswald (55[r]) has commented briefly on the reverberations of the 'Halcion Affair' 10 years on. He argues that the initial incidents were attributable to triazolam being taken in rather large doses by older subjects and that this use had not been adequately explored prior to the marketing of the drug. Furthermore, nighttime triazolam does appear to cause anxiety on the following day, particularly with medium and long-term usage. Oswald makes a strong plea that new compounds should only be marketed after adequate research has been carried out, particularly on longer-term use. Four cases have now been described in which triazolam in overdose was implicated as a possible cause of death (56[c]).

BENZODIAZEPINE ANTAGONISTS *(SED-11, 97; SEDA-12, 45; SEDA-13, 36)*

Flumazenil (flumazepil)

Flumazenil is now quite widely available. Several studies have shown that it is effective. For instance, Ellmauer (57[Cr]) carried out a randomized double-blind study in 57 patients undergoing general surgery and showed that flumazenil was a safe and effective benzodiazepine antagonist with no significant hemodynamic side effects. There were no effects at the site of injection and the side effects noted included *nausea*, *vomiting*, *euphoria*, benign cardiac *arrhythmia* and a state of *excitation*. However, the nausea and vomiting also occurred after placebo. One review (58[R]) suggests that this drug may have many uses, including withdrawal from benzodiazepines. However, it is not without risk. For instance, Short et al (59[c]) suggested that it may precipitate ventricular arrhythmia and Burr et al (60[C]) reported on a patient who died following the use of the drug.

A 31-year-old woman was admitted having take an unknown amount of dothiepin (dosulepin), chlordiazepoxide, temazepam and alcohol. After admission she became deeply unconscious and as she was still so 12 hours after ingestion she was given flumazenil intravenously. She regained consciousness briefly but then had a grand mal seizure followed by status epilepticus. Although the seizures were brought under control, she subsequently developed a cardiac arrest and died despite resuscitation attempts.

The authors suggest that the flumazenil may have precipitated status epilepticus and cardiovascular toxicity, perhaps related to the ingestion of a tricyclic antidepressant as well. They urged that flumazenil should therefore be used with caution and should not be used routinely when drugs other than benzodiazepines have been taken.

NON-BENZODIAZEPINE DRUGS *(SEDA-12, 45; SEDA-13, 37)*

Buspirone *(SED-11, 99; SEDA-12, 45; SEDA-13, 37)*

Buspirone has been available in the Federal Republic of Germany since 1985, the United States since 1987 and the United Kingdom since 1988. Its structure is different from that of other anxiolytics and it does not appear to bind to benzodiazepine receptors. It is a partial agonist of some serotonergic and dopamine receptors but has no effect on muscular relaxation nor does it have any hypnotic or anticonvulsant effects. It has been comprehensively reviewed by Jann (61[R]) who noted that it is indicated in the treatment of generalized anxiety disorders, but that its use in depression and panic disorders requires further investigation. He also noted that the main adverse effects were *headaches*, *dizziness*, *nervousness* and *light-headedeness*. Clearly in view of the furore now surrounding the benzodiazepines an important question will be whether buspirone has any ability to cause dependence. This topic has been comprehensively reviewed by Lader (62[R]) who drew on studies of laboratory animals and evaluation of withdrawal symptoms in human subjects. He noted in particular that so far no 'abstinence syndrome' has been observed clinically following withdrawal of buspirone and that at the moment there is very little other evidence of such a complication with its use. However, some individual side effects have been recorded. Liegghio et al (63[c]) reported 4 patients who developed *jitteriness* when prescribed buspirone, although it is worth noting that the patients all had long-standing symptoms and were receiving other treatment including benzodiazepines and antidepressants. The authors suggest that such jitteriness may be related to buspirone's known actions on various receptors or may be a possible interaction with alprazolam. In view of buspirone's actions on the dopaminergic system a case reported by Strauss (64[c]) is of interest. Although the patient was a very elderly lady with severe progressive dementia who had not responded to a variety of medications, she was prescribed buspirone and within 3 days appeared to have developed an *oral dyskinesia*. This did not remit when the drug was stopped but did lessen over the ensuing 4 months. Buspirone appears to have few interactions with other drugs, and does not interact with benzodiazepines or alcohol (65[R]).

OLDER DRUGS *(SEDA-12, 46; SEDA-13, 38)*

Barbiturates *(SED-11, 97) (see also Chapter 7)*

The barbiturates are rarely used now but do have some specific indications such as the intracarotid sodium amylobarbital (ISA) procedure used in determining cerebral language dominance. Lee et al (66[R]) noted that occasional 'paradoxical' reactions occurred during this procedure. Of 92 patients undergoing ISA evaluation, 5 developed *behavioral disturbances*, including *coma* and *prolonged confusional* state subsequently. All 5 had lesions of some form in the left hemisphere, 4 of them in the frontal region—these lesions included gliomas, arteriovenous malformation and a cyst. Interestingly, no such complications occurred in patients with structural lesions of the right hemisphere. There does seem to be a special role for the left frontal region in the inhibition of affective expression.

Clomethiazole (chlormethiazole) *(SED-11, 99)*

There has been some discussion as to the use of clomethiazole, particularly in the management of delirium tremens. Chick (67[R]) warned that the intravenous use of clomethiazole may lead to *respiratory depression* and subsequent death and suggested that the use of benzodiazepines such as diazepam or chlordiazepoxide would be preferable. In a reply to this Scott (67[c]) argued that respiratory depression occurred very rarely with clomethiazole even when the patients were anesthetized by the drug. He suggested that in capable hands clomethiazole was a safe agent and in view of its rapid clearance may well still be the drug of choice in this condition.

Thalidomide *(SED-11, 100)*

Thalidomide is now rarely used except for certain very specific indications. However, the long-term sequelae of the 'Thalidomide Affair' are still discussed. In two linked papers Warkany (69[R]) and Kelsey (70[R]) discuss respectively why some authorities found it difficult to accept that thalidomide was indeed the cause of phocomelia and the consequences of thalidomide for regulatory procedures for new drugs in general. Clinical findings are still reported. Maouris and Hirsch (71[C]) reported a survey of 35 thalidomide victims who in turn had had children themselves. In all they had had 64 live births and 6 miscarriages. There were no reports of malformation among the viable children so, as is to be expected, thalidomide has no effect upon the offspring of its victims. Generally speaking, the complications of pregnancy seemed to occur at about the normal level, but there was an increased cesarean section rate. The authors also noted other difficulties, including the technical one of recording blood pressure and the effect of episiotomy in mothers who use their feet as a hand substitute.

NEW DRUGS

Modafinil

Speculative reports have appeared from France about modafinil (72[r]). This drug is structurally somewhat similar to the standard antidepressants and has been noted to have a marked effect on increasing vigilance and suppressing sleep in animals and humans. It has been suggested as a treatment for narcolepsy and idiopathic hypersomnia.

REFERENCES

1. Tyrer P, Murphy S, Kingdon D et al (1988) The Nottingham study of neurotic disorder: comparison of drug and psychological treatments. *Lancet, 2*, 235.
2. Lader M, File S (1987) The biological basis of benzodiazepine dependence. *Psychol. Med., 17*, 539.
3. Kraupl Taylor F (1989) The damnation of benzodiazepines. *Br. J. Psychiatry 154*, 697.
4. Tyrer P (1989) Risks of dependence on benzodiazepine drugs: the importance of patient selection. *Br. Med. J., 298*, 102.
5. Ashton H (1989) Risks of dependence of benzodiazepine drugs: a major problem of long term treatment. *Br. Med. J., 298*, 103.
6. Feely MP, Haigh JRM (1988) Differences between benzodiazepines. *Lancet, 1*, 1460.
7. Oswald I (1989) Risks of dependence on benzodiazepine drugs. *Br. Med. J., 298*, 456.
8. Hallstrom C et al (1988), Treatment of tranquillizer dependence by propranolol. *Postgrad. Med. J., 64, Suppl. 2*, 40.
9. Crouch G, Robson M, Hallstrom C (1988) Benzodiazepine dependent patients and their psychological treatment. *Prog. Neuro-Psychopharmacol. Biol. Psychiatry 12*, 503.
10. Onyett SR (1989) The benzodiazepine withdrawal syndrome and its management. *J. R. Coll. Gen. Pract., 39*, 160.
11. Petrillo A, Veillon H, Hofstetter JR (1988) Benzodiazepine withdrawal reactions: implications for the practitioner. *Schweiz. Rundsch. Med., 77*, 601.
12. Brookhuis KA, Borgman AE (1988) De effecten van enkele anxiolytica op het rijgedrag. *TGO Tijdschr. Ther. Geneesm., 13*, 228.
13. Girre C, Facy F, Lagier G et al (1988) Presence of benzodiazepines in the serum of injured persons and its relationship with alcoholism. *Presse Méd., 17*, 1135.
14. Dietch JT, Jennings RK (1988) Aggressive dyscontrol in patients treated with benzodiazepines. *J. Clin. Psychiatry, 49*, 184.
15. Segraves RT (1988) Psychiatric drugs and inhibited female orgasm. *J. Sex Marital Ther., 14*, 202.
16. Cerqueira MJ, Olle C, Bellart J et al (1987) Intoxication by benzodiazepines during pregnancy. *Lancet, 1*, 1341.
17. Poser W, Poser S, Roscher D et al (1983) Do benzodiazepines cause cerebral atrophy? *Lancet, 1*, 715.
18. Lader MH, Ron M, Petursson H (1984) Computed axial brain tomography in long-term benzodiazepine users. *Psychol. Med., 14*, 203.
19. Ron MA, Acker W, Lishman WA et al (1982) Computerized tomography scan changes in chronic alcoholics: a survey and follow-up study. *Brain, 105*, 497.
20. Rickels K (1985) Clinical management of benzodiazepine dependence (Correspondence). *Br. Med. J., 291*, 1649.
21. Schmauss C, Krieg JC (1987) Enlargement of cerebrospinal fluid spaces in long-term benzodiazepine abusers. *Psychol. Med., 17*, 869.
22. Kleinknecht RA, Donaldson D (1975) A review of the effects of diazepam on cognitive and psychomotor performance. *J. Nerv. Ment. Disord., 161*, 399.
23. Vogel JR (1979) Objective measurement of human performance changes produced by antian-

xiety drugs. In: Fielding S, Lal H (Eds.), *Anxiolytics*, Futura, New York.
24. Smith JM, Misiak HC (1976) Critical flicker frequency (CFF) and psychotropic drugs in normal subjects—a review. *Psychopharmacology, 47*, 175.
25. Lucki I, Rickels K, Geller AM (1986) Chronic use of benzodiazepines and psychomotor and cognitive test performance. *Psychopharmacology, 88*, 426.
26. Bergman H, Borg S, Holm L (1980) Neuropsychological impairment and exclusive abuse of sedatives or hypnotics. *Am. J. Psychiatry, 137*, 215.
27. Hendler N, Cimini C, Terrance MA et al (1980) A comparison of cognitive impairment due to benzodiazepines and to narcotics. *Am. J. Psychiatry, 137*, 828.
28. Golombok S, Moodley P, Lader M (1988) Cognitive impairment in long-term benzodiazepine users. *Psychol. Med., 18*, 365.
29. Koeppen D (1984) Memory and benzodiazepines: animal and human studies with 1,4-benzodiazepines and clobazam (1,5-benzodiazepine). *Drug Dev. Res., 4*, 555.
30. Plasky P, Marcus L, Salzman C (1988) Effects of psychotropic drugs on memory. Part 2. *Hosp. Commun. Psychiatry, 39*, 501.
31. Scharf M, Fletcher ACP, Graham JP (1988) Comparative amnesic effects of benzodiazepine hypnotic agents. *J. Clin. Psychiatry, 49*, 134.
32. Hoehn-Saric R, McLeod DR, Zimmerli WD (1988) Differential effects of alprazolam and imipramine in generalized anxiety disorder: somatic versus psychic symptoms. *J. Clin. Psychiatry, 49*, 293.
33. Beitman BD, Basha MI, Trombka LH et al (1988) Alprazolam in the treatment of cardiology patients with atypical chest pain and panic disorder. *J. Clin. Psychopharmacol., 8*, 127.
34. Juergens SM, Morse RM (1988) Alprazolam dependence in seven patients. *Am. J. Psychiatry, 145*, 625.
35. Terrell HB (1988) Behavioural dyscontrol associated with combined use of alprazolam and ethanol. *Am. J. Psychiatry, 145*, 1313.
36. Kales A, Soldatos CR, Bixler EO et al (1988) Diazepam: effects on sleep and withdrawal phenomena. *J. Clin. Psychopharmacol., 8*, 340.
37. Nuotto E, Saarialho-Kere U (1988) Actions and interactions of indomethacin and diazepam on performance in healthy-volunteers. *Pharmacol. Toxicol., 62*, 293.
38. Ancill RJ, Embury GD, MacEwan GW et al (1987) Lorazepam in the elderly—a retrospective study of the side-effects in 20 patients. *J. Psychopharmacol., 2*, 126.
39. Yager JY, Sheshia SS (1988) Sublingual lorazepam in childhood serial seizures. *Am. J. Disord. Child., 142*, 931.
40. Engel WR, Grau A (1988) Drug points: inappropriate secretion of antidiuretic hormone associated with lorazepam. *Br. Med. J., 297*, 858.
41. Khandewal SK (1988) Complete loss of libido with short-term use of lorazepam. *Am. J. Psychiatry, 145*, 1313.
42. El-Sayed S, Symonds RP (1988) Drug points: lorazepam induced pancytopenia. *Br. Med. J., 296*, 1332.
43. White PF (1988) Clinical pharmacology of intravenous induction drugs. *Int. Anesthesiol. Clin., 26*, 98.
44. Kong KL, Willatts SM, Prys-Roberts C (1989) Isoflurane compared with midazolam for sedation in the intensive care unit. *Br. Med. J., 298*, 1277.
45. Editorial (1988) Midazolam—is antagonism justified? *Lancet, 2*, 140.
46. McHugh P, Milligan KA (1989) Use of hospital beds. *Br. Med. J., 298*, 115.
47. Birch B, Miller R (1988) Safety of midazolam. *Lancet, 2*, 683.
48. Grant IS, Davies CA (1989) Use of hospital beds. *Br. Med. J., 298*, 525.
49. Bardhan KD, Hinchliffe RFC et al (1988) Midazolam antagonism. *Lancet, 2*, 388.
50. Malamed SF, Nikchevich Jr D, Block J (1988) Anterograde amnesia as a possible postoperative complication of midazolam as an agent for intravenous conscious sedation. *Anesth. Prog., 35*, 160.
51. Matson AM, Thurlow AC (1988) Hypotension and neurological sequelae following intramuscular midazolam. *Anaesthesia, 43*, 896.
52. Ghilain S, Rijckevorsel-Harmant KV, Harmant J et al (1988) Midazolam in the treatment of epileptic seizures. *J. Neurol. Neurosurg. Psychiatry, 51*, 732.
53. Archer CB, English JSC (1988) Extensive fixed drug eruption induced by temazepam. *Clin. Exp. Dermatol., 13*, 366.
54. Farrell M, Strang J (1988) Misuse of temazepam. *Br. Med. J., 297*, 1402.
55. Oswald I (1989) Triazolam syndrome 10 years on. *Lancet, 2*, 451.
56. O'Dowd JJ, Spragg PP, Routledge PA (1988) Fatal triazolam poisoning. *Br. Med. J., 297*, 1048.
57. Ellmauer S, Muller H, Dick W (1988) Efficacy and safety of the benzodiazepine antagonist Ro 15-1788. *Anaesthesist, 37*, 432.
58. Whitwam J (1988) Flumazenil: a benzodiazepine antagonist. *Br. Med. J., 297*, 999.
59. Short TG, Maling T, Galletly DC (1988) Ventricular arrhythmia precipitated by flumazenil. *Br. Med. J., 296*, 1070.
60. Burr W, Sandham P, Judd A (1989) Drug points: death after flumazenil. *Br. Med. J., 298*, 1713.
61. Jann MW (1988) Buspirone: an update on a unique anxiolytic agent. *Pharmacotherapy, 8*, 100.
62. Lader M (1987) Assessing the potential for buspirone dependence or abuse and effects of its withdrawal. *Am. J. Med., 82, Suppl. 5A*, 20.

63. Liegghio NE, Yeragani VK, Moore NC (1988) Buspirone-induced jitteriness in three patients with panic disorder and one patient with generalized anxiety disorder. *J. Clin. Psychiatry, 49*, 165.
64. Strauss A (1988) Oral dyskinesia associated with buspirone use in an elderly woman. *J. Clin. Psychiatry, 49*, 322.
65. Schuckit MA (1987) Alcohol and drug interactions with antianxiety medications. *Am. J. Med., 82, Suppl. 5A*, 27.
66. Lee GP, Loring DW, Meador KJ et al (1988) Severe behavioural complications following intracarotid sodium amobarbital injection. *Neurology, 38*, 1233.
67. Chick J (1989) Delirium tremens. *Br. Med. J., 298*, 3.
68. Scott DR (1989) Chlormethiazole and treatment of delirium tremens. *Br. Med. J., 298*, 751.
69. Warkany J (1988) Why I doubted that thalidomide was the cause of the epidemic of limb defects of 1959 to 1961. *Teratology, 38*, 217.
70. Kelsey FO (1988) Thalidomide update: regulatory aspects. *Teratology, 38*, 221.
71. Maouris PG, Hirsch PJ (1988) Pregnancy in women with thalidomide induced disability. *Br. J. Obstet. Gynaecol., 95*, 717.
72. Dorozynski A (1989) Sleepless pill. *Br. Med. J., 298*, 1543.

Dolors Capellà and Joan-Ramon Laporte

6 Antipsychotic drugs

PATTERNS OF USE OF ANTIPSYCHOTIC DRUGS

Although much work is being done to evaluate the effects of antipsychotic drugs in the treatment of schizophrenia, little is known about who uses these agents and how they are used. A recent study on the utilization of psychotropic drugs (1[C]) provides an excellent example of how drug use can be characterized, and of the usefulness of this information for the evaluation of reports on adverse effects of drugs.

Half the residents in a random sample of 55 rest homes in Massachusetts were 75 years of age or older, and 26% were 85 or older. Two-thirds (out of a total of 1201 residents) were women, and 45% had never been married. A third had a history of psychiatric hospitalization. The median length of stay at the rest home was 3 years, one-fifth having been residents for 9 or more years. Thirty-nine percent were taking antipsychotic medications, 70% of those who had been admitted from a psychiatric hospital ($n = 360$), and 24% of all other residents ($n = 841$). In most cases the prescriptions had been written in the remote past and were refilled automatically. Eighteen percent of the residents who were taking antipsychotic agents were receiving 2 or more different medications in this class. In a follow-up study focusing on a subset of rest homes in which residents had a high level of psychoactive-drug use, 685 residents [mean age ($\pm$ SD) 64 $\pm$ 12 years] were taking one (84%) or more antipsychotic drugs. Of these, 21% had signs of tardive dyskinesia (17% mild or indeterminate, 4% moderate, and 2% severe). About half the residents had no evidence of participation by a physician in decisions about their mental health during the year of the study. An assessment of staff competence revealed a low level of comprehension of the purpose and side effects of commonly used psychoactive drugs. Although the methods used in this study do not enable us to know whether this high level of medication is truly necessary, its results suggest that some populations may be exposed to antipsychotic drugs without any evidence of efficacy, and with little medical supervision.

Side Effects of Drugs Annual 14
M.N.G. Dukes and L. Beeley, editors

ORGANS AND SYSTEMS

Cardiovascular *Cardiac arrest after haloperidol injection* A case of cardiac arrest associated with haloperidol has recently been reported (2[C]). The patient suffered an asystolic cardiac arrest after an intravenous dose of 7.5 mg of haloperidol given to treat confusion during hospitalization in an intensive care unit because of respiratory insufficiency due to pneumonia caused by *Legionella pneumoniae*. No relation to the administration of haloperidol was suspected, and 2 hours after resuscitation a second dose of 7.5 mg was administered. This was also followed by cardiac arrest. Although no mention is made of alternative explanations (i.e. other drugs used concomitantly, excipients), the positive rechallenge suggests that the administered preparation was the cause. A review of sudden death during neuroleptic treatment (SEDA-7, 63) (which includes 6 cases with haloperidol) discusses the possible mechanisms involved. These may be a cardiac arrhythmia or a nervous reflex affecting cardiac function, or a neuroleptic-induced laryngeal spasm precipitating a vagal reflex which leads to cardiac arrest.

Nervous system *Acute extrapyramidal reactions* The frequency of extrapyramidal reactions to metoclopramide and prochlorperazine has been studied (3[C]). In a prospective study in which cohorts of users of both drugs were identified with the help of community pharmacists, details of patients receiving first prescriptions for prochlorperazine and metoclopramide were obtained. About 4 weeks later the general practitioner who had issued the prescription was contacted and details of the patient, the prescription, the indication, and the occurrence of any adverse event were obtained. A total of 2811 first prescriptions of prochlorperazine were identified, and 57 adverse events were recorded. Of these, 16 involved the extrapyramidal system. There were 4 dystonic-dyskinetic reactions. Contrary to what has been previously suggested (SEDA-12, 50), the incidence was not significantly greater in patients less than 30 years old, compared to those over this age (see Table 1). Of the 8 patients who developed parkinsonism, all but one were aged over 60 years. The incidence in patients over 60 years was significantly greater than in younger patients ($P=0.02$; see Table 1). Akathisia was reported in 2 patients. These results, if representative, provide the most accurate estimate to date of the frequency of these extrapyramidal effects (4[r]).

Neuroleptic-induced acute dystonic reactions are mainly manifested as opisthotonus, torticollis and oculogyric crisis. Two cases of acute upper airway obstruction due to acute supraglottic dystonia have been published, one of them after treatment with prochlorperazine and metoclopramide (5[C]).

Two suppositories of prochlorperazine and 3 injections of metoclopramide were given to a 16-year-old man with anginose infectious mononucleosis. Thirty minutes after the last dose of metoclopramide the patient became agitated and seemed to be choking, having difficulty in speaking and breathing, and coughing frequently to clear his throat. These symptoms persisted for hours; drug dystonia was considered only after he said that he could not control his tongue. Benztropine mesylate 2 mg was given intravenously with immediate and complete resolution of his symptoms. At radiographic examination, the air space between his epiglottis and the posterior pharyngeal wall was 6 mm during the episode and 18 mm after recovery.

Table 1. *Incidence of extrapyramidal reactions to prochlorperazine*

Reaction	Age (yr)	Incidence*
Dystonia	< 30	1 in 464
Parkinsonism	> 30	1 in 707
	< 60	1 in 1555
	> 60	1 in 159 (91–645)
Akathisia		1 in 562 (297–5285)

*95% confidence intervals are given when these can be calculated (3[C]).

The routine use of anticholinergic drugs to reduce the incidence and severity of acute extrapyramidal reactions has been mentioned in previous Annuals (SEDA-12, 50; SEDA-13, 41). A recent review (6[R]) analyzed data from 9 studies, involving a total of 1366 patients. The incidence of acute dystonia induced by neuroleptic agents with and without concomitant use of anticholinergics was compared. The overall effect of prophylaxis was a 1.9-fold reduction of the risk of acute dystonia (from 14.8 to 7.7%). Additional analysis of results from 6 trials involving 330 patients receiving only high-potency neuroleptics (mainly haloperidol) yielded a greater, highly significant overall difference of 51.2 versus 9.5% (a 5.4-fold reduction of risk). In addition, the incidence of dystonia and the efficacy of anticholinergic prophylaxis were inversely related to age. As the authors point out, it is not possible to reliably analyze the relative contribution of factors other than anticholinergic prophylaxis, due to the large variety of unknown and uncontrolled variables among the studies reviewed. Further work is therefore needed to determine the optimal dose and duration of prophylactic treatment as well as the groups of patients who would benefit most (i.e., the younger, men), and to assess the relative cost in terms of side effects. In addition, the use of lower doses of high-potency neuroleptics should be studied as another possible means of reducing the risk of neuroleptic-induced acute dystonia as well as of other neurological side effects of neuroleptics (SEDA-11, 46) (see also page 51).

Akathisia The possible role of β-adrenoceptors in the mechanism of akathisia along with the use of beta-blockers in the treatment of this disorder has been discussed in previous Annuals (SEDA-12, 51; SEDA-13, 41). A double-blind placebo-controlled study suggests that propranolol may be useful in the treatment of neuroleptic-induced akathisia (7[C]).

Twenty neuroleptic-treated schizophrenic patients (22–53 years old, mean age 36 years) were randomly allocated to one of two treatment groups: Group 1 ($n = 10$), 2 days of placebo (1 capsule 3 times daily), followed by 5 days of propranolol (matched capsules, 20 mg 3 times daily); Group 2 ($n = 10$), 2 days of propranolol (20 mg 3 times daily), followed by 5 days of placebo (1 capsule 3 times daily). Previously all patients had been treated for more than 5 days (mean 29 days) with benztropine as tolerated without improvement in akathisia. The average daily doses and the mean duration of previous treatment with benztropine were not significantly different between the two groups of patients. Propranolol at 60 mg daily was well tolerated by all patients. The results of propranolol treatment as compared with placebo suggested improvements in 18 of 26 measures, worsening in 4 of 26 measures, and no change in 4 of 26 measures.

A report describing 4 additional cases is consistent with these findings. Four patients (19–31 years old) with akathisia attributed to neuroleptic treatment showed a marked and significant improvement of their condition after treatment with propranolol 40 mg daily in one patient and 100 mg daily in the others (8[C]). Before propranolol, each patient had a trial of trihexyphenidyl 10–15 mg daily for at least 3 days; after that diazepam 20–30 mg daily was added for another 3 days without success. All 4 patients went on taking propranolol and were followed up for 4–13 months; no akathisia reappeared despite continuous neuroleptic therapy; 3 patients who tried to give up propranolol had a re-emergence of akathisia. There was no effect on blood pressure in any patient; 2 patients presented sinus bradycardia without any other clinical symptom.

More studies are needed (larger, longer, using the same rating scale, without concomitant use of anticholinergics) to confirm these results.

Tardive dyskinesia

Neuroleptic-induced tardive dyskinesia (TD) has been thoroughly discussed and updated in previous volumes of this series (SEDA-6, 46; SEDA-7, 56; SEDA-8, 60; SEDA-11, 44). During the last year many publications on this topic have appeared. The present state of knowledge is presented in several recent reviews (9[R], 10[R]) of its clinical features and diagnosis, epidemiology, risk factors, etiology and pathophysiology, treatment, and clinical management. Various estimates of the prevalence of apparent TD in large series of patients treated with neuroleptics have been published (SEDA-11, 44). According to a review (9[R]), these studies yield average prevalence rates of approximately 20–30%. However, antipsychotic agents are capable of masking the manifestations of the disorder in some patients, and therefore prevalence estimates may need to be corrected for the dyskinesia-suppressing 'artifact' of continued neuroleptic treatment ('false-negative error'). Furthermore, the possibility of false-positive cases (psychiatric patients with abnormal involuntary movements who may never have received neuroleptic drugs) should also be taken into account. In an attempt to estimate the rate of false-negative cases, a sample of 70 patients without evidence of TD while taking neuroleptic drugs were withdrawn from their medication and re-examined at weekly intervals for 3 consecutive weeks (11[R]); 24 (34%) showed emergent dyskinesias; age and total months of neuroleptic treatment were found to be significantly positively related to emergent dyskinesia. On the other hand, the baseline rate of 'spontaneous idiopathic dyskinesias' averages about 5–10%, with a wide range of values (SEDA-11, 45; 9[R], 12[R]). Taking all these data into account, the average prevalence rate of 20–30% has to be reduced by 5–10% to account for the baseline rate of dyskinesia; whether or how to correct the rates upward for cases that appear only on withdrawal of neuroleptics is uncertain, but such increases may be of the order of 30% or more (9[R], 11[R]).

Studying the incidence of TD is still more difficult. A prospective study (11[R]) has been carried out including more than 850 patients; the average age of the cohort was 28 years at entry to the study. One important fact in this study was that for those individuals with a history of neuroleptic exposure at the date of entry, the median duration of exposure was only 12 months; patients were therefore being followed from early in their neuroleptic treatment history. The cumulated incidence of TD was 5% after 1 year, 10% after 2 years, 15% after 3 years, and 19% after 4 years. As the authors point out, these results suggest that the prevalence does increase with increasing duration of neuroleptic exposure and that at least for the first 4–5 years of such exposure the increase is linear. Another follow-

up study of a cohort of 131 patients with an average of 40 years and without any evidence of TD at entry gave a 5-year cumulative incidence rate of 35% (13[C]); among other factors, the older mean age of this population may account for the higher prevalence of TD.

Several reviews have been published on the risk factors for TD. One of them quotes the possibility that hereditary factors could influence the appearance of this disorder (14[R]). In this context, a recent study has been carried out in 14 children of a father with a family history of chronic psychiatric illness, and a mother with a late-onset affective disorder resulting in suicide; out of 12 siblings living to adulthood, 5 had been diagnosed as schizophrenic, 2 had developed an affective disorder in their 6th decade, and 4 died in a psychiatric hospital without a specific diagnosis (there was not enough information to enter the remaining patient to the study). Five of these siblings have been assessed; all had received neuroleptics for periods of 14–26 years and 4 of them showed typical tardive orofacial dyskinesia and had a mental test score lower than the mean of two groups of schizophrenic inpatients of similar age who did not show such movements (15[C]). Could such a high incidence of TD be attributed to a familial predisposition or related to the cognitive impairment? In fact an association between cognitive dysfunction and TD has been suggested (16[C]). More large-scale controlled studies are needed to assess this possible relationship.

Evidence from different studies suggests that affective disorders, particularly depression, are a risk factor for TD. A review of these studies (17[R]) suggests prevalence rates ranging from 30 to 83%, with an average of 44% among neuroleptic-treated patients with affective disorders; these prevalence estimates are higher than those of all neuroleptic-exposed patients. However, several methodological weaknesses of the reviewed studies must be taken into account (i.e., retrospective analysis, small numbers of patients, use of different rating scales, variable criteria for defining movements as abnormal, different demographic and treatment characteristics of patients groups). Although oversimplified, the proposed explanation for this higher rate of TD among depressed patients is that the cyclic mono- and catecholamine activity during mood changes makes the brain more vulnerable to the direct neuroleptic effects or to the compensatory processes initiated by these drugs. In fact, the decreased aminergic activity proposed as the fundamental disturbance underlying depression might result in an increased postsynaptic sensitivity.

A 5-year longitudinal study of a cohort of neuroleptic-treated schizophrenic outpatients focused on the factors related to the subsequent development of TD (13[C]).

In 1975, TD and parkinsonism were assessed in all 256 schizophrenic outpatients; in 1980, 169 of the original cohort of 256 patients (65%) were reassessed; furthermore, 131 patients who did not present TD in 1975 were also reassessed in 1980. The prevalence of TD in the 169 patients assessed in both years increased from 22 to 44% and that of parkinsonism from 33 to 72%, significant differences between the sexes being not recorded. In the cohort of 131 patients without TD in 1975, 35% presented TD in 1980, whilst the prevalence of parkinsonism increased from 32 to 71%. Stepwise multiple logistic regression analysis was used to predict the development of TD. The results suggest that parkinsonism appears to be the best predictor of TD; the authors suggest that two additional factors may be important in the development of TD: poor schizophrenic prognosis and long duration of neuroleptic treatment (over 5 years). Furthermore, 3 additional variables may have acted as uncovering factors of TD: a switch from oral to intramuscular medication in those without parkinsonism (patients were assessed at the end of the injection interval, when blood levels tend to be lower), a neuroleptic dosage reduction, and an increase in antiparkinsonian medication in brain-damaged patients.

The relationship between TD and parkinsonism has been mentioned by other authors (11[R], 18[R]). Kane et al (11[R]) have observed that patients with clinically significant neuroleptic-induced parkinsonism have at least a twofold greater risk of developing TD than patients without such a history. As the authors stress, patients with parkinsonism are more likely to receive anticholinergic drugs and this could result in a potentially false conclusion that the administration of anticholinergics increases the risk of TD. On the other hand, using multivariate statistical analyses, Hansen et al (19[C]) identified risk factors for the development of drug-induced parkinsonism (DIP) in 66 tardive dyskinesia inpatients of whom 12 presented DIP on admission and 25 developed DIP in hospital; the risk factors identified for DIP at admission included older age, TD severity, recent neuroleptic treatment, and fewer years of past neuroleptic exposure. The authors point out that with the exception of TD severity, the other risk factors identified are similar to those reported for the development of DIP in patients without TD. However, shorter duration of past neuroleptic exposure is not usually thought of as a risk factor for DIP, and selection bias cannot be excluded as an explanation for this apparently contradictory finding.

To study the natural history of TD, a cohort of 100 patients with neuroleptic-induced dyskinesia was followed for an average of 41 months from onset of dyskinesia (minimum length of follow-up was 1 year) (20[CR]). After onset of TD, ratings decreased for 4 years, and then stabilized and rose during the 7th year. Longer follow-up is required to confirm the favorable early trend. The discrepancies between different studies [some of them showing improvements while others show aggravation or an increase of the cumulated incidence (13[C])] could be due to the use of different methodologies. As the authors point out, following groups of patients with already manifest TD tends to show overall improvement, while following 'mixed cohorts', e.g. some patients with and some without TD, tends to show exacerbation of TD over time due to the fact that new cases tend to account for the overall TD increases.

Recent observations from human and animal studies suggest that dopamine hypersensitivity is insufficient to explain the pathophysiology of TD. Two additional mechanisms have been proposed: a disturbed balance between D_1- and D_2-dopamine-receptor function and the GABA hypothesis (10[R], 17[R], 21[r]). Studies in animals have revealed that stimulation of D_1-receptors with a partial or a full D_1-agonist causes an oral dyskinesia (22[C]) which looks like TD, especially when D_2-receptor functions are suppressed. These findings suggest that TD is related to a disturbed balance (i.e. an increased ratio) between D_1- and D_2-receptors. Such a hypothesis is in accordance with a similar imbalance between D_1- and D_2-receptor density found in postmortem brains from elderly people. Such reciprocal changes in D_1- and D_2-receptors may explain the increased susceptibility to parkinsonism as well as to the TD seen in elderly people. The GABA hypothesis is based on animal studies in which different GABA neurons projecting from the striatum have been described; one type (from the anterior striatum to the lateral segment of the globus pallidus) is inhibited by dopamine, while another (from the posterior part of the striatum to the reticular zone of the substantia nigra and the medial segment of the globus pallidus) is stimulated by dopamine; neuroleptic drugs stimulate the former type of GABA neurons is linked to Parkinson-like symptoms. On the other hand, it has been shown that an inhibition of the latter type of GABA neurons gives rise to hyperkinetic been shown that an inhibition of the latter type of GABA neurons gives rise to hyperkinetic movements and this could explain, at least in part, the mechanism by which neuroleptics give rise simultaneously to hyperkinetic movements. The final picture of these two actions would depend on the balance between these two opposing effects. In fact, as described above, coexisting parkinsonism and TD is not rare. To test the role of GABA, several placebo-controlled studies have been carried out with different GABA-mimetics (γ-acetylenic GABA, γ-vinyl GABA, and tetrahydroxyisoxazolopyridinol) (18[R]). The main conclusions of these studies suggest that GABA agonists may have some antihyperkinetic effect, but that this effect is limited and might be secondary to an increase in parkinsonism. As Gerlach points out (18[R]), these relatively negative results may be explained by the complexity of GABA functions in the brain. For further clinical pharmacological evaluation of the GABA hypothesis there is a need for more selective GABA agonists.

A satisfactory treatment of TD is not yet available, as shown by a review of the treatment studies published in the 1980s (23[R]). This review included 54 studies, 31 of them double-blind, 6 single-blind, and 17 open. In comparison with a previous review (24[R]), these studies were generally superior to earlier work in terms of methods (more double-blind trials using standardized rating scales), but relatively small sample sizes and short durations of studies were still the main shortcomings. Table 2 presents a summary of this review. It seems that neuroleptic and anticholinergic withdrawal or, when the clinical condition does not allow complete withdrawal, a reduction in neuroleptic and anticholinergic medication to the minimal dosage required by the patient is still the best strategy for prevention. According to this review, if there is no success after this first step of management, several different agents can be tried, with the best evidence existing for propranolol, clonidine, disulfi-

Table 2. Results of studies on the treatment of TD in the 1980s

Treatment	No. of patients included	No. of drugs included	No. of patients/study (range)	Length ($\bar{x} \pm SD$ or range)	Improved (%)
Neuroleptic withdrawal	42	–	6–22	3 mth – 5 yr	55
Neuroleptics	34	4	5–11	3.8 ± 2.9 wk	44
Noradrenergic antagonists	54	4	4–23	8.8 ± 6.6 wk	65
Other catecholamine antagonists	124	5	3–81	2.7 ± 1.6 wk	39
Catecholaminergic drugs	43	4	4–13	2.1 ± 2.2 wk[a]	28
GABAergic drugs	89	5	2–20	4.8 ± 1.4 wk[b]	35
Cholinergic drugs	52	5	9–11	3.5 ± 1.7 wk[c]	21
Anticholinergic drugs	10	2	3–7	4 wk	20
Anticholinergic withdrawal	15	–	3–12	–[d]	60
Miscellaneous	52	6	2–15	9.6 ± 18.8 wk	21
Total	515				38

[a]In 2 studies the length of treatment was not stated.
[b]In 1 study treatment lasted between 1 and 24 weeks.
[c]In 1 study treatment lasted between 6 and 12 weeks.
[d]Length of treatment not stated.

Adapted from Jeste et al (23[R]).

ram and oxypertine. Nevertheless, the variety of drugs included in each pharmacological group, the low number of patients in each study, the short duration of follow-up, and the high frequency of use of concurrent drugs (78% of the studies reviewed) are among the factors that make it difficult to draw definitive conclusions.

Pisa syndrome Pisa syndrome is a form of tardive dystonia that consists of tonic flexion of the trunk to one side accompanied by slight backward rotation in the absence of other dystonic symptoms.

A case has been recently reported of a 25-year-old man with a 5-year history of schizoaffective disorders, treated with haloperidol 8 mg daily plus chlorpromazine 400 mg daily (25[C]). The patient presented a dystonic syndrome consisting of a tonic extension and rigidity of the trunk with the neck flexed towards the right side and rotated backwards. Discontinuation of the drugs resulted in a severe and immediate exacerbation of the schizophrenic symptoms and the appearance of aggressive and impulsive behavior. Treatment with anticholinergic medication did not significantly affect the dystonic symptoms.

Neuroleptic malignant syndrome (NMS) (SEDA-11, 47; SEDA-12, 52; SEDA-13, 43) As described in previous Annuals, many aspects of NMS remain to be elucidated. One of them is the risk of recurrence on rechallenge.

Out of 336 reported cases of NMS, 41 were rechallenged with neuroleptics. NMS was defined by the following major criteria: (1) hyperpyrexia (T > 38°C); (2) extreme muscle rigidity, with or without elevated CPK or hyperpyrexia; and (3) other symptoms such as altered level of consciousness and/or autonomic dysfunction. Twenty-two of these 41 cases fulfilled these criteria, and the remainder (19 cases) were considered possible. Three individuals were rechallenged on a 2nd occasion, bringing the total number of rechallenges to 44. Of the 24 definite cases rechallenged, 6 were positive, 4 were possible, and 14 were negative. Of the 20 cases that were initially possible NMS, on rechallenge 1 was positive, 6 were possible, and 13 were negative (26[CR]).

These retrospective results should be interpreted very cautiously and more studies are needed. Meanwhile, these data suggest that rechallenge following NMS is associated with a risk of recurrence and close monitoring of such patients is mandatory.

The exact constellation of signs by which NMS is manifested is not known. Some authors have suggested that the syndrome may be heterogeneous and show various degrees of severity.

A case of prolonged mild to moderate fever of 9 months duration occurred in a psychotic patient after doubling the oral fluphenazine dose and was accompanied by tachycardia, high blood pressure, diaphoresis and creatine phosphokinase (CPK) elevation at admission (27[Cr]). All signs disappeared after stopping fluphenazine, but fever and CPK elevation recurred on 2 occasions, the 1st one after treatment with lithium and the 2nd after treatment with thioridazine. According to Levenson's diagnostic criteria of NMS, 3 major or 2 major and 4 minor criteria are needed (28[R]). This patient had 2 major (fever, elevated CPK) and 3 minor (tachycardia, abnormal blood pressure, diaphoresis) criteria after exposure to oral fluphenazine and only 2 major criteria after the subsequent exposures.

The diagnosis of NMS in this patient is therefore uncertain, especially as elevated CPK may be caused by other conditions than NMS, such as agitation and psychosis.

Two additional cases of asymptomatic elevation of CPK after neuroleptic treatment have been described (29[Cr]). One patient developed a 1st episode after 3 days of haloperidol treatment and CPK elevation reappeared after 2 days of treatment with thioridazine. The other patient was being treated with perphenazine when CPK levels rose but was then given thiothixene without recurrence. Neither of these cases showed other signs of NMS. As the authors point out, more studies are needed to clarify the distinction between neuroleptic side effects and subclinical myopathy of psychosis.

Several cardiovascular complications of NMS have been described (SEDA-11, 47). A case of myocardial infarction in the absence of risk factors, concurrent with NMS, has been reported (30[C]).

A 32-year-old man developed NMS 48 hours after starting treatment with levomepromazine, 50 mg 3 times daily. Forty-eight hours after stopping medication, while the patient was still febrile and rigid, syncope occurred; ECG showed myocardial infarction which was confirmed by a rise in serum myocardial enzymes and by echocardiography. His past history did not reveal any physical illness, including ischemic heart disease, or any related risk factors such as diabetes mellitus, heavy smoking, obesity, hypertension or hyperlipidemia.

The authors suggest that the increased metabolic demands caused by hyperthermia may produce relative ischemia that affects not only skeletal muscle, but also the myocardium. This might be particularly important in patients at risk for ischemic heart disease.

The incidence of NMS has been discussed in previous Annuals (SEDA-11, 47; SEDA-13, 43). A prospective 6-months study aimed at quantifying the incidence of NMS in a psychiatric inpatient hospital identified only 1 case of NMS among 495 neuroleptic-treated patients (31[C]).

Is intermittent neuroleptic prophylaxis better than continuous treatment in reducing the incidence of extrapyramidal side effects? The efficacy of continuous neuroleptic treatment to prevent exacerbations of schizophrenic illness is supported by a considerable weight of evidence from placebo-controlled trials. However, increasing recognition of the risks, in particular of the risk of tardive dyskinesia, has tempered enthusiasm for this form of treatment. One of the alternative strategies of treatment designed to prevent or attenuate relapse while reducing drug exposure and side effects aims at identifying the earliest signs of decompensation with prompt but time-limited treatment during such periods. It has been suggested that depressive symptoms, which are a frequent accompaniment of schizophrenic illness, form part of the process of decompensation, being more frequent at the onset of acute psychosis and subsiding in parallel with psychotic manifestations. Such affective changes together with the emergence of other neurotic symptoms, are potentially useful in predicting the onset of relapse. A recent clinical trial tested the hypothesis that prompt intermittent neuroleptic treatment in response to the early signs of relapse described above would reduce persistent side effects such as dyskinesia, akathisia, akinesia and sedation, improve social functioning; although it would lead to an increase in the frequency of relapse, such relapses could be attenuated to the point that their negative effects would be outweighed by the potential benefits of the new strategy (32[C]).

Fifty-four stable schizophrenic outpatients in remission were randomized to two groups. Participating clinicians were requested to refer patients whom they thought might benefit from the intermittent treatment approach. The control group ($n=27$) continued to receive fluphenazine decanoate in pretrial doses, whereas in the intermittent treatment group ($n=27$) equivalent doses of placebo injections were substituted under double-blind conditions. After beginning, patients were seen every 4 weeks, and at least weekly during relapse and while prodromal symptoms were present. Additional oral haloperidol (5–10 mg daily, though flexibility was allowed) was given to patients of both groups who developed prodromal symptoms or relapse. Prodromal symptoms were treated for up to 2 weeks, and relapse was treated until 4 weeks after the remission of symptoms. As the authors note, the theoretical rationale for a program of management based on the early detection and treatment of prodromal symptoms is supported by the finding that 8 out of 11 relapses were preceded by such symptoms. After 1 year of follow-up, relapse was significantly more frequent in the intermittent treatment group (8 patients) than in the controls (2 patients), but this difference was not accompanied by any difference in the frequency of admission to hospital (5 patients in each group) and in the regular bimonthly ratings of psychotic symptoms, the global assessments of psychopathology and social functioning, and the mean global assessment. The intermittent treatment group received significantly less total neuroleptic dose than controls. At both 6 and 12 months of follow-up akathisia, retardation, gait abnormality and global parkinsonism had a significantly lower point prevalence in the intermittent treatment group. The point prevalence of tardive dyskinesia rose in the controls and remained comparatively stable in the intermittent treatment group in the 1-year follow-up period.

In conclusion, the results of this study suggest that brief intermittent treatment attenuates psychotic relapses, but these occur more frequently than with continuous prophylaxis. Although intermittent treatment is not as effective in preventing psychotic symptoms, it has the advantages of reduced exposure to drugs and fewer extrapyramidal side effects. The reduced risk of tardive dyskinesia suggested by these results is in conflict with the results of other studies on the relation between tardive dyskinesia and both dosage and duration of neuroleptic treatment, and therefore these results should be interpreted with care. The authors conclude that this approach may prove an acceptable alternative in otherwise cooperative patients who wish to stop prophylactic treatment or are suffering from incipient or established tardive dyskinesia, severe weight gain, or disabling extrapyramidal symptoms.

Endocrine, metabolic *Reduction of bone mineralization* A significant increase in urinary calcium and hydroxyproline levels and a decrease in urinary alkaline phosphatase (ALP) activity were found in 12 schizophrenic patients receiving antipsychotic agents. In these patients the levels of active metabolites of vitamin D_3 were decreased, while the levels of mid-molecule parathyroid hormone were within the normal range, except for 2 cases (33[C]). The results, however, were obtained in only 12 patients (5 men and 7 women, 18–57 years old) who were receiving variable doses of chlorpromazine, levomepromazine, and haloperidol, plus other drugs such as anticholinergic agents and benzodiazepines; the controls were 5 normal men. The authors suggest that chronic neuroleptic treatment alters calcium metabolism by increasing bone resorption and inhibiting bone matrix formation and calcification, although in 2 patients hyperparathyroidism or a calcitonin effect could not be ruled out. These effects are different from those observed in patients chronically treated with antiepileptic drugs, because the latter show reduced serum calcium and phosphorus levels and raised ALP activity, while patients treated with antipsychotic drugs showed increased urinary calcium levels and reduced ALP activity. Although other potential causes of the findings, such as inactivity, were not ruled out, this report is consistent with the increased risk of hip fracture associated with antipsychotic drugs (SEDA-12, 52).

Weight gain In a survey of 226 patients attending depot neuroleptic clinics in London, the prevalence of clinically relevant obesity was found to be 4 times that in the general population (31[C]).

The study involved 226 patients (120 men), the great majority of whom were suffering from chronic schizophrenia. Table 3 shows the prevalence of obesity, as compared with that of the Greater London population. The prevalence of obesity (BMI = 30–39.9) and of crip-

Table 3. *Distribution of BMI[a] by sex and neuroleptic drug*

Sex and BMI	Drugs								All drugs		OPCS study[f]
	FPZ[b]		FPX[c]		FSL[d]		CPX[e]				
	n	%	*n*	%	*n*	%	*n*	%	*n*	%	%
Men											
BMI < 25	21	34	9	23	1	14	5	42	36	30	62
BMI 25–29.9	20	32	19	49	4	57	4	33	47	39	33
BMI 30–39.9	18	29	10	26	2	29	2	17	32	27	6
BMI 40+	3	5	1	2	0	0	1	8	5	4	0
All BMI	62		39		7		12		120		
Women											
BMI < 25	20	37	20	51	4	36	1	50	45	42	68
BMI 25–29.9	15	28	3	8	4	36	0	0	22	21	23
BMI 30–39.9	16	30	13	33	3	27	1	50	33	31	8
BMI 40+	3	5	3	8	0	0	0	0	6	6	1
All BMI	54		39		11		2		106		

[a]BMI = body mass index = weight (kg)/[height (m)]^2. BMI 20–24.9, not obese; 25–29.9, mildly obese; 30–39.9, clinically relevant obesity; 40 and over, crippling obesity.
[b]Fluphenazine decanoate, 12.5 mg 6-weekly to 100 mg weekly (modal value, 25 mg fortnightly).
[c]Flupenthixol decanoate, 10 mg monthly to 100 mg weekly (modal values, 20 mg monthly or 40 mg fortnightly).
[d]Fluspirilene, 2 mg fortnightly to 10 mg weekly.
[e]Clopenthixol, 200 mg 3-weekly to 800 mg weekly.
[f]Office of Population Censuses and Surveys, BMI distribution for Greater London (1981), with a sample of 551 men and 616 women.
Adapted from Silverstone et al (34[C]).

pling obesity (BMI > 40) was much higher among all patients receiving depot medication than in the general population for both men and women. Unfortunately, no analysis of dosage was attempted, because dosage had been changed frequently.

Sexual dysfunction *(SEDA-11, 111)* It is well known that antipsychotic drugs can interfere with male sexual function, producing impotence, retrograde ejaculation, impaired ejaculation, painful ejaculation, decreased libido, and priapism. Their effects on human female sexuality have been studied far less and are generally less appreciated. According to a recent review (35[R]), there have been only a few case-reports of anorgasmia associated with antipsychotic drugs. Orgasmic disturbances have been reported with thioridazine, trifluoperazine, and fluphenazine. Several mechanisms have been suggested, mainly α-adrenergic blockade, but also dopaminergic blockade, because animal studies have suggested that dopaminergic activity may be facilitatory to sexual behavior.

Gastrointestinal *Allergic reactions* A case of acute bilateral swelling of the tongue in a 19-year-old woman with schizophrenia has been reported (36[C]). The patient has been taking 25 mg of trifluoperazine 3 times a day, and after 1 month the dose was reduced to 25 mg twice daily. After 9 days with the new dosage, she reported nausea and vomiting after missing a dose of trifluoperazine, and she was treated with 2 mg of oral benztropine mesylate. One day after she continued to have nausea and vomiting, and it was though that she has 'flu'; the dose of trifluoperazine was further reduced to 20 mg twice daily. The next day the nurse reported that the patient's tongue had suddenly swollen 60–90 min after she had ingested her morning dose of trifluoperazine. There was no evidence of extrapyramidal symptoms, involuntary motor movements or respiratory stridor, and her tongue returned to its normal size within 5 min after being given 50 mg of diphenhydramine. The authors postulate that the reaction was allergic and that it became apparent when the antipsychotic dose was reduced, as a result of loss of the antihistaminic effect of the phenothiazines.

Tumor induction A cohort of 6152 Danish schizophrenic patients was followed from 1957 to 1984, and all patients who had received a diagnosis of cancer during the study period were identified (37[C]). The incidence rate ratio (IRR), i.e. the observed number of cancer patients in the study population divided by the expected number of cases, was calculated. The expected number of cases was calculated on the basis of the cancer incidence rate in the general Danish population, standardized for age. Calculations were performed separately for men and women, but no other potentially confounding variables, such as social class, the use of drugs, or exposure to other known or suspected risk factors, were taken into account. A 24% statistically significant reduction of the incidence of all cancers was found among men, and this reduction was especially marked for respiratory, prostate and bladder cancer. The authors also report a decreased incidence of digestive tract cancer, especially of the pancreas, and a slight increase in the risk of breast cancer among schizophrenic women. Although the possibility of differences in diagnostic accuracy is excluded by the authors, the weakness of the associations found, the fact that the confidence intervals of the IRR values are not presented, the fact that confounding was not reasonably excluded, and the multiple statistical comparisons which increase the likelihood of finding a statistically significant association all tend to cast doubt on the result.

In the Southern Health Care Region of Sweden all cases of male breast cancer ($n=95$) occurring from 1970 to 1986 were identified through the population-based regional cancer registry (38[C]). These patients were compared with two series of controls, i.e. 383 male lung cancer patients and 69 male non-Hodgkin's lymphoma (NHL) patients diagnosed in the same region. The 3 groups were not matched by age or by any other risk factor, including the date of the diagnosis. The information on previous use of drugs known to be associated with plasma prolactin elevations (phenothiazines and derivatives) was abstracted from the patients' hospital records. An odds ratio of 5 for the previous use of prolactin-elevating drugs was found, but the confidence intervals were not presented. The results also suggested that patients with breast cancer had experienced more brain concussions and skull fractures than patients with lung cancer or malignant lymphoma, and it is known that these lesions are associated with an increase in plasma prolactin levels. Selection and information bias cannot be excluded, and although the results are biologically plausible, they should be confirmed by other studies.

Withdrawal effects *(SED-11, 113; SEDA-12, 53; SEDA-13, 45)* A review of non-dyskinetic antipsychotic-withdrawal phenomena (39[R]) focuses on the differential diagnosis between a psychotic relapse and neuroleptic-withdrawal symptoms. As the authors point out, the probability of a psychotic relapse in a previously stable patient is minimal in the first 2 weeks after discontinuing neuroleptics, while withdrawal symptoms generally have their onset within 48 hours of the last dose, and rarely after the 1st week. Other basic questions reviewed reveal that the withdrawal symptoms may be more severe and frequent when anticholinergic-antiparkinsonian agents are simultaneously discontinued. To illustrate the difference between a psychotic relapse and a neuroleptic withdrawal syndrome, the case of a 34-year-old woman has been reported in whom the early relapse on 2 occasions when neuroleptics were stopped abruptly and the lack of relapse when the same drug at the same doses was discontinued very slowly suggested that drug withdrawal, rather than illness relapse, was responsible (40[Cr]).

Parkinsonism is a common extrapyramidal reaction of antipsychotic treatment, but it is more unusual as a withdrawal effect.

Fifteen inpatients on continuous neuroleptic treatment for at least 2 years were selected to investigate the effects of abrupt neuroleptic withdrawal (41[C]). Their mean age was 51 years (range, 41–65 years) and the estimated duration of treatment was at least 12 years. Six of these patients developed parkinsonism 1–4 days after antipsychotic withdrawal. Withdrawal parkinsonism could not be explained by discontinuation of anticholinergic drugs because in 3 of these patients anticholinergics had been discontinued for at least 5 months before antipsychotic withdrawal; in the other 3 subjects, withdrawal of the anticholinergic 5–7 days before the antipsychotic was discontinued produced no motor changes.

INDIVIDUAL AGENTS

Clozapine *(SEDA-4, 40; SEDA-5, 55; SEDA-9, 86)*

Clozapine is unique in that it has a high specificity for limbic rather than striatal dopaminergic receptors, and this seems to be the reason why it causes fewer extrapyramidal side effects than other antipsychotic agents. Clozapine has serotonin (S_2), adrenergic (α_1) and histaminergic blocking activity. It is also a potent muscarinic acetylcholine receptor antagonist. Because of the risk of agranulocytosis associated with th-isdrug, in many countries its use has been limited. The cumulative risk of developing this side effect has been estimated to be 2% (42[R]). However, some countries have allowed continued use of the drug for carefully selected patients who are resistant to other agents, sensitive to extrapyramidal side effects, or dyskinetic.

In order to test the efficacy of clozapine in schizophrenic patients resistant to neuroleptic treatment, a 6-week double-blind treatment trial with either clozapine (up to 900 mg daily) or chlorpromazine and benztropine mesylate (up to 1800 mg daily of chlorpromazine and up to 6 mg daily of benztropine) has been conducted involving 268 patients (43[C]); 30% of the clozapine-treated patients were categorized as responders compared with 4% of chlorpromazine-treated patients. The comparative profile of the most frequently reported adverse drug reactions is presented in Table 4. Fever, salivation and hypertension were more frequent with clozapine.

No cases of agranulocytosis were recorded, but this is probably due to the short duration of this trial and the low number of patients included. Also, the majority of the reported cases of agranulocytosis occurred between the 6th and the 18th week of clozapine treatment. Comparable results have been found in another smaller double-blind clinical trial in schizophrenic non-responders, comparing clozapine to chlorpromazine + benztropine (44[C]).

Table 4. *Most frequently reported adverse drug reactions in a double-blind clinical trial comparing clozapine (up to 900 mg daily) with chlorpromazine (up to 1800 mg daily) + benztropine (up to 6 mg daily)*

	Clozapine		Chlorpromazine + benztropine		P*
	n	%	*n*	%	
Drowsiness	26	21	18	13	0.098
Tachycardia	21	17	16	11	0.218
Constipation	20	16	17	12	0.380
Dizziness	18	14	23	16	0.735
Hypotension	16	13	54	38	< 0.001
Fever	16	13	6	4	0.014
Salivation	17	13	2	1	< 0.001
Hypertension	15	12	7	5	0.045
Headache	13	10	14	10	0.999
Nausea/vomiting	12	10	17	12	0.560
Dry mouth	6	5	28	20	< 0.001

*Based on two-tailed Fisher's exact test.
From Kane et al (43[c]).

REFERENCES

1. Avorn J, Dreyer P, Connelly K, Soumerai SB (1989) Use of psychoactive medication and the quality of care in rest homes. *N. Engl. J. Med., 320*, 227.
2. Huyse F, Van Schijndel RB (1988) Haloperidol and cardiac arrest. *Lancet, 2*, 568.
3. Bateman DN, Darling WM, Boys R, Rawlins MD (1989) Extrapyramidal reactions to metoclopramide and prochlorperazine. *Q. J. Med., 71*, 307.
4. Anonymous (1989) Measuring the therapeutic risk. *Lancet, 2*, 139.
5. Newton-John H (1988) Acute upper airway obstruction due to supraglottic dystonia induced by a neuroleptic. *Br. Med. J., 297*, 964.
6. Arana GW, Goff DC, Baldessarini RJ, Keepers GA (1988) Efficacy of anticholinergic prophylaxis for neuroleptic-induced acute dystonia. *Am. J. Psychiatry, 145*, 993.
7. Kramer MS, Gorkin RA, DiJohnson C, Sheves P (1988) Propranolol in the treatment of neuroleptic-induced akathisia (NIA) in schizophrenics: a double-blind, placebo-controlled study. *Biol. Psychaitry, 24*, 823.
8. Hermesh H, Molcho A, Munitz H (1988) Successful propranolol therapy for neuroleptic-induced akathisia resistant to anticholinergic and benzodiazepine drugs. *Clin. Neuropharmacol., 11*, 369.
9. Baldessarini RJ (1988) A summary of current knowledge of tardive dyskinesia. *Encéphale, 14*, 263.
10. Gerlach J, Casey DE (1988) Tardive dyskinesia. *Acta Psychiatr. Scand., 77*, 369.
11. Kane JM, Woerner M, Lieberman J (1988) Tardive dyskinesia: prevalence, incidence and risk factors. *J. Clin. Psychopharmacol., 8*, 52S.
12. Brion S, Plas J, Chevalier J-F, Dussaux P (1988) Dyskinésies séniles et dyskinésies tardives. *Encéphale, 14*, 215.
13. Chouinard G, Annable L, Ross-Chouinard A, Mercier P (1988) A 5-year prospective longitudinal study of tardive dyskinesia: factors predicting appearance of new cases. *J. Clin. Psychopharmacol., 8*, 21S.
14. Law RM, Jeste SD, Jeste DV (1988) Preventing neuroleptic-induced tardive dyskinesia in adults and children. *Encéphale, 14*, 251.
15. Waddington JL, Youssef HA (1988) The expression of schizophrenia, affective disorder and vulnerability to tardive dyskinesia in an extensive pedigree. *Br. J. Psychiatry, 153*, 376.
16. Waddington JL, Youssef HA (1988) Tardive dyskinesia in bipolar affective disorders: aging, cognitive dysfunction, course of illness, and exposure to neuroleptics and lithium. *Am. J. Psychiatry, 145*, 613.
17. Casey DE (1988) Affective disorders and tardive dyskinesia. *Encéphale, 14*, 221.
18. Gerlach J (1988) Tardive dyskinesia: pathophysiological mechanisms and clinical trials. *Encéphale, 14*, 227.
19. Hansen TE, Brown WL, Weigel RM, Casey DE (1988) Risk factors for drug-induced parkinsonism in tardive dyskinesia patients. *J. Clin. Psychiatry, 49*, 139.
20. Gardos G, Cole JO, Haskell D et al (1988) The natural history of tardive dyskinesia. *J. Clin. Psychopharmacol., 8*, 31S.
21. Waddington JL (1988) The ageing brain, neuroleptic drugs and the enigma of schizophrenia. *Ir. J. Med. Sci., 157*, 135.
22. Johansson P, Levin E, Gunne L, Ellison G (1987) Opposite effects of a D1 and D2 agonist on oral movements in rats. *Eur. J. Pharmacol., 134*, 83.
23. Jeste DV, Lohr JB, Clark K, Wyatt RJ (1988) Pharmacological treatments of tardive dyskinesia in 1980s. *J. Clin. Psychopharmacol., 8*, 38S.
24. Jeste DV, Wyatt RJ (1982) Therapeutic strategies against tardive dyskinesia: two decades of experience. *Arch. Gen. Psychiatry, 39*, 803.
25. Amore M, Cerisoli M, Campanile S, Campanile A (1988) Pisa syndrome: report of a case. *Ital. J. Neurol. Sci., 9*, 273.
26. Wells AJ, Sommi RW, Crismon ML (1988) Neuroleptic rechallenge after neuroleptic malignant syndrome: case report and literature review. *Drug Intell. Clin. Pharm., 22*, 475.
27. Keshavan MS, Krishna Kambhampati R (1989) Prolonged fever without extrapyramidal symptoms during neuroleptic treatment. *J. Clin. Psychopharmacol., 9*, 230.
28. Levenson JL (1985) Neuroleptic malignant syndrome. *Am. J. Psychiatry, 142*, 1137.
29. Pearlman C, Wheadon D, Epstein S (1988) Creatine kinase elevation after neuroleptic treatment. *Am. J. Psychiatry, 145*, 1018.
30. Becker D, Birger M, Samuel E, Floru S (1988) Myocardial infarction: an unusual complication of neuroleptic malignant syndrome. *J. Nerv. Ment. Dis., 176*, 377.
31. Friedman JH, Davis R, Wagner RL (1988) Neuroleptic malignant syndrome: the results of a 6-month perspective study of incidence in a state psychiatric hospital. *Clin. Neuropharmacol., 11*, 373.
32. Jolley AG, Hirsch SR, McRink A, Manchanda R (1989) Trial of brief intermittent neuroleptic prophylaxis for selected schizophrenic outpatients: clinical outcome at one year. *Br. Med. J., 298*, 985.
33. Higuchi T, Komoda T, Sugishita M et al (1987) Certain neuroleptics reduce bone mineralization in schizophrenic patients. *Neuropsychobiology, 18*, 185.
34. Silverstone T, Smith G, Goodall E (1988) Prevalence of obesity in patients receiving depot antipsychotics. *Br. J. Psychiatry, 153*, 214.

35. Segraves RT (1988) Psychiatric drugs and inhibited female orgasm. *J. Sex Marital Ther., 14*, 202.
36. Ward DF, Peters JC (1988) Unusual reaction to trifluoperazine. *Postgrad. Med., 84*, 99.
37. Mortensen PB (1989) The incidence of cancer in schizophrenic patients. *J. Epidemiol. Community Health, 43*, 43.
38. Olsson H, Ramstan J (1988) Head trauma and exposure to prolactin-elevating drugs as risk factors for male breast cancer. *J. Natl. Cancer Inst., 80*, 679.
39. Dilsaver SC, Alessi NE (1988) Antipsychotic withdrawal symptoms: phenomenology and pathophysiology. *Acta Psychiatr. Scand., 77*, 241.
40. Kane GJ (1989) Rebound psychoses following the discontinuation of a high potency neuroleptic. *Can. J. Psychiatry, 34*, 227.
41. Ceccherini Nelli A, Yarden PE, Guazzelli M, Feinberg I (1989) Parkinsonism following neuroleptic withdrawal. *Arch. Gen. Psychiatry, 46*, 383.
42. Bablenis E, Weber SS, Wagner RL (1989) Clozapine: a novel antipsychotic agent. *Drug Intell. Clin. Pharm., 23*, 109.
43. Kane J, Honigfeld G, Singer J et al (1988) Clozapine for the treatment-resistant schizophrenic: a double-blind comparison with chlorpromazine. *Arch. Gen. Psychiatry, 45*, 789.
44. Conley RR, Schulz C, Baker RW et al (1988) Clozapine efficacy in schizophrenic nonresponders. *Psychopharmacol. Bull., 24*, 269.
45. Borison RL, Diamond BI, Sinha D et al (1988) Clozapine withdrawal rebound psychosis. *Psychopharmacol. Bull., 24*, 260.

J.C. Mucklow

7 Anticonvulsant drugs

GENERAL TOPICS

Anticonvulsants and cognitive function *(SED-11, 122; SEDA-11, 62; SEDA-12, 56)* Impaired cognition in children with epilepsy contributes to poor school performance and is an important determinant of intellectual attainment. Holmes (1[R]) has reviewed the factors which can impair cognition and concludes that the cause of the seizures and the child's intelligence quotient before the first seizure are more important than either the type of seizure or the use of anticonvulsant drugs. There is uncertainty about the contribution made by the age of onset and the number of seizures, but he could find no evidence that a single brief seizure, or even a small number of seizures, produces neurological damage. In the large majority of children, intelligence is unaffected.

A controlled study of 13 children aged 5–10 years, who had received phenobarbital 4–5 mg/kg for prevention of febrile convulsions when younger, revealed no effect upon *language development* as judged by assessment of communicative skills (gestural, oral and written), understanding of grammatical structures and auditory memory span (2[C]). In adults, however, Trimble (3[R]) concluded that recurrent tonic-clonic seizures, head injury, the prescription of phenytoin, and low folic acid concentration were the chief factors contributing to a decline in cognitive function.

A comparison, between 2 groups of epileptic patients receiving single drug treatment with phenytoin and a group of matched controls, in which neuropsychological tests of intelligence, vigilance, attention, memory and sensorimotor function were used, revealed that the effect of phenytoin upon cognitive function was greater than that of carbamazepine and independent of serum drug concentration; no legacy of prolonged exposure to these drugs was apparent a year after withdrawal of treatment (4[C]). However, in a larger study of patients taking carbamazepine alone, impaired psychomotor function was related to the serum concentration of carbamazepine and, in particular, to that of its major metabolite, carbamazepine-10,11-epoxide (5[C]).

Endocrine, metabolic *(SED-11, 120; SEDA-11, 63; SEDA-12, 56)* Macphee et al. (6[C]) have examined the *endocrine effects* of different anticonvulsants by measuring circulating sex hormone concentrations and pituitary responsiveness in young epileptic men, compared with untreated age-matched controls. Carbamazepine reduced free testosterone and dehydroepiandrosterone sulfate (DHAS) and increased basal prolactin and luteinizing hormone (LH) as well as the prolactin response to LH-RH, whereas phenytoin reduced only free DHAS, and valproate had no effect. Those receiving more than 1 drug showed the greatest reduction in free testosterone and DHAS, but there was no consistent change in pituitary responsiveness.

Changes in the concentrations of *serum γ-glutamyltranspeptidase (GT)* and *alkaline phosphatase (AP)* are related to the degree of mono-oxygenase enzyme induction by anticonvulsants such as phenytoin and carbamazepine (7[C]). In 54 epileptics receiving phenytoin alone, serum GT and AP were elevated in 91 and 39%, respectively; in 56 receiving carbamazepine alone, the equivalent incidence figures were 64 and 14%: the increases were dose-related, but serum drug concentrations were not measured.

Withdrawal effects With the exception of barbiturates and benzodiazepines, withdrawal of anticonvulsant treatment is not associated with any harmful effects other than an increase in seizure frequency. Duncan et al. (8[C]) have confirmed this in relation to carbamazepine, phenytoin and valproate, in a prospective double-blind placebo-controlled study. However, 2 cases of chronic schizophrenia have been de-

Side Effects of Drugs Annual 14
M.N.G. Dukes and L. Beeley, editors

scribed in whom the abrupt withdrawal of carbamazepine led to an acute exacerbation of their psychoses, characterized by paranoia, hostility and agitation (9[C]).

Second-generation effects *(SED-11, 120; SEDA-12, 57)* It has been stated that *impaired fetal growth*, apparent as reduced body length, body weight and head circumference at birth, can occur if the mother has epilepsy and is receiving anticonvulsant drugs (10[R]). But a historical cohort study carried out by the Italian Multicentre Registry on Birth Defects (11[C]), involving 164 infants of epileptic women and 185 controls, has found intrauterine growth retardation and smaller head circumference but no apparent effect upon body length. They analyzed the effect of separate anticonvulsants where single drug treatment had been used and concluded that only phenobarbital affected birth weight and head circumference; but as no other single drug had been taken by more than 7 mothers, no firm conclusion is possible. The study's most interesting finding was that head circumference was significantly ($P<0.05$) smaller in infants whose mothers were epileptic but had received no anticonvulsant drugs during pregnancy than in the infants of non-epileptic mothers: drug therapy is clearly not the only factor involved.

Annegers et al (12[C]) compared the incidence of *spontaneous abortion* among the pregnancies of women with epilepsy and the wives of men with epilepsy, and found no significant difference; neither epilepsy nor maternal exposure to anticonvulsant drugs was associated with recognized fetal loss.

INDIVIDUAL DRUGS

Carbamazepine *(SED-11, 127; SEDA-11, 63; SEDA-12, 57)*

Cardiovascular A case of unexplained *hypertension* is described in a 20-year-old epileptic woman receiving carbamazepine; a blood pressure of 180/110 mmHg fell to 120/90 mmHg after carbamazepine (800 mg/d) was withdrawn, phenytoin being substituted. Reintroduction of carbamazepine, following an increase in seizure frequency, led to a progressive rise in blood pressure to 180/110 mmHg which fell to normal within 1 week of drug withdrawal. The authors postulate that the effect may have been mediated by an increase in either the release or the action of antidiuretic hormone, but present no supporting evidence (13[C]).

Nervous system Critchley and Phillips (14[C]) describe 2 *unusual neurological reactions* to carbamazepine. A 59-year-old man exhibited bizarre uncontrollable movements of both hands and arms lasting for 12 hours after 2 days treatment with 200 mg twice daily; and a 15-year-old boy developed rigidity, a shuffling gait and repeated attacks of generalized shivering, after 6 months treatment with 100 mg thrice daily, and did not recover completely for a week after drug withdrawal.

Epileptics receiving carbamazepine alone have been found to exhibit *impaired visual contrast sensitivity* (ability to perceive slight differences in luminance between adjacent regions of the visual field) compared with age-matched controls, to an extent which is related to drug concentration (15[C]). The importance of this is uncertain, but age-related loss of visual contrast sensitivity does relate to impaired ability to discriminate between different types of road sign (16).

Other organs and systems The effect of carbamazepine upon *immunoglobulin* (IgG) subclasses has been examined (17[C]): IgG_2 concentration was reduced after 6 weeks treatment, but not below the normal range (the serum drug concentration was in the range 15–45 μmol/l). IgG_1, IgG_3, IgG_4 and total IgG were unaltered and the clinical significance of this observation is unknown.

Overdosage Observations in 4 patients following overdoses of carbamazepine, producing peak serum concentrations of 27–35 mg/l (113–148 μmol/l), suggest that the metabolite carbamazepine-10,11-epoxide (CBZ-E) may have appreciable independent toxic effects. The 2 patients who had the more protracted and serious clinical course had much higher levels of CBZ-E relative to parent drug, as a result of previous regular treatment with carbamazepine (18[C]).

Interactions Carbamazepine and *phenytoin* are known to interact with each other but are usually said to accelerate each other's metabolism with mutual lessening of anticonvulsant effect. However, a detailed investigation using a stable isotope tracer technique, in which carbamazepine was added and its dose increased in patients already receiving phenytoin, has shown a consistent increase in serum phenytoin concentration by an average 35% with resulting neurotoxic effects; the metabolic clearance of phenytoin (via parahydroxyphenylhydantoin) and of phenytoin dihydrodiol decreased and total phenytoin clearance fell by 37%: competitive inhibition by carbamazepine of the enzyme arene oxidase is the likely mechanism (19[C]).

Phenobarbital and primidone *(SED-11, 131, 132; SEDA-11, 64; SEDA-12, 59)*

Depression in adults with epilepsy is more pronounced in those receiving phenobarbital (20[C]) and major depressive disorder and suicidal ideation are much more common in children taking phenobarbital (21[C]). Barabas and Matthews (22[C]) report 2 cases of severe depression, in 15-year-old girls taking phenobarbital and primidone respectively, which resolved promptly after treatment was withdrawn.

Phenytoin *(SED-11, 124; SEDA-11, 64; SEDA-12, 58)*

York and Coleridge (23[C]) report 2 fatal cases of *cardiovascular collapse* occurring after manual infusion of phenytoin 500–880 mg at a rate of 35 mg/min. They conclude that the concentration of phenytoin in the infusion was too high and recommend, if a loading dose cannot be given orally, that a 'piggy-back' infusion be used to ensure an infused drug concentration no greater than 6.7 mg/ml.

Further evidence for *cerebellar atrophy* in epileptics receiving phenytoin comes from high-resolution CT scans of the brain and posterior fossa. In a controlled study, posterior fossa atrophy correlated significantly with both the duration of epilepsy and the total amount of phenytoin ingested during the patient's lifetime, but not with the number of seizures (24[C]).

Phenytoin bioavailability is considerably reduced by an *interaction* with enteral feeding solutions, such as Isocal (25[C]), Osmolite (26[C]) and Ensure (27[C]), all of which contain protein and calcium. When this interaction is unrecognized, correction of a falling serum phenytoin concentration by an increased dose will lead to toxicity after the feeding solution is discontinued.

Sodium valproate *(SED-11, 128; SEDA-11, 65; SEDA-12, 58)*

The effect of valproate upon *haem biosynthesis* has been examined (28[C]): leukocyte 5-aminolaevulinate synthase activity and daily excretion of porphobilinogen and total porphyrins were all higher in epileptics receiving valproate than in age-matched controls; and similar findings emerged from a controlled study of healthy subjects who took valproate for 5 days. The results imply that valproate is porphyrinogenic and should not be used in patients with acute porphyria.

NEW COMPOUNDS

Oxcarbazepine

Oxcarbazepine is closely related to carbamazepine but appears to be more likely to cause *hyponatremia*. In a study of 41 patients treated for 4 weeks or longer, 21 had serum sodium concentrations below 135 mmol/l. The effect was dose-related, but treatment did not have to be stopped. The serum sodium concentration should be checked in patients receiving oxcarbazepine at doses greater than 25–30 mg/kg/d (29[C]).

REFERENCES

1. Holmes GL (1988) Do seizures cause brain damage? *Int. Pediatr., 3*, 158.
2. Hambly G, Frewin C, Dodd B (1988) Effect of anticonvulsant medication in the preschool years on later language development. *Med. J. Aust., 148*, 658.
3. Trimble MR (1988) Cognitive hazards of seizure disorders. *Epilepsia, 29, Suppl. 1*, S19.
4. Gallassi R, Morreale A, Lorusso S et al (1988) Carbamazepine and phenytoin: comparison of cognitive effects in epileptic patients during monotherapy and withdrawal. *Arch. Neurol., 45*, 892.

5. Gillham RA, Williams N, Wiedmann K et al (1988) Concentration–effect relationships with carbamazepine and its epoxide on psychomotor and cognitive function in epileptic patients. *J. Neurol. Neurosurg. Psychiatry, 51*, 929.
6. Macphee GJA, Larkin JG, Butler E et al (1988) Circulating hormones and pituitary responsiveness in young epileptic men receiving long-term anti-epileptic medication. *Epilepsia, 29*, 468.
7. Aldenhövel HG (1988) The influence of long-term anticonvulsant therapy with diphenylhydantoin and carbamazepine on serum gamma-glutamyltransferase, aspartate aminotransferase, alanine aminotransferase and alkaline phosphatase. *Eur. Arch. Psychiatry Neurol. Sci., 237*, 312.
8. Duncan JS, Shorvon SD, Trimble MR (1988) Withdrawal symptoms from phenytoin, carbamazepine and sodium valproate. *J. Neurol. Neurosurg. Psychiatry, 51*, 924.
9. Heh CWC, Sramek J, Herrera J, Costa J (1988) Exacerbation of psychosis after discontinuation of carbamazepine treatment. *Am. J. Psychiatry, 145*, 878.
10. Holmes GL, Flannery DB (1988) The effect of maternal seizures on fetal brain development. *Int. Pediatr., 3*, 86.
11. Mastroiacovo P, Bertollini R, Licata D et al (1988) Fetal growth in the offspring of epileptic women: results of an Italian multicentric cohort study. *Acta Neurol. Scand., 78*, 110.
12. Annegers JF, Baumgartner KB, Hauser WA, Kurland LT (1988) Epilepsy, anti-epileptic drugs, and the risk of spontaneous abortion. *Epilepsia, 29*, 451.
13. Bo G-P, Cocito L, Maffini M et al (1987) Ipertensione arteriosa da carbamazepina. *Riv. Neurol., 57*, 333.
14. Critchley EMR, Phillips M (1988) Unusual idiosyncratic reactions to carbamazepine. *J. Neurol. Neurosurg. Psychiatry, 51*, 1238.
15. Tomson T, Nilsson BY, Levi R (1988) Impaired visual contrast sensitivity in epileptic patients treated with carbamazepine. *Arch. Neurol., 45*, 897.
16. Evans DW, Ginsburg AP (1985) Contrast sensitivity predicts age-related differences in highway-sign discriminability. *Hum. Factors, 27*, 637.
17. Gilhus NE, Lea T (1988) Carbamazepine: effect on IgG subclasses in epileptic patients. *Epilepsia, 29*, 317.
18. Weaver DF, Camfield P, Fraser A (1988) Massive carbamazepine overdose: clinical and pharmacologic observations in five episodes. *Neurology, 38*, 755.
19. Browne TR, Szabo GK, Evans BA et al (1988) Carbamazepine increases phenytoin serum concentration and reduces phenytoin clearance. *Neurology, 38*, 1146.
20. Robertson MM, Trimble MR, Townsend HRA (1987) Phenomenology of depression in epilepsy. *Epilepsia, 28*, 364.
21. Brent DA, Crumrine PK, Varma RR et al (1987) Phenobarbital treatment and major depressive disorder in children with epilepsy. *Pediatrics, 80*, 909.
22. Barabas G, Matthews WS (1988) Barbiturate anticonvulsants as a cause of severe depression. *Pediatrics, 82*, 284.
23. York RC, Coleridge ST (1988) Cardiopulmonary arrest following intravenous phenytoin loading. *Am. J. Emerg. Med., 6*, 255.
24. Botez MI, Attig E, Vezina JL (1988) Cerebellar atrophy in epileptic patients. *Can. J. Neurol. Sci., 15*, 299.
25. Bauer L (1982) Interference of oral phenytoin absorption by continuous nasogastric feedings. *Neurology, 32*, 570.
26. Hooks MA, Longe RL, Taylor AT, Francisco GE (1986) Recovery of phenytoin from an enteral nutrient formula. *Am. J. Hosp. Pharm., 43*, 685.
27. Longe RL, Smith OB (1988) Phenytoin interaction with an oral feeding results in loss of seizure control. *J. Am. Geriatr. Soc., 36*, 542.
28. McGuire GM, Macphee GJA, Thompson GG et al (1988) Effects of sodium valproate on haem biosynthesis in man: implications for seizure management in the porphyric patient. *Eur. J. Clin. Invest., 18*, 29.
29. Nielsen OA, Johannessen AC, Bardrum B (1988) Oxcarbazepine-induced hyponatremia, a cross-sectional study. *Epilepsy Res., 2*, 269.

A.H. Ghodse and B. Ghodse

8 Opioid analgesics and narcotic antagonists

OPIATES *(SED-11, 141; SEDA-12, 61; SEDA-13, 56)*

White (1[R]) has reviewed the use of opioid drugs as intravenous anesthetic agents, pointing out that until the last decade they were not considered to be anesthetics. The more potent and rapidly-acting opiates have now become popular induction agents, particularly when hemodynamic stability is essential, because they do not induce histamine release. However, all opiate analgesics produce dose-dependent CNS and respiratory depression, and use of the potent, rapid-acting opiates for induction of anesthesia may be associated with truncal rigidity, bradycardia, respiratory depression, and postoperative complications (e.g. nausea and vomiting).

Nausea and vomiting are common and familiar side effects of opiate drugs and Kobrinsky's (2[c]) observation that the opiate antagonist naloxone produced a dose-related increase in these symptoms in children receiving cancer chemotherapy is, at first sight, surprising. In a review of this topic (3[R]), he points out that chemotherapy-induced nausea and vomiting are primarily regulated by chemoreceptor trigger zone (CTZ)–vomiting center (VC) pathways. Dopaminergic (D_2), histaminic (H_1) and muscarinic cholinergic (ACh) receptors are present in these sites, and specific receptor antagonists are potent but not 'universal' antiemetics when used alone or in combination. Recently, neurons containing the endogenous opiate enkephalin have been identified near the CTZ and the VC. Kobrinsky suggests that there is a net inhibitory opiate effect acting at the level of the VC during cancer chemotherapy and that naloxone blocks this inhibitory effect, thereby increasing nausea and vomiting. Treatment with low doses of opiates might enhance the inhibitory effect and, contrary to conventional expectations, thereby reduce chemotherapy-induced vomiting.

Side Effects of Drugs Annual 14
M.N.G. Dukes and L. Beeley, editors

Alfentanil *(SED-11, 145; SEDA-12, 61)*

Alfentanil is a short-acting opioid and there have been further reports of its use as an anesthetic agent for outpatient surgical procedures (4[Cr], 5[CR]). When compared with fentanyl, there seems little difference in the incidence of postoperative side effects such as nausea, vomiting, hiccup, hypotension and tachycardia. Although recovery time after alfentanil is slightly shorter than after fentanyl, Enright and Parker (5[CR]) did not find that patients who received alfentanil were 'street-worthy' (assessed by cardiovascular variables and the ability of the patient to walk a straight line) any earlier than those who received fentanyl.

Particular care appears to be needed when alfentanil is used for anesthesia in elderly patients. Lemmens et al (6[Cr]) report high incidences of *muscle rigidity*, *bradycardia* and *hypotension* during induction in 18 elderly patients. Hypotension was dependent on the dose and concentration of alfentanil. Nine patients required naloxone at the end of surgery and ventilatory depression recurred in 3 of these. Kent et al (7[cr]) carried out a pharmacokinetic analysis of alfentanil in 10 elderly patients undergoing anesthesia, and found (by comparing with other studies) that older patients eliminate alfentanil less rapidly than younger patients. Clinical results showed that a small dose of alfentanil in older patients could rapidly depress respiration and even cause *transient apnea*. Depression of systolic blood pressure and pulse rate also occurred. Kent et al conclude that the increased sensitivity of older patients to alfentanil may be partially related to the longer elimination half-life and decreased clearance.

Bradycardia is not however confined to the elderly: Rivard and Lebowitalz (8[c]) report the case of a 51-year-old woman who developed bradycardia and sinus arrest after receiving an intravenous bolus of alfentanil 1.5 mg followed by succinylcholine 100 mg i.v. Nathan (9[R]) has reviewed the cardiovascular effects of inducing anesthesia in patients with coronary artery disease using fentanyl, sufentanil and alfentanil. Whereas the first two drugs appear to provide hemodynamic stability, alfentanil can cause *hemodynamic instability* and *myocardial ischemia*, although it is not clear whether these adverse effects are due to interaction with other drugs, inappropriate dose or rate of administration, or arise because alfentanil actually differs pharmacodynamically from fentanyl and sufentanil.

Drug interaction may also have played a part in the *hypersensitivity reaction* that developed in a 13-year-old girl undergoing anesthesia.

Anesthesia was induced with atropine 0.1 mg, alfentanil 0.2 mg, and thiopental 200 mg after premedication with diazepam 8 mg. The trachea was intubated following vecuronium 4 mg and anesthesia was maintained with isoflurane in oxygen and nitrous oxide. A caudal epidural block was performed with 8 ml of bupivacaine 0.5% and 20 min later a further increment of alfentanil was given. Severe life-threatening bronchospasm developed within minutes and at the same time large urticarial wheals appeared on the perineum, arms, neck and lateral aspects of the chest and abdomen where they formed an almost confluent appearance. Immunological investigation showed the reaction to be non-specific and histaminoid in nature. Plasma IgE levels were 10 times normal at 400–500 U/ml with clinically significant levels of antibodies to both horse and dog dander, indicating an allergic tendency.

Circumstantial evidence in this case appeared to implicate alfentanil as the offending agent, but the reaction may have been modified by agents given subsequently (10[C]).

Alphaprodine *(SEDA-12, 62)*

Alphaprodine is a synthetic opiate used in pediatric dentistry to sedate uncooperative patients because it is rapidly absorbed from oral submucosal injection. It has had a chequered history and has been removed from the market on more than one occasion because of concern about its safety. In a comprehensive review, Currie et al (11[cR]) discuss its pharmacology and describe their experience using alphaprodine in different doses and in different sedation regimes. Some patients developed *hypoxia* (in the mild to moderate range) during the sedation procedures, as demonstrated by pulse oximetry. There was a concomitant *decrease in respiratory rate* during these periods. Postoperative side effects were said to be minimal and limited to transient *nausea and vomiting* as well as *drowsiness* and *lethargy*. Alphaprodine was withdrawn from the market during the course of their study, but the authors believe that longer-acting opiates will be used instead, with the same side effects occurring over a longer period.

Dihydrocodeine

In association with treatment for pharyngitis, a 47-year-old white man developed a systemic illness with fever, myalgia, episcleritis, hemoptysis, pleurisy, eosinophilia and renal impairment. Renal biopsy revealed *granulomatous interstitial nephritis*, which resolved without any specific treatment other than withdrawing all medication. The drugs that may have caused the reaction included dihydrocodeine, phenylpropanolamine, erythromycin and amoxycillin. Although the latter 3 drugs have been previously implicated in the development of interstitial nephritis, there have been no previous reports of granulomatous interstitial nephritis with any of these drugs. The authors comment that both the severe systemic manifestations and spontaneous recovery are unusual in association with drug-induced granulomatous nephritis and suggest that it may have been a combination of drugs that led to the hypersensitivity reaction (12[cr]).

An anaphylactoid reaction developed in a 20-year-old female after an overdose of an unspecified number of dihydrocodeine (DF-118) tablets. She was drowsy and had pinpoint pupils as well as moderate facial edema and a widespread urticarial rash with scratch marks. Within 15–20 min of intravenous naloxone 0.8 mg there was a reduction in vasomotor flushing and the patient reported a marked improvement in pruritus. Facial edema improved over the next few hours. Peripheral blood eosinophil and C-1 esterase inhibitor concentrations were normal. Salicylate and paracetamol were not detected in the blood.

It seems likely, as Panos et al (13[c]) suggest, that naloxone was effective in this situation because it blocked further mast cell degranulation caused by circulating opiates.

Fentanyl *(SED-11, 144; SEDA-12, 62; SEDA-13, 56)*

Muscle rigidity is a well-known side effect of fentanyl, but usually occurs during either the induction period or the immediate postoperative period. Mirenda et al (14[cr]) report a patient who experienced chest wall, truncal, and extremity rigidity more than 24 hours after the induction of anesthesia with a high-dose fentanyl technique. Naloxone 40 μg i.v. was injected with subsequent ablation of rigidity, appearance of spontaneous movement of all extremities, and initiation of spontaneous ventilation, all seen within 45 seconds of administration.

According to Stockham et al (15[Cr]), fentanyl 500 μg, used as pretreatment for anesthetic induction with etomidate, produced a high incidence of apnea (100%) during induction and nausea (67%) and vomiting (47%) postoperatively.

Heroin *(SED-11, 143; SEDA-12, 63)*

When the rates of onset of respiratory depression after heroin 2.5 mg i.v. and morphine 5 mg i.v. were compared, there was no difference in the time taken to achieve 70% of the maximal respiratory depression. For both drugs the rate of onset of depression of tidal volume was more rapid than that of depression of frequency of respiration (16[c]).

Methadone *(SED-11, 143; SEDA-12, 63; SEDA-13, 57)*

The sleep patterns of 13 babies born to opiate addicted mothers were studied (17[cr]). The mothers were all chronically addicted to heroin with a history of drug abuse of more than 1 year, but for most of them methadone (15–30 mg/d) had been substituted for heroin for the last 3 months of their pregnancy and this was the case for all of them during their hospitalization prior to delivery. Sleep samples were recorded and scored within a few days following birth and repeated 4 or 5 weeks later after recovery from the abstinence syndrome. A significant decrease in quiet sleep and increase in active sleep were found. The same alterations, although less marked, were observed in a follow-up recording performed during the second month of life. A clear-cut relation between the severity of the neonatal withdrawal syndrome and the maternal daily dose of opiate was rarely observed, perhaps because the mothers were consuming fairly small doses of methadone.

The authors point out that sleep alterations in addicted newborns could be related to CNS distress caused by withdrawal, but they believe that a derangement of endogenous opiates subsequent to fetal addiction is a more likely cause, because quite a few opiate receptors are located in nuclei which are active in sleep regulation.

Morphine *(SED-11, 142; SEDA-12, 63; SEDA-13, 57)*

Although morphine is a very old drug, it keeps its place in the pharmacopeia despite the advent of many new analogs, and side effects continue to be reported, often related to the method of administration. Patient-controlled analgesia (PCA) is popular and morphine is part of many such treatment regimes. Hodsman et al (18[c]) report two instances where patients using PCA postoperatively had undiagnosed *urinary retention* leading to the consumption of large amounts of morphine. They suggest that the sequence of events for these patients may have been that the central effect of morphine made the patients inattentive to the sensation of urgency from the detrusor muscle. Bladder distention led to discomfort which was not reduced by further doses of morphine, and a cycle was established of increasing bladder volume and distention, increasing discomfort and increased consumption of morphine. The authors point out that there is a risk of undiagnosed bladder distention leading to *respiratory depression* if patients have a large depot of opiate available to them. Thomas and Owen (19[c]) also urge the need for caution in their account of respiratory depression and *oversedation* that occurred during PCA because of a broken syringe barrel.

The administration of morphine by continuous intravenous infusion for postoperative analgesia can also be associated with respiratory depression. When 247 consecutive patients were treated in this way, the infusion had to be discontinued temporarily in 71, mostly because of low respiratory rates. These patients were older ($P < 0.01$), and their mean respiratory rate over the 24 hours was significantly less ($P < 0.001$) than those in whom the infusion was continuous (20[Cr]). When the same technique was used in children aged less than 7 years, the effect of morphine on respiration did not differ from that of adults and Olkkola et al (21[Cr]) found that the pharmacokinetics of morphine in children were similar to those of adults – except in the two youngest patients, aged 11 days and 2.4 months.

When 108 consecutive patients with pain due to advanced cancer requiring parenteral narcotics were treated with a continuous subcutaneous infusion of morphine (62 patients) or hydromorphone (46 patients), *systemic toxicity* consisted of respiratory depression in 2 patients, severe sedation in 6 and confusion in 3; all patients improved upon reduction of the daily dose of opiates. *Local toxicity* consisted of infection in 2 patients, bleeding in 1, and chemical irritation in 6 (22[C]).

Kalso and Vainio (23[c]) give a brief account of patients who *hallucinated* during use of various forms of morphine administration, namely treatment with oral solution, slow-release tablets, intravenous infusion, and intravenous patient-controlled titration. The youngest patient who had hallucinations was 20 years of age and 2 outpatients refused to continue oral morphine because of severe nightmares. When medication was changed to oxycodone, another μ-agonist, none of the patients had hallucinations or nightmares and pain relief was adequate. The authors suggest that the receptor specificity of these two opiates is different and that morphine might have agonistic activity at the putative σ-receptor mediating *hallucinations* and *dysphoria*.

A *purpuric rash* has been reported for the first time in association with morphine sulfate.

A 70-year-old man was prescribed slow release morphine sulfate 20 mg twice daily for stump pain after amputation, his other long-term medication being salbutamol and beclomethasone inhalers for chronic obstructive airways disease. Ten days after starting morphine he developed a purpuric rash on the extensor surface of this thighs, buttocks, and trunk. When investigations were negative, the rash was attributed to morphine, which was stopped, resulting in the disappearance of the rash (24[c]).

Papaverine *(SED-11, 145; SEDA-12, 64; SEDA-13, 57)*

Tamura et al (25[c]) have investigated the mechanism of papaverine-induced *priapism* in 7 cases of functional impotence. Six cases were side effects of papaverine tests and 1 case was self-induced by the use of 80 mg of papaverine without medical guidance. Maintenance inflow rates during erection were low as tested by dynamic cavernography. Blood gas studies in 2 cases showed that there was inadequate circulation in the corpus cavernosum during priapism. The authors suggest that administration of papaverine causes relaxation of the smooth muscles of the corpus cavernosum, thereby compressing venous outflow tracts and reducing venous outflow. In patients with good venous obstructive function, priapism may be due to outflow reduction being severe and prolonged, thus maintaining a high concentration of papaverine in the corpus cavernosum.

Pethidine (meperidine) *(SED-11, 143; SEDA-12, 65; SEDA-13, 57)*

Pethidine and nalbuphine were compared as analgesic components of intravenous conscious sedation in a double-blind, prospective trial of 47 patients undergoing elective oral surgery. Pethidine-treated patients experienced the only notable side effects – a *headache* that responded to additional analgesia, and a *hysterical reaction* that may have been due to diazepam that was part of the treatment regime (26[cr]).

Sufentanil *(SED-11, 145; SEDA-12, 66; SEDA-13, 58)*

Clinically significant *bradycardia* has again been reported when sufentanil (100 μg/kg/h of surgery) has been used in combination with vecuronium for anesthesia, and Dobson et al (27[c]) suggest that patients with a pre-induction bradycardia may not be suitable for this combination of agents.

Cheng et al (28[c]) used much lower doses (0.5–1.0 μg/kg) of sufentanil with or without intravenous lidocaine. They found that when the higher dose was used alone, it was associated with a persistent *apnea rate* and CO_2 *retention* postoperatively in healthy patients undergoing 1.5-hour operations. However, the lower dose of sufentanil in combination with lidocaine blunted the pressor response to laryngoscopy and tracheal intubation while producing minimal respiratory depression.

Henderson et al (29[cr]) administered sufentanil nasally to children for 'pre-induction' of anesthesia. In doses of 4.5 μg/kg, adverse effects such as *rigidity* and *postoperative vomiting* were more common than when doses of 1.5 or 3.0 μg/kg were used. Antagonism of its *respiratory depressant* effect was occasionally necessary. In one case, *tonic-clonic activity* of the left upper extremity which spread rapidly to all other extremities was observed and lasted for 90 seconds. The SPO_2 was 100% and the patient was normocarbic and normotensive at the beginning of this event. Electrolytes and a venous blood gas drawn immediately were also normal.

Tramadol *(SED-11, 145; SEDA-12, 66)*

In a prospective double-blind study to compare the analgesic effects of tramadol and pethidine in 100 patients undergoing laparoscopic sterilization, side effects in both groups were minimal. *Nausea and vomiting* occurred in only 13 patients of the 50 who received tramadol in a dose of 1 mg/kg body wt. (30[cr]).

EPIDURAL AND INTRATHECAL ADMINISTRATION OF OPIATES *(SED-11, 138; SEDA-12, 66; SEDA-13, 58)*

Intrathecal route *(SEDA 12, 66; SEDA-13, 58)*

Despite the introduction of long-acting oral morphine preparations, intrathecal morphine remains a valuable tool in the treatment of chronic, intractable pain due to malignant disease. Technical problems seem to be rare, but catheter occlusion and leakage of cerebrospinal fluid may occur (31[Cr], 32[cr]). Familiar side effects such as *urinary retention, itching, nausea and vomiting, drowsiness* and *constipation* continue to be reported and are usually said to occur more frequently at the onset of therapy and to disappear within a few days (31[Cr], 32[cr], 33[c]).

Madrid et al (31[Cr]) report the development of *respiratory depression* following the injection of 0.5 mg of intrathecal morphine in a patient with carcinoma of the lung and pleural effusion and this side effect was investigated by Fitzpatrick and Moriarty (34[Cr]) when they used intrathecal morphine in the management of pain following cardiac surgery. Postoperative peak expiratory flow rate (PEFR) was significantly better in patients given intrathecal morphine than in those receiving intravenous morphine ($P < 0.01$), but mean $PaCO_2$ was significantly higher in patients given intrathecal morphine 2 mg than in those given only 1 mg or in those given intravenous morphine. Respiratory rate did not differ significantly between the groups

Glavina and Shaw (35[c]) describe *myoclonic spasms* of the legs in a 59-year-old woman receiving intrathecal morphine for intractable pain in the leg caused by infiltration of secondary adenocarcinoma into the body of the L5 vertebra.

Following a 3 mg bolus of morphine, the patient developed episodic spasms, lasting 5–10 s at 30–40 s intervals involving all muscle groups in the upper legs with concurrent spasms of the lower abdominal muscles. There was no evidence of cerebral epileptic activity and intravenous diazepam failed to control the spasms which were eventually abolished by intrathecal bupivacaine.

The authors review reports of this phenomenon in animals and consider whether in their patient it was due to a toxic effect of the preservative *sodium metabisulfite* – a possibility they consider unlikely.

The use of intrathecal pentazocine (5 mg) has been described by Swaraj et al (36[C]); *urinary retention* occurred in 1 patient.

Intracerebroventricular administration of morphine is advocated by Lazorthes (37[CR]) for chronic neoplastic pain of cervicocephalic, thoracic or diffuse origin arising from widespread bone metastases. In a detailed account of his experience with this technique in 55 patients, he comments that minor morphine side effects (*nausea, vomiting, constipation, urinary retention, itching, dizziness, headache, disorientation, euphoria* or *drowsiness*) were initially observed but were always transient: some patients had multiple side effects. Three major central side effects were also observed: in 2 cases, after administration of respectively 1 and 1.5 mg of morphine, the patients progressively developed *drowsiness, miosis* and *respiratory depression.* The third case, after 1 mg, developed *visual hallucination* and behavioral disorders. These 3 central complications were immediately reversed by systemic naloxone administration with a small effect on the induced analgesia. Lazorthes concludes that although the site of administration is central, the side effects – notably central depression – are very moderate, mainly observed in the initial period and rapidly reversible. There is, however, always a potential risk and close surveillance is necessary.

Epidural route *(SEDA-12, 67; SEDA-13, 59)*

Although the intrathecal route is commonly used for the control of pain due to malignant disease, epidural opiates are often used to control acute pain, usually postoperatively. A variety of opiates have been used in this way, including morphine, diamorphine, fentanyl, sufentanil and buprenorphine, sometimes in combination with other drugs such as adrenaline or bupivacaine. The reported side effects are similar whichever drug is used and usually include *urinary retention, itching, nausea and vomiting* and varying degrees of *respiratory depression* (38[CR], 39[cr], 40[CR], 41[CR], 42[Cr], 43[c], 44[cr], 45[cr], 46[Cr]). However, as Dray (47[r]) points out, few clinical studies have critically examined the relationship between different doses of spinal opiates, the intensity of analgesia and the occurrence of side effects, and studies of this kind would be welcome. However, where comparisons between different drugs have been made using equianalgesic doses, clear differences have been observed in the incidence of urinary retention, suggesting that the mechanisms of opiate-induced analgesia and impaired urinary bladder activity are different. Several other factors may also be involved including differences in their pharmacokinetic properties and in their intrinsic pharmacological activity.

Although respiratory depression is a well-recognized risk of epidural opiates in adult patients, Krane (48[cr]) has described it in a $2^1/_2$-year-old child 3.5 hours after administration of 0.1 mg/kg preservative-free morphine in the caudal epidural space, in the absence of known risk factors. The child responded well to intravenous naloxone given by bolus injection followed by continuous intravenous infusion.

The mechanism of some side effects has been explored. Semenikhin (49[c]), for example, has investigated the origin of *skin itch* by studying blood levels of histamine and serotonin before and after epidural administration of narcotic analgesics (morphine, promedol, fentanyl) at a peak of skin itch development and upon its disappearance. A detailed analysis of 53 cases demonstrated a direct correlation between the development of skin itch and an abrupt increase in the blood level of histamine and it is suggested that an allergic-like reaction caused by a high level of histamine in the blood is one of the possible triggering mechanisms of pruritus. However, according to Woodham (50[cr]) non-histamine-releasing opiates also cause pruritus and antihistamines do not reduce opiate-induced itching.

A less common complication is that of *grand mal seizure*, reported by Borgeat et al (51[cr]) when, following an elective cesarean section under extradural anesthesia, a 30-year-old known epileptic woman (gravida 4, para 3) developed a tonic–clonic seizure, 6 hours after the administration of morphine 3 mg into the extradural space.

Dezeros et al (52[Cr]) evaluated the neonatal effects of a bupivacaine–fentanyl mixture (8 ml of bupivacaine 0.25% with 50 μg of fentanyl) in long-duration obstetric epidural analgesia in a series of 40 patients. The maternal side effects of fentanyl (essentially itching) were the same as those found in other studies, but acute fetal suffering was noted in 11 cases, of which 5 required resuscitation. At birth all other newborns had a maximal neurological and Apgar score at 5 min. Average plasma fentanyl concentrations were respectively 0.74 $\pm$ 0.13 ng/ml in mothers and 0.36 $\pm$ 0.04 ng/ml in newborns, the ratio being 0.49. There appeared to be no correlation between acute fetal suffering and newborn plasma fentanyl concentration.

When the epidural route is chosen for the chronic treatment of malignant pain, skin infections may develop at the site of insertion. In addition, long-term epidural infusion leads to fibrosis in the area of the tip of the catheter. This may explain why the amount of drug which penetrates from the epidural space into the cerebrospinal fluid slowly decreases in the course of epidural treatment, leading to a loss of efficacy (33[c]).

NARCOTIC ANTAGONISTS *(SED-11, 146; SEDA-12, 68; SEDA-13, 60)*

Nalmefene

Nalmefene is a new pure opiate antagonist. Its effect on morphine-induced respiratory depression was investigated in 6 healthy male volunteers and was compared with that of naloxone. Three subjects complained of *paraesthesiae* in the midthoracic region following the administration of nalmefene (0.4 mg/70 kg). One had a similar complaint following high dose (1.6 mg/70 kg) naloxone (53[Cr]).

AGONIST/ANTAGONIST OPIOIDS *(SED-11, 148; SEDA-12, 68; SEDA-13, 60)*

Buprenorphine *(SED-11, 149; SEDA-12, 68; SEDA-13, 60)*

Although buprenorphine is more potent than other opiates, its side effects, according to a review by Lober (54[R]), appear to be no greater. The morphine-like effects produced by buprenorphine include *decreased systolic blood pressure, heart rate and stroke volume*, and *constriction of pupils*. Hypotension reportedly occurs in 1–5% of patients and hypertension, tachycardia, or bradycardia in less than 1%. Minor adverse reaction of buprenorphine include *vomiting*, *nausea*, *headache*, *sweating* and *dizziness*, all occurring with varying frequency.

There are varying reports concerning the occurrence of *respiratory depression* after buprenorphine. Some studies have shown some degree of dose-dependent respiratory depression, reversal of which may be difficult because of buprenorphine's extremely strong receptor binding. Thus even very high doses (2.4–16 mg) of the antagonist naloxone may produce only a partial reversal of the depression. However, in clinical practice, respiratory depression has not always been a problem and Lehmann et al (55[CR]) found that a combination of buprenorphine and naloxone gave clinically adequate analgesia without notable impairment of spontaneous respiration. Buprenorphine itself has been found to be as effective as naloxone in antagonizing respiratory rate depression following fentanyl anesthesia (56[C]).

Pruritus developed in a 65-year-old woman who was treated with sublingual buprenorphine for ischemic pain in her left foot. She complained that the buprenorphine caused severe itching which started within 20 min of taking the drug and lasted generally about 4 or 5 hours. Itching was mainly over the back and shoulders and was not associated with a rash. Other opiates (morphine and meptazinol) used to treat the pain did not have this effect. The authors comment that the time course of the symptom fits well with the known duration of action of buprenorphine and tolerance to pruritus did not develop. This appears to be the first time that pruritus has been reported after sublingual buprenorphine (50[cr]).

Butorphanol *(SED-11, 149; SEDA-13, 60)*

Gonzalez et al (57[Cr]) carried out a double-blind study on 18 patients to compare the effects of morphine and butorphanol in patients who presented with pain because of sickle cell crisis. Patients were randomly assigned on each visit to receive either 2 mg i.m. butorphanol or 6 mg i.m. morphine every 30–60 min as needed. Six received only morphine, 6 received only butorphanol, and 6 received each treatment at some time during the study period, resulting in 45 randomizations to treatment. The incidence of adverse effects was 13% and 23% with morphine and butorphanol, respectively ($P = 0.46$). Two patients in the butorphanol group developed *nausea* and became *confused*, a development thought to be drug-related. The same patient became agitated again during butorphanol treatment several months later, but at that time the picture was complicated by family problems.

Nalbuphine *(SED-11, 150; SEDA-12, 69; SEDA-13, 61)*

When nalbuphine was administered orally in a dose of 30 or 60 mg for the treatment of pain after dental extractions, mild side effects – *nausea, drowsiness, light-headedness, itchy nose* – were experienced by a few patients (58[c]). *Nausea and vomiting* were also experienced by 11 patients out of 50 treated with intravenous nalbuphine for the relief of moderate to severe postoperative pain (59[C]). Using the same dose of nalbuphine (20 mg), Schaffer et al (60[CR]) reported a 'significant but tolerable' depression of respiration, with mean arterial PCO_2 raised to a maximum of 55.4 mmHg after 20 min.

Roth et al (61[cr]) investigated the *hemodynamic and respiratory effects* of intravenous nalbuphine in patients (age 65±11 years) with acute myocardial infarction and elevated pulmonary artery wedge pressure. Titration of the nalbuphine dose to lower pulmonary artery wedge pressure by ⩾25% was associated with a reduction in heart rate from 106 ± 20 to 96 ± 19 beats/min ($P < 0.05$) and decreases in mean blood pressure and mean pulmonary artery pressure, without any remarkable change in cardiac index, stroke volume index, stroke work index, or systemic and pulmonary vascular resistances. Nalbuphine also significantly reduced respiratory rate (32 ± 8 to 26 ± 8 resp./min, $P < 0.05$) and pH (7.45 ± 0.04 to 7.41 ± 0.03, $P < 0.05$) and increased arterial PCO_2 (32 ± 6 to 35 ± 6 mmHg, $P < 0.05$) without any major change in arterial PO_2. All these changes were comparable with morphine sulfate and no statistical difference was noted between the effects induced by both drugs. The necessary dose of nalbuphine ranged from 5–30 mg (mean ± standard deviation 17 ± 8 mg).

Because nalbuphine is being used for obstetric analgesia, the investigation by Dadabhoy et al (62[cr]) into its transplacental transfer is timely. They studied 8 patients undergoing cesarean section who received thiopental, succinylcholine and nalbuphine 0.2 ± 0.02 mg/kg i.v. for anesthetic induction/intubations. Nalbuphine serum levels at the time of delivery were found to be 64.1 ± 20.8 ng/ml in the parturient and 89.3 ± 19.3 ng/ml in the umbilical cord ($P < 0.05$). Hence, the umbilical cord/maternal vein ratio was 1.4:1 at delivery, which occurred between 2 and 10 min after nalbuphine injection. Apgar scores at 1 min were 6.6 ± 2.5 and at 5 min 8.5 ± 2.1 which were neither correlated with nalbuphine serum levels nor with the nalbuphine injection–delivery time intervals.

Butsch et al (63[c]) have shown that nalbuphine (20 mg i.v.) causes a statistically significant ($P < 0.01$) elevation in *intrabiliary pressure*. They investigated this in 10 patients undergoing surgery for symptomatic cholelithiasis and choledocholithiasis and found that 30 min after nalbuphine administration, the common duct pressure increased from 11.40 ± 2.74 to 16.75 ± 4.20 cm-H_2O. However, the increase in common duct pressure did not have any apparent deleterious effects, none of the patients experienced any discomfort, and there was no significant alteration in blood pressure, heart rate or respiratory rate.

The safety of nalbuphine for day-case surgery was assessed by Sury and Cole (64[C]) who used doses of nalbuphine of 0.05, 0.1 or 0.2 mg/kg in combination with midazolam 0.05 mg/kg in 18 healthy volunteers. The ventilatory response to carbon dioxide and end-tidal PCO_2 were measured before and after the drugs were administered. A mild degree of *respiratory depression* occurred, which was maximal at 3 and 30 min after intravenous injection. This was not related to dose except that nalbuphine 0.05 mg/kg resulted in the slowest respiratory rates. Dreams and hallucinations were not recalled except for one subject who had an unpleasant hypnopompic sensation several hours later at home. All but 4 volunteers felt tired on the evening following the drugs; nevertheless all agreed that their sedation was pleasant while they were supine. The authors emphasize that their findings should be applied to everyday clinical practice with caution because patients are frequently neither young nor healthy, as their subjects were.

Because nalbuphine has opiate antagonist properties, it has been used to ameliorate the side effects of epidural morphine and fentanyl administered for the relief of post-cesarean section pain. There were no adverse consequences associated with its use in this way and there was no loss of analgesia. The authors attribute the effect of intravenous nalbuphine to its κ-agonist and μ-antagonist properties (65[Cr], 66[cR]).

Picenadol

Picenadol is an *N*-methyl-4-phenylpiperidine derivative, described by Brunelle et al (67[cR]) as unique because it is a racemic mixture whose mixed agonist–antagonist properties are a consequence of the *d*-isomer being a potent opioid whereas the *l*-isomer is an opioid antagonist. In a double-blind study to evaluate the analgesic effect and safety of a single 25 mg oral dose of picenadol, they compared it with a 60 mg dose of codeine and a placebo in patients with postoperative pain. Few side effects were reported. *Drowsiness* was the most frequent, occurring in 10 patients (16%) of the 62 who received picenadol.

REFERENCES

1. White PF (1988) Clinical pharmacology of intravenous induction drugs. *Int. Anesthesiol. Clin., 26*, 98.
2. Kobrinsky NL, Pruden PB, Cheang MS et al (1988) Increased nausea and vomiting induced by naloxone in patients receiving cancer chemotherapy. *Am. J. Pediatr. Hematol./Oncol., 10*, 206.
3. Kobrinsky NL (1988) Regulation of nausea and vomiting in cancer chemotherapy. *Am. J. Pediatr. Hematol./Oncol., 10*, 209.
4. Kallar SK, Keenan RL (1987) Alfentanil and fentanyl for short surgical procedures: evaluation and comparison of recovery time. *Anesthesiol. Rev., 14*, 16.
5. Enright AB, Parker JBR (1988) Double blind comparison of alfentanil N_2O and fentanyl N_2O for outpatient surgical procedures. *Can. J. Anaesth., 35*, 462.
6. Lemmens HJM, Bovill, JG, Burm AGL, Hennis PJ (1988) Alfentanil infusion in the elderly: prolonged computer-assisted infusion of alfentanil in the elderly surgical patient. *Anaesthesia, 43*, 850.
7. Kent AP, Dodson ME, Bower S (1988) The pharmacokinetics and clinical effects of a low dose of alfentanil in elderly patients. *Acta Anaesthesiol. Belg., 39*, 25.
8. Rivard JC, Lebowitz PW (1988) Bradycardia after alfentanil-succinylcholine. *Anesth. Analg., 67*, 907.
9. Nathan HJ (1988) Narcotics and myocardial performance in patients with coronary artery disease. *Can. J. Anaesth. 35*, 209.
10. Coventry DM, Stone P (1988) Hypersensitivity reactions to alfentanil. *Anaesthesia, 43*, 887.
11. Currie WR, Biery KA, Campbell RL, Mourino AP (1988) Narcotic sedation: an evaluation of cardiopulmonary parameters and behaviour modification in pediatric dental patients. *J. Pedodont., 12*, 230.
12. Singer DRJ, Simpson JG, Catto GRD, Johnston AW (1988) Drug hypersensitivity causing granulomatous interstitial nephritis. *Am. J. Kidney Dis., 11*, 357.
13. Panos MZ, Burnett S, Gazzard BG (1988) Use of naloxone in opioid-induced anaphylactoid reaction. *Br. J. Anaesth., 61*, 371.
14. Mirenda J, Tabatabai M, Wong K (1988) Delayed and prolonged rigidity greater than 24h following high-dose fentanyl anesthesia. *Anesthesiology, 69*, 624.
15. Stockham RJ, Stanley TH, Pace NL et al (1988) Fentanyl pretreatment modifies anaesthetic induction with etomidate. *Anaesth. Intensive Care, 16*, 171.
16. Annan FJ, Ray D, Drummond GB (1989) Comparison of rate of onset of respiratory depression after i.v. morphine or diamorphine. *Br. J. Anaesth., 61*, 112.
17. Pinto F, Torrioli MG, Casella G et al (1988) Sleep in babies born to chronically heroin-addicted mothers. A follow up study. *Drug Alcohol Depend., 21*, 43.
18. Hodsman NBA, Kenny GNC, McArdle CS (1988) Patient-controlled analgesia and urinary retention. *Br. J. Surg., 75*, 212.
19. Thomas DW, Owen H (1988) Patient-controlled analgesia – the need for caution. *Anaesthesia, 43*, 770.
20. Ray DC, Drummond GB (1988) Continuous intravenous morphine for pain relief after abdominal surgery. *Ann. R. Coll. Surg. Engl., 70*, 317.
21. Olkkola KT, Maunuksela E-L, Korpela R, Rosenberg PH (1988) Kinetics and dynamics of postoperative intravenous morphine in children. *Clin. Pharmacol. Ther., 44*, 128.
22. Bruera E, Brenneis C, Michaud M et al (1988) Use of the subcutaneous route for the administration of narcotics in patients with cancer pain. *Cancer, 62*, 407.
23. Kalso E, Vainio A (1988) Hallucinations during morphine but not during oxycodone treatment. *Lancet, 2*, 912.
24. Whiston RJ, Griffith CDM, Hopkinson DR (1988) Purpuric rash associated with slow release morphine. *Br. Med. J., 296*, 8.
25. Tamura M, Kawanishi Y, Akiyama K et al (1988) Clinical studies on male sexual dysfunction. Report 7: Priapism caused by intracorporeal papaverine injections. *Nishinihon J. Urol., 50*, 1197.
26. Dolan EA, Murray WJ, Ruddy MP, Durham NC (1988) Double-blind comparison of nalbuphine and meperidine in combination with diazepam for intravenous conscious sedation in oral surgery outpatients. *Oral Surg. Oral Med. Oral Pathol., 66*, 536.
27. Dobson JAR, Davies JM, Hodgson GH (1988) Bradycardia after sufentanil and vecuronium. *Can. J. Anaesth., 35*, S121.
28. Cheng DCH, Chung F, Chapman KR (1988) Optimal sufentanil dosage – haemodynamic control or respiratory depression? *Can. J. Anaesth., 35*, 136.
29. Henderson JM, Brodsky DA, Fisher DM et al (1988) Pre-induction of anesthesia in pediatric patients with nasally administered sufentanil. *Anesthesiology, 68*, 671.
30. Chaturachinda K, Pausawasdi S, Tangtrakul S et al (1988) A comparative study of tramadol and pethidine in laparoscopic interval sterilization. *J. Med. Assoc. Thailand, 71, Suppl. 1*, 55.
31. Madrid JI, Fatela LV, Alcorta J et al (1988) Intermittent intrathecal morphine by means of an implantable reservoir. *J. Pain Symptom Manage., 3*, 67.
32. Dautheribes M, Guerin J (1988) Spinal intrathecal analgesia. A series of 50 cases. *Neurochirurgie, 33*, 194.

33. Muller H, Luben V, Zierski J, Hempelman G (1988) Long term spinal opiate treatment. *Acta Anaesthesiol. Belg., 39, Suppl. 2*, 83.
34. Fitzpatrick GJ, Moriarty DC (1988) Intrathecal morphine in the management of pain following cardiac surgery. *Br. J. Anaesth., 60*, 639.
35. Glavina MJ, Robertshaw R (1988) Myoclonic spasms following intrathecal morphine. *Anaesthesia, 43*, 389.
36. Swaraj, Saxena R, Sabzposh SWA, Shakoor A (1988) Effect of intrathecal pentazocine on postoperative pain relief. *J. Indian Med. Assoc., 86*, 93.
37. Lazorthes Y (1988) Intracerebroventricular administration of morphine for control of irreducible cancer pain. *Ann. N.Y Acad. Sci., 531*, 123.
38. Lee A, Simpson D, Whitfield A, Scott DB (1988) Postoperative analgesia by continuous extradural infusion of bupivacaine and diamorphine. *Br. J. Anaesth., 60*, 845.
39. Verborgh C, Van der Auwera D, Noorduin H, Camu F (1988) Epidural sufentanil for post-operative pain relief: effect of adrenaline. *Eur. J. Anaesthesiol., 5*, 183.
40. Simpson KH, Madej TH, McDowell JM et al (1988) Comparison of extradural buprenorphine and extradural morphine after caesarean section. *Br. J. Anaesth., 60*, 627.
41. Glynn C, Dawson D, Sanders R (1988) A double-blind comparison between epidural morphine and epidural clonidine in patients with chronic noncancer pain. *Pain, 34*, 123.
42. Whiting WC, Sandler AN, Lau LC et al (1988) Analgesic and respiratory effects of epidural sufentanil in patients following thoracotomy. *Anesthesiology, 69*, 36.
43. Noda J, Umeda S, Seki H, Hashida T (1988) Continuous epidural morphine for postoperative pain relief following gynecological surgery. *Hiroshima J. Anaesth., 24*, 21.
44. Blanco J, Blanco E, Carceller JM et al (1987) Epidural analgesia for post-caesarean pain relief: a comparison between morphine and fentanyl. *Eur. J. Anaesthesiol., 4*, 395.
45. Huang F-Y, Tseng S-C, Fan S-Z et al (1988) Epidural morphine for cancer pain control management of pain with implantable portal system. *J. Surg. Assoc. ROC, 21*, 407.
46. Gough JD, Williams AB, Vaughan RS et al (1988) The control of post-thoracotomy pain. A comparative evaluation of thoracic epidural fentanyl infusions and cryo-analgesia. *Anaesthesia 43*, 780.
47. Dray A (1988) Urinary retention following spinal opiates. *Anesthesiology, 69*, 442.
48. Krane EJ (1988) Delayed respiratory depression in a child after caudal epidural morphine. *Anesth. Analg. 67*, 79.
49. Semenikhin AA (1988) On the origin of skin itch upon epidural administration of narcotic analgesics. *Anesteziol. Reanimatol., 3*, 62.
50. Woodham M (1988) Pruritus with sublingual buprenorphine. *Anaesthesia, 43*, 806.
51. Borgeat A, Biollaz J, Depierraz B, Neff R (1988) Grand mal seizure after extradural morphine analgesia. *Br. J. Anaesth., 60*, 733.
52. Dezeros G, Levron JC, Simon A et al (1988) Long duration peridural analgesia in labour by an association of bupivacaine and fentanyl. *Agressologie, 29*, 33.
53. Konieczko KM, Jones JG, Barrowcliffe MP et al (1988) Antagonism of morphine-induced respiratory depression with nalmefene. *Br. J. Anaesth., 61*, 318.
54. Lober C (1988) Buprenorphine. *Conn. Med., 52*, 285.
55. Lehmann KA, Reichling U, Wirtz R (1988) Influence of naloxone on the postoperative analgesic and respiratory effects of buprenorphine. *Eur. J. Clin. Pharmacol., 34*, 343.
56. Boysen K, Herten S, Chraemer-Jorgensen B et al (1988) Buprenorphine antagonism of ventilatory depression following fentanyl anaesthesia. *Acta Anaesthesiol. Scand., 32*, 490.
57. Gonzalez ER, Ornato JP, Ware D et al (1988) Comparison of intramuscular analgesic activity of butorphanol and morphine in patients with sickle cell disease. *Ann. Emerg. Med., 17*, 788.
58. Kay B, Lindsay RG, Mason CJ, Healy TEJ (1988) Oral nalbuphine for the treatment of pain after dental extractions. *Br. J. Anaesth., 61*, 313.
59. Barsoum MW (1988) The safety and efficacy of nalbuphine hydrochloride in postoperative pain. *Emirates Med. J., 6*, 29.
60. Schaffer J, Piepenbrock S, Niekrens E, Panning B (1988) Nalbuphine in comparison with piritramide and placebo for postoperative pain therapy after halothane anesthesia. *Anaesthesist, 37*, 238.
61. Roth AR, Karen G, Gluck A et al (1988) Comparison of nalbuphine hydrochloride versus morphine sulfate for acute myocardial infarction with elevated pulmonary artery wedge pressure. *Am. J. Cardiol., 62*, 551.
62. Dadabhoy ZP, Tapia DP, Zsigmond EK (1988) Transplacental transfer of nalbuphine in patients undergoing cesarean section. *Acta Anaesthesiol. Ital., 39*, 227.
63. Butsch JL, Okoli JA (1988) The effect of nalbuphine on the common bile duct pressure. *Am. Surg., 54*, 253.
64. Sury MRJ, Cole PV (1988) Nalbuphine combined with midazolam for outpatient sedation. *Anaesthesia, 43*, 281.
65. Chalmers PC, Lang CM, Harte FA, Greenhouse BB (1988) Double-blind comparison of intravenous nalbuphine and placebo in the amelioration of side-effects of epidural narcotics. *Pain Clin., 2*, 49.
66. Chalmers PC, Lang CM, Greenhouse BB

(1988) The use of nalbuphine in association with epidural narcotics. *Anesthesiol. Rev., 15*, 21.
67. Brunelle RL, George RE, Sunshine A, Hammonds WD (1988) Analgesic effect of picenadol, codeine, and placebo in patients with postoperative pain. *Clin. Pharmacol. Ther., 43*, 663.

Giancarlo Agnelli

9 Antipyretic analgesics

ACETYLSALICYLIC ACID AND RELATED COMPOUNDS *(SED-11, 158; SEDA-12, 74; SEDA-13, 63)*

Reye's syndrome *(SED-11, 160; SEDA-13, 64)* New information about the association between aspirin usage and Reye's syndrome has been provided by Hall et al (1^C), who reported the findings of a 2-year study based on the 264 cases notified to the British Reye's Syndrome Surveillance Scheme (BRSSS), established in August 1981 in the British Isles. Between April 1984 and August 1985, the parents of 106 children who had had Reye's syndrome were interviewed and then between April 1985 and April 1986, the parents of 185 children who had had febrile illness were also interviewed in order to compare pre-admission medication rates in the 2 groups. Although the overall proportion of cases and controls who had received antipyretics was similar (72% vs 68%), a significant excess of cases (59%) had received aspirin when compared with controls (26%). A significantly higher proportion of control children had received paracetamol (49%) when compared with cases (25%). There was also an excess exposure to aspirin in children under 5 years of age. A significant correlation was also shown between aspirin exposure and the closeness with which cases conformed to the diagnostic criteria of Reye's syndrome. The finding that almost four-fifths of Reye's syndrome cases given aspirin had also been similarly exposed in the past, suggests a complex (multifactorial) etiology of Reye's syndrome. This multifactorial etiology of Reye's syndrome is also suggested by a case-report (2^c) of Reye's syndrome developing in only 1 of 2 11-year-old identical twins who had had the same respiratory illness and who were both given the same preparation of aspirin at the same dosage.

Interactions between viral illness and environmental agents (pesticides, solvents, drugs) have been advanced as possible etiological factors in the development of Reye's syndrome, which is considered a metabolic disorder characterized by mitochondrial injury. Aspirin has been shown to inhibit selectively the mitochondrial oxidation of medium-chain (octanoic acid) and long-chain (palmitic acid) fatty acids in the rat liver mitochondrial-peroxisomal fraction (3^R). This can cause perturbation of the membrane properties of mitochondria due to an excess of free fatty acids. The effect of influenza B virus on a cell gene of human hepatocytes (Hep G2) was observed both in the presence and absence of aspirin (4^R). Aspirin affected neither the kinetics of influenza B virus growth nor the inhibition of protein synthesis of Hep G2 by influenza B virus. The virus was in fact capable of reducing the synthesis of albumin, transferrin and apoprotein B by 40–60% at 12 hours.

Gastrointestinal Three studies provided further evidence of the association of aspirin intake and *upper gastrointestinal bleeding*. A Spanish prospective study of 372 cases of upper gastrointestinal bleeding revealed that 58.1% of cases were associated with previous ASA and/or salicylate intake (5^C). Early upper endoscopy was performed in all patients. A case-control study (6^C) carried out on 230 hospital patients with bleeding gastric ulcer aged 60 or over, and on community controls matched for age and sex, revealed that those who had taken aspirin had a relative risk of 2.2 and 2.9 respectively of admission to hospital for bleeding ulcers as compared with hospital controls and community controls. When aspirin and other NSAIDs were considered together, the overall risk suggested that these medications could account for over a third of the admissions for bleeding peptic ulcers in the elderly. In a re-

Side Effects of Drugs Annual 14
M.N.G. Dukes and L. Beeley, editors

trospective study (7[C]), 1203 gastroscopic investigations performed from 1980–1986 in Austria were analyzed: 47 of these patients had been treated with aspirin for at least 4 weeks, and 39 of them (82.9%) had pathological changes in the gastric and duodenal mucosa. The remaining 1156 patients received no therapy and only 426 of them (36.8%) showed changes in the gastric and duodenal mucosa.

The mechanism of development of *gastric ulceration* due to aspirin is still poorly understood in spite of the more recent acquisition of knowledge stimulated by the concept of gastric 'cytoprotection', i.e. the reduction in susceptibility of the gastric mucosa to noxious stimuli due to a variety of substances. Because of its liposolubility, non-ionized aspirin (pH < 3.5) enters mucosal cells, impairs oxidative phosphorylation in mitochondria, increases membrane permeability and causes necrosis. However, it is the extent of the direct and indirect vascular damage of the superficial capillaries which determines the development of minimal occult bleeding, erosion or deep ulcers. Protective agents such as prostaglandins and sulfhydryl compounds could exert their protective effect by limiting the vascular damage (8[r]).

Although aspirin is a potent inhibitor of the synthesis of protective PGE_2, there is no correlation between the decrease in PGE_2 mucosal content and mucosal damage. There is also a growing body of evidence supporting the involvement of oxygen-derived free radicals (9[r]) in the pathogenesis of gastric ulcerative lesions. While ischemic re-perfusion injury to the gastric vasculature depends on oxygen-free radicals, the epithelial injury is independent of them. Gastric lesions induced by aspirin (200 mg/kg p.o.) were reduced by vitamins A and E which are potent antioxidants (9[r]).

In a study of 14 healthy volunteers (10[C]) who underwent weekly endoscopic assessment, biopsies and gastric wash collections, continuous aspirin administration was found to result in a degree of adaptation in the gastric mucosa. Gastric microbleeding continued to be high during aspirin administration, but there was an improvement in the appearance of the mucosa and a significant increase in DNA acid recovery, taken as an index of cellular exfoliation and regeneration, which almost doubled just before resolution. In the absence of other biochemical and histological changes, these data suggest that gastric adaptation involves increased cellular regulation.

The value of 'cytoprotective' compounds, such as misoprostol, sucralfate and colloidal bismuth subcitrate, in reducing the effects of aspirin on the gastric mucosa is still a matter of debate. A double-blind placebo-controlled study (11[C]) assessed the effectiveness of misoprostol, a synthetic analog of prostaglandin E_1, in preventing gastrointestinal blood loss induced by aspirin in patients with degenerative joint disease.

Forty-five patients were studied. They received 3.9 g of aspirin daily for at least 2 weeks prior to and during the study. Fecal blood loss was evaluated from day 4–7 using ^{51}Cr-labelled red blood cells. Patients with a fecal blood loss of at least 1.5 ml/d were randomly allocated to receive either placebo or misoprostol 200 μg q.i.d. for 7 days. Misoprostol reduced fecal blood loss by 50% compared with baseline values in 11 of the 19 patients who received the drug. There was thus a significant difference in blood loss when compared with placebo. One male patient withdrew from the study because of cramps and abdominal discomfort due to misoprostol.

A double-blind trial examined the effect of misoprostol on the endoscopic appearance of gastroduodenum at the end of 1 week of aspirin ingestion (12[C]).

130 healthy subjects were randomized to take 50, 100 or 200 μg of misoprostol, or placebo along with 975 mg of aspirin 4 times daily. Fewer subjects developed acute endoscopic gastric ulcers in the group taking any dose of misoprostol compared with the placebo group (1% *vs* 43%). No subject taking the 100- or 200-μg dose of misoprostol developed an acute endoscopic duodenal ulcer as compared with 13% of subjects taking placebo ($P < 0.05$). Significantly fewer subjects developed gastric erosions and significantly fewer subjects developed duodenal erosions in each of the 3 groups taking misoprostol compared with the placebo group ($P < 0.01$). There were fewer subjects with a gastric erosion ($P < 0.05$) and fewer subjects with a duodenal erosion ($P < 0.05$) in the group taking the 200-μg dose compared with the group taking the 50-μg dose of misoprostol. The authors conclude that misoprostol can protect the normal gastroduodenum from acute ulceration and reduce the chance of erosion after 1 week of aspirin ingestion.

In another study patients with confirmed rheumatoid arthritis and endoscopically-documented gastroduodenal lesions were randomly assigned to receive 200 μg of misoprostol 4 times daily (123 patients) or placebo (116 patients) (13[C]). Each concurrently received 650–1300 mg of aspirin 4 times a day. After 8 weeks of treatment, misoprostol was statistically superior to placebo in healing gastric mucosal injury (70% *vs* 25%) and duodenal mucosal injury (86% *vs* 53%). Patients with gastric or duodenal ulcers on admission had superior ulcer healing rates with misoprostol (67% *vs* 26%).

Sucralfate, a basic aluminium salt of sulfated disaccharide, has been claimed to exert a cytoprotective action due to stimulation of local prostaglandin production. A placebo-controlled study evaluated the ability of sucralfate, 1 g daily, to reduce aspirin-induced gastric damage in 8 healthy volunteers (14[C]).

Aspirin, 1200 mg, produced endoscopic changes that were significantly inhibited by sucralfate. This protective effect was abolished by indometacin (50 mg) taken 8 h before sucralfate. The authors suggest that the protective action of sucralfate could be due to the stimulation of endogenous prostaglandins, the prevention of mucosal prostaglandin degradation or a prostaglandin-independent mechanism.

The effect of indometacin in the above study seems to suggest a prostaglandin-dependent effect. Indeed, a prostaglandin-independent mechanism has been shown in the protective effect of sucralfate in animal experiments after parenteral aspirin. This prostaglandin-independent effect could be an increase in viscosity of the gastric mucus, stimulation of bicarbonate secretion or blockage of the access to the aspirin binding site on the cyclo-oxygenase molecule. The timing of sucralfate administration seems critical. In fact, in this study it was given 30 min before aspirin, but in other experiments (14[C]), when given simultaneously with aspirin, it failed to show a protective effect.

A second study from the same group evaluated gastric mucosal protection by sucralfate in patients taking a higher dose of aspirin (15[C]):

The ability of sucralfate to prevent gastric mucosal erosions caused by long-term aspirin ingestion was studied in 19 normal human subjects. A placebo-controlled, double-blind, cross-over design was used to study the capacity of 4 g sucralfate daily to lessen the noxious effect on gastric mucosa of 3.6 g aspirin daily for 14 days. Gastric mucosal injury was assessed by endoscopic scoring of erosions. There was no significant difference in mean erosion scores or the degree of partial mucosal protection between the 2 groups. It was concluded that sucralfate lacks a mucosal protection capacity at the dosage studied in human subjects ingesting large doses of aspirin over a 2-week period.

A double-blind, placebo-controlled cross-over trial assessed the effect of colloidal bismuth subcitrate on prostaglandin E_2 generation and gastric mucosal integrity in 10 healthy male volunteers treated with aspirin (16[C]).

Aspirin, 2.5 g, plus placebo produced an 85% reduction of PGE_2 mucosal generation, significant gastric microbleeding, DNA loss, and endoscopic and histological damage of the mucosa. The combination of aspirin and colloidal bismuth subcitrate did not increase PGE_2 mucosal generation, but it reduced both gastric microbleeding and mucosal damage.

Colloidal bismuth subcitrate seems to slow penetration of acid and pepsin by interacting with the adhering mucous gel layer, thus providing a better protection of the underlying epithelial cells. Colloidal bismuth subcitrate was also reported to suppress the production of leukotrienes, in particular leukotriene C4, which participates in vascular injury. There is also increasing evidence that the administration of low concentrations of mild irritants, such as 20% ethanol, 5% NaCl, acetazolamide, bile and hypertonic solutions protect gastric mucosa against noxious agents. This protection was abolished by indometacin, thus indicating a role of endogenous prostaglandins in an 'adaptive cytoprotection'.

A prospective randomized double-blind cross-over trial evaluated the protective effect of low-dose ethanol in aspirin-induced gastric injury (17[C]) in 10 healthy non-drinking volunteers.

Aspirin, 975 mg, was given p.o. 30 min after vodka, 37.5 ml, in tomato juice or in tomato juice alone and endoscopy was performed 1 h later. A significant reduction in antral damage was seen after vodka pretreatment; the trend was similar in the fundus but did not achieve statistical significance. The authors suggest a stimulating effect of a low dose of ethanol on prostaglandin production or on mucosal blood flow, as well as on bicarbonate and mucus secretion.

Five cases of chronic recurrent gastroduodenal ulcers due to the surreptitious use of aspirin were reported (18[C]). All subjects had therapeutic blood levels of salicylates, and all denied use of aspirin. A low serum level of uric acid could also indicate salicylate abuse.

Special senses It is well known that aspirin can induce a temporary *loss of hearing* and a temporary ringing in the ears (*tinnitus*). It has also been speculated that aspirin can produce permanent hearing loss and/or tinnitus. However, the data supporting this effect are weak (19[r]) and there are reports of animal studies that suggest permanent cochlear damage due to aspirin. McFadden and Plattsmier (20[R]) claimed that aspirin enhances the temporary hearing loss produced by moderately intense sound in humans. They observed that subjects treated with both aspirin and sound experienced a greater temporary hearing loss than those exposed to aspirin or to sound alone. More recent data by Long and Tubis (20[R]) suggest that human aspirin intake diminishes the strength of active cochlear mechanisms.

These workers studied 4 subjects before, during and after consumption of 3.9 g of aspirin per day (3 325 mg tablets every 6 h) for 3–4 days. They found evidence that, initially, aspirin modifies the cochlea so that a spontaneous emission is reduced to an evoked emission; changes in the threshold microstructure follow changes in the evoked emissions. They observed a significant reduction of spontaneous otoacoustic emissions within 8 h and then a reduction to the noise floor within 24 h. Evoked otoacoustic emissions and threshold microstructure were also reduced by aspirin but persisted longer and recovered sooner.

The data of Long and Tubis are in keeping with previous reports by Johnsen and Elbenluig in 1982 (19[r]) who reported a reduction in delayed evoked otoacoustic emission by aspirin, and with the data by McFadden and Plattsmier who reported a reversible reduction and subsequent elimination of spontaneous emissions. However, Johnsen and Elbenluig's subjects had taken 10 g of aspirin in 24 hours, while in the study by McFadden and Plattsmier the subjects had taken 3.3 g of aspirin for 3.75 days, making a comparison between the two quite difficult.

The specific mechanism by which aspirin interferes with otoacoustic emissions is not clear. Effects on the synthesis of prostaglandins, reduction of serum calcium levels, interference with membrane ion transport and with energy-demanding functions of hair cells have been hypothesized (20[R]). Aspirin can also reversibly alter the laminated cisternal system responsible for outer-hair-cell motility and for the active and non-linear aspects of cochlear response (20[R]). While stable levels of aspirin in the blood are achieved in 1 week (20[R]), it is not known how much time is necessary to achieve stable levels in the perilymph. Therefore, measurement of the salicylate levels in blood serum will not provide an interpretation of the different effects of aspirin on otoacoustic emissions in different subjects.

Skin A significant positive correlation between the use of aspirin and *vesicular palmar eczema* has been reported in a prospective study of 425 consecutive patch-tested patients, in 153 cases of which (38%) vesicular palmar eczema was found (21[R]).

Liver The potential *hepatoxicity* of aspirin has come to light over the past quarter of a century (22[r]). The hepatotoxic effect of aspirin is due to intrinsic hepatocellular damage which is dose-dependent, related to blood concentration and occurring after a latent period of at least 1 week. Salicylate-related hepatic damage is usually anicteric, mild and reversible after withdrawal of therapy. It is hypothesized that salicylate-related liver toxicity may result from an accumulation of toxic metabolites, since even large single overdoses of aspirin rarely produce significant hepatic injury (22[r]). Monitoring of serum aminotransferase levels at regular intervals during high-dose salicylate therapy probably would preclude the development of permanent hepatic injury (22[r]).

The potential hepatic toxicity of aspirin, ibuprofen and oxaprozin was evaluated in 1468 patients on long-term treatment for rheumatoid arthritis and osteoarthritis (22[C]).

Aspirin dosages ranged from 2600–3900 mg/d ($n=439$), ibuprofen dosages from 1200–2400 mg/d ($n=182$), and oxaprozin from 600–1800 mg/d ($n=847$). The patients were studied for up to 1 year while receiving the test medication. Ibuprofen proved to be the safest; it was not associated with any AST elevation which could be considered drug-related.

Aspirin was associated with significantly more frequent AST elevations than oxaprozin (16% vs. 9%, $P < 0.05$) which were considered to be possibly or probably drug-related.

ANILINE DERIVATIVES *(SED-11, 165; SEDA-12, 67; SEDA-13, 76)*

Paracetamol (acetaminophen) *(SED-11, 165; SEDA-12, 74; SEDA-13, 67)*

Skin A case of *fixed drug eruption* due to paracetamol was reported in Great Britain in a 74-year old-man (23^C). He had taken a single 500 mg tablet of paracetamol and after 12 h several tender areas on the skin of his face developed and faded over a few days. The eruption recurred 2 months later after the intake of another single tablet of paracetamol and faded spontaneously with the discontinuation of the drug. A similar case was observed in an Italian hospital (24^C).

A case of *vascular purpura* due to paracetamol was reported in France (25^C) in a 67-year-old man. He developed a vascular purpura, without other systemic signs or symptoms, during hospitalization for atypical precordialgias. The purpura recurred 2 and 4 months after the first episode concomitantly with the intake of paracetamol which the patient declared to have taken repeatedly during the first episode also. The association between the vascular purpura and paracetamol is based on the absence of other therapeutic changes in this patient and on the disappearance of the purpura following discontinuance of this drug followed by positive rechallenge. It must be stressed that this manifestation developed in a patient with a predisposing immunoallergic background (previous quinidine-induced thrombocytopenia).

REFERENCES

1. Hall SM, Plaster PA, Glasgow JFT, Hancock P (1988) Preadmission antipyretics in Reye's syndrome. *Arch. Dis. Child., 63*, 857.
2. Andreoli A, Bonora G, Luciani L, Perdetti L (1988) Reye's syndrome and aspirin. *Lancet, 2*, 684.
3. Yoshida Y, Fujii M, Brown III FR, Singh I (1988) Effect of salicyclic acid on mitochondrial-peroxisomal fatty acid catabolism. *Pediatr. Res., 23*, 338.
4. Barnard JA, Snyder PN, Werner MJ et al (1988) Protein synthesis by Hep G2 cells infected with influenza B virus. *Pediatr. Res., 23*, 334.
5. Blasco JV, Mouferrer Guardiola R, Simon Marco E (1988) Hemorragia digestiva alta yatrogénica: estudio prospectivo de 372 cases. *An. Med. Intern. (Madrid), 5*, 190.
6. Faulkner G, Prichard P, Somerville K, Longman MJS (1988) Aspirin and bleeding peptic ulcers in the elderly. *Br. Med. J., 297*, 1311.
7. Prochazka E, Pötzi R, Ehringer H, Gangl A (1988) Veränderungen der Magen- und Duodenal-Schleimhaut unter Azetylsalizylsäuretherapie. *Acta Med. Austriaca, 15*, 80.
8. Szabo S (1988) Pathogenesis of gastric mucosal injury. *South Afr. Med. J., 2*, 35.
9. Morgan Smith S, Kvietys PR (1988) Gastric ulcers: role of oxygen radicals. *Crit. Care Med., 16*, 892.
10. Graham DY, Lacey Smith J, Spjut HJ, Torres E (1988) Gastric adaptation: studies in humans during continuous aspirin administration. *Gastroenterology, 95*, 327.
11. Ryan JR, Vargas R, Clay GA, McMahon G (1988) Role of misoprostol in reducing aspirin-induced gastrointestinal blood loss in arthritic patients. *Am. J. Med., 83*, 41.
12. Jiranek GC, Kimmey MB, Saunders DR et al (1989) Misoprostol reduces gastroduodenal injury from one week of aspirin: an endoscopic study. *Gastroenterology, 96*, 656.
13. Roth S, Agrawal N, Mahowald M et al (1989) Misoprostol heals gastroduodenal injury in patients with rheumatoid arthritis receiving aspirin. *Arch. Intern. Med., 149*, 775.
14. Stern AI, Ward F, Hartley G (1987) Protective effect of sucralfate against aspirin-induced damage to the human gastric mucosa. *Am. J. Med., 83*, 83.
15. Stern AI, Ward F, Sievert W (1989) Lack of gastric mucosal protection by sucralfate during long-term aspirin ingestion in humans. *Am. J. Med., 86*, 66.
16. Konturek SJ, Kwiccien N, Obtulouricz W et al (1988) Effects of colloidal bismuth subcitrate on aspirin-induced gastric micro-bleeding, DNA loss and prostaglandin formation in humans. *Scand. J. Gastroenterol., 23*, 861.
17. Cohen MM, Yeung R, Kilcam S, Wang HR (1988) Aspirin-induced human antral injury is reduced by vodka pretreatment. *Dig. Dis. Sci., 33*, 513.

18. Perrault J, Fleming R, Dozois RR (1988) Surreptitious use of salicylates: a cause of chronic recurrent gastroduodenal ulcers. *Mayo Clin. Proc.*, *63*, 337.
19. Brummett RE (1988) Insults to hearing (Interactions). *Pharmindex*, 11.
20. Long GR, Tubis A (1988) Modification of spontaneous and evoked otoacoustic emissions and associated psychoacoustic microstructure by aspirin consumption. *J. Acoust. Soc. Am.*, *84*, 1343.
21. Edman B (1988) Palmar eczema: a pathogenetic role for acetylsalicyclic acid, contraceptives and smoking. *Acta Derm.-Venereol. (Stockholm)*, *68*, 402.
22. Freeland GR, Northington RS, Hedrich DA, Walker BR (1988) Hepatic safety of two analgesics used over the counter: ibuprofen and aspirin. *Clin. Pharmacol. Ther.*, *43*, 473.
23. Meyrick Thomas RH, Murro DD (1986) Fixed drug eruption due to paracetamol. *Br. J. Dermatol.*, *115*, 357.
24. Valsecchi R (1989) Fixed drug eruption to paracetamol. *Dermatologica*, *179*, 51.
25. Dussarat GV, Dalger J, Mafart B, Chagnon A (1988) Purpura vasculaire au paracétémole: une observation. *Presse Méd.*, *17*, 1587.

A. Del Favero

10 Anti-inflammatory analgesics and drugs used in rheumatoid arthritis and gout

NON-STEROIDAL ANTI-INFLAMMATORY DRUGS (NSAID)
(SED-11, 170; SEDA-11, 82; SEDA-12, 79; SEDA-13, 71)

The clinical spectrum of NSAID-induced upper gastrointestinal tract damage

Gastric and duodenal damage by NSAID *Mucosal damage to the upper gastrointestinal (GI) tract is a side effect common to all the NSAID. Despite their obvious benefits, the damage they cause in the GI tract represents a major health problem in current clinical practice. Although a vast amount of information has accumulated on this topic over many years, only the data published in the very recent past provide convincing evidence that NSAID cause severe GI complications and allow the risk to be roughly quantified.*

The renewed attention that this topic is attracting is testified to by the number of reviews and editorials published as well as by the debate on the health impact of upper GI damage caused by NSAID that has engaged various drug regulating agencies (1[R]–13[R]).

Upper GI toxicity occurring after administration of NSAID can present a wide spectrum of clinical expressions ranging from relatively mild, but nonetheless discomforting, conditions such as epigastric pain and dyspepsia, to the more serious and potentially life-threatening states, namely GI ulceration and GI bleeding or perforation.

Endoscopic evaluation of the upper GI tract in patients treated with NSAID reveals a number of lesions that range from simple erythema through diffuse erosions and/or microbleeding to ulceration. The term 'NSAID gastropathy' has recently been proposed by Roth and Bennett to describe those lesions associated with the upper GI tract toxicity that is encountered during NSAID therapy (9[R]).

Damage to the upper GI tract is not limited to the stomach, but can also involve the duodenum and, albeit infrequently, the eosophagus. Parameters for recognizing NSAID gastropathy and classic peptic ulcer disease differ. NSAID gastropathy has a primarily antral or prepyloric localization, it is found especially in the elderly female NSAID user population and its pathogenic mechanism is presumed to be primarily related to the depletion of luminal and tissue prostaglandin (PG) E_2 and gastric prostacyclin, the so-called cytoprotective PGs, brought about by NSAID. In contrast, classic peptic ulcer disease is anatomically primarily duodenal, is found most frequently in younger males and its pathogenesis is primarily acid-mediated (9[R]). However, despite these differences which should permit NSAID-induced ulcers and ordinary peptic ulcers to be distinguished, it is often very difficult to ascertain whether NSAID intake has exacerbated a pre-existing ulcer or caused an ulcer to develop de novo.

Where does the evidence come from? *GI mucosal injury occurring after administration of NSAID has been studied in various ways and evidence on the risks of NSAID treatment has mainly been obtained from 4 sources: (1) endoscopic and microbleeding studies, usually conducted in healthy human volunteers; (2) adverse effects recorded during clinical trials of NSAID therapy; (3) adverse reaction reports to national*

Side Effects of Drugs Annual 14
M.N.G. Dukes and L. Beeley, editors

agencies; (4) 'ad hoc' studies, such as case-control or surveillance studies, or as a by-product of data generated through schemes such as prepayment insurance programs where drug prescriptions can be linked to subsequent events. Each of these sources of information has its merits and limitations.

The endoscopic studies The endoscopic evaluation of gastroduodenal toxicity, most often in comparison with that of acetylsalicylic acid (ASA), has become a must in the evaluation process of any new NSAID. These studies, which are mostly conducted in healthy young volunteers and less frequently in arthritic patients, have clearly demonstrated that NSAID use is associated with gastroduodenal damage ranging from mucosal hemorrhages (petechiae) to simple erosive changes and frank ulceration (SEDA-5, 95). They have been carried out on the hypothesis that analysis of the results of acute NSAID administration in normal volunteers should allow the identification of the propensity of any NSAID to damage the GI mucosa when administered to arthritic patients in daily practice. The underlying assumption of this approach is that there is a relationship between acute mucosal injury and major upper GI tract adverse events associated with the chronic use of these drugs. Unfortunately, such an assumption is far from having been demonstrated to be true. Therefore, short-term studies in normal volunteers and even in arthritic patients are of uncertain value for predicting whether chronic administration of a drug will cause gastroduodenal injury and/or major complications.

The most important information derived from endoscopic studies on volunteers can be summarized as follows: (1) subepithelial hemorrhages, erosions and acute ulcers are the most frequent gastroduodenal lesions; (2) the incidence of duodenal injury is usually lower than that of gastric injury and esophageal damage is even more infrequent; (3) although the dose–response curve for gastrotoxicity of various NSAID has not been systematically investigated, endoscopic studies provide evidence of a dose-related effect for some NSAID (3[r], 14[Cr]); (4) no strict clinical correlation exists between objective findings of gastroscopy and subjective intolerance to medication; (5) NSAID generally cause less gastroduodenal damage than ASA and the differences between various NSAID are usually trivial.

More useful information comes from endoscopic studies conducted in arthritic patients on chronic NSAID therapy.

The findings of the few available studies (15[C]–18[C], 19[R]) show that gastroduodenal damage is frequent in arthritic patients receiving any NSAID. In fact, about 30% of patients treated with a single NSAID develop gastric 'lesions' and more than 10% of patients receiving NSAID have an endoscopically recognizable ulcer on any given day, a point prevalence of ulcer disease 5–10 times higher than in patients who are not taking NSAID. Moreover, if one compares the crude prevalence estimates of gastric ulcer and duodenal ulcer in arthritic NSAID users to that observed in the normal population, it will be found that the users are about 6 times more likely to develop gastric ulcer than duodenal ulcer. However, as these estimates are fraught with uncertainties (e.g. many studies made no clear distinction between erosions and ulcers or acute ulcers and chronic ulcers; ulcer may have antedated the start of NSAID therapy or may have been activated by NSAID; other factors unrelated to NSAID use, such as smoking during the period of NSAID therapy, may not have been taken into due account), the available data must, for the time being, be viewed with caution (19[R]).

Endoscopic studies in arthritic patients have confirmed that there is no strict correlation between clinical symptoms and endoscopic findings. They have also demonstrated that gastric mucosal damage is more common in patients receiving multiple NSAID and ASA, and that recurrence of a healed peptic ulcer is particularly frequent. However, they reach no firm conclusion on the relative toxicity of various NSAID.

Microbleeding studies Most studies that have used the chromium labelling technique, an accurate and sensitive method for quantitating fecal blood loss for evaluating the gastrotoxicity of NSAID, have found that although daily blood loss is increased it is almost always significantly less than in patients taking ASA. There are usually no significant differences between the various NSAID (14[r]).

Blood loss measured with this technique may vary among individuals taking the same NSAID, and a correlation between blood loss and the extent and severity of gastroscopic findings in the stomach has been reported only in some studies

(3[r], 20[c], 21[c]). A possible explanation for the divergence is that radioactive fecal blood loss is an integrated measure of blood loss over the duration of the study, whereas gastroscopy visualizes the state of the gastric mucosa at a specific point in time. In addition, it includes blood loss caused by damage of intestinal mucosa lower than the stomach. A lower-than-expected radioactive fecal blood loss has no predictive value for the ulcerogenesis of NSAID in individual patients. Moreover, there are major drawbacks in evaluating gastrotoxicity by this method. It is time-consuming for the researcher, unpleasant for the patient and requires careful standardization (22[cR]). Fecal blood loss measured by other techniques is even less helpful (23[C]).

The crucial question that emerges from the analysis of information derived from short-term endoscopic or microbleeding studies therefore is: How relevant is the information to the chronic daily use of NSAID in the rheumatic population? Probably the results of these studies should be considered as doing no more than generating hypotheses that need confirmation from appropriate epidemiological studies.

Adverse effects recorded in clinical trials *Data from randomized controlled clinical trials cannot provide sufficient information on the risks of NSAID treatment. In fact, these data have the disadvantage that they may not be applicable to the general arthritic population, the studies are generally too small to produce compelling sets of data, especially on side effects that may be infrequent, the methods of monitoring adverse reactions vary greatly and placebo-treated arthritic patients often have upper GI symptoms that make interpretation of NSAID-associated GI symptoms difficult. Moreover, although abdominal pain, indigestion, nausea, vomiting and heartburn have almost universally been reported with NSAID during short-term clinical trials, whether these reports are predictive of the likelihood of drug-associated major GI side effects (e.g. ulceration, bleeding or perforation) is not clear (24[C]). On the other hand, silent ulcers are particularly common in patients treated with NSAID (25[r], 26[C]).*

Attempts have been made to combine data from many clinical trials in order to provide more useful information. Chalmers et al. (24[C]) performed a meta-analysis of adverse events recorded during 100 placebo-controlled NSAID therapy trials, but, not surprisingly, encountered many difficulties when they attempted to combine the symptom categories in order to obtain a coherent set. Interpreting the data on ulcer occurrence and GI bleeding proved particularly difficult. Of the 5 side effects studied – proven ulcer, GI bleeding, abdominal pain, dyspepsia and unspecified gastric events – only the last presented a statistically significant risk difference for NSAID use.

Adverse reaction reports to national agencies *The information derived from this source provides important clinical evidence on the possible risks of NSAID treatment, but has obvious limitations (27[R]). Such data have well-known inherent biases: reporting rates are low, they are not random samples of events, there is a tendency to collect information on newly marketed rather than standard drugs and the target population may vary with the different marketing strategies. These biases greatly influence the frequency of reported adverse events and make cross-comparison between NSAID almost impossible. Nevertheless, two important facts must be acknowledged: first, NSAID-associated adverse events, mainly affecting the GI tract, are reported to most registration authorities more frequently than adverse reactions for any other drug group (28[R]) and, second, despite intercountry differences in reporting rates, the ordering of drugs in relation to the reporting of adverse effects differs little (4[R]).*

However, although the agencies periodically issue data on the number of serious GI reactions reported for the various NSAID, the true incidence and prevalence remain elusive.

Ad hoc studies *In the last few years a number of formal case-control and cohort studies have been performed to compare GI morbidity in NSAID users and non-users. These studies too have their limitations, but if designed sensibly the information obtained from them is reliable. A formal meta-analysis of such NSAID risk factors studies is impossible since they differ on such points as study design, patient populations and definition of outcome. We shall therefore review only the results of the most important studies.*

Ulcer occurrence *Duggan et al. (29[C]) who conducted a retrospective case-control study on 95 gastric ulcer patients, 85 duodenal ulcer pa-*

tients and 180 matched controls, found a statistically significant association between gastric ulcer but not duodenal ulcer, and NSAID intake. The results agree with those obtained in a similar study conducted in Australia in 104 patients with gastric ulcer and 208 matched controls (30[C]). Estimates of relative risk for gastric ulcer are similar in these two studies, being 5.0 and 4.7 respectively, although confidence intervals for the estimates were wide.

Another case-control study by the same Australian group (31[C]) confirmed that the use of NSAID increases gastric ulcer risk. The researchers examined 225 patients with gastric ulcer and 411 matched controls and found that the odds of having a gastric ulcer were 2.3–5.4 higher in subjects exposed to daily NSAID therapy, irrespective of age. Indometacin was found to be the NSAID most strongly associated with gastric ulcer, with a level similar to that of ASA when used daily. Naproxen, ibuprofen and sulindac also carry the risk of chronic gastric ulcer, but at a lower level than ASA or indometacin. Bleeding from gastric ulcer was more common in NSAID users, but not significantly so.

Other studies support the association between gastric lesions and NSAID use, but because of methodological flaws must be interpreted with caution (32[C]–34[C]). It should be noted that none of these studies was able to reliably discriminate NSAID use that exacerbates pre-existing ulcer from drug use that caused ulcer to develop de novo.

Ulcer complications *Several studies have drawn attention to the high frequency with which previous NSAID use correlated with ulcer complications (bleeding and/or perforation), especially in the elderly (4[R], 35[R], 36[R]). However, many of these studies simply describe series of cases or have serious methodological limitations which make interpretation of their results difficult. More recently, other better-conducted studies have improved our understanding of the problem.*

Collier and Pain (37[C]) compared the number of NSAID users in 269 patients with perforated peptic ulcer and an equal number of inpatient-matched controls and found a highly significant association between NSAID intake and ulcer perforation, both gastric and duodenal, in patients aged ⩾65 years. The relative risk was calculated at 2.3 for patients <65 and 11.5 for those ⩾65 years.

Armstrong and Blower (38[c]) studied 235 patients with life-threatening peptic ulcer complications, who either underwent emergency surgery or died: 137 had perforated ulcers, 5 associated with bleeding, and 98 had bleeding ulcers; 68 patients died, 25 at home. An ulcer inpatient control group was used for comparison. Sixty per cent of the case group and 9% of the control group were recorded as NSAID users. Nearly 80% of the deaths occurred in ulcer patients who used NSAID, suggesting that there is a relationship between NSAID use and life-threatening ulcer complications. This trial has been criticized because it contains unsatisfactory features (4[c]).

In a well-performed case-control study, Sommerville et al. (39[C]) questioned all patients admitted with gastric or duodenal ulcer bleeding to two hospitals serving a single city over a 2-year period. Those ⩾60 years old were matched for both age and sex with a hospital and a community control. Thirty-five per cent of those with bleeding ulcers had been NSAID users compared with 14% of hospital and 16% of community controls (relative risk 3.8 and 2.7). The strong association of bleeding with NSAID use differed little in gastric or duodenal ulcer. The authors calculated that the etiological fraction, the amount of disease directly attributable to NSAID use, assuming causality, was 22%.

Bartle et al. (40[C]), who carried out a case-control study on 57 consecutive patients with GI bleeding and 123 matched controls, found that 42% of the patients were taking NSAID as against 18% of controls. The study confirmed that elderly patients are a group at high risk for developing GI bleeding, probably due to the increased use of NSAID.

In a hospital-based case-control study, Levy et al. (41[C]) also found the risk of a first major upper GI bleeding increased in patients who were regular users of NSAID in the week before onset of complications. The adjusted rate ratio estimate was 9.1, but these data must be interpreted with caution due to the very small number of cases exposed to NSAID.

More recently a preliminary report has been published on the analysis of specific hospitalizations of rheumatoid arthritis patients for GI side effects (42[C]). The data derive from the American Rheumatism Association Medical Information System (ARAMIS). Over a period of 5 years, nearly 2000 consecutive rheumatoid arthritis patients were enrolled in the ARAMIS

Post-Marketing Surveillance Program, which prospectively monitored the side effects experienced by these patients while being treated with salicylates or other NSAID. Patients on NSAID had a hazard ratio for hospitalization due to upper GI ulcer problems that was 9.3 times that of patients not on NSAID.

Two further studies considered the chances of death from peptic ulcer or its complications. The first was a case-control study conducted by Griffin et al (43[C]) on 122 patients aged 60 or more, who died of either gastric or duodenal ulcer or upper GI hemorrhage of unknown cause and 3897 matched controls. The current users of NSAID in this elderly population were 4.7 times more likely to die from peptic ulcer or upper GI hemorrhage than non-users. The persistence of an elevated risk of death from peptic ulcer or bleeding after controlling for co-morbidity indicators, the strength of association, the consistency across most subgroups as defined by the demographic characteristics of the subjects, and the presence of a significant risk associated only with the current users of NSAID argue against potential biases being responsible for the observed increased risk among current NSAID users. A much weaker association was found in the second trial, a smaller cohort study by Guess et al (44[C]). Fatal upper GI hemorrhage and/or perforation in relation to the use of NSAID were identified by using a records linkage system. Death occurred very infrequently in people less than 75 years of age and no significant risk was detected except in female current users aged 75 and older, who were 5 times more likely to die from upper GI hemorrhage than non-users.

It has been suggested that NSAID increase not only the chance of developing fatal ulcer complications, but also the risk of dying from these disorders (38[C]). However, a carefully conducted case-control study indicates that neither NSAID nor ASA are associated with increased case fatality rates from hemorrhage or perforation of peptic ulcers (45[C]).

All the above-mentioned studies contribute to the growing evidence that NSAID can provoke gastric ulcers as well as gastric and duodenal ulcer complications (upper GI hemorrhage or perforation) especially in older patients, but other studies, which have not found them to have any effect, deserve attention (46[C]–49[C]).

Inman (46[C]), with his Prescription Event Monitoring System, found that ulcer complications were recorded only about once every 200 patient-years of treatment with any of 5 NSAID, including 3 which were subsequently withdrawn from the market for other side effects (benoxaprofen, Osmosin and zomepirac) and, apart from dyspepsia and gastritis, he concluded that significant serious risks were not apparent. It should be noted that if the rate of risk of serious adverse events had been of the order of 1 event every 10 000 courses of treatment, the study would not be large enough to detect it. Three other studies (47[C]–49[C]) by Jick and colleagues, all utilizing data from the same population of the Group Health Cooperative of Puget Sound, provided further evidence against a significant increased risk of ulcer complications in NSAID users.

In their first study (47[C]), they performed a follow-up study on the relationship between the use of NSAID and hospitalization for GI bleeding in patients less than 65 years of age. Among some 100 000 members who filled at least one prescription for an NSAID in a 5-year period, only 14 were hospitalized for upper GI bleeding within 90 days of filling a prescription and in only 3 subjects did there seem to be a probable etiological connection. They concluded that the risk attributable to the NSAID studied, if present at all, was very low – less than 1 per million person-days at risk.

In order to evaluate the risks of hospitalization for upper GI bleeding for NSAID users in the elderly, they reviewed the data of members of the same population over the age of 64 years. While the rate of hospitalization in NSAID users was approximately 1.5 times that of non-users, there was some evidence that much, if not all, the discrepancy was due to differences in underlying risk between NSAID users and non-users (48[C]).

In their third study (49[C]) they considered patients of all ages with perforated ulcer. The frequency of hospital admissions for perforated ulcer was low in NSAID users (0.26 per million person-days at risk) and not much different from that of controls who were not current users of NSAID (adjusted rate ratio 1.6, but with confidence intervals overlapping unity).

Finally, Carson et al (50[C]) performed a retrospective cohort study using the Computerized On-line Medicaid Pharmaceutical Analysis and Surveillance System (COMPASS) database, in which the incidence of upper GI bleeding was determined in approximately 50 000 patients exposed to NSAID and in an equal number of un-

exposed matched controls. The risk of developing upper GI bleeding in patients exposed to NSAID was 1.5 times that of the unexposed group (95% confidence intervals 1.2–2.0). These results remained unchanged after examining the effects of many confounding variables. Both dose–response and duration–response relationships were demonstrated, indicating that the higher the dose of drug and the longer the drug is taken, the greater the risk that a patient will develop upper GI bleeding.

At first sight the conclusions reached by individual investigators, which vary from no significant risk to very substantial risks, seem irreconcilable. However, a careful evaluation of the studies suggests that the between-data differences may be largely accounted for by two major factors: (1) differences in study characteristics (2) confounding factors which make the causal relationship between NSAID use and gastropathy difficult to interpret. Differences in the size of the study and the varying inclusions of elderly subjects, who appear at greatest risk, are the most important factors of variability.

It can reasonably be concluded that there is now little disagreement that NSAID damage the gastroduodenal mucosa and cause gastric and, less frequently, duodenal ulcers.

The term 'gastropathy' describes the range of lesions associated with these drugs. As ordinary peptic ulcers are common, some NSAID-associated ulcers (especially duodenal ulcer) will occur on a background of a peptic ulcer predisposition. However, NSAID-induced ulcers often occur in individuals who have never manifested any peptic ulcer diathesis.

In addition, there is little question that NSAID consumption also significantly increases the risk of bleeding and perforation of gastric as well as duodenal ulcers, although the magnitude of this risk is uncertain and fatality rates of these complications seem not to be increased by NSAID therapy.

The extent to which NSAID-associated ulcer complications are due to ulcer caused entirely by NSAID or to exacerbation by NSAID of pre-existing, often asymptomatic, peptic ulcer is not known.

Individual versus population risks *A careful overall interpretation of NSAID risks also demands a clear distinction between individual and population risk. We need to know not only the risk of NSAID use to the individual patient, which from the above data appears to be relatively low, but also its consequences to the general population. Despite the fact that the intrinsic toxicity of NSAID does not seem to be high, their extraordinarily wide use may pose difficulties. The epidemiological problem, at least for the most serious complications, is not the high relative risk of the disease but the high prevalence of the risk factor, and this has important implications in terms of prevention.*

In terms of population the magnitude of the problem of NSAID-associated gastropathy has been assessed from estimates of hospitalization for ulcer complications and excess of GI deaths. In the United Kingdom it has been estimated that 20–30% of all cases of ulcer complications in subjects aged over 60 which result in hospitalization are directly attributable to the use of NSAID, and that 1/10 of these terminate in death (45[c]). That means at least 2000 cases of bleeding induced every year and about 200 deaths (39[c]), in connection with approximately 11 million prescriptions.

The data from the United States are not much different, with the estimate of hospitalization of rheumatoid arthritis patients alone for this cause being 20 000 annually with 2600 deaths (42[c]).

However they are estimated, costs are obviously high (6[R], 51[C]). All these findings lend support to the growing consensus that NSAID-associated gastropathy is a serious medication side effect.

High-risk patients *Once having agreed on the recognition of NSAID gastropathy, it becomes necessary to identify the patients most at risk. Since not everyone treated with NSAID develops ulcers, and even fewer develop complications, it would seem that there must be a subpopulation that suffers from these unwanted reactions. The proposed genetic predisposition to NSAID ulceration remains entirely speculative (52[c]). Both case-control and surveillance studies have identified multiple factors that contribute to the increased vulnerability of certain patients. The most important patient-related factors include age (elderly), history of ulcers and/or gastric bleeding, possibly smoking (18[C], 43[R], 53[r]–55[r]) and combination NSAID therapy with other NSAIDs, including ASA and corticosteroids (15[c], 42[c]). Other suggested potential risk factors are sex (female), the musculoskeletal disease for* which NSAID are used, the nature of the NSAID itself and dosage. The supporting evidence, however, is meagre and/or contradictory. It appears likely that the increased number of serious events in women (33[c], 37[c], 39[c], 44[c]) is simply a consequence of their greater exposure to NSAID. Some data suggest that rheumatoid arthritis itself is a risk factor for GI hospitalization (18[C], 42[Cr]), but other studies provide no evidence that disease is a marker for drug-induced damage (39[c], 55[c]).

Despite the suggestions made by some authors that some NSAID are more (e.g. indometacin, piroxicam) or less (e.g. ibuprofen) gastrotoxic than others (SEDA-12, 91; 31[c], 39[c]) data on individual drugs are at best fragmentary. Carson et al (56[C]) examined this problem using the COMPASS database by creating cohorts of patients exposed to only one NSAID. When 7 NSAID were compared, a significant difference was found only for sulindac, which was associated with more frequent bleeding than the other NSAID. However, considerably larger data sets and more careful analysis for confounding variables are required before one drug is accepted as being more dangerous than any other.

Although the capacity of NSAID to cause chronic ulcers may be dose-related, so far dose–responsiveness has been documented only in the case of acute injury caused by certain NSAID (3[r], 14[Cr], 57[C]) and for the GI bleeding with a number of NSAID (50[C]).

These risk factors are all potentially interactive, but the degree of interdependence has never been established.

In conclusion, the benefit of being able to identify patients who are at risk of developing gastropathy while taking NSAID is obvious, but, unfortunately, a precise risk model to which we can refer to is not at hand.

Reducing the risk of upper GI toxicity: a feasible goal? The increasing awareness of the importance of NSAID-induced gastropathy has stimulated the search for strategies to treat and prevent this problem. There are a few considerations that may be relevant to the understanding of the rationality and limitations of these strategies:

(1) The responsible mechanism or mechanisms of NSAID-mediated gastroduodenal damage remains controversial, but there is a sufficient body of evidence that it is mainly the result of a dual insult. Firstly, direct NSAID-mediated acidic damage, followed almost simultaneously by the deleterious effect of prostaglandin (PG) inhibition (58[R]). The pivotal importance of PG inhibition, which can also occur when the NSAID is administered systemically, in the pathogenic mechanisms of NSAID upper GI toxicity has important implications for prevention and treatment (1[R], 59[R]). However, it should be remembered that some NSAID spare gastric PG synthesis and that there are other ways in which they might induce gastroduodenal damage (e.g. by inhibiting mucus and bicarbonate secretion, by decreasing mucosal permeability, by interfering with active ion transport, by decreasing mucosal blood flow, by causing capillary stasis or even by interfering with upper GI tract motility) (10[R], 58[R]).

(2) There is no clear correlation between either acute and chronic mucosal damage by NSAID or lesions and symptoms. Therefore, a beneficial effect of a preventive therapy on an acute lesion (erosions or even acute ulcer) or in controlling symptoms does not imply the same efficacy in prevention of a chronic ulcer or its complications, which is the problem that really matters (59[R]).

(3) The mechanisms underlying gastric ulceration are probably different from those causing duodenal ulceration and its complications. A prophylactic or a therapeutic measure that is active on one lesion might not protect from the other.

(4) The mechanisms underlying ulcer healing and ulcer prevention are probably not the same. Therefore, a therapeutic approach which may be effective in healing an established ulcer may be ineffective in preventing a NSAID-induced disruption of normal mucosal defense mechanisms.

Keeping these considerations in mind, let us review the published studies that evaluate the capacity of various therapies to prevent or cure NSAID-induced gastroduodenal mucosal damage.

Prevention of NSAID-induced gastropathy Two ways of preventing gastroduodenal damage have been explored: the search for less toxic drugs or formulations and the use of preventive therapy. The concept of a primary role for PG inhibition in NSAID gastric injury prompted the search for compounds with gastric PG-sparing properties theoretically devoid of gastrotoxicity. Only a few of these compounds have been studied in man (e.g. etodolac, carprofen, nabumetone), but data on their sparing properties and on correlation between the degree of PG suppression and endoscopic evidence of mucosal damage are scanty and contradictory (SEDA-13, 81; 58[r], 60[C], 61[c]). Moreover, these compounds have been shown to cause the usual spectrum of upper GI toxicity (SEDA-13, 79, 80, 81).

Awareness of the possible importance of the direct damaging action of the NSAID on the gastric mucosa suggested the use of new formulations and pro-drugs. Parenteral and rectal administration of NSAID does not spare the stomach (62[C]–65[C]). Various new formulations (SEDA-9, 83; SEDA-12, 86; SEDA-13, 81; 66[C]–69[C]) may be less gastrotoxic than standard formulations in short-term studies, but their merits have not yet been proven in long-term use. In the same way, pro-drugs (e.g. sulindac) have not protected against gastric complications (56[c]). It remains to be seen whether the use of a prophylactic therapy is feasible and more effective.

A number of randomized controlled studies have been performed in an attempt to resolve this quandary. The drugs most often used have been the H_2-receptor antagonists and, more recently, the PG analog, misoprostol (see Table 1).

The limited data at present available unanimously indicate that H_2-receptor antagonists cannot prevent NSAID-induced gastric ulcer. Two studies on ranitidine (74[C], 75[C]) reporting that it reduces the incidence of duodenal ulcer contrast with others that do not find it offers any protection against gastroduodenal mucosa lesions (72[C], 73[C], 76[C]). Differences in evaluation parameters and the population studied could explain the discrepancy. In the largest of the two studies (74[C]) which found ranitidine effective, 8 out of 22 ulcers were found in a small subgroup of patients with a history of peptic ulcer disease and 8 out of 12 duodenal ulcers were in patients taking piroxicam. That is to say, avoiding the use of NSAID in a few patients with a history of peptic disease (a frequent and wise suggestion when using NSAID) or using an alternative NSAID in 75 out of 263 patients would have negated any beneficial effect of ranitidine. Or, to put it another way, it would have produced the same beneficial result as ranitidine. We share the author's conclusion that further work is needed to substantiate these findings.

The data on prophylactic use of H_2-receptor antagonists have further limitations: with few exceptions all studies are short-term ($\leqslant$4 weeks duration) and none had sufficient statistical power to detect any effect on ulcer complications.

The studies on misoprostol are even more limited, since only one published clinical trial has been performed in osteoarthritic patients (81[C]). This study showed that coadministration of this synthetic analog of PGs with NSAID significantly reduced the frequency of NSAID-induced gastric ulcer. The numbers of duodenal ulcers were too small for any meaningful comparison. Symptoms (abdominal pain) were not significantly affected by treatment, probably because the great spontaneous pain relief in the placebo group overshadowed any effect of the misoprostol in relieving NSAID-associated abdominal discomfort.

This study too has certain limitations. It included only patients with GI symptoms and one does not know if concurrent therapy in symptom-free patients, who are also at risk of life-threatening GI side effects, would have achieved similar results. The results cannot be generalized to other NSAID with less gastric PG-inhibiting activity. Furthermore, there is evidence that misoprostol may provoke a decrease in the absorption of some NSAID (82[c]), a point that requires clarification.

Pirenzapine has been evaluated in two studies and found efficacious in preventing the occurrence of symptoms in NSAID-treated patients, but the results require confirmation (83[r]).

To extrapolate the data on prophylaxis obtained in clinical trials to general practice usage of NSAID is not straightforward. Two major points should be considered, first of all:

(1) As already pointed out, NSAID are important causes of morbidity and mortality in the community and this is due to their extraordinarily wide use rather than to their intrinsic toxicity. It has been calculated (53[c]) that if, hypothetically, the co-prescription of any mucosal protectant or antisecretory agent halved the risk of serious ulcer complications, it would be necessary to treat an estimated 1000 patients to prevent 3 cases of perforation or bleeding and 10 000 patients to prevent 3 deaths. Thus the main thrust of attempts to reduce risks from NSAID in the community should be to limit their use rather than to attempt to lower relative risk further by widespread co-prescription of agents such as H_2-receptor antagonists, misoprostol, sucralfate or pirenzepine.

Table 1. Prevention of NSAID-induced gastropathy

Drug (daily dosage)	Ref.	Subjects (no./type)	Evaluation time	NSAID	Study design	Control drugs	Findings and comments
Cimetidine 400 mg × 2	70	22 pts. with skeletal disorders	1 wk	indometacin	rdbc	placebo	No. of pts. with mucosal damage not different from placebo Cimetidine significantly prevents gastroduodenal mucosal damage
Cimetidine 300 mg × 4	71	30 volunteers	1 wk	tolmetin	rdbc	placebo misoprostol	No. of pts. with more severe mucosal damage score less in cimetidine group (but misoprostol much more efficacious)
Ranitidine 150 mg × 2	72	9 volunteers	1 wk	indometacin	sbco	placebo misoprostol	Mucosal damage scores not different from that obtained with placebo (misoprostol decreased mucosal damage scores)
Ranitidine 150 mg × 2	73	246 pts. with RA, OA	4 wk	various	rdbc	placebo	No. of pts. with mucosal damage not different from placebo Mucosal gastroduodenal damage scores not different from those obtained with placebo
Ranitidine 50 mg × 2	74	297 symptomatic pts. with RA, OA	8 wk	various	rdbc	placebo	Ranitidine significantly prevented occurrence of DU but not GU Symptoms not ameliorated by treatment
Ranitidine 50 mg × 2	75	144 pts. with RA, OA	8 wk	various	rdbc	placebo	Ranitidine significantly prevented occurrence of DU but not GU
Ranitidine 50 mg × 2	76	110 pts. with musculoskeletal disorders	1 wk	indometacin	rdbc	placebo	No. of pts. with mucosal damage not different from placebo Mucosal damage scores not different from those obtained with placebo Symptoms not ameliorated
Cimetidine 400 mg × 3	77	104 pts. with RA, OA	8 wk	various	rdbc	placebo	Mucosal damage score not different from that obtained with placebo In pts. with lesions, rate of healing not different from placebo
Cimetidine 800 or 400 mg	78	191 pts. with musculoskeletal disorders	1 wk	indometacin	rdbc	placebo	Cimetidine (800 mg) significantly prevented duodenal, but not antral, musocal damage with respect to placebo and cimetidine 400 mg
Misoprostol 200 mg × 2	79	25 volunteers	1 wk	naproxen	rdbc	placebo	Misoprostol significantly prevented mucosal damage
Misoprostol 200 mg × 4	80	60 volunteers	1 wk	tolmetin	rdbc	placebo	Misoprostol significantly prevented mucosal damage
Misoprostol 200 mg × 4	71	30 volunteers	1 wk	tolmetin	rdbc	placebo cimetidine	Misoprostol significantly prevented gastric mucosal damage with respect to placebo and cimetidine Cimetidine and misoprostol not different in prevention of duodenal mucosa damage
Misoprostol 100–200 mg × 4	81	420 OA	3 mth	ibuprofen naproxen piroxicam	rdbc	placebo	GU less frequent in both misoprostol groups Symptoms not reduced

GU = gastric ulcer; RA = rheumatoid arthritis; OA = osteoarthritis; rdbc = randomized double-blind controlled study; sbco = single-blind cross-over study.

Table 2. Therapy of NSAID-induced gastropathy

Drug (daily dosage)	Ref.	Subjects no./type	Evaluation time	NSAID	Study design	Control drugs	Findings and comments
Cimetidine + antacids 400 mg × 3	85	70 GU	12 wk	discontinued	rdbc	antacids	Antacids less effective than combination with cimetidine at 6 wk but not at 12 wk Recurrence 6%/year with cimetidine + NSAID
Cimetidine	86	17 GU or DU	12 wk	continued	open	–	100% DU and 79% GU healed at 12 wk No recurrence (symptomatic)/year with cimetidine + NSAID
Cimetidine + antacids 1.2 g	87	27 GU + DU	6 wk	continued	rdbc	antacids	No significant difference between treatments (trend favoring combination; study short; GU healed slowly) but % healing low
Sucralfate 1 g × 2	88	67 GU or DU	9 wk	continued 50%	rsb	ranitidine 150 mg × 2	No difference in healing in either drug or stopping/continuing NSAID Trend in slower healing or non-healing in GU
Sucralfate 1 g × 4	89	143 symptomatic (60 with GU or erosions)	6 wk	continued	rdbc	placebo	Significant reduction of frequency and severity of symptoms Gastric mucosal healing unaffected
Ranitidine 150 mg × 2	18	56 GU or DU	12 wk	continued	open	–	Healing comparable to that seen in non-NSAID users
Cimetidine 400 mg × 2	90	163 GU or DU 79, erosions 84	8 wk	continued	open	–	Healing comparable to that seen in non-NSAID users (slightly lower for GU) Symptomatic relapse rate with C(400 mg) 12% at 6 mth similar to other ulcers
Cimetidine 400 mg × 2	91	127 lesion-free, symptomatic	4 wk	continued 50%	r. open	placebo	Symptomatic improvement with cimetidine greater than with placebo Maintenance treatment in symptom-free pts. (6 mth) showed no difference in relapse, but symptoms recurred more rapidly Symptom relief quicker in lesion-free patients

Cimetidine 600 mg	*77*	*39 lesions*	*10 mth*	*continued*	*rdbc*	*placebo*	*No difference between cimetidine and placebo in gastroduodenal damage*
Ranitidine 150 mg × 2	*92*	*46 symptomatic with lesions*	*4 wk*	*continued*	*rdbc*	*placebo*	*Total damaging score of gastroduodenal lesions reduced Symptoms significantly reduced*
Ranitidine + antacids 150 mg × 2	*93*	*21 GU or DU*	*3–6 wk*	*continued*	*open*	–	*DU healed but only 50% of GU healed*
Sucralfate 1 g × 4	*94*	*26 symptomatic with lesions*	*6 wk*	*continued*	*rdb comp.*	*cimetidine 800 mg*	*No difference in improvement of gastroduodenal scores between treatments*
Ranitidine 150 mg × 2	*73*	*48 multiple erosions*	*4 wk*	*continued 50%*	*r.open*	*placebo*	*Ranitidine more effective when NSAID discontinued*
Bismuth 300 mg × 4	*73*	*72 DU-GU*	*4 wk*	*continued*	*r.open*	*cimetidine*	*Bismuth and cimetidine similar, but healing rate low when compared with that observed in NSAID non-users*

DU = duodenal ulcer; GU = gastric ulcer; rdbc = randomized double-blind controlled study; rsb = randomized single-blind study; r.open = randomized open; rdb comp. = randomized double-blind comparative study.

(2) Such studies have been based upon the unproven hypothesis that a statistically significant reduction in endoscopically visible mucosal injury would be associated with a reduced frequency of already-rare untoward events of bleeding and perforation. An increasing number of patients are reported to have suffered such complications or even to have died while receiving full doses of H_2-receptor blockers (38[c], 84[c]), which suggests that these drugs can fail to prevent serious GI side effects. Only large-scale clinical trials can establish whether prevention of macroscopic NSAID damage to the gastroduodenal mucosa will result in reduced serious untoward events.

Finally, on the basis of the results of the trials published until now it could be argued that in order to achieve the most effective ulcer prevention, patients taking NSAID should also receive both misoprostol, to prevent gastric ulcer, and ranitidine, to prevent duodenal ulcer (95[R]).

All the above observations suggest that 'protective' co-therapy may have a role only in a limited number of individuals. When NSAID are thought to be important, as in many cases of rheumatoid arthritis, and the patient is in a high-risk group, consideration may be given to using mucosal protective agents as well.

Therapy of NSAID gastropathy *Fifteen studies have been traced in the literature and data are summarized in Table 2. Seven of these studies are blind randomized controlled studies and all but one included H_2-receptor antagonists in the therapeutic regimen studied. Sucralfate and bismuth were also studied. Evaluation end-points varied, but were represented by endoscopically proven healing of ulcer during ongoing NSAID therapy in the majority of studies. A few trials investigated GI symptoms and/or endoscopy proven gastroduodenal 'lesions'. Only 4 trials included follow-up for recurrence of ulcers. Duration varied from 4 to 12 weeks and the different times must be taken into account when examining the healing rate of different studies. Despite clear limitations, the body of data provided by these studies yielded some useful information.*

If NSAID are discontinued most gastric and duodenal ulcers heal with an H_2-receptor antagonist, with or without combined antacids in 12 weeks or less. A recent study (96[C]) has shown that patients with duodenal ulcers who reported previous use of NSAID appeared to have an even more rapid rate of healing than those who had not taken these agents. The enhanced healing could have resulted from the removal of the causative agent allowing the intrinsic protective physiological mechanisms to function normally.

More interesting is the evidence provided that continuing NSAID therapy does not seem to prevent the healing of duodenal ulcers. Gastric ulcers heal less easily and more slowly. This explains the low percentage of healing reported in many short-term (4–6 weeks) studies. Initial ulcer size, also, affects the time required to heal and there is an inverse correlation between ulcer size and early healing. The same efficacy from the H_2-receptor antagonists was found in some studies that had endoscopic lesions and/or GI symptoms as their evaluation end-points (90, 91), even though, in one trial, ranitidine was more efficacious when NSAID were discontinued (73). Sucralfate has been evaluated in only one placebo-controlled study (89[C]) and compared with cimetidine and ranitidine in another two (88[C], 94[C]). Data are insufficient to establish the efficacy of this agent in healing duodenal ulcers; it seems to offer an effective alternative to H_2-receptor antagonists in controlling GI symptoms, but not in healing gastric ulcer.

The one open study that evaluated bismuth subcitrate, a 'mucoprotective' agent, found that it appeared to be as efficacious as cimetidine in treating both gastric and duodenal ulcer, but the healing rate was lower than that usually found in NSAID non-users (73[C]) and the study was too small to reach any firm conclusion.

The only randomized double-blind controlled study that has investigated the efficacy of a maintenance therapy in keeping NSAID-taking patients symptom-free found no difference between cimetidine (400 mg once daily) and placebo when used for 6 months (91[C]).

The results of these studies must not be interpreted as evidence that continuing NSAID therapy during ulcer treatment has no adverse effects in terms of delayed healing or increased risk of complications. In fact, in only two studies were patients properly randomized to continue or discontinue NSAID treatment (73, 88) allowing a reliable comparison of healing rate, and in one of these (73) ranitidine was found to be more effective in healing gastroduodenal erosions when NSAID was discontinued. However, both studies were too small to have enough statistical power to detect any influence of taking NSAID on risk of complications. Caution should also be taken in interpreting the results of symptomatic treatment of these patients. It cannot be denied that regardless of the presence or absence of an ulcer, relief of symptoms, which may be severe, may be desirable so that NSAID therapy can be continued. However, whether suppression of symptoms while continuing NSAID will in the end prove beneficial or hazardous to the patient is not known. Asymptomatic patients may have endoscopically documented severe damage and reports on complications occurring in patients who are being treated with cimetidine therapy have been published. Moreover, a marked amelioration of symptoms with time has been documented in placebo-treated patients, suggesting that patients may develop symptomatic tolerance to NSAID. Therefore, the importance of treating NSAID users with antiulcer drugs solely on the basis of symptoms warrants further large prospective studies.

Clinical implications *Although reduction of the risk of upper GI toxicity remains a major safety issue and improved guidelines have been suggested for achieving this objective (9[R], 19[cR], 53[R], 54[R], 97[R]), the advice offered to prescribing doctors is more like an assembly of common-sense notions than authoritative guidelines founded on reliable scientific data.*

The first step before prescribing a NSAID is to consider whether the drug is really necessary. NSAID therapy can sometimes be avoided, or ended, by using simple analgesics or alternative treatments (e.g. physiotherapy, local treatments, second-line agents, low doses of corticosteroids). This approach is particularly important when faced by factors considered to put a patient at high risk for upper GI toxicity, e.g. elderly females, pre-existing gastroduodenal disease, cigarette smoking, excessive alcohol consumption and concomitant ASA intake. Smoking, excess intake of alcohol and concomitant ASA use are correctable factors. If the drug is really needed, the lowest effective dosage should be preferred. Whether some NSAID are more toxic than others is still a matter of debate, but indometacin and, possibly, piroxicam should perhaps be avoided in high-risk patient groups. Although theoretically attractive, suppositories, pro-drugs, enteric-coated and other types of formulations afford no significant advantage. Data on newer NSAID which spare gastric PGs are still pending.

Due to the fact that the risk of acute bleeding increases to a peak at about 4 months after commencing NSAID and then declines steadily (50[c]), it has been suggested that particular surveillance should be exercised during the early months of therapy. Unfortunately, it is not clear how the patient monitoring should be performed in order to reduce the risk of these complications. Ulcers may be painless and the absence of symptoms is by no means reassuring, fecal occult blood is a poor indicator of the presence of ulcerative lesions and repeated endoscopic examination in all patients taking NSAID is impracticable. Whether patients who start taking NSAID should have prophylaxis with antiulcer drugs is unknown, and the many unresolved controversies on this matter have already been illustrated. Another factor which militates against universal prohylaxis is the cost. It has been calculated (97[c]) that if standard maintenance doses of cimetidine were sufficient to prevent half of the NSAID-associated bleeds occurring once every 500 patient-years, the cost for each life saved would be around one million pounds.

If during treatment the patient becomes symptomatic and the drug cannot be stopped, if he is at risk for upper GI complications or the reaction is severe, a suspected ulcer should be confirmed endoscopically. Otherwise, one should try an alternative NSAID and remember that many patients may develop symptomatic tolerance to NSAID spontaneously.

If the persistence of symptoms would curtail the benefits of NSAID therapy, a short (4-week) full-dose course of an H_2-receptor antagonist, or sucralfate, could prove useful, but maintenance therapy after symptoms have been controlled probably would not.

When an ulcer develops, it is imperative to stop NSAID treatment, if possible, and begin routine antiulcer therapy. If, after having carefully considered the risk/benefit ratio, the NSAID is considered necessary, ulcers should be treated with full doses of H_2-antagonists. Because NSAID may delay the healing of large gastric ulcers, therapy should be continued longer in gastric than in duodenal ulcer patients. Low-dose maintenance therapy after ulcer healing has not been found efficacious.

PYRAZOLONE DERIVATIVES *(SED-11, 176; SEDA-12, 82; SEDA-13, 78)*

Antipyrine (phenazone) *(SED-11, 176)*

Antipyrine is now used only as a marker of hepatic drug-metabolizing activity. Allergic reactions to the drug are very rare (SEDA-6, 92), but a new case-report has been published. A subject participating in a clinical trial employing antipyrine experienced an acute *allergic reaction* to the drug which was characterized by diaphoresis, flushing, swelling of the throat and upper lip, and a diffuse urticarial rash. Although the potential for antipyrine tests to cause an allergic reaction is low, subjects should be informed of the potential risk (98[C]).

Dipyrone *(SEDA-12, 82; SEDA-13, 78)*

The debate on the safety of dipyrone, as well as on the aggressive marketing of dipyrone-containing drugs in the Third World, continues unabated (99[R]). Attention has been drawn to manufacturer-sponsored promotional trials on dipyrone, studies which appear to have no scientific motivations and to be ethically unjustified (100[c], 101[c]).

PHENYLBUTAZONE AND RELATED COMPOUNDS *(SED-11, 173; SEDA-12, 83)*

Azapropazone *(SED-11, 176; SEDA-12, 83)*

Nervous system NSAID have only rarely been implicated in causing extrapyramidal reactions (SEDA-8, 109). An *oculogyric crisis* has been described in a 51-year-old man who was taking indometacin (200 mg/d) for acute gout when azapropazone was added to his therapeutic regimen. The reaction lasted about 1 h and recurred the day after upon rechallenge with azapropazone. Whether azapropazone could have caused extrapyramidal side effects by direct toxicity or by interacting with indometacin is not known (102[Cr]).

Liver Adverse reactions affecting the liver have never been reported in the literature. A 57-year-old woman developed *jaundice* and *erythema multiforme* 2 weeks after having started azapropazone therapy for osteoarthritis. Liver biopsy disclosed a mild non-specific hepatitis with granuloma formation. Recovery was uneventful (103[C]).

INDOMETACIN AND RELATED COMPOUNDS *(SED-11, 178; SEDA-12, 84; SEDA-13, 79)*

Indometacin

Meta-analysis was used to study patients' preference in 37 crossover trials that compared indometacin with newer NSAID. As the most important variable, patients' preference failed to provide any support that, because of their better tolerability, newer NSAID are tending to replace indometacin (104[c]).

Rectal administration of 100 mg of indometacin in solution has as good, and almost as rapid, an effect on renal colic as 50 mg i.v. and causes fewer side effects (105[c]).

Respiratory Indometacin administered orally or rectally can provoke or *aggravate asthma* in hypersensitive patients and cross-sensitivity with aspirin has been demonstrated (SED-11, 178). The hazards of administering topical indometacin to asthmatic patients should also not be ignored. When a patient who suffered from adult onset asthma, received indometacin in ophthalmic solution, his asthma deteriorated so severely that he required hospitalization and mechanical ventilation (106[C]).

Nervous system Indometacin-induced CNS side effects are well known (SED-11, 178), but the psychomotor effects are less well documented. A recent study on objective and subjective effects of single oral doses of indometacin on the performance of healthy volunteers showed that *acute psychomotor effects* are modest and do not alter the psychomotor impairment induced by diazepam in the same subject (107[Cr]). These results are in agreement with those obtained in patients with rheumatic diseases after multiple doses of indometacin (108[C]).

Liver Despite common use, adverse hepatic reactions have rarely been reported (SED-11, 178). A recent report describes a case of indometacin associated primarily *cholestatic liver* *injury*. The reaction was not severe and recovery was rapid and uneventful (109[C]).

Musculoskeletal system The use of NSAID in the routine management of osteoarthritis has been questioned on the basis of a suspected deleterious effect of these drugs on the evolution of the disease, but a causal relationship has by no means been proven (SEDA-11, 87). One recent study compared the effects of a weak (azapropazone) and a strong (indometacin) inhibitor of prostaglandin synthesis on the osteoarthritic process. It was found that *osteoarthritis of the hip progresses more quickly* in patients treated with indometacin, suggesting the wisdom of avoiding the use of the drug in patients with joints severely compromised by osteoarthritis. However, the authors' conclusion should be accepted with caution, as the study was relatively small, lacked a control group of patients who were not receiving NSAID and was not blind (110[C]).

Pregnancy and labor Hazards of the use of indometacin as a tocolytic agent seem to outweight any theoretical advantage (SEDA-12, 84). It has been suggested that when indometacin use is limited to gestations of <35 weeks and for short courses it may be less dangerous, but a recent study has provided evidence that indometacin can cause *constriction of the ductus arteriosus* even after short-term use and several weeks after the start of therapy (111[C]). In premature infants intravenous indometacin promotes closure of the patent ductus arteriosus with a low incidence of adverse events (SEDA-10, 80; 112[C]). However, a recent report suggests that oral indometacin administration may predispose the very-low-weight infant to the development of *sepsis* shortly after therapy is begun. The study is retrospective and uncontrolled and needs confirmation (113[C]).

Gastrointestinal The withdrawal of Osmosin (a controlled-release delivery system) due to safety concerns was primarily based on evidence provided by yellow-card reports received by the U.K. Committee on the Safety of Medicines (CSM) (SEDA-8, 102). CSM data have now been published and provide clear-cut evidence of the peculiar *intestinal toxicity* of Osmosin (114[C]).

Eye There is a great deal of uncertainty regarding the degree to which indometacin can be considered retinotoxic, despite the suggestion that patients undergoing prolonged therapy should be periodically monitored by ophthalmic examinations. A recent report on indometacin *retinopathy* has added more doubts than certainty to this problem (115[Cr]).

Instillation of indometacin ophthalmic solution after implantation surgery seems to delay the *wound healing* process (116[C]).

Risk situations Although the use of NSAID to treat sports injuries is not uncommon, it can be dangerous in some *athletes*, as illustrated by the following case-report:

A 22-year-old athlete in training for a marathon, received 100 mg/d of indometacin for 2 weeks. He complained only of excessive fatigue and a laboratory control showed a *high serum potassium* level (6.4 mmol/l) and an ECG revealed peaked T-waves. Indometacin was withdrawn and serum potassium gradually returned to normal.

Competing in a marathon in warm weather while hyperkalemic could put athletes at risk of serious arrhythmias (117[C]).

Sulindac *(SED-11, 180; SEDA-12, 84; SEDA-13, 79)*

Risk situations *Hyponatremia* has been reported in an elderly patient on a *salt-restricted* diet when treated with sulindac (118[C]). Individuals in a state of sodium depletion are at risk of developing hyponatremia with all NSAID.

ARYLALKANOIC ACID DERIVATIVES AND RELATED COMPOUNDS *(SED-11, 181; SEDA-12, 84; SEDA-13, 79)*

Diclofenac *(SED-11, 184; SEDA-12, 85; SEDA-13, 80)*

Gastrointestinal *Perforation of the terminal ileum* occurred in a patient who had taken an excessive dose (400 mg/d) of controlled-release diclofenac (119[C]).

Fenbufen *(SED-11, 186; SEDA-12, 85; SEDA-13, 80)*

Hematological Several NSAID cause *hemo-*

lytic anemia (120[R]) and a case caused by fenbufen has been reported (121[C]). In some cases hemolytic anemia is accompanied by signs of hypersensitivity (122[C]).

Skin Concern continues to be expressed regarding the high reporting rate of *cutaneous adverse reactions* with fenbufen (123[c], 124[c]), as some of them can be *life-threatening* (SEDA-13, 72).

Hypersensitivity A very severe hypersensitivity reaction has been described in a young woman 4 days after stopping a 10-day course of fenbufen. The reaction was characterized by *generalized erythematous exfoliative rash, fever*, generalized *lymphadenopathy* and *jaundice*. Laboratory investigation revealed eosinophilia, marked elevation of liver enzymes and bilirubin and signs of *autoimmune hemolytic anemia*. Recovery was slow but complete (121[C]).

Fenoprofen *(SED-11, 183; SEDA-12, 85; SEDA-13, 81)*

Skin Two cases of *toxic epidermal necrolysis* have been described. The onset of skin eruption was on the 12th and 16th days of fenoprofen therapy and was accompanied by high fever (125[C]).

Ibuprofen *(SED-11, 182; SEDA-12, 86; SEDA-13, 81)*

Gastrointestinal *Ulcerative proctitis* in a young girl with systemic lupus erythematosus, probably attributable to ibuprofen therapy, has been reported (126[C]).

Skin Two patients on ibuprofen developed a *bullous eruption* limited to non-sun-exposed areas of the lower extremities that resembled limited bullous pemphigoid, a reaction not previously documented to occur with ibuprofen (127[C]).

Hypersensitivity A severe hypersensitivity reaction to ibuprofen has been described in a young woman with systemic lupus erythematosus. The reaction, confirmed by rechallenge, was characterized by *meningitis* (aseptic), *hypotension, fever, conjunctivitis, arthralgias* and *leukopenia*. The patient had been taking ibuprofen for over 2 years without problems (128[C]).

Ketoprofen *(SED-11, 183; SEDA-12, 86; SEDA-13, 81)*

Interactions The risk of acute renal failure from interaction between NSAID and triamterene is well documented (SEDA-12, 80) and this co-administration should be avoided. *Irreversible renal failure* resulting in *death* occurred in an 84-year-old man who received ketoprofen for 7 days along with triamterene (100 mg/d) plus hydrochlorothiazide (50 mg/d (129[C]).

Ketorolac *(SEDA-12, 86)*

Hematological The drug is able to prolong bleeding time in a similar way to aspirin, but when ketorolac is eliminated from the body the effect on hemostasis disappears as well. Injection site ecchymosis seems to be more frequent than with other analgesic drugs (130[c]). Ketorolac crosses the placental barrier and can significantly inhibit the platelet aggregation induced by both collagen and arachidonic acid in neonates whose mother received ketorolac 10 mg i.m. for analgesia during labor (131[c]). Ketorolac should therefore not be used in pregnant patients whose neonates are at risk for hemorrhagic problems.

Gastrointestinal Parenteral administration of ketorolac tromethamine caused *gastric damage* (erosion and ulcers) in healthy volunteers during a short-term endoscopic study (64[c]). Gastric damage appeared to be dose-related.

Naproxen *(SED-11, 184; SEDA-12, 87; SEDA-13, 82)*

Among 586 otherwise healthy rheumatoid arthritis patients receiving 6 months of naproxen therapy at dosages of 750–1500 mg/d, there was no laboratory or clinical evidence which suggested a pattern of adverse hepatic or renal effects (132[c]).

Nervous system *Aseptic meningitis* can occur, albeit rarely, during NSAID therapy, particularly in patients affected by connective tissue disease. A young healthy man suffered from aseptic meningitis 1 week after starting naproxen and cyclobenzaprine therapy for neck pain. Clinically the patient's presentation resembled the majority of the cases of NSAID-induced aseptic meningitis and no cases of cyclobenzaprine-associated aseptic meningitis have been reported. The reaction can therefore probably be attributed to naproxen (133[Cr]).

Tolmetin *(SED-11, 185; SEDA-12, 90; SEDA-13, 82)*

The safety of tolmetin was evaluated in a follow-up study of all patients who were admitted to hospital within 90 days of having a prescription for tolmetin. Almost 25 000 prescriptions were filled for tolmetin during the study period with 692 *hospitalizations*. Tolmetin-induced illness serious enough to cause hospitalization was found in only 2 cases (drug fever and membranous glomerulopathy) (134[C]).

Hypersensitivity Tolmetin has been accused of causing more anaphylactic reactions than do other NSAID (SEDA-7, 134). A retrospective study conducted between 1980 and 1984 evaluated 128 844 subjects receiving 6 different NSAID and found that tolmetin is associated with a *risk of hypersensitivity* reactions similar to that of other NSAID (135[C]).

ANTHRANILIC ACID DERIVATIVES *(SED-11, 190; SEDA-12, 90; SEDA-13, 82)*

Glafenine *(SED-11, 190; SEDA-12, 90; SEDA-13, 82)*

Liver Cases of glafenine kidney stones have been reported (SEDA- 9, 93) and now a case-report on a woman who presented with *choledocholithiases* essentially composed of glafenic acid has been published. The patient had taken glafenine at a dose of 400 mg/d for approximately 12 years (136[c]).

Interactions Interaction with *methotrexate* has been described for many NSAID and glafenine can probably be added to the list (137[C]).

Meclofenamate *(SED-11, 189)*

Steatorrhea has repeatedly been reported after mefenamic acid (SEDA-2, 97). Meclofenamate too seems able to cause this side effect (138[C]).

Mefenamic acid *(SED-11, 189; SEDA-12, 90; SEDA-13, 83)*

Urinary system New cases of *acute renal failure* caused by mefenamic acid have been described. As usual, the presenting symptoms were abdominal pain, diarrhea and vomiting. Renal biopsy showed interstitial nephritis, mesangial proliferation and focal pedicel fusion, a previously undescribed finding (139[C]).

Overdosage Mefenamic acid overdose is characterized by CNS symptoms (SEDA-13, 83). A new case of overdose in an elderly woman who took 50 g of mefenamic acid presenting with *coma* and *brainstem signs* has been described (140[c]).

Niflumic acid *(SED-11, 189; SEDA-13, 83)*

Musculoskeletal Acute *rhabdomyolysis* has been caused by another anthranilic acid derivative, glafenine (SEDA-10, 84), and niflumic acid appears to provoke the same side effect (141[C]).

OXICAM DERIVATIVES *(SED-11, 191; SEDA-12, 91; SEDA-13, 83)*

Piroxicam *(SED-11, 191; SEDA-12, 91; SEDA-13, 83)*

Hematological *Agranulocytosis* due to piroxicam was documented in a 65-year-old woman who was treated with the drug for 3 days. Recovery was complete within 12 days from stopping therapy (142[C]).

Urinary system *Acute renal failure* due to diffuse interstitial nephritis which resulted in *death* has been described in a 32-year-old man who took piroxicam for seronegative arthritis for 3 months (143[c]).

Tenoxicam *(SED-11, 192; SEDA-12, 93; SEDA-13, 83)*

International experience with tenoxicam in comparison with piroxicam has been presented. The side effects profile of both drugs was virtually identical, although tenoxicam seemed to cause slightly fewer serious gastrointestinal side effects (144[R]).

MISCELLANEOUS DRUGS

Diacerein

Experience with this anthraquinone derivative is very limited. The drug is supposed to be free of adverse gastrointestinal effects but, in a comparative study with naproxen in patients with osteoarthritis, *gastrointestinal* side effects (epigastric pain and diarrhea) were the most frequently reported with both drugs (145[c]).

Nimesulide *(SED-11, 193)*

Hematological *Thrombocytopenia* occurred in a patient with HIV infection when nimesulide was administered for a few days for periodontal abscess. Platelet count rapidly increased to normal values when therapy was interrupted (146[C]).

Orgotein *(SED-11, 193; SEDA-12, 94)*

A new case-report on *anaphylactic shock* following a submucosal bladder injection of orgotein has been described (147[C]).

DRUGS USED IN THE TREATMENT OF GOUT *(SED-11, 194; SEDA-12, 94; SEDA-13, 54)*

Allopurinol *(SED-11, 194; SEDA-12, 94; SEDA-13, 84)*

Skin An unusual cutaneous reaction has been described in a 69-year-old man 15 days after having started allopurinol for asymptomatic hyperuricemia. The lesions consisted of *papules* or *plaques* on the neck and trunk and a violaceous indurated nodule on the face. Biopsy showed *benign lymphocytic infiltration.* The lesions disappeared spontaneously after stopping treatment (148[C]).

Hypersensitivity Cutaneous manifestations are a constant finding in the allopurinol hypersensitivity syndrome (SEDA-11, 195), but a syndrome without cutaneous reaction occurred in a patient who was also receiving deoxycoformycin (149[C]).

REFERENCES

1. Soll AH, Kurata J, McGuigan JE (1989) Ulcers, nonsteroidal antiinflammatory drugs, and related matters. *Gastroenterology, 96*, 561.
2. Ivey KJ, Rooney PJ (1989) Nonsteroidal anti-inflammatory drugs and the gastrointestinal tract. In: Rooney PJ (Ed.), *Baillière's Clinical Rheumatology, Vol. 3*, p. 393. Baillière Tindall, London.
3. Butt JH, Barthel JS, Moore RA (1988) Clinical spectrum of the upper gastrointestinal effects of nonsteroidal antiinflammatory drugs. *Am. J. Med., 84 (Suppl. 2A)*, 5.
4. Langman MJS (1989) Epidemiologic evidence on the association between peptic ulceration and antiinflammatory drug use. *Gastroenterology, 96*, 640.
5. Roth SH (1988) Nonsteroidal anti-inflammatory drugs: gastropathy, deaths and medical practice. *Ann. Intern. Med., 109*, 353.
6. Roth SH (1988) NSAIDs: risk–benefit versus cost–benefit. *Drug Inf. J., 22*, 477.
7. Graham DY, Smith JL (1988) Gastroduodenal complications of chronic NSAID therapy. *Am. J. Gastroenterol., 83*, 1081.
8. Roth SH (1988) NSAID and gastropathy: a rheumatologist's review. *J. Rheumatol., 15*, 912.
9. Roth SH, Bennett RE (1987) Nonsteroidal antiinflammatory drug gastropathy. *Arch. Intern. Med., 147*, 2093.
10. Rainsford KD (1988) Gastrointestinal damage from nonsteroidal anti-inflammatory drugs. *Toxicol. Pathol., 16*, 251.
11. Tenenbaum J (1987) Non-steroidal anti-inflammatory drugs (NSAIDs) cause gastrointestinal intolerance and major bleeding – or do they? *Clin. Invest. Med., 10*, 246.
12. Semble EL, Wu WC (1987) Antiinflammatory drugs and gastric mucosal damage. *Semin. Arthritis Rheum., 16*, 271.
13. Ivey KJ (1986) Gastrointestinal intolerance and bleeding with non-narcotic analgesics. *Drugs, 32 (Suppl. 4)*, 71.
14. Katzka DA, Sunshine AG, Cohen S (1987) The effect of nonsteroidal antiinflammatory drugs on upper gastrointestinal tract symptoms and mucosal integrity. *J. Clin. Gastroenterol., 9*, 142.
15. Caruso I, Bianchi Porro G (1980) Gastroscopic evaluation of antiinflammatory agents. *Br. Med. J., 280*, 75.

16. Morris AD, Holt SD, Silvoso GR et al (1981) Effect of anti-inflammatory drug administration in patients with rheumatoid arthritis: an endoscopic assessment. *Scand. J. Gastroenterol., 67 (Suppl.)*, 131.
17. Larkai EN, Smith JL, Lidsky MD et al (1987) Gastroduodenal mucosa and dyspeptic symptoms in arthritic patients during chronic nonsteroidal anti-inflammatory drug use. *Am. J. Gastroenterol., 82*, 1153.
18. Farah D, Sturrock RD, Russell RI (1988) Peptic ulcer in rheumatoid arthritis. *Ann. Rheum. Dis., 47*, 478.
19. McCarthy DM (1989) Nonsteroidal antiinflammatory drug-induced ulcers: management by traditional therapies. *Gastroenterology, 96*, 662.
20. Del Favero A, Patoia L (1989) Non-steroidal antiinflammatory drugs: seven year's experience in preparing an annual review. *Clin. Exp. Rheumatol., 7/S-3*, 171.
21. Hedenbro JL, Wetterberg P, Vallgren S et al (1988) Lack of correlation between fecal blood loss and drug-induced gastric mucosal lesions. *Gastrointest. Endosc., 34*, 247.
22. Lussier A, Arsenault A, Varady J et al (1988) The use of a ^{51}Cr technique to detect gastrointestinal microbleeding associated with nonsteroidal antiinflammatory drugs. *Semin. Arthritis Rheum., 17 (Suppl. 2)*, 40.
23. Collins AJ, DuToit JA (1987) Upper gastrointestinal findings and faecal occult blood in patients with rheumatic disease taking nonsteroidal antiinflammatory drugs. *Br. J. Rheumatol., 26*, 295.
24. Chalmers TC, Berrier J, Hewitt P et al (1988) Meta-analysis of randomized controlled trials as a method of estimating rare complications of non-steroidal antiinflammatory drug therapy. *Aliment. Pharmacol. Ther., 2 (Suppl. 1)*, 9.
25. Doherty M, Hunt RH, Langman MJS et al (1987) Management of NSAID induced gastrointestinal disturbance. *Ann. Rheumatic Dis., 46*, 640.
26. Skander MP, Ryan FP (1988) Non-steroidal antiinflammatory drugs and pain free peptic ulceration in the elderly. *Br. Med. J., 297*, 833.
27. Rossi AC, Hsu JP, Faich GA (1987) Ulcerogenecity of piroxicam: an analysis of spontaneously reported data. *Br. Med. J., 294*, 147.
28. Griffin TP (1986) Survey of the spontaneous adverse reactions reporting schemes in fifteen countries. *Br. J. Clin. Pharmacol., 22 (Suppl. 1)*, 83.
29. Duggan JM, Dobson AJ, Johnson H et al (1986) Peptic ulcer and non-steroidal anti-inflammatory agents. *Gut, 27*, 929.
30. McIntosh JH, Byth K, Piper DW (1985) Environmental factors in aetiology of chronic gastric ulcer: a case control study of exposure variables before the first symptom. *Gut, 26*, 789.
31. McIntosh JH, Fung CS, Berry G et al (1988) Smoking, nonsteroidal anti-inflammatory drugs, and acetaminophen in gastric ulcer: a study of associations and of the effects of previous diagnosis on exposure patterns. *Am. J. Epidemiol., 128*, 761.
32. Taylor RT, Huskisson EC, Whitehouse GH et al (1968) Gastric ulceration occurring during indomethacin therapy. *Br. Med. J., 4*, 734.
33. Gleeson MH (1982) A survey of peptic ulcers associated with NSAIDs. *Eur. J. Rheumatol. Inflammation, 5*, 308.
34. Clinch D, Banerjee AK, Ostick G et al (1983) Nonsteroidal anti-inflammatory drugs and gastrointestinal adverse effects. *J. R. Coll. Physicians London, 17*, 228.
35. Bianchi Porro G, Pace F (1988) Ulcerogenic drugs and upper gastrointestinal bleeding. In: *Baillière's Clinical Gastroenterology, Vol. 2*, 309. Baillière Tindall, London.
36. Kurata JH (1989) Ulcer epidemiology: an overview and proposed research framework. *Gastroenterology, 96*, 569.
37. Collier DStJ, Pain JA (1985) Non steroidal antiinflammatory drugs and peptic ulcer perforation. *Gut, 26*, 359.
38. Armstrong CP, Blower AL (1987) Non-steroidal antiinflammatory drugs and life threatening complications of peptic ulceration. *Gut, 28*, 527.
39. Somerville K, Faulkner G, Langman M (1986) Non-steroidal anti-inflammatory drugs and bleeding peptic ulcer. *Lancet, 1*, 462.
40. Bartle WR, Gupta AK, Lazor J (1986) Non steroidal antiinflammatory drugs and gastrointestinal bleeding: a case control study. *Arch. Intern. Med., 146*, 2365.
41. Levy M, Miller DR, Kaufman DW et al (1988) Major upper gastrointestinal tract bleeding. *Arch. Intern. Med., 148*, 281.
42. Fries JF, Miller SR, Spitz PW et al (1989) Toward an epidemiology of gastropathy associated with nonsteroidal antiinflammatory drug use. *Gastroenterology, 96*, 647.
43. Griffin MR, Ray WA, Schaffner W (1988) Nonsteroidal antiinflammatory drug use and death from peptic ulcer in elderly persons. *Ann. Intern. Med., 109*, 359.
44. Guess HA, West R, Strand LM et al (1988) Fatal upper gastrointestinal hemorrhage or perforation among users and non-users of nonsteroidal anti-inflammatory drugs in Saskatchewan, Canada 1983. *J. Clin. Epidemiol., 41*, 35.
45. Henry DA, Johnston A, Dobson A et al (1987) Fatal peptic ulcer complications and the use of nonsteroidal anti-inflammatory drugs, aspirin, and corticosteroids. *Br. Med. J., 295*, 1227.
46. Inman WHW (1985) Comparative study of five NSAIDs. *PEM News, 3*, 3.
47. Jick H, Feld AD, Perera DR (1985) Certain nonsteroidal antiinflammatory drugs and hospitalization for upper gastrointestinal bleeding. *Pharmacotherapy, 5*, 280.

48. Beard K, Walker AM, Perera DR et al (1987) Nonsteroidal anti-inflammatory drugs and hospitalization for gastroesophageal bleeding in the elderly. *Arch. Intern. Med., 147*, 1621.
49. Jick SS, Perera DR, Walker AM et al (1987) Non-steroidal anti-inflammatory drugs and hospital admission for perforated peptic ulcer. *Lancet, 2*, 380.
50. Carson JL, Strom BL, Soper KA et al (1987) The association of nonsteroidal anti-inflammatory drugs with upper gastrointestinal tract bleeding. *Arch. Intern. Med., 147*, 85.
51. Bloom BS (1988) Direct medical costs of disease and gastrointestinal side effects during treatment for arthritis. *Am. J. Med., 84 (Suppl. 2A)*, 20.
52. Semble EL, Turner RA, Wu WC (1987) Clinical and genetic characteristics of upper gastrointestinal disease in rheumatoid arthritis. *J. Rheumatol., 14*, 692.
53. Champion GD (1988) Therapeutic usage of the non-steroidal anti-inflammatory drugs. *Med. J. Aust., 149*, 203.
54. Doherty M (1989) Non-steroidal anti-inflammatory drugs in patients with peptic ulcer disease: to be considered in certain circumstances. *Br. Med. J., 298*, 178.
55. Malone DE, McCormick PA, Daly I et al (1986) Peptic ulcer in rheumatoid arthritis – intrinsic or related to drug therapy? *Br. J. Rheumatol., 25*, 342.
56. Carson JL, Strom BL, Morse ML et al (1987) The relative gastrointestinal toxicity of the nonsteroidal antiinflammatory drugs. *Arch. Intern. Med., 147*, 1054.
57. Lanza FL (1984) Endoscopic studies of gastric and duodenal injury after the use of ibuprofen, aspirin and other non-steroidal anti-inflammatory agents. *Am. J. Med., 77*, 19.
58. Schoen RT, Vender RJ (1989) Mechanisms of nonsteroidal anti-inflammatory drug-induced gastric damage. *Am. J. Med., 86*, 449.
59. Graham DY (1989) Prevention of gastroduodenal injury induced by chronic nonsteroidal antiinflammatory drug therapy. *Gastroenterology, 96*, 675.
60. Levine RA, Petokas S, Nandi J et al (1988) Effects of nonsteroidal, antiinflammatory drugs on gastrointestinal injury and prostanoid generation in healthy volunteers. *Dig. Dis. Sci., 33*, 660.
61. Taha AS, McLaughlin S, Holland PJ et al (1989) Prevention of NSAID-induced gastric ulcer with prostaglandin analogues. *Lancet, 1*, 52.
62. Redfern JS, Lee E, Feldman M (1987) Effect of indomethacin on gastric mucosal prostaglandins in humans: correlation with mucosal damage. *Gastroenterology, 92*, 969.
63. Biour M, Blanquart A, Moore N et al (1987) Incidence of NSAID-related, severe gastrointestinal bleeding. *Lancet, 2*, 340.
64. Lanza FL, Karlin DA, Yee JP (1987) A double-blind placebo controlled endoscopic study comparing the mucosal injury seen with orally and parenterally administered nonsteroidal analgesic Ketorolac tromethamine at therapeutic and supratherapeutic doses (Abstract). *Am. J. Gastroenterol., 82*, 939.
65. Hansen T, Matzen P, Madsen P (1984) Endoscopic evaluation of the effect of indomethacin capsules and suppositories on the gastric mucosa in rheumatic patients. *J. Rheumatol., 11*, 484.
66. Collins AJ, Davies J, Dixon AStJ (1988) A prospective endoscopic study of the effect of Orudis and Oruval on the upper gastrointestinal tract in patients with osteoarthritis. *Br. J. Rheumatol., 27*, 106.
67. Bluhm GB, MacIlwain HH, Offen WW (1988) Enteric-coated fenoprofen in large-joint osteoarthritis. *Henry Ford Hosp. Med. J., 36*, 56.
68. Trondstad RI, Aadland E, Holler J et al (1985) Gastroscopic findings after treatment with enteric-coated and plain naproxen tablets in healthy subjects. *Scand. J. Gastroenterol., 20*, 239.
69. Patoia L, Clausi G, Farroni F et al (1989) Comparison of faecal blood loss, upper gastrointestinal mucosal integrity and symptoms after piroxicam beta-cyclodextrin, piroxicam and placebo administration. *Eur. J. Clin. Pharmacol., 36*, 599.
70. Rachmilewitz D, Polak D, Eliakim R et al (1986) Cimetidine significantly decreased indomethacin induced gastroduodenal mucosal damage (Abstract). *Gastroenterology, 90*, 1596.
71. Lanza FL, Aspinall RL, Swabb EA et al (1988) Double-blind placebo-controlled endoscopic comparison of the mucosal protective effects of misoprostol versus cimetidine on tolmetin-induced mucosal injury to the stomach and duodenum. *Gastroenterology, 95*, 289.
72. Dammann HG, Simon-Schultz J, Bauermeister W et al (1989) Prevention of NSAID-induced gastric ulcer with prostaglandin analogues. *Lancet, 1*, 52.
73. Bianchi Porro G, Pace F, Caruso I (1987) Why are non-steroid anti-inflammatory drugs important in peptic ulceration? *Aliment. Pharmacol. Ther., 1*, 540S.
74. Ehsanullah RSB, Page MC, Tildesley G et al (1988) Prevention of gastroduodenal damage induced by non-steroidal anti-inflammatory drugs: controlled trial of ranitidine. *Br. Med. J., 297*, 1017.
75. Lanza F, Robinson M, Bowers J et al (1988) A multi-center double-blind comparison of ranitidine vs placebo in the prophylaxis of NSAID induced lesions in gastric and duodenal mucosa (Abstract). *Gastroenterology, 94*, A250.
76. Stalnikowicz R, Goldin E, Fich A et al (1989) Indomethacin-induced gastroduodenal damage is not affected by cotreatment with ranitidine. *J. Clin. Gastroenterol., 11*, 178.
77. Roth SH, Bennett RE, Mitchell CS et al (1987) Cimetidine therapy in nonsteroidal anti-inflammatory drug gastropathy: double-blind long-term evaluation. *Arch. Intern. Med., 147*, 1798.
78. Stalnikowicz R, Pollak D, Eliakim A et al

(1988) Cimetidine decreases indomethacin induced duodenal mucosal damage in patients with acute musculoskeletal disorders. *Gut, 29*, 1578.

79. Aadland E, Fausa O, Vatn M et al (1987) Protection by misoprostol against naproxen-induced gastric mucosal damage. *Am. J. Med., 83 (Suppl. 1A)*, 37.

80. Lanza FL (1986) A double-blind study of prophylactic effect of misoprostol on lesions of gastric and duodenal mucosa induced by oral administration of tolmetin in healthy subjects. *Dig. Dis. Sci., 31 (Suppl. 2)*, 1315.

81. Graham DY, Agrawal NM, Roth SH (1988) Prevention of NSAID-induced gastric ulcer with misoprostol: multicentre, double-blind, placebo-controlled trial. *Lancet, 2*, 1277.

82. Dammann HG, Simon-Schultz J, Bauermeister et al (1989) Prevention of NSAID-induced gastric ulcer with prostaglandin analogues. *Lancet, 1*, 52.

83. Auer IO (1986) Fortschritte und Perspektiven der Prophylaxe und Therapie gastrointestinaler Nebenwirkungen der medikamentösen Therapie mit nichtsteroidalen Antirheumatika. *Aktuel. Rheumatol., 11*, 211.

84. Mitchell WS, Sturrock RD (1982) Ulcers and antiinflammatory agents. *Br. Med. J., 284*, 731.

85. LoIudice TA, Saleem T, Lang JA (1981) Cimetidine in the treatment of gastric ulcer induced by steroidal and nonsteroidal anti-inflammatory agents. *Am. J. Gastroenterol., 75*, 104.

86. Croker JR, Cotton PB, Boyle AC et al (1980) Cimetidine for peptic ulcer in patients with arthritis. *Ann. Rheum. Dis., 39*, 275.

87. Davies J, Collins AJB, Dixon SA (1986) The influence of cimetidine on peptic ulcer in patients with arthritis taking anti-inflammatory drugs. *Br. J. Rheumatol., 25*, 54.

88. Manniche C, Malchow-Miler A, Andersen JR et al (1987) Randomised study of the influence of non-steroidal anti-inflammatory drugs on the treatment of peptic ulcer in patients with rheumatic disease. *Gut, 28*, 226.

89. Caldwell JR, Roth SH, Wu WC et al (1987) Sucralfate treatment of nonsteroidal anti-inflammatory drug-induced gastrointestinal symptoms and mucosal damage. *Am. J. Med., 83 (Suppl. 3B)*, 74.

90. Bijlsma JWJ (1988) Treatment of endoscopy negative NSAID-induced upper gastrointestinal symptoms with cimetidine – an international multicenter collaborative study. *Aliment. Pharmacol. Ther., 2 (Suppl. 2)*, 75.

91. Bijlsma JWJ (1988) Treatment of NSAID-induced gastrointestinal lesions with cimetidine – an international multicenter collaborative study. *Aliment. Pharmacol. Ther., 2 (Suppl. 2)*, 85.

92. Simon B, Beckers K-H, Biewer W et al (1988) Ranitidin in der Therapie NSA-induzierter Schleimhautschäden an Magen und Duodenum. *Z. Gastroenterol., 26*, 310.

93. Stock K-P, Bach GL (1988) Ulkusabheilung unter Ranitidin und Antazida trotz fortgesetzter Therapie mit nichtsteroidalen Antirheumatika. *Z. Rheumatol., 47*, 656.

94. Shepherd HA, Fine D, Hillier K et al (1989) Effect of sucralfate and cimetidine on rheumatoid patients with active gastroduodenal lesions who are taking nonsteroidal antiinflammatory drugs: a pilot study. *Am. J. Med., 86 (Suppl. 6A)*, 49.

95. Anonymous (1988) Misoprostol: ulcer prophylaxis at what cost? *Lancet, 2*, 1293.

96. Reynolds JC (1989) Famotodine therapy for active duodenal ulcers. *Ann. Intern. Med., 111*, 7.

97. Hawkey C (1989) Non-steroidal anti-inflammatory drugs in patients with peptic ulcer disease: rarely justified in terms of cost or patient benefit. *Br. Med. J., 298*, 177.

98. McCrea JB, Vlasses PH, Rocci Jr ML (1989) Allergic reaction to antipyrine, a marker of hepatic enzyme activity. *Ann. Pharmacother., 23*, 38.

99. Anonymous (1989) *Dipyrone: A Drug No One Needs*. Health Action International-Europe and BUKO Pharma Campaign.

100. Kiatboonsri P, Richter J (1988) Unethical trials of dipyrone in Thailand. *Lancet, 2*, 1491.

101. Kiatboonsri P, Richter J (1989) Dipyrone trials in Thailand. *Lancet, 2*, 107.

102. Wood N, Pall HS, Williams AC et al (1988) Extrapyramidal reactions to anti-inflammatory drugs. *J. Neurol. Neurosurg. Psychiatry, 51*, 731.

103. Tcn LO, Dymock IW (1988) Azapropazone induced hepatitis. *Br. Med. J., 297*, 1614.

104. Gotzsche PC (1989) Patients' preference in indomethacin trials: an overview. *Lancet, 1*, 88.

105. Nelson C-E, Nylander C, Olsson AM et al (1988) Rectal v. intravenous administration of indomethacin in the treatment of renal colic. *Acta Chir. Scand., 154*, 253.

106. Sheehan GJ, Kutzner MR, Chin WD (1989) Acute asthma attack due to ophthalmic indomethacin. *Ann. Intern. Med., 111*, 337.

107. Nuotto E, Saarialho-Kere U (1988) Actions and interactions of indomethacin and diazepam on performance in healthy volunteers. *Pharmacol. Toxicol., 62*, 293.

108. Pullar T, Myall O, Haigh JRM et al (1988) The effect of indomethacin on the psychomotor function of patients with rheumatic diseases. *Br. J. Rheumatol., 27*, 227.

109. Cappell MS, Kozicky O, Competiello LS (1988) Indomethacin-associated cholestasis. *J. Clin. Gastroenterol., 10*, 445.

110. Rashad S, Hemingway A, Rainsford K et al (1989) Effect of non-steroidal anti-inflammatory drugs on the course of osteoarthritis. *Lancet, 2*, 519.

111. Moise Jr KJ, Huhta JC, Sharif DS et al (1988) Indomethacin in the treatment of premature labor: effects on the fetal ductus arteriosus. *N. Engl. J. Med., 319*, 327.

112. Walters M (1988) Tolerance of intravenous indomethacin treatment for premature infants with patent ductus arteriosus. *Br. Med. J.*, *297*, 773.
113. Herson VC, Krause PJ, Eisenfeld LI et al (1988) Indomethacin-associated sepsis in very-low-birth-weight infants. *Am. J. Dis. Child.*, *142*, 555.
114. Bem JL, Mann RD, Coulson R (1988) Fatal gastrointestinal damage associated with the use of osmotic mini pump indomethacin (osmosin). *Pharm. Med.*, *3*, 35.
115. Graham CM, Blach RK (1988) Indomethacin retinopathy: case report and review. *Br. J. Ophthalmol.*, *72*, 434.
116. Miyatani H (1988) Indomethacin eyedrops reduce inflammation after ocular lens implantation. *Jpn. J. Clin. Ophthalmol.*, *42*, 419.
117. Johnson RB (1989) Use of NSAIDs in long distance runners: a risk factor for sudden death? *South. Med. J.*, *82*, 95.
118. Chamontin B, Fille A, Salva P et al (188) Does selective inhibition of prostaglandins exist? Concerning a case of hyponatremia with sulindac. *Presse Méd.*, *17*, 2140.
119. Deakin M (1988) Small bowel perforation associated with an excessive dose of slow release diclofenac sodium. *Br. Med. J.*, *297*, 488.
120. Sanford-Driscoll M, Knodell C (1986) Induction of haemolytic anaemia by non-steroidal anti-inflammatory drugs. *Drug Intell. Clin. Pharm.*, *20*, 925.
121. Martland T, Stone WD (1988) Haemolytic anaemia associated with fenbufen. *Br. Med. J.*, *297*, 921.
122. Muthiah MM (1988) Severe hypersensitivity reaction to fenbufen. *Br. Med. J.*, *297*, 1614.
123. Committee on Safety of Medicines (1988) *Current Problems, No. 23.*
124. Edwards IR (1988) Fenbufen: adverse reactions affecting the skin. *NZ Med. J.*, *101*, 550.
125. Stotts JS, Fang ML, Dannaker CS et al (1988) Fenoprofen induced toxic epidermal necrolysis. *J. Am. Acad. Dermatol.*, *18*, 755.
126. Khovry MI (1989) Ulcerative proctitis in juvenile systemic lupus erythematosus after ibuprofen treatment. *J. Rheumatol.*, *16*, 217.
127. Laing VB, Sherertz EF, Flowers FP (1988) Pemphigoid-like bullous eruption related to ibuprofen. *J. Am. Acad. Dermatol.*, *19*, 91.
128. Mandell BF, Raps EC (1987) Severe systemic hypersensitivity reaction to ibuprofen occurring after prolonged therapy. *Am. J. Med.*, *82*, 817.
129. Pazmino PA, Pazmino PB (1988) Ketoprofen induced irreversible renal failure. *Nephron*, *50*, 70.
130. Conrad KA, Fagan TC, Mackie MJ et al (1988) Effects of ketorolac tromethamine on hemostasis in volunteers. *Clin. Pharmacol. Ther.*, *43*, 542.
131. Greer IA, Johnston J, Tulloch I et al (1988) Effect of maternal ketorolac administration on platelet function in the newborn. *Eur. J. Obstet. Gynecol. Reprod. Biol.*, *29*, 257.
132. Turner R (1988) Hepatic and renal tolerability of long-term naproxen treatment in patients with rheumatoid arthritis. *Semin. Arthritis Rheum.*, *17*, 29.
133. Sylvia LM, Forlenza SW, Brocavish JM (1988) Aseptic meningitis associated with naproxen. *Drug Intell. Clin. Pharm.*, *22*, 399.
134. Jick H, Jick SS, Hunter JR et al (1989) Follow-up study of tolmetin users. *Pharmacotherapy*, *9*, 91.
135. Strom BL, Carson JL, Schinnar R et al (1988) The effect of indication on the risk of hypersensitivity reactions associated with tolmetin sodium vs other nonsteroidal antiinflammatory drugs. *J. Rheumatol.*, *15*, 695.
136. Moesch C, Gainant A, Sautereau D (1988) Lithiase biliaire de glafénine: identification par spectrophotométrie infrarouge. *Gastroentérol. Clin. Biol.*, *12*, 387.
137. Dubost JJ, Bauvezie B (1988) Fatal bone marrow toxicity in a patient treated with methotrexate and glafenine for rheumatoid arthritis. *Clin. Exp. Rheumatol.*, *6*, 97.
138. Moeller DD (1987) Steatorrhea associated with meclofenamate sodium therapy. *Am. J. Gastroenterol.*, *82*, 1320.
139. Jenkins DAS, Harrison DJ, MacDonald MK et al (1988) Mefenamic acid nephropathy: an interstitial and mesangial lesion. *Nephrol. Dial. Transplant.*, *2* 217.
140. Hendrickse MT (1988) Mefenamic acid overdose mimicking brainstem stroke. *Lancet*, *2*, 1019.
141. Desvignes V, Fialip J, Palcoux TB et al (1988) Niflumic acid and rhabdomyolysis. *Thérapie*, *43*, 429.
142. Garcia S, Belda J, Linares J et al (1988) Piroxicam-induced agranulocytosis. *Drug Intell. Clin. Pharm.*, *22*, 1003.
143. Sarma PSA (1989) Fatal acute renal failure after piroxicam. *Clin. Nephrol.*, *31*, 54.
144. Bird HA (1988) International experience with tenoxicam: a review. *Scand. J. Rheumatol., Suppl. 73*, 22.
145. Marcolongo R, Fioravanti A, Adami S et al (1988) Efficacy and tolerability of diacerhein in the treatment of osteoarthrosis. *Curr. Ther. Res.*, *43*, 878.
146. Pasticci MB, Menichetti F, Di Candido F (1990) Nimesulide, thrombocytopenic purpura, and human immunodeficiency virus (HIV) infection. *Ann. Intern. Med.*, *112*, 233.
147. Von Maier U, Zechner O (1988) Therapie der Strahlenblase mit Orgotein (Peroxinom). *Z. Urol. Nephrol.*, *61*, 305.
148. Raymond JZ, Goldman HM (1988) An unusual cutaneous reaction secondary to allopurinol. *Cutis*, *41*, 323.
149. Steinmetz JC, DeConti R, Ginsburg R (1989) Hypersensitivity vasculitis associated with 2-deoxycoformycin and allopurinol therapy. *Am. J. Med.*, *86*, 499.

M. Malinge and C. Larousse

11 General anesthetics and therapeutic gases

GENERAL TOPICS

Risk factors *(SED-11, 205; SEDA-12, 101; SEDA-13, 89)* *Underlying disease* The risk of myocardial infarction in surgical patients with *ischemic heart disease* depends on a variety of factors (1[R]). The role of anesthetic technique is unsettled (2[R]). Large prospective studies in subjects undergoing coronary revascularization did not point to the choice of pre-bypass anesthetics as an independent risk factor (3[C], 4[C]). The importance of close pharmacological control of tachycardia (3[C]) and the need for selective trials in patients with steal-prone coronary anatomy (5[C]) have been stressed. The ability of calcium antagonists, when taken chronically, to protect against perioperative myocardial ischemia is questionable (6[C], 7[C]).

The issue of the safety of non-barbiturate hypnotic agents other than propanidid in patients with *hepatic porphyria* is a difficult one. Conflicting data have been presented concerning ketamine, benzodiazepines and etomidate (8[R]). The lack of porphyrogenicity of propofol is debated (8[R], 9[C], 10[C], 11[c]).

Inherited pediatric diseases may have specific anesthetic implications (12[R]). Cardiac involvement should be carefully sought in patients with Friedreich's ataxia (13[Cr]).

Drug interactions The case of a 64-year-old woman treated with *nifedipine* 30 mg/d who experienced 2 sequential cardiac arrests on induction of anesthesia (14[C]) demonstrates further that *calcium antagonists* may interact with anesthetic agents (15[R]).

Malignant hyperthermia *(SED-11, 205; SEDA-12, 101; SEDA-13, 89)* This topic remains a matter of concern (16[C]) and controversy (17[R]). Recent laboratory data suggest that the primary defect of susceptible muscle involves abnormal calcium release channels in the sarcoplasmic reticulum membrane system (18).

Association with myopathic disorders (19[C]–21[C]) and localized muscle weakness (22[c], 23[c]) continues to be noted. Duchenne muscular dystrophy was diagnosed in a 7-week-old infant who developed signs of both malignant hyperthermia and acute rhabdomyolysis following exposure to halothane and succinylcholine (24[C]).

While early recognition of presenting signs (increasing tachycardia, tachypnea and end-tidal CO_2) and prompt institution of dantrolene *therapy* (25[R]) are critical to outcome, not all surgical facilities have dantrolene available (26[C]). The combined use of calcium entry blockers and dantrolene can promote hyperkalemia and myocardial depression (27[Cr]). However, calcium therapy was effective in a 13-year-old boy who had a brief cardiac arrest due to uncontrollable hyperkalemia during malignant hyperthermia (28[C]).

Dantrolene *prophylaxis* can produce unpleasant side effects (29[C]). Limited prospective studies in malignant hyperthermia survivors and susceptible relatives suggest that it is usually not necessary, as long as a 'safe' anesthesia is used and there is close monitoring (30[CR], 31[C], 32[C]). Delayed crisis may occur in the postanesthetic period following dantrolene pretreatment (33[C]); a fatal case has been recently reported in a 5-year-old boy with myotonia congenita (19[C]).

The intrathecal use of contrast media such as metrizamide may be associated with clinical episodes resembling malignant hyperpyrexia (34[C]).

Neuropsychological complications *(SEDA-8, 119)* A within- and between group comparison of early and long-term mental recovery in

(Biomedical Division)
Side Effects of Drugs Annual 14
M.N.G. Dukes and L. Beeley, editors

105 patients randomized to receive either general or spinal/epidural anesthesia failed to detect any difference in the effect on outcome with respect to subjective psychologic status and performance in a range of memory and cognitive tasks (35[CR]).

Hypersensitivity reactions *(SED-11, 206; SEDA-12, 102; SEDA-13, 90)* The National Adverse Anaesthetic Reactions Advisory Service in the United Kingdom recorded 241 severe anaphylactoid responses to anesthesia over a 3-year period ending in 1987. Thiopental sodium and suxamethonium were involved in 79 and 50%, respectively, of the reported cases (36[C]). A fatal hypersensitivity reaction occurred following the thiopental–suxamethonium sequence in a 63-year-old woman. Disseminated intravascular thrombosis was found at postmortem (37[C]). That hypnotics may act in synergy with muscle relaxants to produce anaphylactoid symptoms is also suggested by the prevalence of skin reactions in patients receiving either thiopental (38[C], 39[c]) or propofol (40[C]) in combination with atracurium.

General anesthesia and pregnancy *(SED-11, 206; SEDA-12, 101; SEDA-13, 90)* Birth outcome data from a Swedish registry study for the period 1973–1981 pointed to an increased risk of low birth weight and early neonatal death in the subset of 5405 women operated on during pregnancy, regardless of the type of anesthesia (41[c]). However, general anesthesia emerged as an independent risk factor for low Apgar score and need for resuscitation as compared with regional anesthesia in a survey of 3940 neonates delivered by cesarean section in a general obstetric population (42[CR]).

Anesthetic morbidity and mortality *(SED-11, 207; SEDA-11, 108)* Evidence for an improved anesthesia outcome has been presented (43[C], 44[C], 45[c]). In their 5-year prospective survey of 40 240 pediatric anesthetics from 440 French institutions, Tiret et al (46[Cr]) noted 27 major complications of anesthesia, of which 12 resulted in cardiac arrest (3 per 10 000 cases). One death due to postanesthetic respiratory depression and 2 mild sequelae were noted. Respiratory mishaps during maintenance of anesthesia accounted primarily for the higher complication rate in infants less than 1 year of age (4.3 vs 0.5‰ in children), but anesthetic risk as a whole was closely related to the preoperative condition. Pedersen (47[C]) described 7306 consecutive anesthetics; 967 (i.e. 13%) were spinal or epidural. Regional blocks were involved in 13:43 (i.e. 30%) complications attributable to anesthesia, including 4 of 6 severe adverse outcomes (3 deaths and 3 myocardial infarctions), all in severely ill patients.

Case-analysis studies of rare occurrences in healthy patients may reveal unexpected hazards of anesthetic care. Thus, Caplan et al (48[C]) collected 14 cases of sudden cardiac arrest (all with substantial negative outcome) during spinal anesthesia over an 8-year period. Unsuspected respiratory insufficiency was deemed to be the causative factor. Eichorn (49[C]) analyzed 11 accidents followed by 5 deaths and 4 severe permanent injuries. He classified 8 of them as preventable ventilatory problems and suggested that ventilation monitoring may help in reducing the severity of accidental injury. Nevertheless, inadequate supervision of anesthesia was prominent in most cases.

Toxicity of inhalation anesthetics *(SED-12, 101; SEDA-13, 90)* Additional studies have investigated the potential hazards of anesthetic gases in operating room staff (50[C], 51[c], 52[c]). Stollery et al (53[CR]) found no evidence of acute cognitive dysfunction in 22 anesthetists who completed a variety of psychological tasks on the day of exposure in scavenged theatres by comparison with other places of work. In addition, there was no association between time-weighted exposure levels to either halothane or nitrous oxide and self-reported changes in arousal. The authors also evaluated the role of factors unrelated to exposure. Regular testing of liver function over a 2-year period in an anesthetist aged 54 years suggested that alanine aminotransferase activity varied according to the degree of occupational exposure to halothane (54[C]).

GASES *(SED-11, 206; SEDA-12, 102; SEDA-13, 90)*

Enflurane *(SED-11, 208; SEDA-12, 102; SEDA-13, 90)*

One case of *anaphylactoid* shock due to enflurane has been reported in a 36-year-old female patient. Rechallenge with enflurane was strongly positive and other investigations for drug hypersensitivity revealed a marked allergic tendency (55[c]).

Halothane *(SED-11, 209; SEDA-12, 108; SEDA-13, 91)*

Liver damage A fulminant form of halothane *hepatitis* with a favorable outcome occurred in a 34-year-old atopic man with a history of exposure 9 years previously (56[C]).

Severe post-halothane liver dysfunction has been reported in 2 middle-aged female patients anesthetized with halothane within 2 weeks after enflurane anesthesia (57[c]). An important study by Christ et al (58) demonstrated that the specific serum antibodies from patients with halothane hepatitis recognized the microsomal liver neoantigens induced by either halothane or enflurane in rats, suggesting that the bioactivation of both halogenated agents may produce the same immune response in susceptible individuals.

Isoflurane *(SED-11, 211; SEDA-12, 102; SEDA-13, 91)*

Cardiovascular effects Using intact myocardial tissue, Housmans and Murat (59) stated that the direct depressant effect of isoflurane on muscle contractility is clearly inferior to that of halothane and enflurane at equipotent anesthetic concentrations.

The administration of 1 MAC isoflurane was associated with a profound depression of the *baroresponses* to phenylephrine and nitroglycerine in 8 term neonates (60[C]).

The contention that isoflurane may cause *myocardial ischemia* in patients with critical coronary stenosis (61[R]) has been substantiated by Khambatta et al (62[C]). They compared the effects of 1 MAC isoflurane and halothane in conjunction with etomidate prior to bypass in 20 patients scheduled for coronary artery surgery. Seven out of 10 patients given isoflurane versus none in the halothane group had global or regional lactate production and 4 of them displayed ischemic changes on ECG despite similar reductions in coronary perfusion pressure, myocardial oxygen consumption and regional blood flow. The authors provided convincing evidence for redistribution of myocardial flow due to vasodilatation with isoflurane at equal levels of coronary perfusion pressure.

Miscellaneous *Malignant hyperthermia* occurred following isoflurane anesthesia in a 15-year-old girl who recovered after administration of dantrolene 10 mg/kg (63[C]).

Death following suicidal ingestion of 80 ml isoflurane in the recovery room has been reported in a 37-year-old heroin addict (64[c]).

Nitrous oxide *(SED-11, 207; SEDA-12, 102; SEDA-13, 92)*

A 50-year-old woman with a past history of ear disease developed *hearing loss* associated with bilateral tympanic membrane perforation following general anesthesia supplemented with nitrous oxide (65[C]).

INTRAVENOUS AGENTS *(SED-11, 211; SEDA-12, 103; SEDA-13, 92)*

Barbiturates *(SED-11, 211; SEDA-12, 103; SEDA-13, 92)*

Thiopental sodium A female patient aged 25 years developed progressive hand *ischemia* following intra-arterial injection of thiopental 2.5%. She recovered after a local administration of urokinase (66[Cr]). The use of lignocaine before thiopental injection is likely to reduce accidental arterial damage (67[c]).

Etomidate *(SED-11, 211; SEDA-12, 103; SEDA-13, 92)*

A 13-year-old asthmatic girl receiving prednisolone had a major *anaphylactoid* reaction to etomidate with bronchospasm and cardiac arrest. The outcome was favorable (68[C]).

A further instance of generalized *seizures* on recovery from short-term etomidate anesthesia in 36-year-old female with a past history of epilepsy has been mentioned (69[cr]).

Endocrine effects *(70[r])* The inhibitory effect of etomidate on *steroid* synthesis proved to be dose-dependent in man (71[C], 72[C]). The addition of etomidate 0.04 mg/kg for sedation before thiopental anesthesia flattened the cortisol and aldosterone responses to exogenous

ACTH, as measured 1 hour after induction in 20 patients scheduled for elective cardiac surgery (73[c]). Murat et al (74[CR]) found considerable serum accumulation of both deoxycortisol and deoxycorticosterone throughout 24 hour after etomidate infusion in a comparative study of 12 children given either etomidate (mean overall dose 4.6 mg/kg) or enflurane during epidural block for hypospadias or clubfoot repair.

One case of refractory *hypotension* ascribed to adrenocortical suppression has been reported in a 48-year-old man with alveolar proteinosis who had received 2 induction doses of etomidate within a 18-hour period for bronchial lavage. Blood pressure was restored after hydrocortisone therapy (75[C]). Whether the degree of adrenal suppression produced by single induction doses of etomidate can be detrimental in the context of major surgery is unresolved. In a series of 20 patients anesthetized with etomidate 0.3 mg/kg for colorectal surgery, Stuttmann et al (76[c]) noted less peroperative *volume requirement* in patients receiving hydrocortisone supplements.

Finally, Reddy et al (77[c]) assessed the adrenal response of neonates after administration of etomidate 0.3 mg/kg or thiopental 4 mg/kg to 22 fit women undergoing elective cesarean section. Serum cortisol levels were lower in etomidate-exposed infants at 1 hour post-delivery but no clinical consequences were detected up to 24 hours after birth.

Ketamine *(SED-11, 211; SEDA-12, 103; SEDA-13, 92; 78[R])*

Hamza et al (79[C]) found a significant decrease in the *ventilatory* response to carbon dioxide after induction of anesthesia with ketamine 2 mg/kg i.v. in 9 children aged 6–10 years.

Midazolam and injectable benzodiazepines *(SED-11, 212; SEDA-12, 103; SEDA-13, 92)*

A 67-year-old male patient with a large brain tumor experienced a fall in *blood pressure* and transient dysarthria after administration of midazolam 5 mg by the intramuscular route (80[c]).

Montravers et al (81[C]) studied the effects of midazolam 0.1 mg/kg i.v. on *airway* resistances in 7 healthy volunteers and showed that upper airway obstruction was critically implicated in drug-induced apneas.

When comparing oral midazolam 15 mg and temazepam 20 mg with placebo as premedication in 90 day-surgery patients, Hargreaves (82[C]) found similar anxiolysis in both treatment groups. Midazolam, however, produced marked *amnesia* and delayed recovery of *cognitive* function in comparison with temazepam and placebo.

A case of *seizure* during spinal anesthesia was temporally related to the administration of midazolam 2 mg i.v. in a healthy woman aged 27 years (83[c]). Lobo and Miwa (84[C]) reported a *rage* reaction following combined administration of midazolam 5 mg i.v. and morphine for endoscopy in a 31-year-old man with 'well-suppressed chronic anger'. Abrupt discontinuation of midazolam in a 53-year-old man who had received an average intravenous dose of 22 mg/d for 3 weeks in a postoperative intensive care unit resulted within a few hours in a *withdrawal* syndrome (arthralgias, tachycardia, fever and anxiety) relieved by reintroduction of the drug (85[C]).

A case-report by Brooks (86[c]) lent support to the use of midazolam in patients susceptible to malignant hyperthermia.

Flumazenil Selective placebo-controlled studies have examined the issue of the cardioventilatory safety of benzodiazepine antagonism in anesthesia.

Titrated doses of flumazenil (0.4–1 mg i.v.) did not affect *hemodynamic* variables and serum catecholamine levels in 20 patients sedated with midazolam during regional anesthesia for minor procedures (87[c]). This was confirmed by White et al (88[C]), who in addition found no change in either self-rated anxiety or serum levels of vasopressin and β-endorphin in a comparable patient population. Marty et al (89[C]) reported significant increases in both mean arterial and left ventricular end-diastolic pressures without major alteration of coronary circulation after incremental doses of flumazenil up to 1 mg in 11 patients with coronary artery disease who had received flunitrazepam for cardiac catheterization.

Flumazenil proved to be only partially effective in reversing the depressant effect of benzodiazepines on the *ventilatory* response to both isocapnic hypoxia (90[C]) and hypercarbia (91[C]). In addition, recurrent depression in carbon dioxide responsiveness was noted at 60–90 min after reversal of midazolam-induced sedation by 1 mg flumazenil (91[C], 92[C]).

Propofol *(SED-11, 212; SEDA-12, 103; SEDA-13, 93)*

Recent studies on the *cardiovascular* and *ventilatory* effects of intravenous anesthetics have focused on propofol (93[R]).

A 66-year-old male patient developed signs of *anaphylactic* shock on induction of anesthesia with propofol. True anaphylaxis was subsequently inferred from both histamine release testing and the serum titers of IgE antibodies to propofol; prick tests produced positive responses to propofol emulsion and propofol but not to the lipid solvent (94[C]). Serious delayed hypersensitivity reactions to propofol have been suspected in a 31-year-old man with a history of allergy (95[c]) and in a 48-year-old asthmatic woman (96[c]), but no laboratory support for drug allergy was provided.

When comparing propofol 18 mg/kg/h and enflurane 2.5% in 42 children undergoing strabismus surgery, Queinnec et al (97[C]) found a higher incidence of *oculocardiac reflex* in the propofol group (9:21 vs. 3:21).

Generalized *seizure* occurred during recovery from propofol anesthesia (total dose 5 mg/kg) in a healthy young man (98[c]). However, cross-over comparisons of low-dose propofol (1.3–1.6 mg/kg) and methohexital (1 mg/kg) in depressed patients requiring electroconvulsive therapy showed that propofol consistently reduced the clinical duration of fits (99[C], 100[C]) as well as the resulting hypertension (100[C]).

The *recovery* characteristics of propofol compared favorably with those of enflurane (101[C]) and isoflurane (102[C]) in the short outpatient setting. Korttila et al (103[C]) found similar emergence times in 60 unpremedicated patients given either propofol 100–200 μg/kg/min or enflurane 0.5–2% for major gynecological surgery. Propofol was associated with less *emetic* sequelae (23 vs. 63%) and dizziness in the recovery room; in addition, fewer patients in the propofol group complained of sadness, difficulty in concentrating and hunger in the 48 hours after anesthesia. By contrast, propofol did not provide any advantage over isoflurane in 40 patients undergoing major abdominal surgery (102[C]).

Hallucinations and sexual *disinhibition* have been occasionally reported following propofol anesthesia (104[r]).

Propofol was used safely in a patient with proven susceptibility to malignant hyperthermia (105[c]).

Interactions *Cholinergic drugs* may be hazardous in patients anesthetized with propofol:

A 54-year-old hypertensive woman taking a beta-blocker and a 46-year-old man susceptible to malignant hyperthermia, both without conduction defect, had intermittent episodes of ventricular asystole with persisting atrial activity when given suxamethonium and neostigmine, respectively, during propofol anesthesia. Sinus rhythm and blood pressure were restored after administration of anticholinergic drugs (106[C]). Induction of anesthesia with propofol followed by suxamethonium was associated with severe sinus bradycardia in 2 healthy unpremedicated female patients (107[C]).

REFERENCES

1. Haagensen R, Steen PA (1988) Perioperative myocardial infarction. *Br. J. Anaesth.*, *61*, 24.
2. Mangano DT (1989) Anesthetics, coronary artery disease, and outcome: unresolved controversies (Editorial). *Anesthesiology*, *70*, 175.
3. Slogoff S, Keats AS (1989) Randomized trial of primary anesthetic agents on outcome of coronary artery bypass operations. *Anesthesiology*, *70*, 179.
4. Tuman KJ, McCarthy RJ, Spiess BD et al (1989) Does choice of anesthetic agent significantly affect outcome after coronary surgery? *Anesthesiology*, *70*, 189.
5. Buffington CW, Davis KB, Gillespie S et al (1988) The prevalence of steal-prone coronary anatomy in patients with coronary artery disease: an analysis of the coronary artery surgery study registry. *Anesthesiology*, *69*, 721.
6. Slogoff S, Keats AS (1988) Does chronic treatment with calcium entry blocking drugs reduce perioperative myocardial ischemia? *Anesthesiology*, *68*, 676.
7. Chung F, Houston PL, Cheng DCH et al (1988) Calcium channel blockade does not offer adequate protection from perioperative myocardial ischemia. *Anesthesiology*, *69*, 343.
8. Blanloeil Y, Deybach JC, Portier D et al (1989) Anesthesia for hepatic porphyrias. *Ann. Fr. Anesth. Réanim.*, *8*, 109.

9. Richard T, Haberer JP (1988) Using propofol (Diprivan) in a pregnant patient with intermittent acute porphyria (Correspondence). *Ann. Fr. Anesth. Réanim., 7*: 442.
10. Weir PM, Hodkinson BP (1988) Is propofol a safe agent in porphyria? *Anaesthesia, 43*, 1022.
11. McLouglin C (1989) Use of propofol in a patient with porphyria (Correspondence). *Br. J. Anaesth., 62*, 114.
12. Hamza J (1988) Maladies familiales de l'enfant ayant une implication anesthésique spécifique. In: Balagny E, Clergue F, Conseiller C et al (Eds.), *Journées d'Enseignement Post-Universitaire d'Anesthésie et de Réanimation*, p. 225. Arnette, Paris.
13. Campbell AM, Finley GA (1989) Anaesthesia for a patient with Friedreich's ataxia and cardiomyopathy. *Can. J. Anaesth., 36*, 89.
14. Plotkin CN, Eckenbrecht PD, Waldo DA (1989) Consecutive cardiac arrests on induction of anesthesia associated with nifedipine-induced carotid sinus hypersensitivity. *Anesth. Analg., 68*, 402.
15. Adnet P, Krivosic-Horber R (1988) Calcium-channel blockers and anaesthesia. *Ann. Fr. Anesth. Réanim., 7*, 494.
16. Jacquot C, Stieglitz P, Kozak-Reiss G et al (1988) Register of french cases of anaesthetic malignant hyperthermia: an update. *Ann. Fr. Anesth. Réanim., 7*, 524.
17. Gronert GA (1989) Malignant hyperthermia. *Curr. Opin. Anaesthesiol., 2*, 357.
18. Nelson TE (1988) SR function in malignant hyperthermia. *Cell Calcium, 9*, 257.
19. Haberer JP, Fabre F, Rose E (1989) Malignant hyperthermia and myotonia congenita (Thomsen's disease) (Correspondence). *Anaesthesia, 44*, 166.
20. Houvenaeghel M, Achilli-Cornesse E, Jullian-Papouin H et al (1988) Preoperative oral dantrolene for a pregnant malignant hyperthermia susceptible patient with myotonia atrophica. *Ann. Fr. Anesth. Réanim., 7*, 408.
21. Pippin LK, Armstrong J, Schreiber T (1988) Malignant hyperthermia in a patient with King syndrome. *AANA J, 56:* 234.
22. Nègre F, Caujolle JP, Ghenassia C et al (1988) Malignant hyperthermia in ophthalmologic surgery. *J. Fr. Ophthalmol., 11*, 753.
23. Schwartz N, Eisenkraft JB (1988) Malignant hyperthermia and sleep apnea (Correspondence). *Anesthesiology, 69*, 433.
24. Wilhoit RD, Brown RE, Bauman LA (1989) Possible malignant hyperthermia in a 7-week-old infant. *Anesth. Analg., 68*, 688.
25. Harrison GG (1988) Dantrolene – Dynamics and kinetics. *Br. J. Anaesth., 60*, 279.
26. Hein HAT (1988) Lack of avaibility of dantrolene in American surgical facilities: an estimate of associated mortality. *Anesthesiology, 69*, A726.
27. Yoganathan T, Casthely PA, Lamprou M (1988) Dantrolene-induced hyperkaliemia in a patient treated with diltiazem and metoprolol. *J. Cardiothorac. Anesth., 2*, 363.
28. Murakawa M, Hatano Y, Magaribuchi T et al (1988) Should calcium administration be avoided in treatment of hyperkaliemia in malignant hyperthermia? (Correspondence). *Anesth. Analg., 67*, 596.
29. Allen GC, Cattran CB, Peterson RG et al (1988) Plasma levels of dantrolene following oral administration in malignant hyperthermia-susceptible patients. *Anesthesiology, 69*, 900.
30. Mauritz W, Hackl W, Sporn P et al (1988) Malignant hyperthermia in Austria. III. Anesthesia in 16 MH-susceptible patients. *Anaesthesist, 37*, 522.
31. Wackym PA, Abdul-Rasool IH (1988) Prospective management of malignant hyperthermia in the otolaryngological patient. *J. Laryngol. Otol., 102*, 513.
32. Dubrow TJ, Wackym PA, Abdul-Rasool IH et al (1989) Malignant hyperthermia: experience in the prospective management of eight children. *J. Pediatr. Surg., 24*, 163.
33. Welfringer P, Cornet C (1988) is preventing anaesthetic malignant hyperthermia with dantrolene justified? (Correspondence). *Ann. Fr. Anesth. Réanim., 7*, 437.
34. Ong RO, Rosenberg H (1989) Malignant hyperthermia-like syndrome associated with metrizamide myelography. *Anesth. Analg., 68*, 795.
35. Ghoneim MM, Hinrichs JV, O'Hara MW et al (1988) Comparison of psychologic and cognitive functions after general or regional anesthesia. *Anesthesiology, 69*, 507.
36. Watkins J (1989) Second report from an anaesthetic reactions advisory service. *Anaesthesia, 44*, 157.
37. Wright PJ, Shortland JR, Stevens JD et al (1989) Fatal haematopathological consequences of general anaesthesia. *Br. J. Anaesth., 62*, 104.
38. Lynas AGA, Clarke RSJ, Fee JPH et al (1988) Factors that influence cutaneous reactions following administration of thiopentone and atracurium. *Anaesthesia, 43*, 825.
39. Radford P (1988) Flushing between thiopentone and atracurium (Correspondence). *Anaesthesia, 43*, 798.
40. Naquib M (1989) Anaphylactoid reactions following propofol–atracurium sequence (Correspondence). *Can. J. Anaesth., 36*, 358.
41. Mazze RI, Kallen B (1988) Adverse reproductive outcomes following anesthesia and operation during pregnancy: a swedish registry study, 1973–1981. *Anesthesiology, 69*: A661.
42. Ong BY, Cohen MM, Palahniuk RJ (1989) Anesthesia for cesarean section-Effects on neonates. *Anesth. Analg., 68*: 270.
43. Buck N, Devlin HS, Lunn JN (1987) *Report of the Confidential Enquiry into Perioperative Deaths.* Nuffield Provincial Hospitals Trust and the King's Fund for Hospitals, London.

44. Olsson GL, Hallén B (1988) Cardiac arrest during anaesthesia: a computer-aided study in 250 543 anaesthetics. *Acta Anaesthesiol. Scand., 32*, 653.

45. Zeitlin GL (1989) Possible decrease in mortality associated with anaesthesia: a comparison of two time periods in Massachussets, USA. *Anaesthesia, 44*, 432.

46. Tiret L, Nivoche Y, Hatton F et al (1988) Complications related to anaesthesia in infants and children. *Br. J. Anaesth., 61*, 263.

47. Pedersen T (1989) Serious morbidity attributable to anaesthesia: considerations for prevention. *Anaesthesia, 44*, 504.

48. Caplan RA, Ward RJ, Posner K et al (1988) Unexpected cardiac arrest during spinal anesthesia: a closed claims analysis of predisposing factors. *Anesthesiology, 68*, 5.

49. Eichorn JH (1989) Prevention of intraoperative anaesthesia accidents and related severe injury through safety monitoring. *Anesthesiology, 70*, 572.

50. Lamberti L, Bigatti P, Ardito G et al (1989) Chromosome analysis in operating room personel. *Mutagenesis, 4*, 95.

51. Ziv Y, Shohat B, Baniel J et al (1988) The immunologic profile of anesthetists. *Anesth. Analg., 67*, 849.

52. Moral V, Blanco D, Pérez R et al (1988) Professional toxicity due to volatile agents. *Rev. Esp. Anestesiol. Reanim., 35*, 199.

53. Stollery BT, Broadbent DE, Lee WR et al (1988) Mood and cognitive functions in anaesthetists working in actively scavenged operating theatres. *Br. J. Anaesth., 61*, 446.

54. Lings S (1988) Halothane related liver affection in an anesthetist. *Br. J. Ind. Med., 45*, 716.

55. Ganzuka A, Tohdoh Y, Murakami S (1988) A case of anaphylactoid reactions to enflurane. *Jpn. J. Anesthesiol., 37*, 1382.

56. Vallet B, Cortot A, Darras J et al (1988) Hépatite grave après anesthésie à l'halothane. *Cah. Anesthésiol., 36*, 317.

57. Watanabe A, Kumeta Y, Ohguro S et al (1988) Case reports of postoperative liver dysfunction following halothane anesthesia within a short period after enflurane anesthesia. *Jpn. J. Anesthesiol., 37*, 1112.

58. Christ DD, Kenna JG, Kammerer W et al (1988) Enflurane metabolism produces covalently bound liver adducts recognized by antibodies from patients with halothane hepatitis. *Anesthesiology, 69*, 833.

59. Housmans PR, Murat I (1988) Comparative effects of halothane, enflurane, and isoflurane at equipotent anesthetic concentrations on isolated ventricular myocardium of the ferret. I. Contractility. *Anesthesiology, 69*, 451.

60. Murat I, Lapeyre G, Saint-Maurice C (1989) Isoflurane attenuates baroreflex control of heart rate in human neonates. *Anesthesiology, 70*, 395.

61. Priebe HJ (1988) Disadvantages of isoflurane in coronary artery disease. *Acta Anaesthesiol. Belg., 39, Suppl. 2*, 189.

62. Khambatta HJ, Sonntag H, Larsen R et al (1988) Global and regional myocardial blood flow and metabolism during equipotent halothane and isoflurane anesthesia in patients with coronary artery disease. *Anesth. Analg., 67*, 936.

63. Lapeyre G, Egu JF, Raynaud P et al (1989) Hyperthermie maligne peranesthésique et isoflurane. *Ann. Fr. Anesth. Réanim., 8*, 13A.

64. Dooper PhMM, Beerens J, Brenninkmeijer VJ et al (1988) Fatal intoxication after ingestion of isoflurane. *Neth. J. Med., 33*, 74.

65. Bailie R, Restall J (1988) Otic barotrauma due to nitrous oxide (Correspondence). *Anaesthesia, 43*, 888.

66. Vangerven M, Delrue G, Brugman E et al (1989) A new therapeutic approach to accidental intra-arterial injection of thiopentone. *Br. J. Anaesth., 62*, 98.

67. McKinney MS, Bali IM (1988) Concealed intra-arterial injection of thiopentone (Correspondence). *Anaesthesia, 43*, 612.

68. Fazackerley EJ, Martin AJ, Tolhurst-Cleaver CL et al (1988) Anaphylactoid reaction following the use of etomidate. *Anaesthesia, 43*, 953.

69. Hansen HC, Drenck NE (1988) Generalized seizures after etomidate anaesthesia (Correspondence). *Anaesthesia, 43*, 805.

70. Du Cailar J (1989) Etomidate: Why not tell all? (Editorial). *Ann. Fr. Anesth. Réanim., 8*, 83.

71. Crozier TA, Beck D, Wuttke W et al (1988) In vivo suppression of steroid synthesis by etomidate is concentration-dependent. *Anaesthesist, 37*, 337.

72. Sear JW, Edwards CRW, Atherden SM (1988) Dual effect of etomidate on mineralocorticoid biosynthesis. *Acta Anaesthesiol. Belg., 39*, 87.

73. Diago MC, Amado JA, Otero M et al (1988) Anti-adrenal action of a subanaesthetic dose of etomidate. *Anaesthesia, 43*, 644.

74. Murat I, Estève C, Delleur MM et al (1989) Hormonal changes during the 24 hours following etomidate infusion in children. *Ann. Fr. Anesth. Réanim., 8*, 102.

75. McGrady EM, Wright IH (1989) Cardiovascular instability following bolus dose of etomidate. *Anaesthesia, 44*, 404.

76. Stuttmann R, Allolio B, Becker A et al (1988) Etomidate versus etomidate plus hydrocortisone in major abdominal surgery. *Anaesthesist, 37*, 576.

77. Reddy BK, Pizer B, Bull PT (1988) Neonatal serum cortisol suppression by etomidate compared with thiopentone, for elective caesarean section. *Eur. J. Anesthesiol., 5*, 1.

78. Reich DL, Silvay G (1989) Ketamine: an update on the first twenty-five years of clinical experience. *Can. J. Anaesth., 36*: 186.

79. Hamza J, Ecoffey C, Gross JB (1989) Ventila-

tory response to CO_2 following ketamine in children. *Anesthesiology, 70*, 422.
80. Matson AM, Thurlow AC (1988) Hypotension and neurological sequelae following intramuscular midazolam (Correspondence). *Anaesthesia, 43*, 896.
81. Montravers Ph, Dureuil B, Desmonts JM (1988) Effects of midazolam on upper airway resistances. *Anesthesiology, 69*, A824.
82. Hargreaves J (1988) Benzodiazepine premedication in minor day-case surgery: comparison of oral midazolam and temazepam with placebo. *Br. J. Anaesth., 61*, 611.
83. Engstrom RH, Cohen SE (1989) A complication associated with the use of midazolam (Correspondence). *Anesthesiology, 70*, 719.
84. Lobo BL, Miwa LJ (1988) Midazolam desinhibition reaction. *Drug Intell. Clin. Pharm., 22*, 725.
85. Finley PR, Nolan PE (1989) Precipitation of benzodiazepine withdrawal following sudden discontinuation of midazolam. *Ann. Pharmacother., 23*, 151.
86. Brooks JH (1989) Midazolam in a malignant hyperthermia-susceptible patient. (Correspondence). *Anesthesiology, 70*, 167.
87. Ritter JW, Flacke WE, Norel E et al (1988) Adrenergic and hemodynamic response to flumazenil (Ro 15-1788) reversal of midazolam sedation. *Anesthesiology, 69*, A109.
88. White PF, Shaffer A, Boyle WA et al (1989) Benzodiazepine antagonism does not provoke a stress response. *Anesthesiology, 70*, 636.
89. Marty J, Nitenberg A, Philip I et al (1988) Coronary hemodynamic responses following reversal of benzodiazepine induced sedation with flumazenil in patients with coronary artery disease. *Anesthesiology, 69*, A110.
90. Mora CT, Torjman M, White PF (1989) Effects of diazepam and flumazenil on sedation and hypoxic ventilatory response. *Anesth. Analg., 68*, 473.
91. Barakat T, Lechat JP, Laurent P et al (1988) Ventilatory effects of flumazenil on midazolam-induced sedation. *Anesthesiology, 69*, A817.
92. Dailland Ph, Lirzin JD, Jugan E et al (1988) Effects of Ro 15-1788 (flumazenil) on the CO_2 responsiveness after midazolam–fentanyl anesthesia. *Anesthesiology, 69*, A815.
93. Coates DP (1988) Cardioventilatory effects of intravenous anaesthetics. *Curr. Opin. Anaesthesiol., 1*, 182.
94. Laxenaire MC, Gueant JL, Bermejo E et al (1988) Anaphylactic shock due to propofol. *Lancet, Sept. 24*, 739.
95. Dold M, Konarzewski WH (1989) Delayed allergic response to propofol (Correspondence). *Anaesthesia, 44*, 532.
96. Kumar CM, McNeela BJ (1989) Ocular manifestation of propofol allergy. (Correspondence). *Anaesthesia, 44*, 266.
97. Queinnec MC, De Dieuleveult C, Chupin AM et al (1989) Continuous propofol infusion vs enflurane for squint surgery in the child: comparative study of anaesthetic and recovery conditions. *Ann. Fr. Anesth. Réanim., 8*, 37.
98. Victory RAP, Magee D (1988) A case of convulsion after propofol anaesthesia. (Correspondence). *Anaesthesia, 43*, 904.
99. Simpson KH, Halsall PJ, Carr CME et al (1988) Propofol reduces seizure duration in patients having anaesthesia for electroconvulsive therapy. *Br. J. Anaesth., 61*, 343.
100. Rampton AJ, Griffin RM, Stuart CS et al (1989) Comparison of methohexital and propofol for electroconvulsive therapy: effects on hemodynamic response and seizure duration. *Anesthesiology, 70*, 412.
101. Millar JM, Jewkes CF (1988) Recovery and morbidity after daycase anaesthesia: a comparison of propofol with thiopentone–enflurane with and without alfentanil. *Anaesthesia, 43*, 738.
102. Doze VA, Shafer A, White PF (1988) Propofol–nitrous oxide versus thiopental–isoflurane–nitrous oxide for general anesthesia. *Anesthesiology, 69*, 63.
103. Korttila K, Östman PL, Faure E et al (1989) Randomized comparison of outcome after propofol or enflurane anesthesia. *Anesth. Analg., 68*, S150.
104. Lienhart A (1989) Love advances after propofol: a British fantasy or reality? (Correspondence). *Ann. Fr. Anesth. Réanim., 8*, 79.
105. Cartwright DP (1989) Propofol in patients susceptible to malignant hyperpyrexia (Correspondence). *Anaesthesia, 44*, 173.
106. James MFM, Reyneke CJ, Whiffler K (1989) Heart block following propofol: a case report. *Br. J. Anaesth., 62*, 213.
107. Baraka A (1988) Severe bradycardia following propofol–suxamethonium sequence. *Br. J. Anaesth., 61*, 482.

Yves Le Normand and Claude Larousse

12 Local anesthetics

GENERAL TOPICS

Little new has been published in the past year about local anesthetics and no new drugs have appeared in the past few years. Moreover, local and regional anesthesia are carried out following well-known procedures.

The general toxicity of local anesthetic agents has been recently reviewed by Covino (1[R]). He deals with the opinion that these drugs are relatively free of side effects if they are administered in an appropriate dosage and in the appropriate anatomical location. Two categories of toxic reactions may be encountered: systemic toxic reactions due usually to an accidental intravascular or subarachnoid injection, and local tissue toxicity.

In other reviews, the problem of sudden and severe complications that occur in regional anesthesia is discussed (2[R], 3[R]). Vagal syncope, 'allergic reactions', CNS and cardiovascular toxicity may occur, as total spinal, and is usually unexpected.

Allergy *(SED-11, 217; SEDA-12, 107; SEDA-13, 98)* It is well recognized that allergic reactions to local anesthetic agents are extremely rare and difficult to investigate (SEDA-13, 98). Nevertheless, severe anaphylactic reactions can occur. In a case of hypotension, tachycardia and coma from which the patient recovered after adrenaline, a human basophil degranulation test was positive for lidocaine and negative for other amide local anesthetic agents and preservatives (4[C]). Recently, it was suggested that local anesthetic sensitization should be tested with a mixture of several drugs, and not with benzocaine alone, as usually practiced in the United Kingdom: 52.5% of allergic subjects have a positive patch test to amethocaine or cinchocaine, but not to benzocaine (5[c]).

© 1990 Elsevier Science Publishers B.V.
(Biomedical Division)
Side Effects of Drugs Annual 14
M.N.G. Dukes and L. Beeley, editors

Methemoglobinemia *(SEDA-13, 98)* No important new information has appeared on this topic. One case of acute cyanosis and methemoglobinemia requiring tracheal intubation and mechanical ventilation after cetacaine topical spray was reported (6[c]). Neonatal cyanosis, methemoglobinemia and hemolytic anemia after inadvertent injection of prilocaine were also observed in 2 cases (7[c]).

Malignant hyperthermia The use of local anesthetics in dental patients presumed to be susceptible to malignant hyperthermia is controversial. In a study of 307 malignant-hyperthermia-susceptible patients, symptoms which apparently lifted with the administration of amide local anesthetics were reported in 1 case only. This supports the conclusion that they may be administered to these patients without significant risk (8[C]).

Influence of patient's condition on toxicity Cardiotoxicity due to bupivacaine seems to be worsened by pregnancy. In the fetus and newborn, toxicity gives the same clinical picture as in the adult. In the elderly patient, the elimination half-life is increased for both lidocaine and bupivacaine. Hyperkalemia, acidosis, severe hypoxia and myocardial ischemia increase the depressive effects of bupivacaine (9[r]).

Drug interactions Co-administration of adrenaline with local anesthetics for epidural anesthesia in obstetrics has been reviewed by Abboud (10[r]).

The addition of dextran to a lidocaine–adrenaline solution administered in infiltration anesthesia significantly reduces the absorption of both adrenaline and lidocaine (11[C]).

As bupivacaine inhibits the inward current of calcium in cardiac tissues, beta-blockers and calcium blockers may potentiate its cardiotoxicity (9[r]). This has been observed in patients on both lidocaine and a β-adrenoceptor blocking agent (12[c]).

EFFECTS RELATED TO DIFFERENT MODES OF USE

Epidural and spinal anesthesia *(SED-11, 219; SEDA-12, 107; SEDA-13, 99)*

In a study of analgesia following epidural blockade in 30 patients with either postoperative or chronic low back pain, a high incidence of *headache* (53%) and *nausea* (35–40%) was observed 9 hours after surgery (13[c]).

Lower limb compression using inflatable splints significantly reduces the frequency and severity of hypotension during spinal anesthesia for cesarean section (14[C]). The incidence of cardiac arrest during spinal anesthesia is extremely low, but a case of progressive *bradycardia* and sudden *cardiac arrest* during spinal anesthesia has been reported: this happened immediately after the patient was moved from the 15° Trendelenburg to the supine horizontal position (15[c]).

Intraoperative *penile erection* may be observed, sometimes followed by prolonged *priapism*, after spinal, intradural or epidural anesthesia (16[c], 17[c]).

Spinal analgesia is sometimes used in obstetric practice, as an alternative to epidural analgesia. Though spinal analgesia leads rapidly to a satisfactory distribution of analgesia, the incidence of *hypotension* is important (40–50%). Another disadvantage is the unpredictable response in some patients (18[R]).

Obstetric extradural analgesia

The most common side effect observed during extradural anesthesia with bupivacaine or lidocaine is *hypotension* which occurs in 36% of patients. Significantly more patients receiving the first injection of local anesthetic agent in the sitting position require ephedrine to correct maternal hypotension than those who receive the drug in the lateral position (19[c]).

Retrobulbar block and facial block *(SED-11, 218; SEDA-12, 107; SEDA-13, 99)*

Additional studies confirm the risk of cardiorespiratory complications after retrobulbar block: *respiratory arrest* is rare, but always possible (20[c]). It has been recently suggested that the proximity of the subdural and subarachnoid space surrounding the optic nerve facilitates bupivacaine diffusion towards the CSF: this phenomenon is possibly involved in the mechanism of *cardiac toxicity* during retrobulbar block (21[c]).

Headache following the use of bupivacaine before eye operations has been shown to be related to the vasoconstrictor additive. It occurs more frequently with noradrenaline than with adrenaline (22[c]).

The first 3 cases of *dysphagia* and *respiratory distress* after a Nadbath block have been reported (23[c]), following administration of a 1:1 mixture of bupivacaine and lidocaine.

Retinal vascular occlusion is a rare complication after retrobulbar injection of local anesthetics, but it can occur in patients with severe vascular disease, without retrobulbar or optic nerve sheath hemorrhage (24[c]). The mechanism of this complication remains uncertain.

Hematoma blocks

Injection of local anesthetics into the fracture hematoma after Colle's fractures is considered satisfactory by patients, but may lead to toxic concentrations of lidocaine in the arterial circulation (25[c]).

Rectal administration

In a controversy about the contents of data sheets, a case of convulsions was attributed to topical use of a lidocaine ointment in the treatment of an anal fissure (26[c]). This problem was later attributed to rectal absorption of lidocaine (27[c]).

Local anesthesia

Inadvertent injection of prilocaine into a child's scalp has been shown to produce neonatal cyanosis, methemoglobinemia and hemolytic anemia. This happened in 2 cases when the mother's perineum was injected prior to episiotomy (7[c]).

Gargling with normal doses of 0.5% solution of tetracaine before endoscopic procedures may lead to rapid tetracaine absorption and serious *systemic toxicity*, possibly fatal (28[c]).

Local dental anesthesia *(SED-11, 219; SEDA-13, 99)*

Facial paralysis after local dental anesthesia is a rare complication, the origin of which is generally unclear. Vascular spasm has been considered as a possible mechanism in a 15-year-old patient (29[c]).

EFFECTS RELATED TO INDIVIDUAL COMPOUNDS

Bupivacaine *(SED-11, 221; SEDA-12, 108; SEDA-13, 100)*

From the results of a study concerning normal term infants delivered by cesarean section whose mothers received peridural anesthesia, it was suggested that the combination of bupivacaine and oxytocin increased the incidence of *jaundice* without affecting the severity (30[c]). In this study, lidocaine did not produce the same effect.

Chloroprocaine *(SED-11, 221; SEDA-12, 109; SEDA-13, 100)*

Although chloroprocaine has a low potential for systemic toxicity, localized neural irritation has been reported in some patients in whom large amounts of this drug were administered epidurally or intrathecally. The *local neural toxicity* of chloroprocaine is attributed to the low pH and the inclusion of sodium bisulfite in these particular solutions (31[r]).

Lidocaine *(SED-11, 220; SEDA-12, 109; SEDA-13, 100)*

Using premedication with diazepam or hyoscine+morphine or no premedication before rapid intravenous injection of lidocaine 1 mg/kg in healthy volunteers, no correlation was observed between premedication and the degree of severity or numbers of CNS symptoms (32[c]).

In a study of 60 patients, a significant reduction of the *decrease in respiratory rate* caused by intravenous lidocaine was obtained by naloxone treatment (33[c]).

Oxybuprocaine

Fibrinous iritis and moderate corneal swelling has been recently reported after topical application of oxybuprocaine. This seems to be caused by inadvertent entry of the drug into the anterior chamber (34[c]).

Prilocaine *(SED-11, 221)*

Neonatal methemoglobinemia was observed in 2 cases and attributed to inadvertent injection of prilocaine hydrochloride (7[c]). In adults with chronic anemia, prilocaine should be considered as a safe local anesthetic, since methemoglobin levels are within the ranges measured in healthy patients (35[c]).

Tetracaine *(SED-11, 221; SEDA-12, 109)*

The use of a pneumatic tourniquet during spinal anesthesia induces pain in a significant number of patients: the incidence of *tourniquet pain* is greater in patients given tetracaine (60%) than in patients given bupivacaine (25%) (36[c]).

REFERENCES

1. Covino BG (1988) Toxicity of local anesthetic agents. *Acta Anaesthesiol. Belg., 39, Suppl. 2*, 159.
2. Gribomont BF (1988) Sudden complications in regional anesthesia. *Acta Anaesthesiol. Belg., 39, Suppl. 2*, 165.
3. Berlin J, Erdmann W, Cartellieri S (1989) Lokalanesthetika: Unerwünschte Wirkungen und ihre Behandlung. *Fortschr. Med., 107*, 288.
4. Bonnet MC, Du Cailar G, Deschot J (1989) Anaphylaxie à la lidocaïne. *Ann. Fr. Anesth. Réanim., 8*, 127.
5. Beck MH, Holden A (1988) Benzocaine – an unsatisfactory indicator of topical local anaesthetic sensitization for the U.K. *Br. J. Dermatol., 118*, 91.
6. Ferraro L, Zeichner S, Greenblott G, Groeger JS (1988) Cetacaine-induced acute methemoglobinemia. *Anesthesiology, 69*, 614.
7. Menahem S (1988) Neonatal cyanosis, methaemoglobinaemia and haemolytic anaemia. *Acta Paediatr. Scand., 77*, 755.
8. Minasian A, Yagiela JA (1988) The use of local anesthetics in patients susceptible to malignant hyperthermia. *Oral Surg. Oral Med. Oral Pathol., 66*, 405.

9. Chauvin M (1988) Toxicité aigué des anesthésiques locaux en fonction du terrain. *Ann. Fr. Anesth. Réanim.*, *7*, 216.
10. Abboud T (1988) Vasopressors and local anesthetics. *Acta Anaesthesiol. Belg.*, *39*, *Suppl. 2*, 195.
11. Adams HA, Biscoping J, Kafurke H et al (1988) Influence of dextran on the absorption of adrenaline-containing lignocaine solutions: a protective mechanism in local anaesthesia. *Br. J. Anaesth.*, *60*, 645.
12. Wyse DG, Kellen J, Tam Y, Rademaker AW (1989) Increased efficacy and toxicity of lidocaine in patients on beta-blockers. *Int. J. Cardiol.*, *21*, 59.
13. Raj PP, Knarr D, Vigdorth E et al (1988) Difference in analgesia following epidural blockade in patients with postoperative or chronic low back pain. *Pain*, *34*, 21.
14. Goudie TA, Winter AW, Ferguson DJM (1988) Lower limb compression using inflatable splints to prevent hypotension during spinal anaesthesia for caesarean section. *Acta Anaesthesiol. Scand.*, *32*, 541.
15. Nishikawa T, Anzai Y, Namiki A (1988) Asystole during spinal anaesthesia after change from Trendelenburg to horizontal position. *Can. J. Anaesth.*, *35*, 406.
16. Dávila Muñoz PA, Martin Bermejo P, Madrid Arias JL (1988) Erección del pene: complicación de la cirugia transuretral. Estudio de un caso tratado con metoxamina. *Rev. Esp. Anestesiol. Reanim.*, *35*, 159.
17. Vásques Pérez MJ, Sánchez del Mazo MT, Pose Cambeiro MP, Fraga Garcia M (1988) Priapismo prolongado tras anesthesia locorregional. *Rev. Esp. Anestesiol. Reanim.*, *35*, 157.
18. Crawford JS (1988) There is only a limited place for spinals in obstetrics. *Acta Anaesthesiol. Belg.*, *39*, 181.
19. Reid JA, Thorburn J (1988) Extradural bupivacaine or lignocaine anaesthesia for elective caesarean section: the role of maternal posture. *Br. J. Anaesth.*, *61*, 149.
20. Ruusuvaara P, Setälä K, Tarkkanen A (1988) Respiratory arrest after retrobulbar block. *Acta Ophthalmol. (Copenh.)*, *66*, 223.
21. Le Normand Y, De Dieuleveult C, Athouël A et al (1989) Pharmacokinetics of lidocaine and bupivacaine in retrobulbar and facial block. *Fundam. Clin. Pharmacol.*, *3*, 95.
22. Pilz J (1988) Kopfschmerz bei ophthalmologischer Lokalanästhesie in Abhängigkeit von der Art des Vasokonstriktorzusatzes. *Folia Ophthalmol.*, *13*, 133.
23. Koenig SB, Snyder RW, Kay J (1988) Respiratory distress after a Nadbath block. *Ophthalmology*, *95*, 1285.
24. Cowley M, Campochiaro PA, Newman SA, Fogle JA (1988) Retinal vascular occlusion without retrobulbar or optic nerve sheath hemorrhage after retrobulbar injection of lidocaine. *Ophthalmic Surg.*, *19*, 859.
25. Quinton DN (1988) Local anaesthetic toxicity of haematoma blocks in manipulation of Colle's fractures. *Injury*, *19*, 239.
26. Medawar C (1988) Data sheets: a consumer perspective. *Lancet*, *1*, 777.
27. Pottage A, Scott DB (1988) Safety of 'topical' lignocaine. *Lancet*, *1*, 1003.
28. Patel D, Chopra S, Berman MD (1989) Serious systemic toxicity resulting from use of tetracaine for pharyngeal anesthesia in upper endoscopic procedures. *Dig. Dis. Sci.*, *34*, 882.
29. Rives JM, Flocard F, Ribot C et al (1989) Paralysie faciale périphérique après anesthésie locale dentaire. *Presse Méd.*, *18*, 729.
30. Procianoy RS, Ossanai Jr J, Ossanai JN (1988) Relação entre ictericia neonatal e anestesia peridural materna. *J. Pediatr.*, *64*, 291.
31. Covino BG (1988) Is there a need for chloroprocaine 3% and bupivacaine 0.75%? *Acta Anaesthesiol. Belg.*, *3*, 151.
32. Haasio J, Hekali R, Rosenberg PH (1988) Influence of premedication on lignocaine-induced acute toxicity and plasma concentrations of lignocaine. *Br. J. Anaesth.*, *61*, 131.
33. Ackerman WE, Colclough GW, Martin ST, Hiett AK (1987) Naloxone treatment of intravenous lidocaine-induced central nervous system depression. *Anesthesiol. Rev.*, *14*, 21.
34. Haddad R (1989) Fibrinous iritis due to oxybuprocaine. *Br. J. Ophthalmol.*, *73*, 76.
35. Wald-Oboussier G, Viell B (1989) Supraklavikulare Plexusblockade mit Prilocain bei Patienten mit chronischer Anämie. *Reg. Anaesth.*, *12*, 31.
36. Conception MA, Lambert DH, Welch KA, Covino BG (1988) Tourniquet pain during spinal anesthesia: a comparison of plain solutions of tetracaine and bupivacaine. *Anesth. Analg.*, *67*, 828.

F.J. Richardson and S. Agoston

13 Neuromuscular blocking agents and skeletal muscle relaxants

GENERAL INTERACTIONS

Doxapram, a drug used as a respiratory stimulant, has not been reported as affecting neuromuscular transmission before. A recent study using the rat phrenic nerve–diaphragm preparation (1) demonstrates that *doxapram on its own augments neuromuscular transmission* at concentrations below those which inhibit acetylcholinesterase. However, *partial neuromuscular blockade by d-tubocurarine and pancuronium was increased* by the addition of doxapram. The effects were dose-related. The investigators reconcile these different actions by suggesting that doxapram has both a presynaptic facilitatory action at the neuromuscular junction and an inhibitory action which is probably postsynaptic. The facilitatory action may be reduced or lost in the presence of drugs which have a significant presynaptic action such as tubocurarine. The concentrations at which the effects were seen were 5 or more times greater than those obtained with usual dosage in clinical practice. It remains to be seen if doxapram produces clinically important actions on neuromuscular transmission in man and, if it does, if the interaction with neuromuscular blocking agents is influenced by the balance between pre- and postjunctional effects of the individual drugs.

The effect of *ketamine* on the action of neuromuscular blocking drugs is controversial. Three recent publications (2^r, 3^r, 4^C) lend support to those investigators who have claimed that *ketamine potentiates suxamethonium and non-depolarizing neuromuscular blocking agents.* In the human study (4^C), the duration of *atracurium* block (0.5 mg/kg) was longer when ketamine (2 mg/kg bolus followed by an infusion of 2 mg/kg/h) was added to the anesthetic regime. The median duration to 25% recovery of the twitch height was only 8 min longer in the ketamine group, so clinical problems are not to be expected on the basis of this investigation. An effect of lighter anesthesia in the group not receiving ketamine cannot be excluded. Monkeys (*Macaca cyclopis*) under light O_2/halothane anesthesia were used in the other two studies. In the first of these, bolus doses of ketamine (2.5 or 10 mg/kg) were found to potentiate, in a dose-related manner, a steady-state 50% neuromuscular blockade maintained by the infusion of *d-tubocurarine, atracurium, vecuronium or pancuronium* (2^r). The maximum effect took 5–10 min to develop and, with the highest dose, the potentiation lasted 32–61 min, depending on the relaxant used. The ketamine dose–neuromuscular response curves for the different relaxants were not parallel. There was a statistically significant potentiation in all cases except for the combination of the lowest ketamine dose with pancuronium. At the highest ketamine dose the twitch height decreased from 50% to about 10–25% of control depending on the relaxant studied. The authors suggest that the differences seen with the various relaxants are due to the 'difference in relative importance of their prejunctional and postjunctional (receptor-occupying and channel-blocking) effects' and to 'the different dose–response curves for the various neuromuscular actions of ketamine' – a good diplomatic attempt to reconcile their findings with those of earlier studies. In the second animal study (3^r) *ketamine was shown to enhance both Phase I and Phase II neuromuscular blockade with suxamethonium.* While the methodology might raise some eyebrows, the ED_{90} for suxamethonium was reduced by a prior dose of 2 mg/kg ketamine from 0.99 mg/kg ($\pm$ 0.13) to

Side Effects of Drugs Annual 14
M.N.G. Dukes and L. Beeley, editors

0.74 mg/kg (± 0.13). The Phase II block (maintained with a steady infusion rate) was potentiated to a greater extent than that seen with the non-depolarizing drugs described above.

DEPOLARIZING NEUROMUSCULAR BLOCKING AGENTS

Suxamethonium *(SED-11, 226; SEDA-11, 120; SEDA-12, 112; SEDA-13, 102)*

Neuromuscular *An increase in serum creatine kinase (CPK)* associated with the use of suxamethonium in 4 *young children with 'muscle, eye and brain disease'* has been reported (5[C]). The children were anesthetized on several occasions and substantial rises in CPK occurred only following those anesthesias which included intravenous suxamethonium. Elevated CPK levels have, however, been frequently measured after suxamethonium, particularly in children and with halothane anesthesia (SED-11, 227; SEDA-10, 107; SEDA-11, 121). The dangers of using suxamethonium in another form of muscular dystrophy, the Duchenne type, have already been stressed (SEDA-11, 121). The use of suxamethonium should be avoided in all forms of *muscular dystrophy*.

Endocrine, metabolic The syndrome of malignant hyperthermia (MH) is most frequently triggered by suxamethonium. *Dantrolene* is used in the treatment of the syndrome and also for prophylaxis in patients who are suspected of being susceptible to MH. When used for the treatment of spasticity (in daily doses of up to 400 mg), one of the commonest side effects is weakness which often improves with continued use. *Postoperative muscle weakness resulting in respiratory depression* requiring mechanical assistance has recently been described in a patient who already had a diminished respiratory reserve (VC of 900 ml and an FVC of 41%) and was given dantrolene 4 mg/kg/d orally for 2 days as MH prophylaxis (6[Cr]). Although other factors probably contributed to this situation, such as possible myopathy and pancuronium [prophylactic dantrolene has been associated with prolongation of a vecuronium block (SEDA-11, 126)], the plasma levels of dantrolene measured (2.5–3.5 μg/ml) indicate that the dantrolene could certainly have produced significant weakness. Flewellen et al. (7), administering intravenous bolus doses of dantrolene, found a correlation between similar blood levels and a 65–70% depression of adductor pollicis twitch height with significant diminution of grip strength; respiratory parameters remained normal, but his subjects were healthy volunteers. This case illustrates the danger of using dantrolene in patients with compromised respiratory function or pre-existing muscle weakness. Peak plasma concentrations after a single 100 mg oral dose of dantrolene are reached at various times 1–12 hours after ingestion, and the half-life ranges between 4 and 22 hours (8), so that giving dantrolene in divided doses orally over a 2-day period as MH prophylaxis could produce either inadequate blood levels at the time of operation or clinically important side effects, even preoperatively. Intravenous prophylaxis immediately prior to anesthesia would not only obviate problems arising from preoperative weakness and minimize unpleasant side effects such as nausea, but would also produce more predictable blood levels (7). The problem of post-operative muscle weakness remains.

Mineral and fluid balance One of the most insidious side effects of suxamethonium is the potentially lethal rise in serum potassium which can occur in certain circumstances, e.g. following trauma and burns. A case-report of a *high serum potassium level* (7.3 mmol/l) associated with *ventricular dysrhythmias and fibrillation* in a patient with *metastatic embryonal rhabdomyosarcoma* (9[C]) is suggestive that suxamethonium (20 mg for 18 kg) may have been responsible. The association is not entirely clear-cut, since atropine (0.05 mg i.v.) was given at the same time and the blood sample was obtained after defibrillation. It is also possible that pyrexia coupled with halothane, atropine, stress and intubation provoked the dysrhythmias. Biopsies showed partly necrotic tumor filling the bone marrow spaces. This rare condition should, perhaps, be added to the long list of contraindications to the use of suxamethonium.

Interactions *Bambuterol (carbamylated terbutaline) has been shown to inhibit plasma cholinesterase and prolong the action of suxamethon-*

ium (10[C]). Bambuterol is used to relieve bronchospasm. The active drug terbutaline is slowly freed as the *carbamate* groups are cleaved from the compound. Like organophosphorus compounds, carbamates are commonly used as insecticides and inhibit plasma (and acetyl-) cholinesterase. Unlike organophosphorus compounds they bind reversibly to the enzymes. Nevertheless, in the present investigation a single 30 mg oral dose of bambuterol was still capable of inhibiting plasma cholinesterase to a significant extent some 10–12.5 hours later. The plasma cholinesterase activity at that time was between 9 and 73% of the control values measured before the drug was given (in 13 patients). The duration of action of a 1 mg/kg dose of suxamethonium, as measured by recovery of adductor pollicis twitch tension to 90% of control, was 24.9 $\pm$ 12 min (mean $\pm$ SD) in the patients given bambuterol as against 11.2 $\pm$ 3.7 min in a control group given a placebo. Train-of-four fade developed in the patients with the lowest plasma cholinesterase activities and the longest blocks. Edrophonium was found to be effective in these patients for reversal. Neuromuscular function should be monitored in patients taking this drug even if the last dose was ingested more than 12 hours earlier. In asthmatic patients edrophonium and other anticholinesterases are better avoided if possible, so it may be simpler to use a non-depolarizing relaxant instead of suxamethonium in order to avoid the possible development of a Phase II block.

Cimetidine has in the past (SEDA-12, 113; 11[C]) been claimed to be responsible for doubling the duration of action of suxamethonium. Subsequently, it has been shown that usual doses of cimetidine do not inhibit plasma cholinesterase activity in patients and only concentrations much higher than those achieved therapeutically inhibit the cholinesterases in vitro (SEDA-13, 103). Several recent publications (12[Cr], 13[C], 14[C]) throw doubt on the accuracy of the initial claim, *the action of suxamethonium not being prolonged after cimetidine* 300–400 mg (*or ranitidine* 150 mg) given orally the evening before operation and again 1–2 hours prior to anesthesia (with suxamethonium 1 or 1.5 mg/kg). The most detailed study (12[Cr]) demonstrates once again that plasma cholinesterase inhibition is not produced by cimetidine or ranitidine and introduces the suggestion that the original paper (11[C]) may have included patients given *metoclopramide* which has since been shown to inhibit plasma cholinesterase (15) and prolong the action of suxamethonium (16[C]). Is this the solution to the conundrum?

Metoclopramide has been shown to *inhibit plasma cholinesterase activity* in vitro in human plasma (15). The authors of this short communication suggest that the inhibition could be of clinical importance if very high doses of metoclopromide are given, as in the treatment of vomiting resulting from cancer chemotherapy, or if other factors are present which also reduce plasma cholinesterase activity such as pregnancy. In another paper (16[C]) metoclopramide was shown to inhibit the hydrolysis of suxamethonium by plasma cholinesterase in vitro and, in patients, a 10 mg intravenous dose of metoclopramide was found to *prolong the duration of action of suxamethonium* (a third dose) given 1 min later. The unusual methodology in the clinical part of this study precludes any prediction of the degree of prolongation which might be expected under more usual clinical circumstances.

NON-DEPOLARIZING NEUROMUSCULAR BLOCKING AGENTS *(SED-11, 234; SEDA-11, 122; SEDA-12, 114; SEDA-13, 103)*

General There have been several publications involving one or more non-depolarizing neuromuscular blocking agents which can probably be applied to a greater or lesser extent to the group as a whole.

Neuromuscular/respiratory systems *Respiratory-induced acid–base changes*, in the rat phrenic nerve–diaphragm preparation, have once again been examined (17[r]). An increase in CO_2 from 2.5 to 7.5% on its own resulted in a 5% decrease in the indirectly elicited contractions of the diaphragm whereas a change of similar magnitude in the opposite direction produced a 2% increase in contraction. When similar changes in CO_2 were introduced in the presence of a 50% neuromuscular blockade by *d-tubocurarine or vecuronium*, the higher CO_2 concentration potentiated the block significantly and the low CO_2 level significantly antagonized it. In contrast, the actions of *metocu-*

rine, pancuronium and alcuronium were affected to a lesser degree and in the opposite direction. The authors of this paper provide a well-reasoned view of a very complicated subject on which conflicting claims have been made by distinguished researchers over many years. In their detailed discussion they postulate that the difference seen in the effect of respiratory acidosis on the neuromuscular blocking actions of d-tubocurarine and vecuronium on the one hand and the other relaxants examined on the other lies in the *monoquaternary* nature of the first two drugs. They suggest that the increased formation of pseudo-bisquaternary compounds at lower pH leads to a greater affinity of d-tubocurarine and vecuronium for the receptor. The lesser effects seen in the case of bisquaternary relaxants may be due to alterations in receptor affinity caused by changes in their ionization.

Interactions *Ciclosporin* has previously been shown to potentiate neuromuscular blockade induced by vecuronium or alcuronium in cats (SEDA-12, 118; 18). Two cases have now been reported which are strongly suggestive of *prolongation of neuromuscular blockade in patients* treated with this immunosuppressive agent. In one case the relaxant used was *pancuronium* (19^{C}) and in the other *vecuronium* (20^{C}). The dosage of both relaxants was 0.1 mg/kg and after 4 hours and 1 hour, respectively, both patients required reversal which needed supplementation, both neostigmine and edrophonium being used in doses that would normally have been sufficient. The pancuronium-treated patient was then detubated but later required re-intubation for a further 4 hours. The vecuronium-treated patient was considered to have adequate neuromuscular function for detubation only 3 hours and 20 min after the vecuronium had been given. In both patients the ciclosporin level was within the therapeutic range. Although these patients both had a minor degree of renal dysfunction the ciclosporin seems most likely to be the agent responsible for the prolonged neuromuscular blockade described. The solvent in ciclosporin preparations, cremophor-EL, may also contribute to the effect. Monitoring of neuromuscular function seems essential for patients on ciclosporin therapy and particular care should be taken post-operatively that residual curarization does not later become manifest again when the initially adequate reversal wears off.

Disopyramide has previously been reported to have its neuromuscular blocking actions potentiated by low concentrations of d-tubocurarine in animal experiments (SED-11, 238). Failure of neostigmine to reverse disopyramide-induced neuromuscular blockade has been described in other animal experiments (SEDA-13, 102). In a case-report (21^{Cr}) *residual impairment of neuromuscular transmission in a patient after reversal of a vecuronium block by neostigmine* is described. Disopyramide had been given preoperatively (250 mg twice daily) and during the operation three 10 mg i.v. doses were given followed by an infusion of 25 mg/h for supraventricular extrasystoles. At the end of the operation the disopyramide plasma concentration was 5.1 μg/ml. Neostigmine (40 μg/kg) was given and the twitch height and train-of-four response returned to 100 and 85%, respectively. However, 15 min after the neostigmine was given, tetanic stimulation demonstrated marked fade to 45% at 50 Hz and to 10% at 100 Hz. The authors of this article suggest that therapeutic levels of disopyramide may impair the antagonism of vecuronium paralysis by neostigmine. In view of the earlier animal reports (SED-11, 238; SEDA-13, 102) this may well be true, although it is not proven since this patient was also receiving other drugs. However, it seems likely that disopyramide can delay the reversal of competitive neuromuscular blocking agents. The interaction is unlikely to be of major clinical significance unless a patient's neuromuscular function is already compromised.

Testosterone enanthate, given intramuscularly in a dose of 200 mg twice monthly, has been *associated with resistance to the neuromuscular blocking action of vecuronium* (22^{C}). The patient had used testosterone in this way for 10 years and associated changes of virilization were present. She weighed 150 lb and was only 5′ 1’ tall. The last dose had been 2 weeks before. After intubation with suxamethonium, vecuronium 0.1 mg/kg was given. This resulted in only 50% blockade of the twitch response and 15 min later there was no fade in the train-of-four or with tetanic stimulation of the ulnar nerve at 50 and 100 Hz. More vecuronium was given with again much less effect than expected. Further doses from different batches were administered to a total dose of 22 mg over 50 min. The patient was not taking any other medication and no explanation for the apparent resistance to vecuronium can be deduced from the case history presented other than that which the authors suggest, namely that the prolonged use of testosterone enanthate was in some way responsible. Salt and water retention leading to an increased volume of distribution, increase in muscle mass associated with an increased number of acetylcholine receptors (though this is unproven) and enhanced neuromuscular transmission (as has been described for ACTH and corticosteroids) are possible explanations proffered by the authors. Is the next step a double-blind trial of the effectiveness of muscle relaxants in athletes who have or who have not built up their muscles with anabolic steroids?

Atracurium *(SED 11, 243; SEDA-11, 122; SEDA-12, 115; SEDA-13, 105)*

Cardiovascular system *Slight tachycardia* is occasionally seen after the injection of atracurium and up to now this has been attributed to histamine release. An alternative explanation is offered in a recent publication (23) examining *the effects of atracurium and laudanosine (atracurium's major metabolite) on the release of ^{3}H-noradrenaline* from sympathetic axon terminals in isolated right atria of guinea-pigs. The results suggest that *atracurium may possess antimuscarinic activity* which is probably clinically unimportant, whereas laudanosine does not. Of more importance, the authors measured a several-fold *increase in release of ^{3}H-noradrenaline* after perfusion with high concentrations of atracurium which, they contend, was probably caused primarily by *laudanosine*. Furthermore, the concentrations of laudanosine associated with increased evoked release of noradrenaline in this study were within the range measured during the prolonged use of atracurium in intensive care patients (1.9–5.1 μg/ml). This is the only study so far that has reached these conclusions and only minor degrees of tachycardia have been reported up to now. Nevertheless, the possibility of increased noradrenaline release in situations where higher-than-usual plasma concentrations of laudanosine are to be expected should be borne in mind.

Vecuronium *(SED-11, 242; SEDA-11, 125; SEDA-12, 118; SEDA-13, 105)*

Anaphylactoid reactions These are extremely rare with vecuronium. One case of hypotension and another of bronchospasm and circulatory collapse (SED-11, 242) have been reported in the past. Two new cases originating in the Antipodes have been described in letter form. In the first of these (24[C]) a healthy 55 kg patient became peripherally *pulseless* following intubation with 6 mg vecuronium. The ECG showed sinus rhythm at 50–60 per minute. There was no bronchospasm. After resuscitation with crystalloids and adrenaline (100 μg) a red blush and periorbital edema were noted. Postoperatively the plasma histamine was elevated (6.5 ng/ml) though C3 and C4 complement fractions and IgE remained normal. The hematocrit was increased despite the infusion of 3 liters of crystalloid fluids. Skin testing at 6 weeks was positive for vecuronium. This appears to be a genuine anaphylactoid reaction to vecuronium. The second letter (25[c]) describes *bronchospasm and hypotension* following intubation with 6 mg vecuronium. Periorbital edema and flushing of the face and trunk were later noted. Resuscitation was also successful here with intravenous fluids and adrenaline (0.5 mg i.v.). Intradermal testing at 1 month was positive for both vecuronium and pancuronium. The patient had received pancuronium in the past and the authors suggest that the reaction was an example of cross-sensitivity, although there is no further evidence for this. Indeed, the only evidence presented that this second case was an anaphylactoid reaction to vecuronium is the positive skin test and it remains, therefore, inconclusive.

REFERENCES

1. Pollard BJ, Randall NPC, Pleuvry BF (1989) Doxapram and the neuromuscular junction. *Br. J. Anaesth., 62*, 664.
2. Tsai SK, Lee C (1989) Ketamine potentiates nondepolarizing neuromuscular relaxants in a primate. *Anesth. Analg., 68*, 5.
3. Tsai SK, Lee C, Tran B (1989) Ketamine enhances phase I and phase II neuromuscular block of succinylcholine. *Can. J. Anaesth., 36*, 120.
4. Toft P, Helbo-Hansen S (1989) Interaction of ketamine with atracurium. *Br. J. Anaesth., 62*, 319.
5. Karhunen U (1988) Serum creatine kinase levels after succinylcholine in children with 'muscle, eye and brain disease'. *Can. J. Anaesth., 35*, 90.
6. Hara Y, Kato A, Horikawa H et al (1988) Postoperative respiratory depression thought to be due to oral dantrolene pretreatment in a malignant hyperthermia-susceptible patient. *Masui (Jpn. J. Anesthesiol.), 4*, 483.
7. Flewellen EH, Nelson TE, Jones WP et al (1983) Dantrolene dose response in awake man: implications for management of malignant hyperthermia. *Anesthesiology, 59*, 275.
8. Meyler WJ, Mols-Thürkow HW, Wesseling H (1979) Relationship between plasma concentration and effect of dantrolene sodium in man. *Eur. J. Clin. Pharmacol., 16*, 203.
9. Krikken-Hogenberg LG, de Jong JR, Bovill JG (1989) Succinylcholine-induced hyperkalemia in a patient with metastatic rhabdomyosarcoma. *Anesthesiology, 70*, 553.
10. Fisher DM, Caldwell JE, Sharma M, Wirén JE (1988) The influence of bambuterol (carbamylated terbutaline) on the duration of action of succinylcholine-induced paralysis in humans. *Anesthesiology, 69*, 757.
11. Kambam JR, Dymond R, Krestow M (1987) Effect of cimetidine on duration of action of succinylcholine. *Anesth. Analg., 66*, 191.
12. Woodworth GE, Sears DH, Grove TM et al (1989) The effect of cimetidine and ranitidine on the duration of action of succinylcholine *Anesth. Analg., 68*, 295.
13. Stirt JS, Sperry RJ, DiFazio CA (1988) Cimetidine and succinylcholine: potential interaction and effect on neuromuscular blockade in man. *Anesthesiology, 69*, 607.
14. Bogod DG (1989) The effect of H_2 antagonists on duration of action of suxamethonium in the parturient. *Anaesthesia, 44*, 591.
15. Kambam JR, Parris WCV, Franks JJ, Sastry BVR (1988) The inhibitory effect of metoclopramide on plasma cholinesterase activity. *Anesth. Analg., 67*, S107.
16. Kao YJ, Turner DR (1989) Prolongation of succinylcholine block by metoclopramide. *Anesthesiology, 70*, 905.
17. Ono K, Ohta Y, Morita K, Kosaka F (1988) The influence of respiratory-induced acid–base changes on the action of non-depolarizing muscle relaxants in rats. *Anesthesiology, 68*, 357.
18. Gramstad L, Gjerlow JA, Hysing ES, Rugstad HE (1986) Interaction of cyclosporine and its solvent, cremophor, with atracurium and vecuronium. *Br. J. Anaesth., 58*, 1149.
19. Crosby E, Robblee JA (1988) Cyclosporine–pancuronium interaction in a patient with a renal allograft. *Can. J. Anaesth., 35*, 300.
20. Wood GG (1989) Cyclosporine–vecuronium interaction. *Can. J. Anaesth., 36*, 358.
21. Baurain M, Barvais L, d'Hollander A, Hennart D (1989) Impairment of the antagonism of vecuronium-induced paralysis and intraoperative disopyramide administration. *Anaesthesia, 44*, 34.
22. Reddy P, Guzman A, Robalino J, Shevde K (1989) Resistance to muscle relaxants in a patient receiving prolonged testosterone therapy. *Anesthesiology, 70*, 871.
23. Kinjo M, Nagashima H, Vizi ES (1989) Effect of atracurium and laudanosine on the release of ^{3}H-noradrenaline. *Br. J. Anaesth., 67*, 683.
24. Thacker MA, Boon von Ochssee D (1988) Anaphylactoid reaction to vecuronium. *Anaesth. Intens. Care, 16*, 129.
25. Holt AW, Vedig AE (1988) Anaphylaxis following vecuronium. *Anaesth. Intens. Care, 16*, 378.

Inga Lunde

14 Drugs affecting autonomic functions or the extrapyramidal system

DRUGS STIMULATING BOTH α- AND β-ADRENERGIC RECEPTORS *(SED-11, 259; SEDA-12, 122; SEDA-13, 108)*

Adrenaline (epinephrine) *(SED-11, 259; SEDA-12, 122; SEDA-13, 108)*

Episodes of facial swelling have been reported in connection with the use of an adrenaline inhaler in a woman with asthma (1[C]).

The patient had a history of perennial asthma of 20 years duration. Her symptoms were controlled by the use of adrenaline inhaler. The episodes of facial swelling began 12 years earlier, and consisted of paroxysmal painless swelling of one or both sides of the face. The episodes always occurred during or immediately after meals. More recently the patient noted swelling of the upper eyelids and the cheeks, and these symptoms occurred more frequently during exacerbation of her asthma, and they were associated with increased use of adrenaline. A gallium-67 citrate scan suggested a diagnosis of drug-induced *sialadenosis*. The patient discontinued her use of adrenaline and was treated with amoxicillin, antihistamines, decongestants and prednisone. Her asthma was treated with theophylline, beclometasone and flunisolide. Complete resolution of her sinusitis and marked improvement of asthmatic and nasal symptoms were noted at 5 months follow-up. Inhaled adrenaline was again used on 2 occasions with recurrence of facial swelling in both instances.

DRUGS PREDOMINANTLY STIMULATING β-ADRENERGIC RECEPTORS *(SED-11, 268; SEDA-12, 122; SEDA-13, 109)*

Side Effects of Drugs Annual 14
M.N.G. Dukes and L. Beeley, editors

Dopamine *(SED-11, 263)*

Local coronary spasm at the site of balloon dilatation is a known complication of percutanous transluminal angioplasty (PTCA) (2[C]).

A PTCA procedure which was complicated by diffuse *coronary artery spasm*, distant from the site of dilatation while the patient was receiving infusions of dopamine, has been reported (3[C]). The authors conclude that dopamine used for hypotension during PTCA may be associated with the development of diffuse coronary spasms, and that it therefore should be used with caution, particularly if high doses are required.

DRUGS STIMULATING DOPAMINERGIC RECEPTORS *(SED-11, 267; SEDA-12, 123; SEDA-13, 111)*

Bromocriptine *(SED-11, 267; SEDA-12, 123; SEDA-13, 111)*

Three cases of *contractures of the extremities* which were possibly caused by bromocriptine have been reported (4[C]).

The patients were all females and suffering from Parkinson's disease. In all 3 patients the contractures developed over a 2-week period in the absence of any precipitating local pathology or trauma. In all cases the contractures involved the hands; in one case both feet were also involved. Two of the patients had been taking bromocriptine for more than 2 years prior to the development of the contractures, but in one case they developed within 2 weeks of starting the drug. Two of the patients also received other antiparkinson drugs.

The authors are not at all certain that bromocriptine was the causative agent in these cases. They do however feel that awareness of this possibility may permit the association to be confirmed or refuted. A further report by Kyriakides and Langton Hewer (5[C]), describing 3 similar cases in which bromocriptine was *not* administered, has been published. Bromocriptine has been reported to induce *trigeminal attacks* in a patient suffering from ophthalmic trigeminal neuralgia as an isolated symptom of a non-invasive pituitary tumor (6[C]). Bromocriptine appeared to provoke the attacks within hours. The provocation could be prevented by domperidone. After adenomectomy both the spontaneous and the bromocriptine-induced attacks disappeared. The authors suggest that bromocriptine seems to have an early tumor-volume-increasing effect, presumably as a result of a transient cell swelling, and that this may explain the neuralgic attacks.

DRUGS PREDOMINANTLY STIMULATING β_2-ADRENERGIC RECEPTORS *(SED-11, 268; SEDA-12, 122; SEDA-13, 109)*

Fenoterol *(SED-11, 270)*

The use of fenoterol by metered dose inhaler (MDI) has come under suspicion in association with the increasing mortality of asthma patients in New Zealand in the late 1970s. Fenoterol was introduced in New Zealand in April 1976, and the epidemic began the same year. By 1983 fenoterol accounted for almost 30% of the total MDI β-agonist sales in New Zealand. A case-control study to examine the hypothesis that fenoterol by MDI increases the risk of deaths in patients with asthma was therefore carried out and the results have been published (7[C]).

The case group comprised 117 patients aged 5–45 who died of asthma during a two-year period (1981–1983). For each case, 4 controls, matched for age and ethnic group, were selected from asthma admissions to hospitals to which the cases themselves would have been admitted, had they not died.

The relative risk of asthma death in patients prescribed fenoterol by MDI was 1.55. The fenoterol MDI relative risks were similar in males (1.44) ad females (1.65), and in Europeans (1.72) and non-Europeans (1.42). The fenoterol MDI relative risk was greater in subjects aged less than 20 years (2.08) than in subjects aged 20 years or more (1.34).

The relative fenoterol risk factors were also higher for patients prescribed 3 or more asthma drugs (2.21), patients hospitalized because of asthma during the previous 12 months (2.16), and patients prescribed oral corticosteroids at the time of death or admission (6.45). The highest relative risk of asthma death (13.29) occurred in patients prescribed fenoterol by MDI who had severe asthma, defined as a history of hospitalization in the previous year and a prescription of oral corticosteroids.

None of the other asthma treatments examined (salbutamol, oral theophylline, sodium cromoglycate, inhaled and oral corticosteroids) was associated with such high risks of asthma death, particularly in severe asthma.

The authors conclude that no single case-control study may be regarded as conclusive, because not all sources of bias can be definitely excluded. They feel however, that the results, when taken together with other epidemiological and experimental evidence, are consistent with the hypothesis that the unsupervised self-administration of fenoterol by inhalation in severe asthma *increases the risk of death*.

This study was subsequently strongly criticised:

Persons who were closely involved with the original descriptive study of asthma mortality in New Zealand have given their comments (8[C]):

Based on remarks regarding study design, controls, drug information, matching for severity, biological plausibility and market share, they clearly state that they do not concur with the conclusion that the study shows that fenoterol given by MDI increases the risk of severe asthma. They interpret the data as showing that in 1981–1983 long-term fenoterol, which was at that time promoted as a more potent longer-acting bronchodilator than others available, was more commonly prescribed for patients with severe unstable asthma, i.e. the association between fenoterol and asthma mortality was secondary rather than causal.

Another group who previously had been independently approached by the producer of fenoterol to comment on the study presented, has also commented (9[C]):

They argue that the study has 3 fundamental flaws: confusion about the underlying clinical question, inadequate classification of and misleading adjustment for asthma severity, and poor standardization of methods for collecting data from cases and controls.

The effect of fenoterol on *plasma potassium* compared to salbutamol and terbutaline has been investigated in another study (10[C]). The drugs were given as metered dose-inhalers.

All 3 drugs caused a significant, dose-dependent decrease in plasma potassium. The decrease was more pronounced for fenoterol and salbutamol than for terbutaline. The effect on plasma potassium seemed to be related to the structure of the drugs: the more lipophilic the drug, the more pronounced the effect.

The authors suggest that although β_2-agonists continue to be a cornerstone in the treatment of asthma, they carry a risk of overdosing and hypokalemia. They think this could explain the increasing incidence of sudden deaths in asthmatics, which continue to be reported in the literature.

Tulobuterol *(SED-11, 270)*

Tulobuterol is a relatively new β_2-adrenergic stimulant (11[C]). The drug has been compared to salbutamol in 20 patients with asthma in a randomized, cross-over, blinded study. The effects of the two drugs were found to be similar. The side effects were reported to be mild and included *palpitations, tremor and nervousness.*

DRUGS BLOCKING α-ADRENERGIC RECEPTORS *(SED-11, 271; SEDA-13, 113)*

Indoramin

Indoramin is an α-blocking agent which has been compared to dihydroergotamine in the long-term treatment of migraine in a recently published study (12[C]). The study was performed double-blind; 82 patients were included in the trial and received either 50 mg daily of indoramin or 10 mg daily of dihydroergotamine. Seven patients from the dihydroergotamine group and 2 patients from the indoramin group dropped out due to lack of effect.

The pattern of side effects was the same for the two drugs: 18 side effects were related to indoramin and 14 to dihydroergotamine. They included *dryness of the mouth* and *sedation.*

THE ERGOT ALKALOIDS AND RELATED AGENTS *(SED-11, 272; SEDA-12, 124; SEDA-13, 113)*

Codergocrine

A double-blind randomized placebo-controlled study has been undertaken to investigate the effectivenes of codergocrine in improving cognitive functions and behavioral symptoms associated with learning disorders in children (13[C]).

Forty children of either sex participated. Twenty of them were given an increasing dose of codergocrine mesylate and followed for 12 weeks whilst 12 were treated with placebo.

The most frequently reported side effect was *nasal stuffiness* which occurred in 60% of the codergocrine-treated children and which accounted for 2 drop-outs from the group. The other main side effect was *anorexia* (in 40%) which tended to be overcome as treatment continued. *Headache* was reported in 2 of the children in the codergocrine-group and one reported *giddiness.*

Dihydroergotamine in combination with heparin

A case of *severe vasospasm* producing *ischemia* associated with the use of dihydroergotamine and heparin for prophylaxis of deep venous thrombosis has been reported (14[C]).

The patient, a 31-year-old female, had been severely injured in a motor vehicle accident and received heparin and dihydroergotamine after surgical operation of the lower extremities following the accident. The vasospasm that developed was refractory to treatment with intra-arterial vasodilators and necessitated amputation.

Several factors in addition to heparin/dihydroergotamine may have acted synergistically to produce refractory vasospasm in this patient. The authors do however feel that heparin/dihydroergotamine should not be used in trauma patients as prophylaxis for deep vein thrombosis. It is their view that the risk of refractory vasospasm exceeds the slight benefit of improved prophylaxis of the combination compared to heparin alone.

Ergotamine *(SED-11, 272; SEDA-12, 124; SEDA-13, 113)*

Protracted *coronary spasm* due to the use of ergotamine has been reported (15[C]). This complication occurred in two women aged 49 and 55 years. They were hospitalized because of symptoms of acute extensive anterior wall infarction. In both patients the protracted coronary spasm was considered to be caused by ergotamine which had been given for erroneously diagnosed migraine. The left ventricular function returned to normal in both patients, indicating that the reaction was due to myocardial ischemia and not necrosis.

AGENTS WITH CHOLINERGIC EFFECTS *(SED-11, 274)*

Methacholine

Methacholine has been compared to histamine inhalation challenge for measuring bronchial activity (16[C]). Side effects were reported to be mild with both agents. Histamine caused more *voice change* than methacholine (18 vs. 10%). The frequency of *cough* was similar with both drugs (30 vs. 34%).

AGENTS WITH ANTICHOLINERGIC EFFECTS *(SED-11, 275; SEDA-12, 125; SEDA-13, 114)*

Atropine *(SED-11, 276)*

Anaphylactic shock has been reported following intravenous injection of atropine (17[C]).

The reaction occurred in a 38-year-old woman with no history of allergy or atopy who was scheduled for varicose vein surgery under spinal anesthesia. Shortly after being given atropine intravenously she became anxious and developed generalized urticaria and pruritus followed by intense abdominal pain and vomiting. Peripheral pulses became impalpable and the heart rate increased to 170 beats/min. She was treated intensively and recovered completely. Intradermal testing gave a strong positive response.

The patient had taken an oral analgesic compound containing atropine 1 year before the reported event. The authors think that this exposure could have produced IgE antibodies in the patient. The serious reaction was provoked when the patient received the intravenous injection of atropine which resulted in much higher levels of atropine than would have been reached after oral intake.

Ipratropium bromide *(SED-11, 277)*

The development of *urinary retention* in 3 elderly patients during treatment with ipratropium bromide has been described (18[C]).

A dose of 40 mg 3 times daily for 3 days has been reported to have no effect on the flow and volume characteristics of micturition in middle-aged and elderly patients with chronic bronchitis (19[C]). Larger doses are however increasingly being used. In the present cases the dose was 0.5 mg 5 times daily.

Many of the patients using ipratropium bromide are elderly males who may have prostatic hypertrophy even in the absence of urinary symptoms. The authors advise that ipratropium bromide should be used with caution in these patients.

Orphenadrine *(SED-11, 279)*

Orphenadrine *abuse* has been described (20[C]).

A 24-year-old man had been using tetrahydrocannabinols non-medically at age 14, and at 18 he began using intravenous heroin and other drugs. After an hallucinatory episode resulting from massive overdose of amphetamine, he was admitted to hospital. On discharge haloperidol and orphenadrine hydrochloride were prescribed. He persisted in his abuse of amphetamines, and self-prescribed haloperidol to control the hallucinatory episodes. About 2 months later he returned to the hospital insisting on the prescription of orphenadrine. He admitted that he had progressively increased the dose of orphenadrine to as much as 1500 mg/d. During the period of abuse he was experiencing *dizziness* and *tremor* as well as *euphoria* and *visual hallucinations*. The patient stopped taking the drug because it was difficult to obtain and resumed his abuse of amphetamines and cocaine.

The authors comment that orphenadrine did not cause potentially life-endangering anticholinergic effects in this patient and they think that this may be due to liver enzyme induction leading to increased hepatic metabolism.

They believe that extreme caution should be taken in prescribing antiparkinson drugs having anticholinergic activity together with neuroleptic agents, when there is a suspected history of drug abuse.

REFERENCES

1. Loria RC (1989) Facial swelling secondary to inhaled bronchodilator abuse: catecholamine-induced sialoadenitis. *Ann. Allergy, 62*, 289.
2. Cowley MJ, Dorros G, Kelsey SF et al (1984) Acute coronary events associated with percutaneous coronary angioplasty. *Am. J. Cardiol., 53*, 12C.
3. McEniery PT, Hollmann J (1988) Coronary artery spasm during balloon angioplasty in a patient receiving dopamine infusion. *Cleveland Clin. J. Med., 55*, 464.
4. Quinn NP, Ring H, Honavar M, Marsden CD (1988) Contractures of the extremities in Parkinsonian subjects: a report of three cases with a possible association with bromocriptine treatment. *Clin. Neuropharmacol., 11*, 268.
5. Kyriakides T, Langton Hewer R (1988) Hand contractures in Parkinson's disease. *J. Neurol. Neurosurg. Psychiatry, 51*, 1221.
6. Ferrari MD, Haan J, Van Seters AP (1988) Bromocriptine-induced trigeminal neuralgia attacks in a patient with a pituitary tumor. *Neurology, 38*, 11482.
7. Crane J, Flatt A, Jackson R et al (1989) Prescribed fenoterol and death from asthma in New Zealand, 1981–1983: case-control study. *Lancet, 1*, 817.
8. O'Donnell TV, Rea HH, Holst PE, Sears MR (1989) Fenoterol and fatal asthma. *Lancet, 1*, 1070.
9. Buist S, Burney PGJ, Feinstein AR et al (1989) Fenoterol and fatal asthma. *Lancet, 1*, 1071.
10. Deenstra M, Haalboom JRE, Struyvenberg A (1987) Decrease of plasma potassium due to inhalation of beta-2-agonists: absence of an additional effect of intravenous theophylline. *Eur. J. Clin. Invest., 18*, 162.
11. Aguero R, Dal-Re R (1988) Comparative trial of tulobuterol, a new beta-2 agonist, and salbutamol in adult asthmatic patients. *Clin. Trials J., 25*, 109.
12. Pradalier A, Dry J, Loisy B et al (1988) Etude comparative indoramine versus dihydroergotamine dans le traitement préventif de la migraine. *Thérapie, 43*, 292.
13. Tareen KI, Bashir A, Saeed K, Hussain T (1988) Clinical efficacy of codergocrine mesylate in children with learning difficulties. *J. Int. Med. Res., 16*, 204.
14. Shackford SR, Davis JW (1988) Refractory vasospasm occurring in a trauma patient receiving dihydroergotamine and heparin. *Crit. Care Med., 16*, 909.
15. Slob J, Burgersdijk C, Ruiter JH (1988) Ergotamine: van hoofdpijn naar hartpijn. *Ned. Tijdschr. Geneeskd., 132*, 927.
16. Higgins BG, Britton JR, Chinn S et al (1988) Comparison of histamine and methacholine for use in bronchial challenge tests in community studies. *Thorax, 43*, 605.
17. Aguilera L, Martinez-Bourio R, Cid C, Arino JJ (1988) Anaphylactic reaction after atropine. *Anaesthesia, 43*, 955.
18. Lozewicz A (1989) Bladder outflow obstruction induced by ipratropium bromide. *Postgrad. Med. J., 65*, 260.
19. Molkenboer JFWM, Lardenoye JG (1979) The effect of Atrovent in micturition function: double blind cross-over study. *Scand. J. Respir. Dis., 103*, 154.
20. Schifano F, Marra R, Magni G (1988) Orphenadrine abuse. *South. Med. J.*, 81, 546.

Anton C. de Groot and Johan P. Nater

15 Dermatological drugs, topical agents and cosmetics

ORAL PHOTOCHEMOTHERAPY (PUVA) *(SED-11, 284; SEDA-12, 130; SEDA-13, 119)*

There have been occasional published reports of *leukemia* developing during PUVA therapy (SEDA-4, 130; SEDA-10, 125), and a recent paper presents what may be a new aspect of the issue:

A patient with stable chronic myelomonocytic leukemia was treated with PUVA for erythrodermic psoriasis (1[Cr]). After 4 months, transformation to acute myeloid leukemia occurred. Although this patient had a substantial risk of spontaneous malignant transformation, the authors suggest that the possibility that PUVA was responsible cannot be ruled out. Therefore, they urge caution in the uncommon event of PUVA therapy being considered for use in patients who have preleukemic disorders (1[Cr]).

RETINOIDS *(SED-11, 285; SEDA-12, 131; SEDA-13, 120)*

An excellent review article on the adverse effects of retinoids was published by David et al in 1988 (2[R]). Ocular effects of oral retinoids have also been reviewed (3[R]).

Hepatotoxicity of retinoids *(SED-11, 286; SEDA-10, 124; SEDA-13, 122)* Animal and human studies of liver function tests suggest some abnormalities in the liver in about 25% of patients treated with etretinate or isotretinoin. The liver toxicity of retinoid therapy has been reviewed (4[R]) by assessing isolated case reports, 2 retrospective and 1 prospective liver biopsy studies.

Side Effects of Drugs Annual 14
M.N.G. Dukes and L. Beeley, editors

In the prospective study (5[CR]) 20 psoriatic patients who had an increased risk of hepatotoxicity (alcohol, previous use of methotrexate, persistent abnormalities of liver function tests, clinical findings of liver abnormalities, liver biopsy abnormalities) were treated with etretinate for 3 years. Liver biopsies were evaluated prospectively. Twelve patients had abnormal liver biopsy specimens before starting therapy. Of 17 evaluable patients, 15 had no change or improved, and 2 had deterioration of liver biopsy results manifested by progressive liver cell injury and deterioration of class (5[CR]). From this study and a literature review it is concluded that retinoids do not produce consistent toxic liver abnormalities (4[R]).

Etretinate (Tigason, Tegison) *(SEDA-12, 127; SEDA-13, 121)*

Whereas mucocutaneous side effects such as erythema, dryness and desquamation occur in most patients treated with etretinate, hypersensitivity drug eruptions are rare. Two patients have been described in whom *erythema-multiforme-like eruptions* appeared several days after oral intake of etretinate. In 1 patient (the second refused) etretinate rechallenge again produced the skin eruption (6[Cr]).

Isotretinoin has also been implicated as the cause of erythema multiforme in 2 patients (7[c]).

Muscle damage *(SEDA-9, 133; SEDA-12, 136)* Three patients showing clinical and electromyographic (EMG) signs of skeletal muscle damage while undergoing treatment with etretinate have been reported previously (8[Cr]). To investigate whether etretinate may cause subclinical muscle damage, neuromuscular evaluation including electromyographic studies and serum muscle enzyme level determinations were performed in 13 patients who had received etretinate for 1–2.5 years (9[Cr]).

None of the patients had complained of muscle pains or weakness. In 3 of 13 patients the EMG studies showed low amplitude and short duration action potentials. Mild muscular weakness was detected in 1. The levels of serum muscle enzymes were within the normal range in all patients. The results suggest that etretinate may cause subclinical muscle damage. The authors are of the opinion that neuromuscular evaluation should be part of the routine follow-up of patients receiving long-term therapy with etretinate (9[Cr]).

CONTACT ALLERGY *(SED-11, 287; SEDA-12, 136; SEDA-13, 128)*

Every year 'new' allergens (i.e. chemicals which have not previously caused contact allergy) are described in the literature. These allergens and updated information on chemicals which are already known to be sensitizers are presented in Table 1 (topical drugs) and Table 2 (cosmetic ingredients).

Table 1. *Contact allergy to topical drugs*

Drug	Use	Test concentration and vehicle	No. of patients	Cross-reactions	Comments	Ref.
Aciclovir	antiviral drug	1-5% pet.	1		Urticarial reaction 15 min after intravenous aciclovir infusion	11[Cr]
	antiviral drug	5% aqua	1		First report of contact allergy; no controls performed, but report reliable	12[Cr]
Ambroxol hydrochloride	mucolytic drug	0.0125–0.75% aqua	1	not to bromhexine, from which it is metabolite 8	First report of contact allergy; 20 controls negative to 0.75% aqua	13[C]
3-(Aminomethyl)-pyridyl salicylate	analgesic	1% aqua	2	Para-compounds: benzocaine, *p*-phenylenediamine, diaminodiphenylmethane	Lymphocyte transformation test positive; 35 controls were negative; see SEDA-13, 124	10[Cr]
Befunolol	beta-blocker in eye drops for glaucoma	1% aqua	6	not to other beta-blockers: timolol, carteolol		14[cr]
Clindamycin phosphate	antibiotic	1% aqua	1		The patient presented with flare of rosacea	15[Cr]
Clobetasol propionate	corticosteroid	5% pet.	2	not to other fluorinated corticosteroids	Contact allergy to corticosteroids occurs more often than reported in literature	16[CR]
Dexpanthenol	wound/eczema treatment	5% pet.	11		The patients (esp. with leg ulcers) often have other allergies as well	17[CR]
Diisopropanolamine	emollient (?)	1% aqua	1		Of 12 controls, 1 had a ?+ reaction	18[Cr]
Dipicolinic acid (2,6-pyridine dicarboxylic acid)	disinfectant	0.1% pet.	2		No reactions when tested in water; first report; 33 controls were negative	19[Cr]

(continued)

Table 1. *(continued)*

Drug	Use	Test concentration and vehicle	No. of patients	Cross-reactions	Comments	Ref.
Econazole	antifungal	comm. prep.	1	miconazole and sulconazole cream	No cross-sensitivity to clotrimazole, which differs structurally	21[Cr]
	antifungal	2% pet.	2	miconazole (2), isoconazole (2)	Imidazoles may be tested 1–2% alcohol	20[CR]
Estradiol	hormone in transdermal therapeutic system	??	1		Most contact allergic reactions to the estradiol TTS are caused by the adhesive	22[Cr]
Gentamicin	intravenous antibiotic	20% pet.	1	neomycin, amikacin, kanamycin, tobramycin	The patient had been presensitized to neomycin	23[Cr]
Gentamicin sulfate	antibiotic	20% pet.	1	neomycin sulfate	Diffuse drug rash after intravenous injection of gentamicin	24[CR]
Heparin	anti-clotting drug	sodium heparin 20,000 IU/ml	1	other commercial heparin prep. (beef, pork)		25[Cr]
	anti-clotting drug	> 25 U/ml calcium heparin sol.	1		Patch test negative; prick test positive at 20 min and after 48 h	26[Cr]
Isoconazole	antifungal	2% pet.	5	miconazole (4), econazole (2)	Imidazoles may be tested 1–2% alcohol	20[CR]
Miconazole	antifungal	2% pet.	1	isoconazole, econazole, sulconazole, tioconazole	No cross-reactions to clotrimazole and ketoconazole, which differ structurally	27[Cr]
	antifungal	2% pet.	6	econazole (1), isoconazole (1)	Imidazoles may be tested 1–2% alcohol	20[CR]
Naftifine hydrochloride	antifungal	1% pet	2		*See* SEDA-13, 126	28[Cr]
Nonoxynol-10	non-ionic surfactant	0.04% aqua	1		First report of contact allergy; 20 controls were negative	29[Cr]
Prednisolone	corticosteroid	comm. prep.	1		Pustular drug rash after intravenous injection of prednisolone succinate; *see* SEDA-13, 126	30[Cr]
Propyl gallate	antioxidant	1% pet.	2		*See under* Photosensitivity; *see* SEDA-13, 126	31[Cr]
Scopolamine	for prevention of motion sickness in TTS	no patch tests performed	16		10% of men treated were affected; placebo patches did not cause skin reactions.	32[cr]

Table 1. *(continued)*

Drug	Use	Test concentration and vehicle	No. of patients	Cross-reactions	Comments	Ref.
Scopolamine *(continued)*					*See also under* Transdermal therapeutic systems; *see* SEDA-11, 139	
Sodium cromoglycate	mast cell stabilizer	2% aqua	1		First report of contact allergy; 15 controls were negative	33[Cr]
Thimerosal	preservative in eye drops and contact lens fluids	0.1% pet.	36		The patients usually have negative reactions to the eye drops themselves; *see* SEDA-11, 140	34[Cr]
Thymol	antiseptic	1% pet.	1		3 controls were negative; no reaction to thymol-containing mouthwash	35[Cr]
Tioconazole	antifungal	2% pet.	1	miconazole, isoconazole, clotrimazole (?)	Imidazoles may be tested 1–2% alcohol	20[CR]
Tixocortol pivalate	corticosteroid	1% pet.	83		Tixocortol pivalate appears to be a marker for corticosteroid sensitivity; *see* SEDA-12, 133 *and* SEDA-10, 129	36[c]

alc. = alcohol; comm. prep. = commercial preparation; pet. = petrolatum; sol. = solution.

Table 2. *Contact allergy to cosmetic ingredients*

Ingredient	Cosmetic/use	Test concentration and vehicle	No. of patients	Cross-reactions	Comments	Ref.
Butyl methoxydibenzoylmethane	UV-filter	2% pet.	4	definitely from isopropyl-dibenzoylmethane, and possibly to isopropyldibenzoylmethane	Also photoallergic reactions reported (*see under* Photosensitivity); *see* SEDA-12, 135)	37[Cr]
Chloroxylenol	antiseptic in soap	2% pet.	1		*see* SEDA-11, 139 *and* SEDA-12, 135.	38[Cr]
1,2-Dibromo-2,4-dicyanobutane	preservative	0.004–0.1% aqua	2		Present in the commercial preparation Euxyl K 400 together with phenoxyethanol; first report of contact allergy	39[Cr]

(continued)

Table 2. *(continued)*

Ingredient	Cosmetic/use	Test concentration and vehicle	No. of patients	Cross-reactions	Comments	Ref.
Glyceryl stearate	emollient in body lotion	20% pet.	1		Rare cosmetic sensitizer; *see* SEDA-12, 135	40[Cr]
4-Isopropyl-dibenzoyl-methane	UV-filter	2% pet.	14	butyl methoxy-dibenzoylmethane	Also photoallergic reactions reported (*see under* Photosensitivity); *see* SEDA-12, 135.	37[Cr]
3-(4-Methyl-benzylidene)-camphor	UV-filter	5% pet.	8	often concomitant sensitization to isopropyl-dibenzoylmethane, the other UV-filter in the commercial preparation Eusolex 8021	Also photoallergic reactions reported (*see under* Photosensitivity); *see* SEDA-12, 135	37[Cr]
Methylionone	fragrance	0.04% alc.	1		Patch testing with various isomers suggested that the allergen was γ-methylionone	41[Cr]
Myristyl alcohol	emollient in cosmetic cream	5% pet.	3		First report of sensitization to myristyl alcohol from cosmetic source	42[Cr]
Oleamidopropyl dimethylamine	cationic emulsifier in baby body lotion	0.4% aqua	13	other amide-amine type surfactants, notably ricinoleamidopropyl dimethylamine lactate, tallowamidopropyl dimethylamine, lauramidopropyl and myristamidopropyl dimethylamine		43[Cr]
2-Phenyl-5-methylbenzoxazol (Witisol)	UV-filter	1% isopropylmyristate	2		Also photoallergic reactions reported (*see under* Photosensitivity)	37[r]
Phenyl-benzimidazole-5-sulfonic acid	UV-filter	1% aqua	4		First report of contact allergy	37[Cr]

Table 2. *(continued)*

Ingredient	Cosmetic/use	Test concentration and vehicle	No. of patients	Cross-reactions	Comments	Ref.
Potassium coco-hydrolyzed animal protein	anionic detergent in shampoo	5% and 30% aqua	1	TEA-coco-hydrolyzed animal protein; potassium undecylenoyl-hydrolyzed animal protein; TEA-oleyl-hydrolyzed animal protein	The patient had been presensitized to TEA-oleyl-hydrolyzed animal protein in ear drops; first report of contact allergy	44[Cr]
Propyl gallate	antioxidant in body lotion	1% pet.	6		*See* SEDA-13, 126; *see* Table 1	45[Cr]
	antioxidant in lipbalm	2% pet.	1			46[Cr]
	antioxidant in cosmetic cream	0.1% pet.	1			47[Cr]
Pyrocatechol	dye in cream dye for eyelashes and eyebrows	0.1% and 0.5% pet.	1	weak cross-reaction to the isomeric benzenediol hydroquinone	First report of contact allergy; no controls performed, but report undoubtedly reliable	48[Cr]
Quinophthalone (D&C Yellow no. 11)	color in hair stick	0.0001–0.1% pet.	1		*See* SEDA-13, 127	49[CR]
Stearic acid	emollient in facial moisturizer	5% pet.	1		Rare cosmetic sensitizer	40[Cr]
Toluenesulfonamide/formaldehyde resin (TSFR)	resin in nail hardener	10% pet.	8		TSFR is the usual allergen in nail lacquers; first report of contact allergy in nail hardeners	50[CR]

For explanation of abbreviations, see Table 1.

PHOTOSENSITIVITY *(SED-10, 131; SED-11, 296)*

Compared to contact allergic reactions, photocontact dermatitis is reported infrequently. This may partly be explained by the removal from general use of known photosensitizers such as the halogenated salicylanilides, which caused many cases of photosensitivity in the 1960s. However, photocontact dermatitis is probably underreported, as photopatch testing is not a standard procedure in most dermatological clinics.

From 1980–1985 16 dermatology departments in Scandinavia performed photopatch testing on 1993 patients with suspected photodermatosis (51). Photocontact dermatitis was confirmed in 217 of the subjects (10.9%). The substances tested and the number of photocontact reactions are shown in Table 3. Musk ambrette (20%), *p*-aminobenzoic acid (16%) and the phenothiazines promethazine (13%) and chlorpromazine (12%) were the principal photosensitizers. The reactions to the phenothiazines were often phototoxic.

The most frequent diagnosis in the group of 1993 patients was polymorphic light eruption ($n = 749$). In this group, 50 photocontact allergic reactions and 77 contact allergic reactions were observed, notably to sunscreens

Table 3. *Number of positive reactions in the Scandinavian photopatch test tray (n = 1993)*

Substance	Concentration and vehicle	Positive reactions
Antimicrobial agents		
Trichlorcarbanilide	1% pet.	0
Tribromsalicylanilide	1% pet.	9
Tetrachlorsalicylanilide	0.1% pet.	12
Bithionol	1% pet.	11
Hexachlorophene	1% pet.	6
Fentichlor	1% pet.	25
Trichlosan	2% pet.	3
Chlorhexidine gluconate	0.5% pet.	2
Plant derivatives and cosmetic ingredients		
Balsam of Peru	25% pet.	13
Wood mixture	20% pet.	2
Lichen mixture	16% pet.	7
Musk ambrette	1% pet.	54
6-Methylcoumarin	1% alc.	4
Perfume mixture	6% pet.	10
Therapeutic agents		
Promethazine	1% pet.	37
Chlorpromazine hydrochloride	0.1% pet.	33
p-Aminobenzoic acid	5% alc.	43

For explanation of abbreviations, see Table 1.

(among which were 8 reactions to oxybenzone). This emphasizes the importance of patch and photopatch testing of all photodermatoses, even when the primary photodermatosis diagnosis has already been established (51). The importance of sunscreens as photosensitizers also comes to the fore in a German report (37). The new group of dibenzoylmethanes, which are (next to the benzophenones) the only effective UV-A filters available, appears to be responsible for most cases of photocontact dermatitis: 18 patients were photoallergic to 4-isopropyl-dibenzoylmethane, and 7 to butyl methoxydibenzoylmethane. Sporadic cases of photosensitization were also observed to other sunscreens: 3-(4-methylbenzylidene)-camphor ($n = 4$), and 1 reaction to 2-phenyl-5-methylbenzoxazol (Witisol). Contact allergic reactions were also observed to various sunscreens (Table 1).

The results of photopatch testing performed at the Mayo Clinic from 1980 – 1985 (52) are similar to the Scandinavian experience (51).

70 patients were photopatch-tested. Photocontact dermatitis was confirmed in 14 (20%). Most reactions were observed to the phenothiazines chlorpromazine ($n = 13$) and promethazine ($n = 8$); these reactions were usually phototoxic in nature. Next came musk ambrette ($n = 9$), fentichlor and 6-methylcoumarin ($n = 5$), and hexachlorophene ($n = 4$). It is remarkable that there was only one reaction to *p*-aminobenzoic acid, whereas this UV-filter was one of the most important causes of photocontact dermatitis in Scandinavia (51); the cause remains obscure. Other recent reports have implicated fentichlor (53), benzydamine (54), and oxybenzone (55) as causes of photoallergic contact dermatitis. Photosensitivity in one patient after the use of topical desoximetasone (56) was probably caused by phototoxicity rather than photocontact allergy.

TRANSDERMAL THERAPEUTIC SYSTEMS *(SED-11, 302, 308; SEDA-11, 141)*

Scopolamine *(SED-11, 308)*

The so-called Scopolamine Transdermal Therapeutic System (TTS) is widely used for the prophylaxis and treatment of motion sickness. The principal pharmacological actions of

Table 4. *Side effects of transdermal scopolamine (59[CR])*

CNS effects	Urinary retention
Confusion	
Disorientation	Dry mouth
Dizziness	
Drowsiness	Constipation
Excitability	
Hallucinations	Cutaneous effects
Memory disturbances	Irritant dermatitis
Restlessness	Allergic contact dermatitis
Ocular effects	Withdrawal symptoms
Cycloplegia	Disturbances of equilibrium
Mydriasis	Dizziness
Acute narrow-angle glaucoma	Headaches
Impaired ocular accommodation	Nausea
	Vomiting

scopolamine are related to its anticholinergic effects. The ability of scopolamine to prevent motion-induced nausea is thought to be related to the depressant effect on the central nervous system (CNS); more specifically there is inhibition of vestibular input into the CNS resulting in inhibition of the vomiting reflex. Furthermore, scopolamine may have a direct action on the vomiting center within the reticular formation of the brainstem (57[r]). The most common side effects with the TTS are *dry mouth* (occurring in approximately 67%), *drowsiness* (about 16%), *mydriasis*, and *impaired ocular accommodation* (58[Cr]). Side effects of transdermal scopolamine reported are listed in Table 4.

The effects of single and repeated patches of scopolamine TTS upon psychological task performance were investigated in 12 normal volunteer subjects (60[CR]).

Transdermal scopolamine produced psychological and autonomic effects which are traditionally found with muscarinic acetylcholine antagonists. Alertness, sleep, memory, and attention were affected, while dry mouth, blurred vision, and bradycardia were also evident. Repeated intermittent patch applications did not produce a consistent level of performance change, but there was no evidence of either systematic increases or decreases in the psychological effects. Visual problems did, however, increase in frequency following repeated patches (60[CR]).

Several cases of psychosis due to transdermal scopolamine have recently been reported (58[Cr], 59[CR], 61[c]). Advanced age, pre-existing psychiatric disease, decline in renal function, and concurrent treatment with medications that possess anticholinergic activity (notably antihistamines) appear to predispose to this adverse reaction. The scopolamine TTS should be used with particular caution in the elderly (58[Cr]); it should not be given to children (57[R]), who are particularly sensitive to the central effects of anticholinergic drugs.

Contact dermatitis associated with transdermal therapeutic systems In an excellent article by Holdiness (62[R]), the literature has been reviewed for contact dermatitis associated with transdermal therapeutic systems. Most cutaneous reactions are limited to localized dermatitis; however, generalized systemic effects may occur. Investigators are reporting skin-related side effects in up to 50% of patients using transdermal clonidine. With the other agents (nitroglycerin, scopolamine, estradiol and testosterone), this is demonstrated much less frequently. Reactivation of the dermatitis via oral medication, following sensitization to the patch, has been noted in rare instances. Unexpectedly, of 164 naval crew members treated with scopolamine TTS for 1.5 to 15 months, 16 developed skin reactions under the patches suggestive of allergic contact dermatitis. Patch tests were not performed, but application of placebo patches did not cause skin reactions (32[c]).

Ageusia associated with transdermal nitroglycerin 'Ageusia' is the term used to describe drug-induced absence of taste.

A patient on transdermal nitroglycerin after 2 weeks reportedly lost the ability to detect bitter and salty tastes (63[C]); over the next 4 weeks, the sense of taste was lost completely. The patient reported complete return of taste perception within 1 week of discontinuing transdermal nitroglycerin. A rechallenge 3 months later again resulted in renewed loss of bitter and salty taste sensation. Although the patient's sense of taste was never tested objectively, and he was never determined to have any condition, such as a cold or sinus congestion, that may have impaired taste sensation, there is probably an association between the ageusia and the transdermal nitroglycerin.

The manufacturer of the nitroglycerin preparation had up to January 1987 received 2 complaints of altered taste perception associated with its use (63[C]).

MISCELLANEOUS SIDE EFFECTS

Anaphylaxis due to chlorhexidine gluconate Six patients who developed *urticaria, dyspnea* and *anaphylactic shock* due to topical application of chlorhexidine gluconate solution have been described (64[CR]). Using intradermal, scratch, and epicutaneous tests, the disinfectant was shown to be the causative agent of Type I hypersensitivity. To prevent life-threatening adverse reactions, the authors recommend using chlorhexidine gluconate on wound surfaces at the lowest bactericidal concentration (0.05%). Application to mucous membranes is discouraged (64[CR]). Contact urticaria to chlorhexidine was also observed in a veterinarian with hand dermatitis (65[Cr]).

Diphencyprone Diphencyprone (2,3-diphenylcyclopropenone-1) is a potent contact allergen that has been used for the treatment of alopecia areata and resistant warts. Of 10 patients treated with diphencyprone for verrucae, 2 had to discontinue treatment because of serious adverse reactions (66[C]). One patient developed a *generalized dermatitis*. In addition, she experienced palpitations, which ECG recordings showed to be caused by *ventricular extrasystoles*. The other patient developed *generalized urticaria* after 5 weekly applications of diphencyprone 0.1–1% in hydrous emulsifying cream. The urticaria resolved 4 days after the diphencyprone was discontinued (66[C]). In Greece, 45 patients were treated with diphencyprone for alopecia areata (67[Cr]). Three (6.7%) developed *vitiligo*. None of these patients had a personal or family history of vitiligo. The vitiligo appeared 3–5 months after the onset of treatment. It was localized to the areas of application in 2 patients. In the 3rd, vitiliginous areas also developed elsewhere. Mitochondrial autoantibodies were found in one case. Vitiligo and alopecia areata are both autoimmune disorders, and up to 9% of patients with alopecia areata also suffer from vitiligo. The authors suggest that their 3 patients had subclinical vitiligo, which was triggered (Koebner-phenomenon) by the repeated contact dermatitis which resulted from diphencyprone applications (67[Cr]).

Carcinogenicity of topical mechlorethamine hydrochloride Topical applications of mechlorethamine hydrochloride (nitrogen mustard) have been used for the treatment of cutaneous T cell lymphomas for more than 30 years. However, the drug is a known carcinogen, and administration for long periods might be expected to induce cancers in the skin and perhaps other organs if sufficient mechlorethamine were absorbed into the general circulation. 331 patients with cutaneous T cell lymphoma were treated with topical mechlorethamine in 2 large USA centers between 1968 and 1982 (68[CR]). When compared with the general population of the USA, these patients were at an 8.6-fold and a 1.8-fold increased risk for the development of squamous cell carcinoma and basal cell carcinoma of the skin, respectively. In addition, their risk was significantly enhanced for Hodgkin's disease and colon cancer but not for systemic cancers known to be induced by systemic administration of alkylating drugs. In contrast to the skin cancers, these malignancies were not attributed to mechlorethamine. Both Hodgkin's disease and colon cancer have been linked to cutaneous T-cell lymphomas before; genetic factors and related pathogenic mechanisms may account for these associations rather than the carcinogenic action of therapeutic agents such as mechlorethamine hydrochloride (68[CR]).

REFERENCES

1. Sheehan-Dare RA, Cotterill JA, Barnard DL (1989) Transformation of myelodysplasia to acute myeloid leukaemia during psoralen photochemotherapy (PUVA) treatment of psoriasis. *Acta Derm.-Venereol., 69,* 262.
2. David M, Hodak E, Lowe NJ (1988) Adverse effects of retinoids. *Med. Toxicol., 3,* 273.
3. Lebowitz MA, Berson DS (1988) Ocular effects of oral retinoids. *J. Am. Acad. Dermatol., 19,* 209.
4. Roenigk HH Jr. (1988) Liver toxicity of retinoid therapy. *J. Am. Acad. Dermatol., 19,* 199.
5. Roenigk HH Jr, Gibstine C, Glazer SD et al (1985) Serial liver biopsies in psoriatic patients receiving long-term etretinate. *Br. J. Dermatol., 112,* 77.
6. David M, Sandbank M, Lowe NJ (1989) Erythema multiforme-like eruptions associated with etretinate therapy. *Clin. Exp. Dermatol., 14,* 230.
7. Bigby M, Stern RS (1988) Adverse reactions to isotretinoin. *J. Am. Acad. Dermatol., 18,* 547.
8. Hodak E, David M, Gadoth N et al (1987) Etretinate-involved muscle damage. *Br. J. Dermatol., 116,* 623.
9. David M, Hodak E, Sandbank M (1988) Electromyographic abnormalities in patients undergoing long-term therapy with etretinate. *J. Am. Acad. Dermatol., 19,* 273.
10. Camarasa JG, Lluch M, Serra-Baldrich E et al (1989) Allergic contact dermatitis from 3-(aminomethyl)-pyridyl salicylate. *Contact Derm., 20,* 347.
11. Gola M, Francalanci S, Brusi C et al (1989) Contact sensitization to acyclovir. *Contact Derm., 20,* 394.
12. Camarasa JG, Serra-Baldrich E (1988) Allergic contact dermatitis from acyclovir. *Contact Derm., 19,* 235.
13. Mancuso G, Berdondini RM (1989) Contact allergy to ambroxol. *Contact Derm., 20,* 154.
14. Kanzaki T, Kato N, Kabasawa Y et al (1988) Contact dermatitis due to the beta-blocker timolol in eyedrops. *Contact Derm., 19,* 388.
15. De Kort WJA, De Groot AC (1989) Clindamycin allergy presenting as rosacea. *Contact Derm., 20,* 72.
16. Cox NH (1988) Contact allergy to clobetasol propionate. *Arch. Dermatol., 124,* 911.
17. Schulze-Dirks A, Frosch PJ (1988) Kontaktallergie auf Dexpanthenol. *Hautarzt, 39,* 375.
18. Fujimoto K, Hashimoto S, Kozuka T et al (1989) Contact dermatitis due to isopropanolamine. *Contact Derm., 21,* 56.
19. Hums R (1988) Dipicolinsäure – ein Allergen? *Dermatol. Monatsschr., 174,* 333.
20. Jelen G, Tennstedt D (1989) Contact dermatitis from topical imidazole antifungals: 15 new cases. *Contact Derm., 21,* 6.
21. Carmichael AJ, Foulds IS (1988) Imidazole cross-sensitivity to sulconazole. *Contact Derm., 19,* 237.
22. McBurney EI, Boustany Noel S, Collins JH (1989) Contact dermatitis to transdermal estradiol system. *J. Am. Acad. Dermatol., 20,* 508.
23. Guin JD, Phillips D (1989) Erythroderma from systemic contact dermatitis: a complication of systemic gentamicin in a patient with contact allergy to neomycin. *Cutis, 43,* 564.
24. Ghadially R, Ramsay CA (1988) Gentamicin: systemic exposure to a contact allergen. *J. Am. Acad. Dermatol., 19,* 428.
25. Korstanje MJ, Bessems PJMJ, Hardy E et al (1989) Delayed-type hypersensitivity reaction to heparin. *Contact Derm., 20,* 383.
26. Young E (1988) Allergy to subcutaneous heparin. *Contact Derm., 19,* 152.
27. Motley RJ, Reynolds AJ (1988) Contact allergy to 2,4-dichlorophenylethyl imidazole derivatives. *Contact Derm., 19,* 381.
28. Senff H, Tholen S, Stieler W et al (1989) Allergic contact dermatitis to naftifine. *Dermatologica, 178,* 107.
29. Kabasawa Y, Kanzaki T (1989) Allergic contact dermatitis from the surfactant in Hibitane. *Contact Derm., 20,* 378.
30. Voss M (1988) Eine Prednisolon-Allergie mit pustulosem Exanthem. *Dermatol. Monatsschr., 174,* 221.
31. Valsecchi R, Cainelli T (1988) Contact allergy to propyl gallate. *Contact Derm., 19,* 380.
32. Gordon CR, Shupak A, Doweck I et al (1989) Allergic contact dermatitis caused by transdermal hyoscine. *Br. Med. J., 298,* 1220.
33. Kudo H, Tanaka T, Miyachi Y et al (1988) Contact dermatitis from sodium cromoglycate eyedrops. *Contact Derm., 19,* 312.
34. Tosti A, Tosti G (1988) Thimerosal: a hidden allergen in ophthalmology. *Contact Derm., 18,* 268.
35. Fisher AA (1989) Allergic contact dermatitis due to thymol in Listerine for treatment of paronychia. *Cutis, 43,* 531.
36. Dooms-Goossens A, Andersen KE, Burrows D et al (1989) A survey of the results of patch tests with tixocortol pivalate. *Contact Derm., 20,* 158.
37. Schauder S, Ippen H (1988) Photoallergisches und allergisches Kontaktekzem durch Dibenzoylmethan-Verbindungen und andere Lichtschutzfilter. *Hautarzt, 39,* 435.
38. Libow LF, Ruszkowski AM, DeLeo VA (1989) Allergic contact dermatitis from para-chloro-metaxylenol in Lurosep soap. *Contact Derm., 20,* 67.
39. Senff H, Exner M, Gortz J, Goos M (1989) Kontaktallergie auf einen neuen Konservierungsstoff. Dermatosen *37,* 45.

40. De Groot AC, van der Meeren HLM, Weyland JW (1988) Cosmetic allergy from stearic acid and glyceryl stearate. *Contact Derm., 19,* 77.
41. Bernaola G, Escayol P, Fernandez E et al (1989) Contact dermatitis from methylionone fragrance. *Contact Derm., 20,* 71.
42. De Groot AC, Bruynzeel DP, van Joost Th et al (1988) Contact allergy from myristyl alcohol. *Contact Derm., 19,* 76.
43. De Groot AC, Jagtman BA, van der Meeren HLM et al (1988) Crossreaction pattern of the cationic emulsifier oleamidopropyl dimethylamine. *Contact Derm., 19,* 284.
44. Dooms-Goossens A, Debusschere K, Dupre K et al (1988) Can eardrops induce a shampoo dermatitis? A case study. *Contact Derm., 19,* 143.
45. Heine A (1988) Contact dermatitis from propyl gallate. *Contact Derm., 18,* 313.
46. Wilson AGMcT, White IR, Kirby JDT (1989) Allergic contact dermatitis from propyl gallate in a lip balm. *Contact Derm., 20,* 145.
47. Bardazzi F, Misciali C, Borrello P et al (1988) Contact dermatitis due to antioxidants. *Contact Derm., 19,* 385.
48. Andersen KE, Carlsen L (1988) Pyrocatechol contact allergy from a permanent cream dye for eyelashes and eyebrows. *Contact Derm., 18,* 306.
49. Komamura H, Kozuka T, Ishii M et al (1989) Allergic contact sensitivity to quinophthalone. *Contact Derm., 20,* 177.
50. De Wit FS, De Groot AC, Weyland JM et al (1988) An outbreak of contact dermatitis from toluenesulfonamide formaldehyde resin in a nail hardener. *Contact Derm., 18,* 280.
51. Thune P, Jansen C, Wennersten G et al (1988) The Scandinavian multicenter photopatch study 1985–1985: final report. *Photodermatology, 5,* 261.
52. Menz J, Muller SA, Connolly SM (1988) Photopatch testing: A six-year experience. *J. Am. Acad. Dermatol., 18,* 1044.
53. Norris PG, Hawk JLM, White IR (1988) Photoallergic contact dermatitis from fentichlor. *Contact Derm., 18,* 318.
54. Motley RJ, Reynolds AJ (1988) Photodermatitis from benzydamine cream. *Contact Derm., 19,* 1.
55. Knobler E, Almeida L, Ruzkowski AM (1989) Photoallergy to benzophenone. *Arch. Dermatol., 125,* 801.
56. Stierstorfer MB, Baughman RD (1988) Photosensitivity to desoximetasone emollient cream. *Arch. Dermatol., 124,* 1870.
57. Nairn JG (1988) Transdermal therapeutic systems: Scopolamine. *Can. J. Hosp. Pharm., 41,* 201.
58. Mego DM, Omori DJM, Hanley JF (1988) Transdermal scopolamine as a cause of transient psychosis in two elderly patients. *South. Med. J., 81,* 394.
59. Ziskind AA (1988) Transdermal scopolamine-induced psychosis. *Postgrad. Med., 84,* 73.
60. Parrott AC (1987) Transdermal scopolamine: effects of single and repeated patches upon psychological task performance. *Neuropsychobiology, 17,* 53.
61. Rozzini R, Inzola M, Trabucchi M (1988) Delirium from transdermal scopolamine in an elderly woman. *J. Am. Med. Assoc., 260,* 478.
62. Holdiness MR (1989) A review of contact dermatitis associated with transdermal therapeutic systems. *Contact Derm., 20,* 3.
63. Ewing RC, Janda SM, Henann NE (1989) Ageusia associated with transdermal nitroglycerin. *Clin. Pharm., 8,* 146.
64. Okano M, Nomura M, Hata S et al (1989) Anaphylactic symptoms due to chlorhexidine gluconate. *Arch. Dermatol., 125,* 50.
65. Fisher AA (1989) Contact urticaria from chlorhexidine. *Cutis, 43,* 17.
66. Lane PR, Hogan DJ (1988) Diphencyprone. *J. Am. Acad. Dermatol., 19,* 364.
67. Hatzis J, Gourgiotou K, Tosca A et al (1988) Vitiligo as a reaction to topical treatment with diphencyprone. *Dermatologica, 177,* 146.
68. Vonderheid EC, Tan ET, Kantor AF et al (1988) Long-term efficacy, curative potential, and carcinogenicity of topical mechlorethamine chemotherapy in cutaneous T cell lymphoma. *J. Am. Acad. Dermatol., 20,* 416.

Inga Lunde

16 Antihistamines

GENERAL TOPICS

The use of antihistamines in patients with asthma The American Academy of Allergy and Immunology (AAAI) has published a position statement on the use of antihistamines in patients with asthma (1^{R}). They state that although antihistamines have been considered to be ineffective in asthma, they have been demonstrated to produce modest bronchdilatation in patients with asthma. In addition, they have been demonstrated to increase the threshold for bronchoconstriction after challenge.

They further state that histamines have a place in the treatment of allergic rhinitis which is especially important in patients with asthma to facilitate filtration, warming and humidification of inspired air. There are however reports of hydroxyzine, brompheniramine and diphenhydramine causing *airway obstruction* in some patients with asthma. Patients with a history of breathing difficulty after antihistamine administration should therefore be carefully evaluated. Only pulmonary function testing before and after the administration of antihistamines to patients (who should not be receiving bronchodilators) can objectively identify those patients who are subject to this adverse effect.

Although antihistamines are not first-line drugs for the treatment of asthma, they should not be withheld from patients with asthma who require treatment for concomitant disorders such as allergic rhinitis, allergic dermatoses, and urticaria.

The traditional labelling for antihistamines in the United States includes the statement 'antihistamines should not be used to treat lower respiratory tract symptoms including asthma'. The AAAI recommends that this labelling be revised to reflect current knowledge that antihistamines are not contraindicated in patients with asthma unless adverse reactions to this treatment have previously been demonstrated.

INDIVIDUAL DRUGS

Acrivastine

Acrivastine is one of the recently introduced antihistamines claimed to have a low sedating potential. The product has been studied in a randomized, double-blind trial (2^{C}). Seventy patients with seasonal allergic rhinitis were included. They received either 8 mg of acrivastine or placebo twice daily for 10 days. Acrivastine was significantly better than placebo in reducing the severity of the symptoms of allergic rhinitis. *Drowsiness* was reported by 5 of the patients receiving acrivastine; one of them also reported *dizziness*. None of the patients receiving placebo complained of drowsiness.

Astemizole *(SED-11, 316, 317; SEDA-12, 142)*

Overdose A 15-year-old girl with a history of allergic rhinitis, who stated that she had been treated with astemizole 10 mg daily for 10 weeks, has been reported to develop *torsade de pointes* (3^{C}).

The last dose of astemizole was taken 28 hours before admission to hospital. She collapsed outdoors, and after emergency admission, she collapsed again. ECG showed *multiform premature ventricular contractions* and *prolonged QT interval with first-degree atrioventricular block*. She was admitted to intensive care for monitoring and 5 hours later she had 2 episodes of torsade de pointes associated with loss of consciousness. No further arrhythmias occurred and the QT interval returned to normal over the next 6 days.

The patient gave a history of recurrent *syncope* for 3 days preceding admission. She denied astemizole overdose and did not use any other medication and had no history of smoking, drinking or substance

Side Effects of Drugs Annual 14
M.N.G. Dukes and L. Beeley, editors

abuse. There was no history of cardiac problems, seizures or sudden death in her family.

The distribution plasma half-life of 13.4 hours and the elimination-phase half-life of 13.5 days for astemizole plus hydroxylated metabolites in this patient were similar to values in another adolescent previously reported to develop cardiac problems after overdose of astemizole.

Although the patient denied overdose, the authors think that the data are more consistent with ingestion of a 200–300 mg single dose than with chronic ingestion of 10 mg daily for 10 days in this patient who had normal liver function and no predisposition to drug accumulation.

Azatadine *(SED-11, 317)*

The results of two separate randomized double-blind studies indicate that *sedation* occurs only very rarely in patients treated with azatadine.

Azatadine maleate (1 mg twice daily) was compared to pheniramine maleate (25 mg 3 times daily) in 50 patients with allergic rhinitis in one of the studies. The treatment period was 7 days (4[C]). None of the patients taking azatadine in this study experienced side effects. Nearly half of the patients (48%) treated with pheniramine complained of drowsiness and epigastric discomfort.

The same design was used in the other study, but here the 50 patients were suffering from urticaria and the total treatment period was 14 days (5[C]). *Drowsiness* was the only reported side effect in this study. It was recorded in only 1 patient (4%) taking azatadine compared to 16 patients (64%) taking pheniramine.

No details are given as to how the side effects were recorded in these two studies.

Cinnarizine and flunarizine *(SED-11, 391; SEDA-13, 131)*

Cinnarizine and flunarizine are piperazine derivatives with antihistamine properties and calcium-channel blocking activity. Several recent reports have described *extrapyramidal reactions* and *depression* associated with their use. (6[C]–10[C]).

In Spain a system of spontaneous reporting of side effects has been operating since 1983 and around 5000 reports have been received: 86 of these refer to cinnarizine as the suspected drug, 25 refer to flunarizine, and 5 to both drugs taken simultanously (11[R]). Of these 116 reports, 87 described *extrapyramidal symptoms* or *depression* or both; cinnarizine had been taken in 70 cases, flunarizine in 13, and both drugs in 4 cases.

Seventy patients developed tremor and parkinsonism while being treated with cinnarizine. Only 3 patients were taking other drugs likely to induce parkinsonism. Eight additional patients developed parkinsonism and 3 developed tremor while being treated with flunarizine. Four additional patients developed parkinsonism while being treated with both drugs simultaneously.

Four patients developed *depression* whilst taking flunarizine. The patients improved when the treatment stopped. None of them had taken any other drug which could have contributed to their depression.

The authors have started a case-control study with the aim of quantifying the risk of extrapyramidal disorders associated with these drugs.

Loratadine *(SEDA-12, 143)*

This new H_1-receptor antagonist has been devoid of significant CNS effects in experimental studies carried out so far.

The efficacy and safety of single oral doses (10, 20, 40 and 80 mg) of loratadine in suppressing formation of histamine-induced wheals have been assessed in a cross-over study in 29 healthy male subjects. Measurements of resulting wheal areas showed that loratadine suppressed wheal formation significantly better than placebo. *Sedation* was reported by only 1 subject in the 40 mg loratadine group, 3 in the 80 mg loratadine groups and one in the placebo group. No anticholinergic effects were reported (12[C]).

The effect of loratadine on task performance has also been studied in 12 male subjects in 2 separate experiments (13[C]).

In the 1st experiment the subjects were treated with loratadine 10 mg, clemastine 1 mg, terfenadine 60 mg, or placebo. In the 2nd experiment 5 mg diazepam was given together with each of the 4 treatments used in the 1st experiment. The subjects were tested at weekly intervals in this study which was carried out double-blind with a latin square design.

The performance of the subjects was evaluated by reaction time and a tracking task after treatment. The tracking task was performed initially and then repeated together with a continuous memory task. In addition, the subjects graded their mental status on visual analog rating scales.

Task performance was not generally impaired after treatment with loratadine or terfenadine in these experiments. The concomitant administration of diazepam in the 2nd experiment did not appear to affect the performance of the subjects. Clemastine caused a decrease in the performance in both experiments.

As a conclusion of both experiments *sleepiness* was reported by more subjects when treated with clemastine than with loratadine, terfenadine or placebo.

Terfenadine *(SED-11, 317; SEDA-12, 143; SEDA-13, 132)*

Severe exacerbation of psoriasis possibly due to terfenadine has been reported (14[C]).

The patient had suffered from unstable psoriasis for 20 years, requiring repeated hospital admissions and intermittent systemic therapy. He was admitted for treatment during an active phase of the disease. His only systemic therapy at the time of admission was terfenadine 60 mg twice daily which had been started 10 days previously. He was given ciclosporin which initially improved his condition. Twenty days after admission he developed severe exacerbation of his psoriasis, progressing to generalized erythrodermia. Ciclosporin and terfenadine were discontinued, and he received intensive treatment for his condition. The severe reaction was initially attributed to ciclosporin. However, it was decided to exclude terfenadine as a causative factor and 3 months later the patient was rechallenged with terfenadine under hospital supervision. Within 36 hours of starting terfenadine 60 mg daily, an urticarial eruption appeared. The histology showed similar features to those found in a skin biopsy done at the time of the first reactions suggesting that terfenadine had been responsible for the exacerbation of his psoriasis.

Overdose A retrospective study has been carried out to determine the incidence, severity and outcome of accidental terfenadine ingestion in children aged 1–5 years.

Twenty-eight cases were identified: One child (2 years of age, 900 mg terfenadine ingested) received hospital treatment with the administration of activated charcoal and sorbitol; 2 children (21 months old, 120 mg; 2 years old, 300 mg) received ipecac huana at home; and 25 children (14 months–4 years old, 60–180 mg) received home management with observation alone. In all of the cases followed up the patients remained asymptomatic.

Based on these results, the authors propose that terfenadine ingestion of up to 120 mg in small children may be managed at home with observation, but until sufficient data have been collected on larger doses, 'children who ingest more than 120 mg or who are less than one year old should be referred to a health care facility for evaluation and treatment' (15[C]).

A *quinidine-like effect on the myocardium with convulsions* has been reported in a patient with terfenadine toxicity (16[C]).

A healthy 21-year-old woman developed generalized convulsions before admission to hospital. The patient had been given terfenadine for pruritus 7 days earlier. Two tablets per day had been prescribed (120 mg), but she had taken 4 tablets daily, except for the day when the convulsion occurred when she took none. Although 56 tablets had been prescribed, only 3 remained in the packet; the patient claimed she had thrown the rest away.

On admission there were no abnormal physical signs and blood pressure was normal. An ECG showed prolonged QT-intervals, however, with widened notched and inverted T-waves and a single premature beat. These changes later reversed to normal.

The high levels of metabolized and unmetabolized terfenadine in the plasma on admission with lowered levels 9 hours later pointed to overdose, although delayed metabolic clearance could not be excluded.

The authors note that 771 reactions to terfenadine have been reported to the U.K. Committee on Safety of Medicines since 1981, including 1 case of arrhythmia, 1 of extrasystole, and 1 of cardiac arrest. CNS effects include 1 report of convulsions and 2 cases of aggravated epilepsy. Cardiotoxic effects may be more common than realized because ECGs are not routinely performed.

REFERENCES

1. Sly RM, Kemp JP (1988) The use of antihistamines in patients with asthma. *J. Allergy Clin. Immunol., September*, 481.
2. Leonhardt L, Gale NM, Gibbs TG (1988) Placebo-controlled, randomized evaluation of acrivastine in seasonal allergic rhinitis. *Acta Ther.* 14, 241.
3. Simons FER, Kesselman MS, Giddens NG et al (1988) Astemisole-induced torsade de pointes. *Lancet, 2*, 624.
4. Tepan MG, Sharma SD (1988) Azatadine vis-a-vis pheniramine in allergic rhinitis. *Med. Surg.*, 19.
5. Dhurandhar MW, Sharma SD (1988) Azatadine versus pheniramine in chronic urticaria. *Med. Surg.*, 15.
6. Marti Masso JF, Carrera N, and De la Puente E (1985) Posible parkinsonismo por cinaricina. *Med. Clin. (Barc.), 85*, 614.
7. Chouza C, Scaramelli A, Caamano JL, De Medina O (1986) Parkinsonism, tardive dyskinesia, akathisia, and depression induced by flunarizine. *Lancet, 1*, 1303.
8. Meyboom RHB, Ferrari MD, Dieleman BP (1986) Parkinsonism, tardive dyskinesia, akathisia, and depression induced by flunarizine. *Lancet, 2*, 292.
9. Joint Formulary Committee (1987) *British National Formulary, No. 14*, p. 60. British Medical Association and the Pharmaceutical Society of Great Britain, London.
10. Laporte JR, Capella D (1986) Useless drugs are not placebos. *Lancet, 2*, 853.
11. Capellà D, Laporte JR, Castel JM et al (1988) Parkinsonism, tremor, and depression induced by cinnarizine and flunarizine. *Br. Med. J., 297*, 722.
12. Kassem N, Roman I, Gural R et al (1988) Effects of loratadine (SCH 29851) in suppression of histamine-induced skin wheals. *Ann. Allergy, 90*, 505.
13. Gaillard AWK, Gruisen A, De Jong R (1988) The influence of antihistamines on human performance. *Eur. J. Clin. Pharmacol., 35*, 249.
14. Harrison PV, Stones RN (1988) Severe exacerbation of psoriasis due to terfenadine. *Clin. Exp. Dermatol., 13*, 275.
15. Spiller HA, Picciotti M, Perez E (1989) Accidental terfenadine ingestion in children. *Vet. Hum. Toxicol., 31*, 154.
16. Davies AJ, Harindra V, McEwan A, Ghose RR (1989) Cardiotoxic effect with convulsions in terfenadine overdose. *Br. Med. J., 298*, 325.

F.A. Nelemans

17 Antiallergic and antitussive drugs

Editorial note *Several drugs used in bronchial asthma and cough are dealt with in other chapters. These include xanthine compounds (Chapter 1), the opiates and derivatives such as dextromethorphan (Chapter 8), sympathomimetic and parasympatholytic agents (Chapter 14), the antihistamines (Chapter 16) and the corticosteroids (Chapter 41).*

DRUGS USED IN BRONCHIAL ASTHMA *(SED-11, 322; SEDA-12, 144; SEDA-13, 134)*

Tranilast (Rizaben) *(SED-11, 325; SEDA-12, 145)*

Bladder biopsy performed on 6 of 8 patients with cystitis probably caused by tranilast showed an eosinophilic cystitis in 3 cases. In the lymphocyte stimulation test using tranilast as an antigen, 1 positive and 1 false-positive reaction were seen (1).

MUCOLYTIC AGENTS *(SED-11, 328; SEDA-12, 145)*

Acetylcysteine *(SED-11, 328; SEDA-12, 145)*

Conventional treatment of patients with meconium ileus equivalent in cystic fibrosis consists of the oral and rectal administration of acetylcysteine and hypertonic solutions of sodium diatrizoate. No changes in plasma sodium, potassium or calcium were observed, but in all 7 patients acute decreases in plasma *magnesium* (< 0.70 mmol/l) occurred (2[c]).

Side Effects of Drugs Annual 14
M.N.G. Dukes and L. Beeley, editors

Carbocisteine *(SEDA-10, 138)*

An extensive literature review shows that carbocisteine is a safe drug. Serious adverse events associated with its use have not been reported. It is not known if carbocysteine can be used safely in pregnancy and lactation (3[r]).

Stepronine lysine

Stepronine taken orally at a dose of 810 mg daily (3 times 270 mg) by 12 healthy volunteers for 10 days) had no adverse effects on the gastric mucosa (4[c]).

COUGH REMEDIES *(SED-11, 329; SEDA-12, 145; SEDA-13, 135)*

Benylin expectorant

A 77-year-old retired publican woke at 05.00 h with a grossly swollen tongue after gargling with Benylin expectorant for 20 min the previous evening. Intubation for 48 h was necessary. He was also receiving chemotherapy for a centroblastic/centrocytic lymphoma and had been in remission for some time. The etiology of the *edema* is discussed. It may have occurred because of a reaction to one of the constituents of Benylin expectorant (Ponceau 4RE124?, benzoate?) (5[c]).

MISCELLANEOUS

Almitrine bimesilate *(SED-11, 330; SEDA-12, 145; SEDA-13, 136)*

A 1-year study of 701 patients (344 on almitrine and 357 on placebo) showed that almitrine improves hypoxemia in a high percentage of patients with chronic obstructive pulmonary diseases. 20% of the patients did not respond. Side-effects (mainly *paresthesia*) are generally related to high almitrine plasma levels. It is now recommended that treatment should be stopped for 1 month out of every 3. It must be stressed that almitrine is treatment for hypoxemia and not for chronic bronchitis (6^c).

REFERENCES

1. Kuwabara T, Kase T, Kuroda K et al (1988) Cystitis in 8 patients treated with tranilast. *Acta Urol. Jpn., 34*, 874.
2. Godsen C, Ryan MP, Brady HR (1988) Acute hypomagnesemia complicating the treatment of meconium ileus equivalent in cystic fibrosis. *Scand. J. Gastroenterol., 23, Suppl. 143*, 148.
3. Brown DT (1988) Carbocysteine. *Drug Intell. Clin Pharm., 22*, 603.
4. Grislandi M, Barbieri P, Gaiani P et al (1988) Non-involvement of gastric mucus in the mucolytic effect of stepronine lysine salt. *Int. J. Clin. Pharm. Res., 8*, 223.
5. Self F, Bates GJEM, Drake-Les A (1988) Severe angioneurotic oedema causing acute airway obstruction, *J. R. Soc. Med., 81*, 544.
6. Weitzenbeum E, Kessler R, Apprill M et al (1988) Place de l'almitrine dans le traitement de l'insufficience respiratoire chronique. *J. Med. Strasbourg, 19*, 377.

J.K. Aronson

18 Positive inotropic drugs and drugs used in dysrhythmias

POSITIVE INOTROPIC DRUGS *(SED-11, 333; SEDA-12, 148; SEDA-13, 138)*

The actions of positive inotropic drugs in heart failure have recently been reviewed (1[R]).

CARDIAC GLYCOSIDES *(SED-11, 333; SEDA-12, 148; SEDA-138)*

The clinical manifestations and treatment of digitalis toxicity have again been reviewed (2[R], 3[R]).

The clinical pharmacology of cardiac glycosides which are predominantly eliminated via hepatic metabolism has been extensively reviewed in a monograph in which much German-language literature, previously scantily reviewed, has been discussed (4[R]). The principal drugs covered are digitoxin, gitoxin, pengitoxin (16-acetylgitoxin), and gitoformate.

The use of digoxin compared with other drugs in heart failure in sinus rhythm

In recent years there have appeared several reports of studies in which the effects of digoxin in heart failure in sinus rhythm have been compared with those of other types of drugs, both positive inotropic drugs (β_1-adrenoceptor agonists and inhibitors of phosphodiesterase type III) and vasodilators (calcium antagonists, angiotensin-converting enzyme (ACE) inhibitors, and other vasodilators). Some of these studies have been briefly reviewed elsewhere (5[R]). In this account I shall deal only with direct comparisons of digoxin with other drugs. I shall not review these reports in detail, but shall outline only those features of greatest interest.

DIGOXIN VERSUS OTHER POSITIVE INOTROPIC DRUGS

β_1-Adrenoceptor agonists

Dobutamine *The acute hemodynamic effects of digoxin and dobutamine have been compared in an open study in 6 patients with acute myocardial infarction (6[C]). The effects of dobutamine on left ventricular filling pressure (LVFP), cardiac index, and stroke work index were all greater than those of digoxin, the effects of which were small.*

Xamoterol *Xamoterol is a β_1-adrenoceptor agonist with partial antagonist activity. While it therefore has a positive inotropic effect in patients with mild heart failure, it acts as a beta-blocker in patients with high sympathetic tone and may therefore worsen moderate or severe heart failure. The current list of contraindications in the Data Sheet, which ICI have published in the United Kingdom, is extensive, and includes patients with breathlessness at rest or on minimal exercise, those who have or have had pulmonary edema, those with tachycardia or hypotension, those taking more than 40 mg furosemide per day, and those taking an ACE inhibitor.*

In a double-blind comparison of xamoterol with digoxin in 433 patients with moderate chronic heart failure xamoterol produced very similar clinical effects to those of digoxin (7[C]). Although the authors stressed the differences between the two drugs, which were in favor of xamoterol, the differences were small, except in the case of subjective tiredness. Furthermore, the patients on digoxin were underdigitalized, judging by the mean plasma digoxin concentration of 1.2 nmol/l (0.87 ng/ml), which is at the lower end

Side Effects of Drugs Annual 14
M.N.G. Dukes and L. Beeley, editors

of the therapeutic range. One is justified in concluding from this study that xamoterol is not more effective than digoxin.

Most of the adverse drug effects in this study were cardiovascular, and there was no overall difference between the two drugs. However, digoxin caused more nausea and vomiting.

Inhibitors of phosphodiesterase III

Milrinone has been compared with digoxin in a double-blind study in 230 patients with chronic heart failure (8^C). Both drugs had similar effects in increasing exercise time, but the effects of the combination were no greater than with either drug alone. Additional treatment was required more often in the patients taking milrinone alone compared with digoxin or the combination. Furthermore, there was a trend to an increased mortality at 3 months and a significantly higher incidence of palpitation and arrhythmias in those taking milrinone. The authors concluded that no benefit would be gained by substituting milrinone for digoxin in patients already stable on digoxin.

DIGOXIN VERSUS VASODILATORS

Calcium antagonists

Hemodynamic responses to nifedipine and digoxin have been compared in 12 patients with congestive cardiac failure (9^C). Both drugs reduced left ventricular (LV) filling pressure equally and a greater effect was achieved with a combination of the two. There were no adverse drug effects during this short-term study.

ACE inhibitors

The clinical and hemodynamic effects of captopril have been compared with those of digoxin in patients with congestive heart failure in 3 studies (10^C–12^C).

The first two of these studies were small. In 8 patients both drugs reduced LV filling pressure and increased cardiac index (10^C). The effects of the two drugs were similar and the combination produced a greater effect than either drug alone. In 16 patients the two drugs had similar effects on systolic time intervals and exercise tolerance (11^C). No adverse effects were seen over a period of a month.

The third study (12^C) was much larger. In 300 patients captopril significantly improved exercise time; the effect of digoxin was larger than that of placebo, but not significantly so. Digoxin significantly increased LV ejection fraction and captopril did not. Captopril reduced the frequency of ventricular extra beats and digoxin did not. More adverse effects were attributed to captopril than to digoxin, and the excess was largely accounted for by mild and transient dizziness and light-headedness. The interpretation of the results of this study is complicated by the fact that 65% of the patients had been on digoxin before the study began and patients in whom digoxin withdrawal could not be tolerated were not included.

Other vasodilators

The clinical and hemodynamic effects of other vasodilators have been compared with those of digoxin in patients with congestive heart failure in 7 studies (13^c, 14^c, 15^C–19^C).

Hydralazine *There have been 3 small studies (13^c, 14^c, 15^C) and one large study (16^C) in which digoxin and hydralazine have been compared.*

In 18 patients hydralazine, in combination with a nitrate (n=14) or prazosin (n=4), significantly increased LV ejection fraction. Digoxin had a similar effect and the effect was larger when the drugs were combined (13^c). In 8 patients the addition of digoxin to a diuretic reduced pulmonary capillary wedge pressure, increased cardiac output during exercise, and reduced heart size (14^c). The addition of hydralazine further improved these effects.

In 14 patients with congestive heart failure the acute hemodynamic effects of digoxin, hydralazine, and their combination were studied (15^C). Both drugs increased cardiac output and stroke volume and reduced pulmonary wedge pressure, both at rest and during exercise. The effects of hydralazine alone on cardiac output and stroke volume were greater than those of digoxin at rest, although not during exercise. The effects of the combination were greater still both at rest and during exercise.

In 186 patients hydralazine plus isosorbide dinitrate were added to digoxin therapy (16^C). The addition of the vasodilators increased LV ejection fraction and reduced cumulative mortal-

ity over 36 months. Adverse effects were significantly more frequent in those on vasodilators and digoxin (19%) than in those on digoxin alone (4%). The chief adverse effects were headache and dizziness.

Nitroprusside *In 11 patients with congestive heart failure after acute myocardial infarction the acute hemodynamic effects of digoxin were compared with those of digoxin plus nitroprusside (17^C^). Nitroprusside increased cardiac index and this effect was greater when nitroprusside was combined with digoxin. The beneficial effect of nitroprusside on pulmonary wedge pressure was not enhanced by digoxin. Nitroprusside had no effect on stroke work index, but the combination increased it significantly.*

Isosorbide dinitrate *A study in which digoxin has been compared with a combination of hydralazine and isosorbide dinitrate (16^C^) is referred to above.*

Prazosin *A comparison of prazosin with digoxin is mentioned above (13^c^). In another study mentioned above (16^C^) 183 patients were given prazosin in addition to digoxin (16^C^). The addition of prazosin had no effect on LV ejection fraction or on cumulative mortality over 42 months, in contrast to the effect of adding hydralazine and isosorbide (see above). The reasons for this difference were not clear; they may have been due to tachyphylaxis in response to the effects of prazosin, or to the need for venous and arteriolar vasodilatation, rather than one of those alone, or to some other difference dependent on the modes of action of the different drugs. Adverse effects were significantly more frequent in those on prazosin and digoxin (11%) than in those on digoxin alone (4%). The chief adverse effects were headache and dizziness.*

From the time of its earliest use in patients with aortic regurgitation (18^C^) it has been believed that digitalis may not be beneficial and may even make cardiac function worse in these patients. In a study of 8 patients digoxin increased systemic vascular resistance but did not alter other hemodynamic measurements (19^C^). In contrast, prazosin caused significant improvement in cardiac index and pulmonary wedge pressure.

Various *The acute hemodynamic effects of intravenous digoxin were studied in 11 patients with congestive heart failure who had already been treated with diuretics and vasodilators (nifedipine, captopril, nitroprusside, isosorbide dinitrate, and prazosin, either alone or in combinations) (20^C^). In all cases heart failure scores fell with the vasodilators and in all cases heart failure was stable before the administration of digoxin. Digoxin then increased cardiac index, LV stroke work index, and LV ejection fraction, and reduced pulmonary wedge pressure. These effects occurred principally in those in whom there were persistent hemodynamic abnormalities despite diuretics and vasodilators.*

CONCLUSIONS

Combinations of positive inotropic drugs *There is little theoretical rationale for combining two drugs with positive inotropic actions in chronic congestive heart failure, unless it were in order to reduce adverse effects by using low doses of each drug. However, this approach has not been tested, and what little evidence there is suggests that it is not beneficial to combine ordinary doses of digoxin with other positive inotropic drugs. Furthermore, there is little evidence that other such drugs alone are any better than digoxin alone, although it may be that in some cases their adverse effects are fewer.*

The use of digoxin alone in acute heart failure after myocardial infarction is controversial, and requires separate review. However, if a positive inotrope is required in such circumstances it is probably wise not to use digoxin, particularly since dobutamine seems to be more effective.

Combinations of digoxin with vasodilators *The rationale for combining digoxin with a vasodilator in the treatment of heart failure is thoroughly discussed in most of the papers quoted above. Briefly, by so doing it is possible to affect simultaneously the 3 important factors determining cardiac output: contractility, pre-load, and after-load. Furthermore, a vasodilator will oppose the small effect which digoxin has in increasing peripheral resistance, and which may reduce the beneficial effect of digoxin on cardiac output.*

The clinical studies outlined above confirm the potential value of such a combination both in acute heart failure after myocardial infarction and in chronic heart failure in which there is severely impaired left ventricular function. However, this does not apply to those circumstances in which digoxin is either contraindicated or not generally beneficial, including aortic valvular disease and hypertrophic congestive cardiomyopathy.

The use of digoxin compared with other drugs in chronic uncomplicated atrial fibrillation

Digitalis has long been looked on as the drug of choice in the treatment of chronic atrial fibrillation, ever since its introduction for this purpose at the beginning of the century by Sir James Mackenzie (21[C]). However, a major disadvantage of digoxin is that during exercise it does not control the heart rate, which may rise well above the rate expected in subjects in sinus rhythm (22[C]). This is because its action is mainly via vagal stimulation, which is overcome during exercise, rather than via a direct action on the AV node. The theoretical disadvantage of this is that exercise tolerance during exercise may be poor, because of impaired filling of the left ventricle during diastole.

Recently alternatives to digitalis have been studied, including amiodarone, the calcium antagonists verapamil and diltiazem, and β-adrenoceptor antagonists. The results have been briefly reviewed elsewhere (23[R]).

Amiodarone

Amiodarone may be effective in patients whose atrial fibrillation has not responded to other treatment (24[C]), but its long-term adverse effects rule it out as a first-line measure.

Calcium antagonists

Verapamil Verapamil acts directly on the AV node in atrial fibrillation, and would therefore be expected to enhance the action of digitalis on ventricular rate and to prevent the exercise-induced tachycardia which digitalis does not prevent. These effects have been shown in several studies (25[C]–31[C], 32[R], 33[C]). However, verapamil alone is not better than digoxin in improving exercise tolerance (30[C], 31[C], 32[R]). Furthermore, while some studies show that the combination of verapamil with digoxin increases maximum exercise capacity (25[C]–27[C]), others have not shown this to happen (29[C], 33[C]). On the other hand, in 3 studies there was less palpitation when verapamil was added to digoxin (25[C], 28[C], 29[C]).

It should also be noted that adverse effects have been reported to be more frequent during therapy with the combination of verapamil and digoxin (28[C]). In this study 6 of 8 patients had adverse effects, mostly worsening edema and dyspnea. This is not unexpected, since verapamil has a negative inotropic effect on the heart. Furthermore, it increases steady-state plasma digoxin concentrations and may precipitate digoxin toxicity (see SEDA-10, 145 and below).

Diltiazem Diltiazem has less of a negative inotropic effect on the heart than verapamil, and it has little or no effect on plasma digoxin concentrations (SEDA-11, 154). Therefore, if it had the same beneficial effect in atrial fibrillation as verapamil, it might be of use instead of or as an adjunct to digoxin therapy.

Diltiazem has been shown to reduce heart rate at rest and during exercise, both alone and when combined with digoxin (31[C], 32[R], 34[C]–36[C]), the combination being more effective than either alone (35[C], 36[C]). However, there is no evidence that diltiazem improves exercise tolerance when added to digoxin (31[C], 32[R], 36[C]). Furthermore, adverse effects may be frequent during combined diltiazem and digoxin therapy. In one study 9 of 12 subjects had adverse effects, leg and/or periorbital edema occurring in 6 cases (34[C]). In another study 3 out of 14 subjects were withdrawn because of adverse effects before the main study began (36[C]). On the other hand, diltiazem may not have the same adverse electrophysiological effects as verapamil (37[C]), and there are fewer ventricular extra beats during treatment with diltiazem alone than with digoxin (38[C]).

β-Adrenoceptor antagonists

Conventional β-adrenoceptor antagonists prevent the increase in exercise heart rate in atrial fibrillation which digoxin does not (33[C], 39[C]-41[C]). However, they can cause excess bradycardia at rest and they have a negative inotropic ef-

fect, which can impair cardiac function. Impaired exercise tolerance has been reported in patients taking atenolol with digoxin compared with digoxin alone (33[C]).

The beta-blockers which have previously been studied have been either full antagonists or antagonists with slight partial agonist activity. In contrast, xamoterol is an agonist with about 45% partial antagonist activity. It is therefore a β-adrenoceptor ***agonist*** *when sympathetic nervous system activity is low, but is a partial antagonist and therefore acts as a* ***beta-blocker*** *during exercise, when sympathetic nervous system activity is increased. It might therefore be effective as a beta-blocker in preventing the increase in heart rate during exercise, but without the adverse effects of full beta-blockers.*

Two studies have shown that xamoterol does indeed reduce heart rate in atrial fibrillation both at rest and during exercise when added to digoxin (33[C], 42[C]). In one study exercise capacity was increased by xamoterol (42[C]), but in the other it was reduced (33[C]). The hazards of using xamoterol in patients with moderate or severe heart failure have been mentioned above.

Conclusions

Digoxin remains the drug of first choice for slowing the ventricular rate in uncomplicated atrial fibrillation. The addition of a calcium antagonist might be justified in those in whom either digoxin was not completely effective or in whom symptoms, such as palpitation, persisted, despite adequate digitalization. Diltiazem would probably be preferred to verapamil in these circumstances, since it has less of a negative inotropic effect and since it has little effect on the pharmacokinetics of digoxin. Conventional beta-blockers cannot be recommended in these circumstances, but they are of value in patients with atrial fibrillation secondary to hyperthyroidism. It is too soon to comment on the potential usefulness of xamoterol.

In patients with atrial fibrillation secondary to an anomalous conduction pathway (e.g. Wolff-Parkinson-White syndrome), in most of whom digitalis is contraindicated, a calcium antagonist would be the treatment of choice. Paroxysmal atrial fibrillation is often refractory to digitalis, as well as to other drugs, and its treatment is problematic.

Long-term treatment with cardiac glycosides

Since this topic was reviewed in SEDA-4 (p.123) several other studies of the effect of digoxin withdrawal after long-term therapy in cardiac failure in sinus rhythm have appeared (43[C]-51[C]) and some have been reviewed (52[R], 53[R]).

In the last of these studies (51[C]) placebo was substituted for digoxin for 8 weeks and digoxin was then reintroduced in 44 patients in stable heart failure in sinus rhythm. There was no evidence of clinical deterioration in 64% of the patients after digoxin withdrawal. In another 11% deterioration occurred despite the continued presence of digoxin. In only 25% was there deterioration attributable to digoxin withdrawal. The results of an earlier study (45[C]) suggested that those most likely to benefit from long-term digoxin therapy are those with poor left ventricular function. However, in the later study (51[C]) deterioration could not be predicted *a priori* from the systolic time intervals or from echocardiographic measurements made before withdrawal.

Currently the following recommendations seem sensible for deciding on whether or not to continue digoxin therapy in patients who are in a stable condition in heart failure in sinus rhythm (51[C]):

(a) If the plasma digoxin concentration is below 1.0 nmol/l (0.8 ng/ml), withdrawal is very likely not to produce deterioration. [This also applies to patients in atrial fibrillation.]
(b) If a patient's condition is stable with a plasma digoxin concentration above 1.0 nmol/l and at little risk of toxicity, withdrawal is probably not worth while, because of the risk of deterioration.
(c) However, if there is an increased risk of toxicity (e.g. because of renal impairment or if potassium balance is difficult to maintain) careful withdrawal of digoxin may be worth attempting.
(d) In those patients who have evidence of poor left ventricular function it may be better to continue therapy, even if there is an increased risk of toxicity. In such cases careful monitoring of therapy may help reduce that risk.

Cardiovascular Two cases of parasystolic accelerated idioventricular rhythm, resulting in

ECG patterns of *bidirectional tachycardia*, have been attributed to digitalis toxicity (54[C]).

Nervous system Another study has confirmed the finding (SEDA-5, 176) that cardiac glycosides can *impair color vision* to an extent detectable by sensitive tests (55[C]). There was no difference in this study between the effects of digoxin and digitoxin.

Interactions Pharmacokinetic interactions with digoxin have again been reviewed (56[R]). *Calcium antagonists* Further reports confirm (SEDA-11, 154) that *diltiazem* has little effect on steady-state serum digoxin concentrations (34[C]-36[C]). Furthermore, digoxin has no effect on diltiazem concentrations (34[C]).

Israpidine has been reported to have no effect on the clearance of digoxin (57[C]) or on steady-state plasma digoxin concentrations (58[C]), although it does increase its apparent volume of distribution slightly (57[C]). This interaction is probably of no clinical importance.

Nitrendipine has been reported to increase the AUC of digoxin at steady state without altering its clearance (59[C]), implying that it reduces its apparent volume of distribution. In support of this there was also an increase in C_{max}. The change in systolic time intervals caused by digoxin was not affected by nitrendipine. This interaction is probably of no clinical significance, although the authors of this report suggest that it may cause toxicity in some patients.

Felodipine did not alter steady-state plasma digoxin concentrations in a study of 12 patients with heart failure (60[C]).

Adverse effects of antidigoxin antibody fragments

The common adverse effects of the Fab fragments of antidigoxin antibody result from the effects of reversing the actions of digitalis, namely heart failure and potassium depletion (SEDA-12, 148). Direct adverse immunological effects have not been reported. In a recently reported case of digitoxin overdose (61[C]) 960 mg of antidigoxin antiserum was given without any evidence of immunological reactions. In vitro studies suggested that digitoxin in high nanomolar concentrations inhibits immune responses and might therefore protect against any such reactions. However, it is difficult to interpret the results of these in vitro experiments, since in vivo digitoxin is highly protein-bound and the in vitro incubations contained only 20% serum. Indeed, the concentrations of ouabain which inhibit mitogen-induced lymphocyte proliferation (62, 63) are similar to those of digitoxin used in these experiments, and ouabain is poorly protein-bound.

OTHER POSITIVE INOTROPIC DRUGS

The possibility that long-term treatment with cardiac glycosides might prove deleterious to the patient with heart failure was discussed in SEDA-10 (p. 142). The same question has now been reviewed in relation to the inhibitors of phosphodiesterase type III (64[R]–66[R]).

Amrinone *(SEDA-11, 340; SEDA-13, 139)*

Amrinone has been used in high doses in the treatment of 16 patients with cardiogenic shock (67[C]). In 11 of the patients amrinone was thought to have produced a beneficial effect. In only 1 case was there evidence of an adverse effect, a *paroxysmal supraventricular tachycardia*, which resolved on withdrawal of amrinone.

DRUGS USED IN DYSRHYTHMIAS *(SEDA-11, 340; SEDA-12, 151; SEDA-13, 139)*

The ability of antidysrhythmic drugs to cause or worsen cardiac dysrhythmias has again been reviewed (68[R]) and has been the subject of 3 further reports (69[C]–71[C]).

The ability of 14 antidysrhythmic drugs, either alone or in combination, to worsen pre-existing ventricular dysrhythmias has been evaluated electrophysiologically in 801 investigations in 314 patients who were taking steady-state therapy (69[C]). Prodysrhythmic effects of 4 different types were described and overall occurred in 122 (39%) of the patients in at least one investigation and in 193 (24%) of the investigations. The drugs which most commonly caused dysrhythmias were indecainide (37% of studies), flecainide (33%), amiodarone (30%), amiodarone + procainamide (30%), quinidine + mexiletine (30%), and procainamide + mexiletine (22%). Significantly lower rates occurred with single-drug therapy with mexiletine (19%), procainamide (19%) and quinidine (15%). There was no difference in the incidence of dysrhythmias between single-drug regimens and combinations. There were no differences in plasma drug concentrations between those who developed a dysrhythmia and those who did not, except in the case of quinidine (3.8 versus 2.9 μg/ml respectively). Dysrhythmias occurred more frequently in patients with a lower LV ejection fraction.

In a smaller study of 56 patients, worsening of dysrhythmias was studied electrocardiographically during treatment with antidysrhythmic drugs (70[C]). Worsening of dysrhythmias was noted in 7 (8.3%) of the patients.

Discrepancies of this kind between electrophysiological results and clinical results may be due to the fact that prodysrhythmic effects detected by relatively sensitive electrophysiological methods may have little clinical relevance (69[C]).

The observation that a lower LV ejection fraction may predispose to a prodysrhythmic effect of antidysrhythmic drug treatment has been confirmed in a small retrospective study (71[C]), in which 26 patients who had ventricular fibrillation during therapy with either quinidine, procainamide, or disopyramide were compared with 62 patients who were on similar treatment but did not have ventricular fibrillation. Other findings were that the patients with dysrhythmias were older, had a longer baseline QT_c interval, and were more likely to be taking digitalis, a diuretic, or a potassium supplement. The last observation presumably relates to the generally increased likelihood of dysrhythmias when there is potassium depletion, which also promotes the dysrhythmogenic effects of a long QT interval.

Acecainide (*N*-acetylprocainamide) *(SED-11, 342; SEDA-13, 140)*

The actions, clinical pharmacology, and adverse effects of acecainide have been reviewed (72[R]).

Cardiovascular Acecainide prolongs the QT interval, and this has been associated with dysrhythmias (SEDA-11, 155). In a recent study acecainide was shown to *prolong the QT_c interval* in 5 subjects after acute administration (73[C]), and this prolongation was related to plasma acecainide concentrations. However, the QT_c interval did not predict torsades de pointes in one patient with a relatively short QT_c interval nor the absence of dysrhythmias in another patient with relatively long QT_c interval.

Interactions Drugs which inhibit the renal tubular secretion of other drugs may inhibit the renal clearance of acecainide, as has been shown in two studies of the effects of *cimetidine* (74[C]) and *trimethoprim* (75[C]) on the pharmacokinetics of acecainide after the administration of procainamide. However, the effect is quite small, and it is not clear whether it would be of clinical importance if these drugs were given together with acecainide itself.

Ajmaline *(SED-11, 342)*

Despite the facts that ajmaline is well known as a cause of *liver damage* and *agranulocytosis*, that the risks are high, and that other drugs are safer and at least as effective, reports of these adverse effects continue to appear (76[C], 77[C]).

Amiodarone *(SED-11, 342; SEDA-12, 151; SEDA-13, 140)*

It is not clear to what extent adverse effects of amiodarone are dose-related and to what extent they may be immunological in origin. Anti-amiodarone antibodies were sought in the serum of 33 patients taking amiodarone for various tachydysrhythmias (78[C]). The antibodies were either absent or present in low amounts in those without adverse effects. They were found in higher amounts in those with a variety of adverse effects, mostly related to thyroid function, but also vasculitis, erythroderma, polyserositis, photosensitivity, epididymitis, pleuritic pain, and liver damage. There was no correlation between serum amiodarone concentration and the amount of antibody detected. Of 16 patients without adverse effects 11 had detectable antibody, but in only 1 case was the amount of antibody raised. In contrast, 9 of 17 patients with adverse effects had raised amounts of antibody. The authors therefore suggested that although the generation of antibody *per se* might not determine the occurrence of adverse effects, the quantity of antibody generated might be important in some patients. It is also possible that anti-amiodarone antibodies might distinguish between autoimmune thyroid disease and iodine-induced thyroid disease secondary to amiodarone.

Monitoring therapy The usefulness of plasma amiodarone and desethylamiodarone concentration measurement in monitoring amiodarone therapy has been reviewed (79[R]). The minimum effective plasma concentration of amiodarone is around 1–2.5 μg/ml and there is no clear limit to the concentration above which toxicity starts to become important. Further discussion will be found in previous volumes (SEDA-9, 165; SEDA-10, 146; SEDA-12, 151; SEDA-13, 142).

Cardiovascular The incidence of *prodysrhythmias* has been assessed clinically in 107 patients at steady state taking amiodarone in a low dose (80[C]). The incidence was 2.8%, which (even allowing for differences in dosage) confirms the discrepancy between electrophysiological evidence of prodysrhythmia and its clinical manifestations, as mentioned above. One case was of torsades de pointes, which has been previously reported with amiodarone (SEDA-9, 164).

Respiratory The role of amiodarone in the generation of *lung damage* has recently been reviewed (81[R]).

The diagnosis of amiodarone-induced lung damage can be difficult. The presentation of symptoms and clinical signs, the changes on chest radiography, and abnormalities of lung function tests are all non-specific. The presence of CD8+ lymphocytes and foamy (i.e. phospholipid-laden) macrophages or pneumocytes in bronchial lavage fluid is suggestive, as is the presence of phospholipidosis in a lung biopsy. Resolution of the damage on withdrawal of the drug would be supporting evidence.

Scintiscanning with gallium-67 has been investigated as a diagnostic tool in 54 patients, 22 with clinically suspected amiodarone-induced lung damage (including 13 with foamy macrophages and/or pneumocytes on lavage), 19 with other causes of lung symptoms, and 13 with no signs or symptoms of lung disease (82[C]). Of the patients with suspected amiodarone-induced damage 18 had abnormal scans, in contrast to only 1 subject in each of the other groups. In the group with abnormal scans there was a correlation between dosage and degree of abnormality, and the patients with abnormal scans were taking a significantly higher dosage of amiodarone.

Gallium-67 scanning was also used in a study of 11 out of 15 patients with amiodarone-induced lung disease (83[C]). Ten of the 11 patients had abnormal scans. In 12 other patients with symptoms attributed to other causes the scans were normal.

Carbon monoxide diffusing capacity was also measured in these studies. In the first study (82[C]) the extent of reduction of diffusion capacity correlated with the extent of abnormality on the gallium scan. In the second study (83[C]) 6 out of 8 patients had a reduction in diffusing capacity of 30% or greater and all 8 had a reduction of at least 15%. In contrast, in patients without toxicity only 4 out of 211 tests were 30% or greater and only 24 out of 211 tests were 15% or greater. The role of lung function testing in the diagnosis of amiodarone-induced lung damage has been discussed in the light of the results of the second of these studies (84[r]).

Endocrine It has been suggested that amiodarone-induced *thyroid disease* may occur either because of a direct effect on thyroid function of the iodine that amiodarone contains or because amiodarone affects autoimmunity through its iodine content or through some other facet of its structure. However, the relationship between amiodarone-induced thyroid disease and autoimmunity is not clear. Although some have reported an association between the presence of autoantibodies in patients with amiodarone-induced thyroid disease (85[C], 86[C]), others have not (SEDA-12, 152; 87[C]-89[C]). It has been reported that amiodarone can modulate pre-existing antibody titers (87[C]).

In a patient who had amiodarone-induced lung damage and hyperthyroidism a positive gallium lung scan (see above) also showed abnormal thyroid uptake (90[c]). The pathology of the thyroid abnormality in this case was not clear.

There has been another report of the effects of amiodarone on thyroid function in the fetus (SEDA-13, 141). An infant who had been exposed to amiodarone during the last trimester was born with hyperthyroxinemia without autoantibodies and without clear clinical evidence of hyperthyroidism (91[c]).

Metabolic The effects of amiodarone on *serum lipid concentrations* (SEDA-9, 166; SEDA-12, 152) have been confirmed in another study (92[C]). In 21 patients with normal total serum cholesterol before the study amiodarone caused an increase from 4.6 to 5.4 mmol/l. Ten patients had rises to above the 75th percentile for their age and sex and those 10 had increases in serum glucose and triglyceride concentrations as well as higher plasma concentrations of desethylamiodarone than those who did not have such high rises in plasma cholesterol. Thyroid function was not reported in this study, and the question still remains of the extent to which changes in lipids are associated with changes in thyroid function in patients taking amiodarone.

Liver *Pseudoalcoholic changes* in the liver have been reported in patients taking amiodarone (SEDA-9, 166; 93[C], 94[R]). In one series of 13 patients 4 had such changes attributable to amiodarone and 7 had changes attributable to other causes (93[C]). However, in all cases there was phospholipidosis, stressing that liver damage in the presence of phospholipidosis in a patient taking amiodarone is not necessarily indicative of an adverse effect of amiodarone.

Amiodarone may cause *acute hepatitis* (SEDA-9, 166), as another report of 2 cases confirms (95[c]). However, in both cases amiodarone was given intravenously, and one cannot therefore rule out the possibility that this adverse reaction may have been due to the vehicle, Tween 80, rather than the drug.

Skin Phototoxicity is well known as an adverse effect of amiodarone (SEDA-7, 205; SEDA-9, 166). There has now been a report that it can occur in conjunction with a syndrome resembling porphyria cutanea tarda, with more severe *photosensitivity* than is normally associated with amiodarone, resulting in bullous lesions (96[c]). However, the authors relied for their diagnosis on clinical description, and did not back it up with histological examination.

Exfoliative dermatitis has been attributed to amiodarone in 2 cases (97[c]).

Risk situations The non-cardiac adverse effects of amiodarone in 61 elderly patients have been reported (98[C]). Hypothyroidism occurred in 15%, but there were no cases of hyperthyroidism. Increases in serum AsT occurred in 26% and photosensitivity in 10%. Corneal deposits occurred in 77% of those studied, but caused symptoms in only 1 patient. In 12 patients amiodarone had to be withdrawn because of adverse effects.

These data may represent an increased risk of hypothyroidism in the elderly. However, the study was too small to be conclusive, and the results of a previous large study in the elderly (reported in detail in SEDA-8, 177) do not allow an accurate calculation of the incidence of hypothyroidism.

Second-generation effects There have been 2 recent case-reports of the birth of normal children after exposure to amiodarone, in one case perhaps for the whole of pregnancy (the wording is not clear) (89[C]) and in the other for the last 5 weeks (99[cR]). In their literature review the authors of the second paper reported the adverse effects of amiodarone on fetal thyroid function (mentioned above). They also concluded that there is no risk of teratogenicity, that there is QT prolongation in infancy without an increased risk of dysrhythmias, and that infant bradycardia may occur.

Interactions The interaction of amiodarone with *anesthesia* has been studied in 37 patients (100[Cr]). In 8 patients undergoing non-cardiac operations 2 had postoperative atrial fibrillation and 1 transient worsening of cardiac failure. In the other 29 patients, all of whom underwent cardiac surgery, postoperative dysrhythmias (atrial fibrillation, sinus bradycardia, atrioventricular block, ventricular dysrhythmias, and junctional rhythm) occurred in 52%, in addition to other postoperative complications, including cardiogenic shock (of which 1 patient died) or severe heart failure in 21%. A pacemaker was necessary in 24% of the patients.

Since the authors did not report the incidence of dysrhythmias in a group undergoing cardiac surgery but not taking amiodarone, it is not possible to say to what extent amiodarone contributed to the dysrhythmias. However, the incidence they have reported is certainly very high, and others have reported severe hypotension, myocardial depression, and atropine-resistant bradycardia in patients undergoing cardiac surgery having taken amiodarone. Nor is it clear whether the interaction of amiodarone with anesthesia is with anesthetic agents or with catecholamines released during anesthesia. It is not clear whether or not amiodarone should be withdrawn in patients about to undergo cardiac surgery. Certainly its long half-life would make effective withdrawal difficult.

Encainide *(SED-11, 346; SEDA-13, 143)*

The clinical use of encainide in patients with supraventricular dysrhythmias has been the subject of a symposium (101[CR]). Adverse effects were not infrequent and were similar to those previously reported (SEDA-10, 149). The non-cardiac effects of encainide most commonly affected the *central nervous system*, and included abnormal or blurred vision (10.6%), dizziness (7.3%), headache (6.0%), nausea (4.3%), vertigo (2.3%), insomnia and fatigue. The figures in parentheses are taken from a review of 349 patients with supraventricular dysrhythmias treated with encainide (102[CR]).

Cardiovascular *Prodysrhythmic effects* were reported not uncommonly in the same symposium, and it was notable that in some patients with no previous history of ventricular dysrhythmias encainide reportedly precipitated ventricular tachycardia (103[C]–105[C]). The review of 349 patients with supraventricular dysrhythmias treated with encainide reported an incidence of ventricular dysrhythmias of 1.4% (102[CR]). The dosages in all these studies were very similar.

In two other studies of patients taking encainide for ventricular dysrhythmias similar cardiac and non-cardiac adverse effects were reported (106[C], 107[C]). However, in the larger of these two studies the incidence of prodysrhythmias (mostly ventricular) was much higher (21%) than in patients being treated for supraventricular dysrhythmias (107[C]). In addition 2 patients had sick sinus syndrome which was attributed to the drug.

Risk situations In one study it was reported that children under the age of 6 months may be more liable to the prodysrhythmic effects of encainide than older children (108[C]).

Flecainide *(SED-11, 347; SEDA-12, 153; SEDA-13, 143)*

The clinical use of flecainide in patients with supraventricular dysrhythmias has been the subject of a symposium (109[CR]). Adverse effects were similar to those previously reported (SEDA-11, 156). The non-cardiac adverse effects of flecainide were most commonly on the *central nervous system*, and included paraesthesiae (7.1%), visual disturbances (3.0%), dizziness, drowsiness, oral paraesthesiae, and headache. The figures in parentheses are taken from a review of 1371 courses of treatment in 1289 patients with supraventricular dysrhythmias treated with flecainide (110[CR]).

Cardiovascular In the same symposium *hypotension* (1.7%) was not uncommonly reported (110[CR]). *Prodysrhythmic effects* occurred occasionally (4%) (110[R], 111[C]–113[C]), but in contrast to encainide (see above) flecainide rarely precipitated ventricular tachycardia, there being only one report in the whole symposium (112[C]). Flecainide was also reported to cause conduction disturbances in 2.2% of patients (110[R], 111[C], 114[C]). Flecainide has also been reported to have caused T-wave changes (flattening and notching) in 2 patients, but not in association with other adverse effects (115[c]).

Despite these relatively negative reports in relation to prodysrhythmic effects of flecainide, there is now evidence that flecainide increases the risk of death from cardiac dysrhythmias and cardiac arrest in patients with asymptomatic ventricular dysrhythmias after myocardial infarction (152[r]). Further analysis has suggested that this effect was confined to those with a history of multiple previous myocardial infarctions, although since this conclusion was based on an analysis of subgroups it presumably requires confirmation. Patients with poor left ventricular function are also said to be particularly at risk. The U.K. Committee on Safety of Medicines has therefore recommended that treatment with flecainide should be initiated only in hospital. The Committee has also published a list of suggested indications and contraindications. The recommended indications are: (a) AV nodal reciprocating tachycardia, (b) symptomatic sustained ventricular tachycardia, and (c) extra ventricular beats and/or non-sustained ventricular tachycardia which are causing disabling symptoms. In the last category it is recommended that flecainide be used only if other drugs have proved ineffective or have not been tolerated. It is suggested that flecainide is contraindicated in patients with a history of myocardial infarction who have either asymptomatic ventricular extra beats or asymptomatic non-sustained ventricular tachycardia.

Skin A psoriasiform eruption in an 82-year-old man has been attributed to flecainide (116[c]).

Interactions Flecainide prolongs conduction in the His-Purkinje system (117[R]) and might therefore be expected to interact with other drugs which affect conduction. Two anecdotal reports suggest that the combination of flecainide with *amiodarone* may result in reduced conduction. In one case there was right bundle branch block (114[C]) and in another recurrent ventricular tachycardia associated with a prolonged QRS interval and left bundle branch block (118[c]).

Risk situations The effects of flecainide have been reported in 16 children aged 21 months to 13 years (119[C]). Adverse effects (nausea, vertigo, and blurred vision) occurred in only 1 patient.

Flecainide is cleared partly by metabolism and partly unchanged via the kidneys. One would therefore expect impairment of renal and hepatic function to reduce its clearance, and this has now been reported. In 12 patients with severe renal impairment the total body clearance of flecainide was reduced and its half-life prolonged, as compared with previously reported results in healthy volunteers (120[C]). In another study 6 patients with hepatic impairment were compared directly with 6 controls. Hepatic impairment caused a 5-fold increase in the half-life of flecainide, associated with a reduction in total clearance and a small increase in apparent volume of distribution (121[C]). Clearly, maintenance dosages of flecainide should be reduced in patients with either renal or hepatic impairment.

Lidocaine (lignocaine) *(SED-11, 347)*

Interactions *Propranolol* has been reported to reduce the clearance of lidocaine (122[C], 123[C]), and one would therefore expect this combination to increase the chance of adverse effects of lidocaine.

A recent comparison of lidocaine and placebo in 103 patients already taking *β-adrenoceptor antagonists* and 108 patients not taking β-adrenoceptor antagonists showed that there was a trend to a greater risk of some minor non-cardiac adverse events (dizziness, numbness, somnolence, confusion, slurred speech, and nausea and vomiting) in those taking the combination, although the differences did not reach statistical significance. There was no difference at all in the incidence of cardiac dysrhythmias in those taking the combination compared with lidocaine alone (124[C]).

In this study the efficacy of the combination in reducing the frequency of cardiac dysrhythmias was greater than with either drug alone, and this suggests that there may be a beneficial interaction between the two types of drugs. However, there was no significant change in the plasma concentrations of lidocaine and its two chief metabolites in patients taking β-adrenoceptor antagonists, and it may be that the interaction described here is as much pharmacodynamic as pharmacokinetic. The authors suggested that the pharmacokinetic interaction might become more important after 24 h, when the serum concentration of α_1-acid glycoprotein, the main binding protein of lidocaine, rises.

Mexiletine *(SED-11, 348; SEDA-12, 153)*

The adverse effects of mexiletine have been compared with those of quinidine in a randomized double-blind comparison in 491 patients (125[C]).

The commonest adverse effects in the 246 patients given mexiletine were upper *gastrointestinal distress* (38%), *lightheadedness* (20%), *tremor* (12%), and *co-ordination difficulties* (11%). These all occurred more frequently than with quinidine. However, quinidine more often caused diarrhea (35% vs. 7%) and dysrhythmias (19 vs. 12 patients). The other reported adverse effects, associated in equal frequency with the two drugs, were *fatigue, changes in sleep habit, weakness, headache, angina-like pain,* and *rash. Visual problems* (7% vs. 3%) and nervousness (6% vs. 2%) occurred slightly more often on mexiletine.

Procainamide *(SED-11, 348; SEDA-12, 153; SEDA-13, 143)*

Nervous system In a patient with a pre-existing peripheral neuropathy attributed to amiodarone, procainamide caused severe *weakness of the respiratory muscles*, thought to be due to neuromuscular blockade, with consequent respiratory failure (126[c]).

Skin *Lichen planus* has been attributed to procainamide as part of a lupus-like syndrome in a 57-year-old man (127[c]).

Lupus-like syndrome Drug-induced lupus has been reviewed in the context of immunological mechanisms in autoimmune disease (128[R]).

The presence of specific anti-histone antibodies and of anti-guanosine antibodies in procainamide-induced lupus may help to distinguish it from idiopathic lupus and from lupus due to other drugs (SEDA-12, 154; SEDA-13, 143). In a series of 51 patients taking procainamide, 20 asymptomatic and 31 with evidence of a lupus-like syndrome, all the symptomatic patients had increased IgG antibodies to histones H2A-H2B, in contrast to only 2 asymptomatic patients (129[C]). Antibodies of this type were not found in patients with lupus associated with hydralazine or quinidine. However, antiguanosine antibodies were increased in both the symptomatic (65%) and asymptomatic (61%) patients.

Anti-dDNA and antiphospholipid antibodies in patients with lupus may act as anticoagulants, and thrombotic problems in procainamide-induced lupus associated with such antibodies continue to be reported (130[c]). However, lupus anticoagulants may be detected in individuals taking procainamide but without clinical evidence of lupus (131[c]).

The main metabolite of procainamide, *N*-acetylprocainamide (acecainide), is not associated with lupus, and this suggests that procainamide-induced lupus is due either to procainamide itself or to some other metabolite (SEDA-7, 198; SEDA-9, 163). Several candidate metabolites have been described in bacteria in vitro (132) and there is also published evidence that such metabolites may be formed by human hepatic microsomes and leukocytes (133[C], 134[C]). It is also possible that such metabolites may be responsible for the neutropenia which sometimes occurs during procainamide administration (SEDA-12, 154).

Interactions *Cimetidine* (74[C]) and *trimethoprim* (75[C]), both of which can inhibit the tubular secretion of other drugs, have both been reported to reduce the renal clearance of procainamide (see also 'Acecainide' above).

Propafenone *(SED-11, 349; SEDA-12, 154; SEDA-13, 144)*

The pharmacology, clinical pharmacology, and clinical use of propafenone have again been reviewed (135[R]).

The adverse effects of propafenone in 774 patients have been reviewed (136[CR]). At least one adverse effect occurred in 58% of the patients, but most were mild and dose-related and did not necessitate drug withdrawal. The most common adverse effects were *cardiovascular* (27.1%), *central nervous* (20.7%), and *gastrointestinal* (19.9%). Other adverse effects occurred in less than 6% of cases.

Among the cardiovascular adverse effects the most common were increased angina, AV block, bundle branch block, congestive cardiac failure, and ventricular tachydysrhythmias. Among the CNS adverse effects the most common were dizziness or lightheadedness, altered mental status, paraesthesiae or numbness, headache and ataxia. Among the gastrointestinal adverse effects the most common were nausea and vomiting, dysgeusia, constipation, and dyspepsia or abdominal discomfort. In addition to these, skin rashes were reported in 3.6%, blurred vision and other visual disturbances in 3.5%, and non-specific muscle pain in 2.5% of patients.

All these adverse effects were dose-related. At 300 mg/d the incidence was 10.7%, at 450 mg/d it was 22.1%, at 600 mg/d 32.8%, and at 900 mg/d 47.9%. In the 99 patients in whom the plasma propafenone concentrations were measured there was a relationship between adverse effects and concentration. The elderly were at greater risk of adverse effects than the young.

Similar frequencies of these adverse effects have been reported in other studies (137[C], 138[R], 139[C], 140[C]).

In one large study of the use of propafenone in the treatment of ventricular extra beats, adverse effects in patients taking propafenone occurred less often than in patients taking quinidine (137[C]).

Cardiovascular *Sinus node dysfunction* has been attributed to propafenone in 7 cases (141[c], 142[c]).

Risk situations The use of propafenone in a dosage of 300 mg 3 times a day has been reported in a pregnant woman from the 5th month to term (143[c]). Her dysrhythmias responded satisfactorily, minimum steady-state plasma concentrations of propafenone and its hydroxylated metabolite were 96 and 63 ng/ml respectively, and the fetus was healthy at birth with a normal heart rate and no dysrhythmias. The plasma concentrations of propafenone and its metabolite in umbilical cord blood at the time of delivery were 21 and 39 ng/ml respectively, suggesting some transplacental transfer.

Quinidine *(SED-11, 350; SEDA-12, 155; SEDA-13, 144)*

The actions, clinical use, interactions, and adverse effects of quinidine have again been reviewed (144[R]).

The results of a comparative study of mexiletine and quinidine have been mentioned above (125[C]). The most common adverse effects among the 245 patients treated with quinidine were *diarrhea* (35%), *upper gastrointestinal distress* (22%), and *lightheadedness* (15%). Other common adverse effects included *fatigue* (7%), *palpitation* (7%), *headache* (7%), *angina-like pain* (6%), *weakness* (5%), and *rash* (5%). *Prodysrhythmic effects* were observed in 19 patients in all. Withdrawal of quinidine because of adverse effects was required in 33% of cases.

In a small comparative study of moricizine and quinidine (145[C]) the incidence of adverse effects was much higher in the 27 patients taking quinidine (63%) than in the 28 taking moracizine (moricizine, ethmozin) (25%). *Diarrhea* (14 cases) was the most common adverse effect of quinidine. Prodysrhythmic effects occurred in 2 patients on quinidine and 1 moricizine on.

Cardiovascular Cases of *torsades de pointes* in patients taking quinidine continue to be reported, in one case in association with a normal QT_c interval (146[c]) and in another without associated symptoms (147[c]).

Hematological The effects of quinine, quinidine, 8 of their metabolites, and 4 structurally related analogs on platelets in patients with thrombocytopenia have been reported (148[C]). Quinine and quinidine were 10–300 times more potent in promoting *antibody-mediated platelet lysis* than the other compounds studied. However, quinidine-mediated lysis was partially inhibited by the metabolite desmethylquinidine, and the authors suggested that the metabolites of quinine and quinidine might have a protective role in some individuals.

Musculoskeletal *Polyarthropathy* has been reported in 7 patients taking quinidine (149[c]). In 4 cases it could be attributed to a lupus-like syndrome, on the basis of antinuclear and antihistone antibodies. However, no such association was found in the other 3 cases, which were milder than the others. Polyarthropathy may therefore occur as a distinct syndrome unassociated with lupus.

Tocainide *(SED-11, 351; SEDA-12, 155; SEDA-13, 145)*

Respiratory *Interstitial pneumonitis* has previously been reported in patients on tocainide (SEDA-7, Refs. 85 and 90; 150[c]), and it has reportedly resolved on withdrawal of tocainide and the addition of corticosteroids. However, more recently a case has been reported in which an acute interstitial pneumonitis was rapidly fatal, despite drug withdrawal and prednisone therapy (151[c]).

REFERENCES

1. Sanders MR, Kostis JB (1989) The use of inotropic agents in acute and chronic congestive heart failure. *Med. Clin. North Am.*, *73*, 283.
2. Buchanan JF, Olson KR (1988) Current management of digitalis toxicity: clinical manifestations. *Pract. Cardiol.*, *14*, 75.
3. Buchanan JF, Olson KR (1988) Current management of digitalis toxicity: treatment of digitalis intoxication. *Pract. Cardiol.*, *14*, 92.
4. Rietbrock N, Woodcock BG (1989) *Handbook of Renal-Independent Cardiac Glycosides: Pharmacology and Clinical Pharmacology*. Ellis Horwood, Chichester.
5. Kelly RA (1988) Role of digitalis in the management of congestive heart failure. *Pract. Cardiol.*, *14*, 57.
6. Goldstein RA, Passamani ER, Roberts R (1980) A comparison of digoxin and dobutamine in patients with acute infarction and cardiac failure. *N. Engl. J. Med.*, *303*, 846.
7. The German and Austrian Xamoterol Study Group (1988) Double-blind placebo-controlled comparison of digoxin and xamoterol in chronic heart failure. *Lancet*, *1*, 489.
8. DiBianco R, Shabetai R, Kostuk W et al (1989) A comparison of oral milrinone, digoxin, and their combination in the treatment of patients with chronic heart failure. *N. Engl. J. Med.*, *320*, 677.
9. Cantelli I, Pavesi PC, Parchi C et al (1983) Acute hemodynamic effects of combined therapy with digoxin and nifedipine in patients with chronic heart failure. *Am. Heart J.*, *106*, 308.
10. Cantelli I, Vitolo A, Lombardi G et al (1984) Combined haemodynamic effects of digoxin and captopril in patients with congestive heart failure. *Curr. Ther. Res.*, *36*, 323.
11. Alicandri C, Fariello R, Zaninelli A et al (1987) Captopril versus digoxin in mild-moderate chronic heart failure: a crossover study. *J. Cardiovasc. Pharmacol.*, *9*, *Suppl. 2*, S61.
12. The Captopril–Digoxin Multicenter Research Group (1988) Comparative effects of therapy with captopril and digoxin in patients with mild to moderate heart failure. *J. Am. Med. Assoc.*, *259*, 539.
13. Taylor SH (1979) Clinical and haemodynamic evaluation of treatment with diuretics, digitalis and vasodilator drugs in chronic heart failure (Abstract). *R. Soc. Med. Int. Congr. Symp. Ser.*, *10*, 35.
14. Rosenfeld SP, Carney MS, Waggoner AD et al (1981) Maximal improvement in ventricular performance during rest and exercise in chronic severe cardiac failure by combined inotropic and vasodilator therapy compared to either modality alone (Abstract). *Am. J. Cardiol.*, *47*, 390.
15. Ribner HS, Zucker MJ, Stasior C et al (1987) Vasodilators as first-line therapy for congestive heart failure: a comparative hemodynamic study of hydralazine, digoxin, and their combination. *Am. Heart J.*, *114*, 91.
16. Cohn JN, Archibald DG, Ziesche S et al (1986) Effect of vasodilator therapy on mortality in chronic congestive heart failure. *N. Engl. J. Med.*, *314*, 1547.
17. Raabe DS (1979) Combined therapy with digoxin and nitroprusside in heart failure complicating acute myocardial infarction. *Am. J. Cardiol.*, *43*, 990.
18. Corrigan DJ (1832) On the patency of the mouth of the aorta, or inadequacy of the aortic valves. *Edin. Med. Surg. J.*, *37*, 225.
19. Hockings BEF, Cope GD, Clarke GM, Taylor RR (1980) Comparison of vasodilator drug prazosin with digoxin in aortic regurgitation. *Br. Heart J.*, *43*, 550.
20. Gheorghiade M, St Clair J, St Clair C, Beller GA (1987) Hemodynamic effects of intravenous digoxin in patients with severe heart failure initially treated with diuretics and vasodilators. *J. Am. Coll. Cardiol.*, *9*, 849.
21. Mackenzie J (1905) New methods of studying affections of the heart (in 5 parts). *Br. Med. J.*, *1*, 519, 587, 702, 759, 812.
22. Beasley R, Smith DA, McHaffie DJ (1985) Exercise heart rates at different serum digoxin concentrations in patients with atrial fibrillation. *Br. Med. J.*, *290*, 9.
23. Lewis R, McClay J (1988) Clinical pharmacology of chronic atrial fibrillation. *J. R. Coll. Physicians London*, *22*, 252.
24. Fricke G, Mattern H, Runkel W (1983) Clinical efficacy of amiodarone in refractory supraventricular and ventricular arrhythmias. In: Breithardt G, Loogen F (Eds.), *New Aspects in the Medical Treatment of Tachyarrhythmias*, p. 216. Urban and Schwarzenberg, Munich.
25. Klein HO, Pauzner H, DiSegni E et al (1979) The beneficial effects of verapamil in chronic atrial fibrillation. *Arch. Intern. Med.*, *139*, 747.
26. Lang R, Klein HO, Weiss E et al (1983) Superiority of oral verapamil therapy to digoxin in treatment of chronic atrial fibrillation. *Chest*, *83*, 491.
27. Lang R, Klein HO, DiSegni E et al (1983) Verapamil improves exercise capacity in chronic atrial fibrillation: double-blind crossover study. *Am. Heart J.*, *105*, 820.
28. Johansson P-A, Olsson SB (1984) Long-term oral treatment with high doses of verapamil in lone atrial fibrillation. *Clin. Cardiol.*, *7*, 163.
29. Channer KS, Papouchado M, James MA, Russell Rees J (1987) Towards improved control of atrial fibrillation. *Eur. Heart J.*, *8*, 141.
30. Lewis R, Lakhani M, Moreland TA, McDevitt DG (1987) A comparison of verapamil and digoxin in the treatment of atrial fibrillation. *Eur. Heart J.*, *8*, 148.

31. Lewis RV, Irvine N, McDevitt DG (1988) Relationships between heart rate, exercise tolerance and cardiac output in atrial fibrillation: the effects of treatment with digoxin, verapamil and diltiazem. *Eur. Heart J.*, *9*, 777.
32. Lewis RV, McDevitt DG (1988) Factors affecting the clinical response to treatment with digoxin and two calcium antagonists in patients with atrial fibrillation. *Br. J. Clin. Pharmacol.*, *25*, 603.
33. Lewis RV, McMurray J, McDevitt DG (1989) Effects of atenolol, verapamil, and xamoterol on heart rate and exercise tolerance in digitalised patients with chronic atrial fibrillation. *J. Cardiovasc. Pharmacol.*, *13*, 1.
34. Roth A, Harrison E, Mitani G et al (1986) Efficacy and safety of medium- and high-dose diltiazem alone and in combination with digoxin for control of heart rate at rest and during exercise in patients with chronic atrial fibrillation. *Circulation*, *73*, 316.
35. Maragno I, Santostasi G, Gaion RM (1988) Low- and medium-dose diltiazem in chronic atrial fibrillation: comparison with digoxin and correlation with drug plasma levels. *Am. Heart J.*, *116*, 385.
36. Lewis RV, Laing E, Moreland TA et al (1988) A comparison of digoxin, diltiazem and their combination in the treatment of atrial fibrillation. *Eur. Heart J.*, *9*, 279.
37. Mitchell LB, Jutzy KR, Lewis SJ et al (1982) Intracardiac electrophysiologic study of intravenous diltiazem and combined diltiazem–digoxin in patients. *Am. Heart J.*, *103*, 57.
38. Lewis RV, McDevitt DG (1988) The relative effect of digoxin and diltiazem upon ventricular ectopic activity in patients with chronic atrial fibrillation. *Br. J. Clin. Pharmacol.*, *26*, 327.
39. Yahalom J, Klein HO, Kaplinsky E (1977) Beta-adrenergic blockade as adjunctive oral therapy in patients with chronic atrial fibrillation. *Chest*, *71*, 592.
40. David D, DiSegni E, Klein HO, Kaplinsky E (1979) Inefficacy of digitalis in the control of heart rate in patients with chronic atrial fibrillation: beneficial effect of an added beta adrenergic blocking agent. *Am. J. Cardiol.*, *44*, 1378.
41. Zoble RG, Brewington J, Olukotun AY, Gore R (1987) Comparative effects of nadolol–digoxin combination therapy and digoxin monotherapy for chronic atrial fibrillation. *Am. J. Cardiol.*, *60*, 39D.
42. Molajo AO, Coupe MO, Bennett DH (1984) Effect of Corwin (ICI 118587) on resting and exercise heart rate and exercise tolerance in digitalised patients with chronic atrial fibrillation. *Br. Heart J.*, *52*, 392.
43. Sommers De K, Reitz CJ, Kock K, Avenant JC (1981) Digoxin withdrawal in patients with sinus rhythm. *South Afr. Med. J.*, *60*, 239.
44. Griffiths BE, Penny WJ, Lewis MJ, Henderson AH (1982) Maintenance of the inotropic effect of digoxin on long-term treatment. *Br. Med. J.*, *284*, 1819.
45. Lee DC-S, Johnson RA, Bingham JB et al (1982) Heart failure in outpatients: a randomized trial of digoxin versus placebo. *N. Engl. J. Med.*, *306*, 699.
46. Fleg JL, Gottlieb SH, Lakatta EG (1982) Is digoxin really important in treatment of compensated heart failure? A placebo-controlled crossover study in patients with sinus rhythm. *Am. J. Med.*, *73*, 244.
47. Arnold SB, Byrd RC, Meister W et al (1983) Long-term digitalis therapy improves left ventricular function in heart failure. *N. Engl. J. Med.*, *303*, 143.
48. Boman K (1983) Digoxin and the geriatric patient: a randomized trial of digoxin versus placebo. *Acta Med. Scand.*, *214*, 353.
49. Gheorghiade M, Beller G (1983) Effects of discontinuing maintenance digoxin therapy in patients with ischemic heart disease and congestive heart failure in sinus rhythm. *Am. J. Cardiol.*, *51*, 1243.
50. Taggart AJ, Johnston GD, McDevitt DG (1983) Digoxin withdrawal after cardiac failure in patients with sinus rhythm. *J. Cardiovasc. Pharmacol.*, *5*, 229.
51. Pugh SE, White NJ, Aronson JK et al (1989) Clinical, haemodynamic, and pharmacological effects of withdrawal and reintroduction of digoxin in patients with heart failure in sinus rhythm after long term treatment. *Br. Heart J.*, *61*, 529.
52. Fleg JL, Lakatta EG (1984) How useful is digitalis in patients with congestive heart failure and sinus rhythm? *Int. J. Cardiol.*, *6*, 295.
53. Mulrow CD, Feussner JR, Velez R (1984) Reevaluation of digitalis efficacy: new light on an old leaf. *Ann. Intern. Med.*, *101*, 113.
54. Castellanos A, Shin E-K, Luceri RM, Myerburg RJ (1988) Parasystolic accelerated idioventricular rhythms producing bidirectional tachycardia patterns. *J. Electrophysiol.*, *2*, 296.
55. Horst H-A, Kolenda K-D, Duncker G et al (1988) Häufigkeit and Ausmass digitalisinduziertier Farbsehstörungen: eine vergleichende Studie bei subtoxischen und toxischen Digoxin- und Digitoxinserumkonzentrationen. *Med. Klin.*, *83*, 541.
56. Rodin SM, Johnson BF (1988) Pharmacokinetic interactions with digoxin. *Clin. Pharmacokinet.*, *15*, 227.
57. Johnson BF, Wilson J, Marwaha R et al (1987) The comparative effects of verapamil and a new dihydropyridine calcium channel blocker on digoxin pharmacokinetics. *Clin. Pharmacol. Ther.*, *42*, 66.
58. Rodin SM, Johnson BF, Wilson J et al (1988) Comparative effects of verapamil and israpidine upon steady-state digoxin kinetics. *Clin. Pharmacol. Ther.*, *43*, 668.
59. Kirch W, Logemann C, Heidemann H et al (1987) Nitrendipine/digoxin interaction. *J. Cardiovasc. Pharmacol.*, *10*, *Suppl. 10*, S74.

60. Dunselman PHJM, Scaf AHJ, Kuntze CEE et al (1988) Digoxin–felodipine interaction in patients with congestive heart failure. *Eur. J. Clin. Pharmacol., 35*, 461.
61. Bruserud Ø, Skadberg BT, Ohm OJ (1988) Combined intoxication with digitoxin and verapamil: the possible inhibition of sensitisation to digitalis-specific antiserum by toxic drug concentrations. *J. Lab. Clin. Immunol., 25*, 167.
62. Quastel MR, Kaplan JG (1970) Inhibition by ouabain of human lymphocyte transformation induced by phytohaemagglutinin. *Nature (Lond.), 219*, 198.
63. Stoeck M, Northoff H, Resch K (1983) Inhibition of mitogen-induced lymphocyte proliferation by ouabain: influence with interleukin 2 production and interleukin 2 action. *J. Immunol., 131*, 1433.
64. Cody RJ (1988) Do positive inotropic agents adversely affect the survival of patients with chronic congestive heart failure? I. Introduction. *J. Am. Coll. Cardiol., 12*, 559.
65. Packer M (1988) Do positive inotropic agents adversely affect the survival of patients with chronic congestive heart failure? II. Protagonist's viewpoint. *J. Am. Coll. Cardiol., 12*, 562.
66. Collucci WS (1988) Do positive inotropic agents adversely affect the survival of patients with chronic congestive heart failure? III. Antagonist's viewpoint. *J. Am. Coll. Cardiol., 12*, 566.
67. Bichel T, Steinbach G, Olry L, Lambert H (1988) Utilisation de l'amrinone intraveineux dans le traitement du choc cardiogénique. *Agressologie, 29*, 187.
68. Hohnloser SH, Meinertz T, Zehender M et al (1988) Auslösung und Verstärkung von Herzrhythmusstörungen durch Antiarrhythmika. *Aktuel. Ther., 29*, 338.
69. Rae AP, Kay HR, Horowitz LN et al (1988) Proarrhythmic effects of antiarrhythmic drugs in patients with malignant ventricular arrhythmias evaluated by electrophysiologic testing. *J. Am. Coll. Cardiol., 12*, 131.
70. Lanza GA, Tamburi S, Malvestiti FMPM et al (1988) Aggravamento di aritmie ventricolari all'ECG dinamico in pazienti trattati con farmaci antiaritmici. *Cardiologia, 33*, 613.
71. Minardo JD, Heger JJ, Miles WM et al (1988) Clinical characteristics of patients with ventricular fibrillation during antiarrhythmic drug therapy. *N. Engl. J. Med., 319*, 257.
72. Atkinson AJ, Ih Ruo T, Piergies AA (1988) Comparison of the pharmacokinetic and pharmacodynamic properties of procainamide and *N*-acetylprocainamide. *Angiology, 39*, 655.
73. Piergies AA, Ih Ruo T, Jansyn EM et al (1987) Effect kinetics of *N*-acetylprocainamide-induced QT interval prolongation. *Clin. Pharmacol. Ther., 42*, 107.
74. Somogyi A, McLean A, Heinzow B (1983) Cimetidine–procainamide pharmacokinetic interaction in man: evidence of competition for tubular secretion of basic drugs. *Eur. J. Clin. Pharmacol., 25*, 339.
75. Kosoglou T, Rocci ML, Vlasses PH (1988) Trimethoprim alters the disposition of procainamide and *N*-acetylprocainamide. *Clin. Pharmacol. Ther., 44*, 467.
76. Narciso V, Tedesco A, Russo E et al (1988) Su di un caso di epatite colestatica da feniletilbarbiturato di ajmaline. *Quad. Med. Chir., 4*, 69.
77. Yamamoto M, Katsuno M, Toyota T et al (1988) Three cases of drug-induced agranulocytosis: identifying offending drugs by CFU-GM assay. *Saishin-Igaku, 43*, 1314.
78. Pichler WJ, Schindler L, Stäubli M et al (1988) Anti-amiodarone antibodies: detection and relationship to the development of side effects. *Am. J. Med., 85*, 197.
79. Maling T (1988) Amiodarone therapeutic plasma concentration monitoring: is it practical? *Clin. Pharmacokinet., 14*, 321.
80. Kerin NZ, Blevins RD, Kerner N et al (1988) A low incidence of proarrhythmia using low-dose amiodarone. *J. Electrophysiol., 2*, 289.
81. Martin WJ, Rosenow EC (1988) Amiodarone pulmonary toxicity: recognition and pathogenesis. *Chest, 93*, 1067 (Part 1), 1242 (Part 2).
82. Yu YZ, Botvinnick E, Dae M et al (1988) Gallium lung scintigraphy in amiodarone pulmonary toxicity. *Chest, 93*, 1126.
83. Magro SA, Lawrence EC, Wheeler SH et al (1988) Amiodarone pulmonary toxicity: prospective evaluation of serial pulmonary function tests. *J. Am. Coll. Cardiol., 12*, 781.
84. Horowitz LN (1988) Detection of amiodarone pulmonary toxicity: to screen or not to screen, that is the question! *J. Am. Coll. Cardiol., 12*, 789.
85. Monteiro E, Gatrao-Teles A, Santos ML et al (1986) Antithyroid antibodies as an early marker for thyroid disease induced by amiodarone. *Br. Med. J., 292*, 227.
86. Rabinowe SL, Larsen PR, Antman EM et al (1986) Amiodarone therapy and autoimmune thyroid disease. *Am. J. Med., 81*, 53.
87. Weetman AP, Bhandal SK, Burrin JM et al (1988) Amiodarone and thyroid autoimmunity in the United Kingdom. *Br. Med. J., 297*, 33.
88. Safran M, Martino E, Aghini-Lombardi F et al (1988) Effect of amiodarone on circulating thyroid antibodies. *Br. Med. J., 297*, 456.
89. Bordalo ADB, Ribiero C (1988) Clinical safety of long-term amiodarone therapy. *N. Trends Arrhythm., 4*, 841.
90. Ling MCC, Dake MD, Okelund MD (1988) Gallium uptake in the thyroid gland in amiodarone-induced hyperthyroidism. *Clin. Nucl. Med., 13*, 258.
91. Tubman R, Jenkins J, Lim J (1988) Neonatal hyperthyroxinaemia associated with maternal

amiodarone therapy: case report. *Ir. J. Med. Sci.*, *157*, 243.
92. Pollak PT, Sharma AD, Carruthers G (1988) Elevation of serum total cholesterol and triglyceride levels during amiodarone therapy. *Am. J. Cardiol.*, *62*, 562.
93. Guigui B, Perrot S, Berry JP et al (1988) Amiodarone-induced hepatic phospholipidosis: a morphological alteration independent of pseudoalcoholic liver disease. *Hepatology*, *8*, 1063.
94. Freneaux E, Larrey D, Pessayre D (1988) Phospholipidose et lésions pseudoalcoöliques hépatiques médicamenteuses. *Rev. Fr. Gastro-entérol.*, *24*, 879.
95. Pye M, Northcote RJ, Cobbe SM (1988) Acute hepatitis after parenteral amiodarone administration. *Br. Heart J.*, *59*, 690.
96. Parodi A, Guarrera M, Rebora A (1988) Amiodarone-induced pseudoporphyria. *Photodermatology*, *5*, 146.
97. Moots RJ, Banerjee A (1988) Exfoliative dermatitis after amiodarone treatment. *Br. Med. J.*, *296*, 1332.
98. Hyatt RH, Sinha B, Vallon A et al (1988) Noncardiac side-effects of long-term oral amiodarone in the elderly. *Age Ageing*, *17*, 116.
99. Foster CJ, Love HG (1988) Amiodarone in pregnancy: case report and review of the literature. *Int. J. Cardiol.*, *20*, 307.
100. Van Dyck M, Baele P, Rennotte MT et al (1988) Should amiodarone be discontinued before cardiac surgery? *Acta Anaesth. Belg.*, *39*, 3.
101. Naccarelli GV, Wellens HJJ (Eds.) (1988) A symposium: the use of encainide in supraventricular tachycardias. *Am. J. Cardiol.*, *62*, 1L.
102. Soyka LF (1988) Safety considerations and dosing guidelines for encainide in supraventricular arrhythmias. *Am. J. Cardiol.*, *62*, 63L.
103. Miles WM, Zipes DP, Rinkenberger RL et al (1988) Encainide for treatment of atrioventricular reciprocating tachycardia in the Wolff-Parkinson-White syndrome. *Am. J. Cardiol.*, *62*, 20L.
104. Rinkenberger RL, Naccarelli GV, Miles WM (1988) Encainide for atrial fibrillation associated with Wolff-Parkinson-White syndrome. *Am. J. Cardiol.*, *62*, 26L.
105. Naccarelli GV, Jackman WM, Akhtar M et al (1988) Efficacy and electrophysiologic effects of encainide for atrioventricular nodal reentrant tachycardia. *Am. J. Cardiol.*, *62*, 31L.
106. Bongiorni MG, Levorato D, Arlotta C et al (1988) Long-term efficacy of oral encainide in frequent and repetitive ventricular arrhythmias. *Eur. Heart J.*, *9*, 765.
107. The Encainide-Ventricular Tachycardia Study Group (1988) Treatment of life-threatening ventricular tachycardia with encainide hydrochloride in patients with left ventricular dysfunction. *Am. J. Cardiol.*, *62*, 571.
108. Strasburger JF, Smith Jr RT, Moak JP et al (1988) Encainide for resistant supraventricular tachycardia in children: follow-up report. *Am. J. Cardiol.*, *62*, 50L.
109. Anderson JL, Pritchett ELC (Eds.) (1988) International symposium on supraventricular arrhythmias: focus on flecainide. *Am. J. Cardiol.*, *62*, 1D.
110. Anderson JL, Jolivette DM, Fredell PA (1988) Summary of efficacy of flecainide for supraventricular arrhythmias. *Am. J. Cardiol.*, *62*, 62D.
111. Hellestrand KJ (1988) Intravenous flecainide acetate for supraventricular tachycardias. *Am. J. Cardiol.*, *62*, 16D.
112. Kim SS, Smith P, Ruffy R (1988) Treatment of atrial tachyarrhythmias and preexcitation syndrome with flecainide acetate. *Am. J. Cardiol.*, *62*, 29D.
113. Ziegler V, Gillette PC, Hammill B et al (1988) Flecainide for supraventricular tachycardia in children. *Am. J. Cardiol.*, *62*, 41D.
114. Chouty F, Coumel P (1988) Oral flecainide for prophylaxis of paroxysmal atrial fibrillation. *Am. J. Cardiol.*, *62*, 35D.
115. Stoltz JP, Weingrod M, Leroy G et al (1988) Anomalies des ondes T induites par le flécaïnide. *Arch. Mal. Coeur*, *81*, 1009.
116. Mancuso G, Tampieri E, Berdondini RM (1988) Eruzione psoriasiforme da flecainide. *G. Ital. Dermatol. Venereol.*, *123*, 171.
117. Mehta D, Camm J, Ward DE (1988) Clinical electrophysiologic effects of flecainide acetate. *Cardiovasc. Drugs Ther.*, *1*, 599.
118. Saoudi N, Galtier M, Hidden F et al (1988) Bundle-branch reentrant ventricular tachycardia: a possible mechanism of flecainide proarrhythmic effect. *J. Electrophysiol.*, *2*, 365.
119. Musto B, D'Onfrio A, Cavallaro C (1988) Electrophysiologic effects and clinical efficacy of flecainide in children with recurrent paroxysmal supraventricular tachycardia. *Am. J. Cardiol.*, *62*, 229.
120. Williams AJ, McQuinn RL, Walls J (1988) Pharmacokinetics of flecainide acetate in patients with severe renal impairment. *Clin. Pharmacol. Ther.*, *43*, 449.
121. McQuinn RL, Pentikäinen PJ, Chang SF, Conard GJ (1988) Pharmacokinetics of flecainide in patients with cirrhosis of the liver. *Clin. Pharmacol. Ther.*, *44*, 566.
122. Ochs HR, Carstens G, Greenblatt DJ (1980) Reduction in lidocaine clearance during continuous infusion and by co-administration of propranolol. *N. Engl. J. Med.*, *303*, 373.
123. Bax NDS, Tucker GT, Lennard MS et al (1984) The impairment of lignocaine clearance by propranolol: major contribution from enzyme inhibition. *Br. J. Clin. Pharmacol.*, *19*, 597.
124. Wyse DG, Kellen J, Tam Y, Rademaker AW (1988) Increased efficacy and toxicity of lidocaine in patients on beta-blockers. *Int. J. Cardiol.*, *21*, 59.

125. Morganroth J, for the Mexiletine-Quinidine Research Group (1987) Comparative efficacy and safety of oral mexiletine and quinidine in benign or potentially lethal ventricular arrhythmias. *Am. J. Cardiol., 60*, 1276.
126. Miller B, Skupin A, Rubenfire M, Bigman O (1988) Respiratory failure produced by severe procainamide intoxication in a patient with preexisting peripheral neuropathy caused by amiodarone. *Chest, 94*, 663.
127. Sherentz EF (1988) Lichen planus following procainamide-induced lupus erythematosus. *Cutis, 42*, 51.
128. Smiley JD, Moore SE (1988) Molecular mechanisms of autoimmunity. *Am. J. Med. Sci., 295*, 478.
129. Totoritis MC, Tan EM, McNally EM, Rubin RL (1988) Association of antibody to histone complex H2A-H2B with symptomatic procainamide-induced lupus. *N. Engl. J. Med., 318*, 1431.
130. Weber MT, Hocking WG (1988) Procainamide induced lupus anticoagulant. *Wisc. Med. J., 87*, 30.
131. Heyman MR, Flores RH, Edelman BB, Carliner NH (1988) Procainamide-induced lupus anticoagulant. *South. Med. J., 81*, 934.
132. Uetrecht JP, Freeman RW, Woosley RL (1981) The implications of procainamide metabolism to its induction of lupus. *Arthr. Rheum., 24*, 994.
133. Uetrecht J, Sweetman B, Woosley R, Oates J (1984) Metabolism of procainamide to a hydroxylamine by rat and human hepatic microsomes. *Drug Metab. Disposit., 12*, 77.
134. Uetrecht J, Zahid N, Rubin R (1988) Metabolism of procainamide to a hydroxylamine by human neutrophils and mononuclear leucocytes. *Chem. Res. Toxicol., 1*, 74.
135. Somberg JC, Tepper D, Landau S (1988) Propafenone: a new antiarrhythmic agent. *Am. Heart J., 115*, 1274.
136. Ravid S, Podrid PJ, Novrit B (1987) Safety of long-term propafenone therapy for cardiac arrhythmia – experience with 774 patients. *J. Electrophysiol., 1*, 580.
137. Hodges M (1987) Role of propafenone in the treatment of ventricular premature beats. *J. Electrophysiol., 1*, 536.
138. Hammill SC (1987) Use of propafenone in patients with supraventricular tachycardia. *J. Electrophysiol., 1*, 561.
139. Klein RC, Marcus FI (1987) Efficacy of propafenone when used in combination antiarrhythmic therapy. *J. Electrophysiol., 1*, 575.
140. Antman EM, Beamer AD, Cantillon C et al (1988) Long-term oral propafenone therapy for suppression of refractory symptomatic atrial fibrillation and atrial flutter. *J. Am. Coll. Cardiol., 12*, 1005.
141. Casariego Roson JR, Moreno Roldan A, Velasco L et al (1988) Disfunción sinusal inducida por propafenona: presentación de un caso. *Med. Intens., 12*, 89.
142. Lee P-K, Kerr CR, Vorderbrugge S et al (1988) Symptomatic sinus node dysfunction associated with the use of propafenone. *Am. J. Cardiol., 62*, 480.
143. Brunozzi LT, Meniconi L, Chiocchi P et al (1988) Propafenone in the treatment of chronic ventricular arrhythmias in a pregnant patient. *Br. J. Clin. Pharmacol., 26*, 489.
144. Malcolm AD, David GK (1987) Quinidine in cardiology. *Acta Leidens., 55*, 87.
145. Kennedy HL, DeMaria AN, Sprague MK et al (1988) Comparative efficacy of moricizine and quinidine for benign and potentially lethal ventricular arrhythmias. *Am. J. Noninvas. Cardiol., 2*, 98.
146. Fields CD, Ezri MD, Denes P (1988) 'Quinidine syncope' without lengthening of Q-Tc interval in the presence of left bundle branch block: role of programmed ventricular stimulation studies. *Chest, 94*, 111.
147. Schieman G, Blacky AR, Nicod PH, Dittrich HC (1988) Prolonged asymptomatic torsade de pointes. *J. Electrophysiol., 2*, 46.
148. Christie DJ, Diaz-Arauzo H, Cook JM (1988) Antibody-mediated platelet destruction by quinine, quinidine, and their metabolites. *J. Lab. Clin. Med., 112*, 92.
149. Cohen MG, Kevat S, Prowse MV, Ahern MJ (1988) Two distinct quinidine-induced rheumatic syndromes. *Ann. Intern. Med., 108*, 369.
150. Braude AC, Downar E, Chamberlain DW et al (1982) Tocainide-associated interstitial pneumonitis. *Thorax, 37*, 309.
151. van Natta B, Lazarus M, Li C (1988) Irreversible interstitial pneumonitis associated with tocainide therapy. *West. J. Med., 149*, 91.
152. Committee on Safety of Medicines (1989) Revised indications for flecainide. *Curr. Probl., 27*.

M.N.G. Dukes

19 β-Adrenoceptor antagonists and antianginal drugs

β-ADRENOCEPTOR ANTAGONISTS *(SED-11, 360; SEDA-13, 149)*

Cardiovascular system The fact that β-adrenergic blockers can produce symptoms of peripheral ischemia is long known, but as a rule the effect is uncomfortable rather than serious, with complaints of Raynaud-like coldness of the extremities. Just occasionally, in patients predisposed to this effect, the impairment of peripheral circulation may be sufficient to produce gangrene; a recent case from France is apparently the ninth on record:

A man of 48 sought medical advice because of necrotic changes in all 10 toes. He had always suffered from poor peripheral circulation, most marked in cold weather, and for 2 years he had been treated for hypertension with diuretics and timolol 10 mg daily by mouth. After 7 months of treatment he had noted onset of intermittent claudication, but had not reported this to the doctor. Six months later after exposure to snow he had suffered severe pain and edema of the toes with generalized pyrexia. Despite supportive treatment distal amputation of the toes proved necessary (1[CR]).

Nervous system In a paper dealing primarily with seizures induced by esmolol and discussed below, Das and Ferris provided in 1988 a short but clear review of the way in which β-adrenoceptor antagonists may induce *seizures*. It is sufficient to remark here that seizures have generally followed the ingestion of excessively high doses, though in a few cases normal doses caused seizures in susceptible individuals. The effect might in some cases be attributable to some better-known pharmacological effects of these compounds, such as the induction of bradycardia or hypoglycemia or to the membrane-stabilizing properties of these substances. In the esmolol case reported by these authors, however, none of these explanations seem to hold good (18[cr], 19[c]).

Skin and appendages Alongside a general literature overview by Heng and Heng of the incidence of psoriatic eruption during beta-blocker therapy which generally confirms existing impressions (2[R]), 1988 saw a new study of the actual frequency in a population of 588 psoriasis patients who had in the past received ultra-violet light therapy for their condition.

After examining the histories of all 588 cases, 73 were selected as being likely or potential users of beta-blockers in view of a history of cardiovascular disorders or migraine, and they received a questionnaire. Of the 47 who provided evaluable responses, 25 had indeed received one or more beta-blockers, and one current case of psoriasis flare associated with metoprolol was also noted. In the group as a whole, exacerbation of psoriasis had occurred in 9 of 13 patients on propranolol, 4 of 4 on nadolol, 6 of 8 on atenolol and 2 of 3 on metoprolol. One patient claimed that the psoriasis had improved during the beta-blockade (3[Cr]).

This work makes it fairly clear that about two thirds of patients on a beta-blocker are likely to experience a flare-up of existing psoriasis, irrespective of the agent employed.

Risk situations A child with the *tetralogy of Fallot* is clearly likely to be highly sensitive to the effects of some drugs with cardiac effects. Clark et al in 1989 presented a case of a girl of 18 months with this condition who received propranolol 5 mg 3 times daily to treat attacks of acute cyanosis. The drug appeared to be effective but during a severe episode she was admitted to hospital and the dose was raised to 8 mg

Side Effects of Drugs Annual 14
M.N.G. Dukes and L. Beeley, editors

daily. Thereafter she suffered a series of episodes of near syncope which were traced to extreme bradycardia and paroxysmal sinus arrest. These new episodes disappeared when the propranolol was discontinued (4[C]).

Withdrawal effects See propranolol below.

Interactions The fact that beta-blockers can interact violently with *epinephrine (adrenaline)*, as one would expect from their pharmacology, is still overlooked in practice. While it has become fairly generally appreciated that a catecholamine analog will derange antihypertensive therapy with a beta-blocker, the fact that a non-selective beta-blocker can greatly increase the pressure response to epinephrine and lead to hypertension and reflex bradycardia seems to be forgotten. Gandy has described a typical case in which a man on long-term propranolol maintenance therapy was admitted with severe pharyngeal and uvular edema and was given 0.3 ml of a 1:1000 solution of epinephrine subcutaneously. Severe headache and acute hypertension occurred with sinus bradycardia, though with emergency treatment the patient recovered (5[Cr]).

Since the ability of *non-steroidal anti-inflammatory drugs* to counter the effects of beta-blockers was first discussed (SED-11, 369), research groups have been anxious to find evidence that their own particular non-steroidal agent does not have this effect to any significant degree. The Boots company was able to show that 1600 mg/d ibuprofen did not significantly affect blood pressure control by propranolol (6[c]). In fact the effect was first demonstrated with indometacin and it seems increasingly doubtful whether it plays any real role in practice; one should simply bear in mind that if an NSAID is added to existing beta-blocker therapy it will be sensible to monitor the effects of the antihypertensive treatment more frequently for a while to exclude any interference.

Beta-blockers can obviously potentiate or buttress *one anothers' effects*, and this would hardly be worth recording were it not for the fact that a systemic beta-blocker prescribed in general medicine may have at least an additive effect with one prescribed for topical use by the ophthalmologist, the possibility of the interaction having been missed by both parties. That ophthalmic beta-blockers can produce severe systemic effects, e.g. involving the nervous or cardiovascular systems, has been discussed repeatedly in Chapter 49 of these volumes, and documented particularly with respect to timolol and more recently as regards betaxolol (7[c], 8[C], 9[R]). A classic interaction between the 2 forms of treatment has also been reported for betaxolol and labetalol, the joint treatment resulting in confusion, bronchospasm and congestive heart failure in an elderly woman in intensive care (10[c]).

INDIVIDUAL β-ADRENOCEPTOR ANTAGONISTS

Propranolol (*SED-11, 360; SEDA-12, 159*)

Respiratory Precipitation of *asthma* in susceptible individuals is a classic risk with the non-selective beta-blockers, though cases still occur where the attendant clinician overlooks the onset of wheezing as an early warning sign (11[C]). The risk is not always one which can be avoided in advance, since in much of the developing world low-cost propranolol may be the only beta-blocker available.

Less typical is a report of what seems to have been *hypersensitivity pneumonitis* reflecting an immune lung reaction of cell-mediated type.

A man of 59 with a long history of exposure both to asbestos and to pigeons and doves was treated for 30 months with propranolol (40 mg/d) and pentaethyl tetranitrate because of coronary disease. He now presented with mild fever, loss of weight, cough and dyspnea of effort. Although the clinical lung examination detected no abnormalities, there were small interstitial opacities at the lung bases on X-ray, a hypergammaglobulinemia and marked lymphocytosis. Bronchoalveolar lavage showed 3 asbestos bodies per ml, 30.3% macrophages, 18.6% neutrophils, 4.6% eosinophils, 44.9% lymphocytes and a CD4/CD8 lymphocyte ratio of 0.58.

Withdrawal of propranolol produced progressive improvement in the symptoms, X-ray and cytology, whereas rechallenge with propranolol caused recurrence (12[CR]).

This case points to the fact that where other risk or complicating factors are present – in this instance a suspicion of both asbestosis and psittacosis – one may need both rechallenge and bronchoalveolar lavage to make the diagnosis.

Withdrawal reactions There has for a long time been some doubt as to the reality of withdrawal reactions following beta-blocker treatment; clearly sometimes one is simply dealing with a recurrence of the original condition which may in the meantime have become more severe. The 'overshoot' effect on the *blood pressure* seems to be reasonably clear and continues to be documented with new cases (13[CR]); it would seem that the beta-receptors have as a result of the drug treatment become oversensitive to circulating agonists. Sequelae can be serious, even including myocardial infarction. The withdrawal effects are not limited to the cardiovascular system; headaches, tremulousness and anxiety are common, and one sometimes also sees an acute *psychic derangement* when treatment is stopped, rather as one may when a short-acting benzodiazepine is withdrawn. It now seems very likely that (just as with the benzodiazepines) a minority of individuals, commonly with a history of normal mental function, are unable to tolerate the sudden loss of supportive treatment.

A woman of 68 with no history of psychiatric problems had been treated for 10 years with 160 mg propranolol daily for essential tremor. When she ceased to take the drug, she developed over the course of a week increasing paranoid delusions, insomnia and auditory and tactile hallucinations. In the acute phase she required neuroleptic treatment, but she recovered after propranolol treatment was progressively resumed.

A man of 52 with no history of mental disorder had been treated for some weeks with 80 mg propranolol daily for hypertension. He discontinued it abruptly of his own accord and began to suffer severe nightly confusion. In this case too, recovery followed reinstitution of propranolol treatment. (14[C])

If it is true that one is dealing with a question of particular sensitivity in a minority group this would explain why a study in 30 healthy volunteers failed to show any evidence of a CNS withdrawal syndrome after the use of practolol (15[C]).

Celiprolol *(SEDA-12, 162; SEDA-13, 154)*

On present data, the adverse reaction profile of celiprolol still appears relatively favorable. Since it has both β_1 selectively and intrinsic agonist activity it is distinct from the older and most widely-used beta-blockers; in that respect one would expect its reaction pattern to be most closely similar to those of epanolol and xamoterol. The comparisons published so far are with older drugs including atenolol and propranolol, and celiprolol has proved to be free of the headache, dizziness, fatigue and bradycardia produced by these other compounds (16[R]). It appears to have a more favorable effect on bronchial reactivity than metoprolol, which is cardioselective but has no agonist activity (17[c]). The only reservation one must make is that one is still in the early phases. Work examined earlier in these volumes related to a dose of 200 mg daily, whereas recent studies use some 400 mg daily. Only once one is sure of the optimal dose range and has used the drug over the same length of time as some of the classic products have been employed will one be able to draw firm conclusions.

Esmolol *(SED-11, 371; SEDA-13, 154)*

The most characteristic feature of esmolol continues to be its extremely short half-life, so brief that it has little opportunity to cause adverse effects of interactions. That might be its main virtue, since when used for the treatment of conditions such as supraventricular tachyarrhythmias one needs only a brief corrective effect, after which the field should be free for the use of other agents (e.g. calcium antagonists) without the prospect of beta-blocker interactions (18[C]). On the other hand, this short and intensive treatment is not without its problems, one perhaps being induction of seizures, a recognized problem with excessively high doses of beta-blockers:

A very old man received esmolol i.v. for atrial tachycardia at a rate of a dose of 25 g/kg/min, doubled after 5 min and again after 10. Four minutes after the final infusion was started, the patient appeared drowsy and sleepy and he soon developed generalized tonic-clonic seizures. The infusion was terminated and the seizures abated in less than 1 min. After 5 min, when the patient had fully recovered, the infusion was restarted and within 3 min the patient again became drowsy and hyporesponsive; the infusion was stopped and no infusion occurred (19).

NITRATE DERIVATIVES *(SED-11, 371; SEDA-13, 154)*

Skin and appendages Further cases of contact dermatitis with nitroglycerine patches continue to be reported, and it seems evident that both the nitroglycerine itself and one or more components of the delivery system may be involved (20[C], 21[C]). A clinically important finding in the former of these two reports is that as the allergic contact dermatitis developed the resorption of the active component through the inflamed area apparently declined, resulting in deterioration of the cardiovascular condition.

Special senses When a man of 61 was given follow-up treatment for myocardial infarction using a nitroglycerine transdermal patch he complained that after 2 weeks he lost the sensation of bitter and salty taste, and by the sixth week his *sense of taste* had disappeared completely. When the patch was withdrawn the full sense of taste returned. Rechallenge seemed to confirm the effect, bitter and salt sensations vanishing within 5 days, and returning a week after final withdrawal (22[C]). The patient was also being treated with sublingual nitroglycerine as required, as well as diltiazem, aspirin and metoprolol, but the time frame and rechallenge strongly suggest that the nitroglycerine patch was responsible for the loss of taste.

Effects of excipients Demey et al have provided experimental evidence in a series of 28 patients that propylene glycol, used as a solvent in a commercially available intravenous nitroglycerine solution, can cause hyperosmolarity (and hence intracranial hypertension), hemolysis and lactic acidosis. The finding may in particular explain the neurological complications which sometimes occur during nitrate treatment. The risk of problems seems to be greatest where kidney function is impaired, causing the solvent to accumulate, but it is removed by hemodialysis (23).

CALCIUM ANTAGONISTS *(SED-11, 373; SEDA-13, 155)*

Cardiovascular Many of the recurrent troubles with calcium antagonists reported in the adverse reaction literature in fact reflect insufficiently close monitoring of their potent effects when they are used in high-risk patients. It is sufficiently well known that if they are used in severe congestive heart failure in old people they may produce circulatory collapse with renal failure (24[C]) and that they may cause cardiogenic shock in patients with a recent myocardial infarct (25[Cr]). These are not contraindications, but risk situations demanding great caution in the use of these drugs.

Endocrine, metabolic Calcium antagonists usually do not interfere with *carbohydrate metabolism* and cause no problems in most diabetic patients. One of the occasional exceptions which prove the rule may have been described by Heyman et al (26[C]); in their 60-year-old patient who was receiving both oral antihyperglycemic agents and insulin, nifedipine deranged the control of blood sugar. What one may note in this case, however, is that there was an earlier long history of maintenance therapy on beta-blockers (which have a known hypoglycemic effect), and from the time sequence it looks as if the increase in blood sugar levels was associated as much with the withdrawal of the beta-blockers as with the introduction of nifedipine treatment.

Interaction Ever since the severe interaction between calcium antagonists and *β-adrenoceptor blockers* (resulting in severe hypotension or even cardiac failure) became recognized the question has been whether one calcium antagonist is in this respect less risky than another. Intravenous verapamil has been regarded as notorious and it has been suggested (SED-13, 160) that nifedipine might be safer. Maclean's group, working with ICI, have studied the effects and tolerability of combined treatment with atenolol and nifedipine in 25 patients treated for 4 weeks with each of various dose levels; their conclusion is that tolerability was actually better than that of atenolol alone (27[C]). However when one looks at the vast number of relevant reports one must conclude that the risk of a serious interaction is still present, as stressed by Stockley, in discussing some recent cases in which nifedipine caused precisely the same problems when used alongside propranolol, alprenolol or atenolol (28[R]). The conclusion must still be that one should not lightheartedly use beta-blockers and calcium antagonists together; there must be a good reason for it.

INDIVIDUAL CALCIUM ANTAGONISTS

Nifedipine

Respiratory Since *pulmonary edema* in the category of patients eligible for calcium antagonist therapy is most likely to be a manifestation of heart failure, the physician may look no further for an explanation. However it looks as if it might also occur as an allergic reaction to some formulations of nifedipine:

A man of 76 with multiple disorders including poorly controlled hypertension was treated with 20-mg tablets of controlled-release nifedipine ('Adalat L®'). Within 3 days he developed severe and symptomatic pulmonary edema. The condition normalized after withdrawal of all the drugs which he was receiving. Subsequent lymphocyte-stimulating tests using all the products which he had been taking showed positive results only with Adalat L, the highest score being noted with the substance used for coating the tablets (20[C]).

Hematological Nifedipine may very occasionally have caused blood dyscrasias, and a report of purpura suggests this mechanism; however in the patient described by Oren et al in 1989, a women of 63 clearly developed an acute and extensive *non-thrombocytopenic purpuric reaction* to nifedipine which persisted throughout the 4 weeks of treatment and then disappeared within a few days after the drug was withdrawn. One should add that she was also receiving quinidine, but this had been given for a longer period and she appeared to tolerate it well (30[C]).

Skin and appendages A lichenoid reaction presenting clinically as an *exfoliative dermatitis* must be added to the list of skin reactions known with nifedipine (31); the reaction recurred twice on subsequent rechallenges with the drug.

Cases of *gingival hyperplasia* attributable to nifedipine continue to be reported (32[c], 33[CR]), though the absolute incidence must be very low.

Miscellaneous A somewhat unclear report has associated the use of nifedipine with *epistaxis* in a middle-aged alcoholic man (34[c]). Bearing in mind that epistaxis can be a complication of hypertension, which was the patient's principal disorder, and that epistaxis occurred on one occasion following the use of nifedipine but on another following its withdrawal one would not be inclined to conclude that there was a link with the drug.

Interactions Since calcium antagonists have been known to interfere with the effect of dantrolene it is not entirely surprising to note a recent report of what may have been a potentiating effect on the neuromuscular blockade produced by *magnesium sulfate*, when using both agents as tocolytic agents in premature labor.

A woman of 22 experienced uterine contractions at the 32nd week of pregnancy and was given 60 mg nifedipine over a 3-hour period, followed by a maintenance dose of 20 mg every 8 h. Since after an initial response the contractions nevertheless recurred and it was considered unwise to raise the nifedipine dose any further, intravenous magnesium sulfate was given (300 mg in all). The patient developed jerky movements of the limbs and respiratory apparatus and found it difficult to swallow or raise her head because of marked muscular weakness. The effect wore off 25 min after magnesium sulfate was discontinued (35).

Whether one is dealing here with true potentiation or a simple additive effect is not clear; the authors of the report recommend against using the 2 agents together for tocolysis, and at the very least cases where 1 drug alone proves insufficient should be very closely monitored if 2 are given together.

Risk situations An interaction of calcium antagonists with volatile anesthetic agents was discussed in SEDA-13. One must now add a later case of cardiac arrest on 2 occasions apparently due to the influence of nifedipine in a woman in whom anesthesia was induced primarily with thiopental sodium; she was also receiving succinylcholine. The case was regarded as one of *carotid sinus syndrome*, a condition in which the induction of anesthesia can trigger cardiovascular collapse; under normal conditions the patient was asymptomatic and she had previously tolerated general anesthesia several times, but the syndrome was considered to have been rendered more severe under the influence of nifedipine. Follow-up study showed that while carotid sinus massage produced a normal response so long as she was not taking nifedipine, sublingual use of the drug in a 10 mg dose was sufficient to cause sinus arrest and a fall in systolic blood pressure (36[Cr]).

Calcium antagonists are sometimes used as vasodilators in *pulmonary hypertension*. A case reported by Pohar et al suggests that this may not be without risk in some cases. In their 55-year-old patient with known primary pulmonary hypertension the severity of the condition increased 2 hours after a 10 mg sublingual dose of nifedipine. Since no other treatment proved effective she was ultimately stabilized under careful control on nifedipine in the form of 10 mg sustained-release tablets 4 times daily. What appears to have happened here is that the sublingual dose was initially effective, but that the rapid decline in circulating levels of nifedipine which followed its use produced some sort of withdrawal reaction. The prolonged moderate blood levels produced with the long-acting product evaded this risk (37[C]). This is perhaps one of the instances where slow-release preparations are entirely meaningful from the point of view of drug safety.

Diltiazem *(SED-11, 373; SEDA-13, 160)*

Hypersensitivity reactions Three recent case reports of *angioneurotic edema* from a single source seem incontrovertible; 2 concerned diltiazem, 1 verapamil. The cases occurred 2, 4 and 8 weeks after starting on diltiazem, and in all cases the symptoms receded completely 48–72 hours after the drug was withdrawn (38[C]). Most calcium inhibitors have been associated with a range of allergic reactions and angioneurotic edema can probably be expected from time to time with any of them.

Cardiovascular As noted above, the most troublesome 'adverse' effects of calcium antagonists are a consequence of their desired effect when it is exerted to excess or in high-risk situations. In a post-marketing surveillance programme, Waller and Inman in 1989 studied the incidence of heart block in a total of 10 119 patients taking the drug for at least 12 months. Atrioventricular block occurred in 22 cases, the dose of diltiazem being taken at the time averaging 180 mg. Third degree heart block occurred in 8 patients. Nine of the 22 were at the time concurrently receiving a beta-blocker, pointing to the special risk of this combination considered above and below (39[C]).

Nervous system In a mentally stable woman of 72 described by Bushe in 1988, treatment with 60 mg diltiazem 3 times daily apparently induced a florid *organic psychosis* within 2 days. The condition, characterized particularly by auditory and visual hallucinations and paranoid delusional ideas, rapidly receded over 3 days after withdrawal of the drug, and after a week she was fully normal (40[cR]). Rechallenge was not attempted, and she was treated thereafter with nifedipine which she tolerated well. Such a complication has been reported on one occasion before (by Polat in 1984, though with negative rechallenge (41[C])) and it is possible that like some of the other nervous system complications discussed in this Chapter it represents an event to which a small minority of users are peculiarly susceptible.

Hematological Leukopenia has been described earlier with diltiazem and in 1989 there was a case report of *thrombopenia* occurring acutely within 2 days of starting diltiazem treatment in a man of 61. The condition was marked by fever, hepatomegaly and rash, and resolved progressively over 8 days following withdrawal of the drug (42[C]).

Skin and appendages For at least 5 years there has been evidence that diltiazem may cause *erythema multiforme* (SED-11, 376), and in 1988 the Federal German Health Authorities actually issued a warning as to this and other serious skin effects (SEDA-13, 161). What was claimed in 1989 to be the first report of the problem is thus not by any means unprecedented but it is well documented. The 67-year-old woman concerned had previously tolerated isosorbide dinitrate well for some years, but within 2 weeks of starting treatment with diltiazem she developed over much of the body a very typical erythema multiforme confirmed by biopsy. The condition normalized rapidly when diltiazem was withdrawn (43[C]).

Interaction The interaction between calcium antagonists and beta-blockers is discussed elsewhere in this Chapter. A well-documented case involving diltiazem was reported by Partanen et al:

A middle-aged man with a long history of angina pectoris and more recent atrial fibrillation had long been receiving atenolol and digoxin. Diltiazem 60 mg 3 times daily was added because of deterioration in his condition. Atrioventricular conduction was still normal. He tolerated the combination well for nearly 3 months but then omitted his morning medication and took all the drugs in the course of a few hours later in the day. Sinus node arrest developed and he required emergency treatment (44^C).

Although in this case there was a clear degree of overdosage which undoubtedly raised the risk, 2 other cases in elderly people have been reported in which compliance was adequate (45^C); the suggestion of the authors concerned that nifedipine or nicardipine are less likely to cause an interaction with *β*-adrenergic blockers must, as pointed out above, be treated with much reserve.

Nicardipine *(SED-11, 378; SEDA-13, 161)*

Skin and appendages Levesque et al have described a case of *erythromelalgia* which was so closely associated in time with the use of nicardipine that the cause and effect relationship seems very likely. The 67-year old hypertensive patient began to experience typical symptoms (intermittent attacks of redness, heat and pain in the fingers, relieved by immersing the hands in cold water) 3–4 weeks after starting treatment. The symptoms were more frequent in warm weather and bed at night. The diagnosis was made only after a year and the drug was withdrawn, after which the symptoms quickly disappeared (40^C).

Verapamil *(SED-11, 374)*

Liver Mild hepatic reactions are known with verapamil and seem to be allergic in nature. An unusually severe reaction in a woman of 56 involved 2 episodes of jaundice, pruritus and upper abdominal pain with transaminase elevated up to 6-fold and alkaline phosphatase up to 4-fold when she was inadvertently rechallenged with the drug. The liver biopsy showed marked cholestasis (47^C).

ACKNOWLEDGEMENT

The author would like to acknowledge the support which he received in the preparation of this Chapter from a specialized section of the Working Group on Human Toxicological Assessment at the University of Copenhagen.

REFERENCES

1. Dompmartin A, Le Maitre M, Letessier D et al (1988) Nécrose digitales sous bêta-bloquants. *Ann. Dermatol. Venerol., 115,* 593.
2. Heng MCY, Heng MK (1988) Beta-adrenoceptor antagonist-induced psoriasiform eruption. *Int. J. Dermatol., 27,* 619.
3. Gold MH, Holy AK, Roenigk Jr HH (1988) Beta-blocking drugs and psoriasis. A review of cutaneous side effects and retrospective analysis of their effects on psoriasis. *J. Am. Acad. Dermatol., 19,* 837.
4. Clark DJ, Chan KC, Gibbs JL (1989) Propranolol-induced bradycardia in tetralogy of Fallot. *Br. Heart J., 61,* 378.
5. Gandy W (1989) Severe epinephrine–propranolol interaction. *Ann. Emerg. Med., 18,* 98.
6. Davies JG, Rawlins DC, Busson M (1988) Effect of ibuprofen on blood pressure control by propranolol and bendrofluazide. *J. Int. Med. Res., 16,* 173.
7. Chamberlain TJ (1989) Myocardial infarction after ophthalmic betaxolol. *N. Engl. J. Med., 321,* 1342.
8. Cohn JB (1989) A comparative study of the central nervous system effects of betaxolol *vs* timolol. *Arch. Ophthalmol., 107,* 633.
9. Lynch MG, Whitson JT, Brown RH et al (1988) Topical *β*-blocker therapy and central nervous system side effects. *Arch. Ophthalmol., 106,* 908.
10. Herschman Z, Kaufman B (1989) Complications arising from the use of ophthalmic medications in an intensive care unit patient. *NY State J. Med., 89,* 537.
11. Oppenheim EB (1988) An asthmatic woman given the wrong antihypertensive drug. *Cardiovasc. Rev. Rep., 9,* 70.
12. Akoun GM, Milleron BJ, Mayaud CM et al (1989) Provocation test coupled with bronchoalveolar lavage in diagnosis of propranolol-induced hypersensitivity pneumonitis. *Am. Rev. Respir. Dis., 139,* 247.

13. Houston MC, Hodge R (1988) Beta-adrenergic blocker withdrawal syndromes in hypertension and other cardiovascular diseases. *Am. Heart J.*, *116*, 515.
14. Golden RN, Hoffman J, Falk D (1989) Psychoses associated with propranolol withdrawal. *Biol. Psychiatry*, *25*, 351.
15. Al-Qassab H, Cleeves LA, Francis PL et al (1988) Is there a central nervous withdrawal syndrome associated with discontinuing long-term treatment with propranolol? *Hum. Toxicol.*, *7*, 249.
16. Lamon KD (1988) Safety profile of celiprolol. *Am. Heart J.*, *116*, 1438.
17. Bruschi C, Casali L, Cerveri I (1988) Effects of celiprolol on the bronchial reactivity in asthma. *Am. J. Cardiol.*, *61*, 53C.
18. Das G, Ferris J (1988) Esmolol in the treatment of supraventricular tachyarrhythmias. *Can. J. Cardiol.*, *4*, 177.
19. Das G, Ferris JC (1988) Generalized convulsions in a patient receiving ultrashort-acting betablocker infusion. *DICP Ann. Pharmacother.*, *22*, 484.
20. Carmichael AJ, Foulds IS (1989) Allergic contact dermatitis from transdermal nitroglycerin. *Contact Derm.*, *21*, 113.
21. Di Landro A, Valsecchi R, Cainelli T (1989) Contact dermatitis from Nitroderm. *Contact Derm.*, *21*, 115.
22. Ewing RC, Janda SM, Henann NE (1989) Ageusia-associated with transdermal nitroglycerin. *Clin. Pharm.*, *8*, 146.
23. Demey HE, Daelemans RA, Verpoorten GA et al (1988) Propylene glycol-induced side effects during intravenous nitroglycerine therapy. *Intens. Care Med.*, *14*, 221.
24. Eicher JC, Morelon P, Chalopin JM et al (1988) Acute renal failure during nifedipine therapy in a patient with congestive heart failure. *Crit. Care Med.*, *16*, 1163.
25. Shettigar UR, Loungani R (1989) Adverse effects of sublingual nifedipine in acute myocardial infarction. *Crit. Care Med.*, *17*, 196.
26. Heyman SN, Heyman A, Halperin I (1989) Diabetogenic effect of nifedipine. *DICP Ann. Pharmacother.*, *23*, 236.
27. Maclean D, Mitchell ET, Coulson RR et al (1988) Atenolol-nifedipine combinations compared to atenolol alone in hypertension: efficacy and tolerability. *Br. J. Clin. Pharmacol.*, *25*, 425.
28. Stockley IH (1989) Are β-blockers and nifedipine safe? *Br. Med. J.*, *296*, 1584.
29. Hasebe N, Fujikana T, Watanabe M et al (1988) A case of acute respiratory failure precipitated by long-acting nifedipine. *Kokyu To Junkan*, *36*, 1255.
30. Oren R, Polak A, Goldenhersch M et al (1989) Nifedipine-induced non-thrombocytopenic purpura. *DICP Ann. Pharmacother.*, *23*, 88.
31. Reynolds NJ, Jones SK, Crossley J et al (1989) Exfoliative dermatitis due to nifedipine. *Br. J. Dermatol.*, *121*, 401.
32. Ferrés E, López Colomés JL, Moreno A et al (1989) Gingival hyperplasia associated with nifedipine. (in Spanish) *Rev. Clin. Esp.*, *184*, 341.
33. Zlotgorski A, Nyska M, Sela M et al (1989) Nifedipine-induced gingival hyperplasia: case reports and literature review. *Isr. J. Med. Sci.*, *25*, 453.
34. Martinez MR, Gasulla G, Lafuente A (1989) Nifedipine and recurrent epistaxis. (in Spanish) *Med. Clin.*, *92*, 476.
35. Snyder SW, Cardwell MS (1989) Neuromuscular blockade with magnesium sulphate and nifedipine. *Am. J. Obstet. Gynecol.*, *161*, 35.
36. Plotkin CN, Eckenbrecht PD, Waldo DA (1989) Consecutive cardiac arrests on induction of anaesthesia associated with nifedipine-induced carotid sinus hypersensitivity. *Anesth. Analg.*, *63*, 402.
37. Pohar B, Grad A, Mozina M et al (1989) Paradoxical elevation of pulmonary vascular resistance after nifedipine in primary pulmonary hypertension. *Cor Vasa*, *31*, 238.
38. Sadick NS, Katz AS, Schreiber TL (1989) Angioedema from calcium channel blockers. *J. Am. Acad. Dermatol.*, *21*, 132.
39. Waller PC, Inman WHW (1989) Diltiazem and heart block. *Lancet*, *1*, 617.
40. Bushe CJ (1988) Organic psychosis caused by diltiazem. *J. R. Soc. Med.*, *81*, 296.
41. Polat GK, Hooker EA, Movaked M (1984) Secondary mania associated with diltiazem. *Clin. Cardiol.*, *7*, 611.
42. Lahav M, Arav R (1989) Diltiazem and thrombocytopenia. *Ann. Intern. Med.*, *16*, 327.
43. Berbis P, Alfonso MJ, Levy JL et al (1989) Diltiazem associated erythema multiforme. *Dermatologica*, *179*, 90.
44. Partanen J, Pellinen TJ (1989) Diltiazem and sinus arrest in connection with atenolol and digoxin. *Arch. Intern. Med.*, *149*, 223.
45. Hassell AB, Creamer JB (1989) Profound bradycardia after the addition of diltiazem to a β-blocker. *Br. Med. J.*, *298*, 675.
46. Levesque H, Moore N, Wolfe LM et al (1989) Erythromelalgia induced by Nicardipine (inverse Raynaud's phenomenon?) *Br. J. Med.*, *298*, 1252.
47. Burgunder J-M, Abernethy DR, Laurerburg BH (1988) Liver injury due to verapamil. *Hepatogastroenterology*, *35*, 169.

R. Verhaeghe and M. Verstraete

20 Drugs acting on the cerebral and peripheral circulation

Buflomedil *(SED-11, 391; SEDA-13, 169)*

Orally administered buflomedil is usually well tolerated and reported side effects are minor. Intravenous administration of vasoactive substances is practised in a number of European centers in patients with critical leg ischemia in whom surgery or percutaneous reopening procedures appear impractial. Evidence from controlled clinical trials that such therapy is efficacious in terms of limb salvage or healing of ischemic ulcers is almost non-existent. A Milanese center now reports 4 patients who developed *acute coronary incidents* during intravenous infusion of buflomedil (400 mg/d divided over 2 short infusions at a rate of 70 mg/h and with a free interval of 10 h) for critical leg ischemia (1[c]). Two patients suffered a myocardial infarction, one of whom eventually died from refractory heart failure. All patients were asymptomatic when buflomedil therapy was started. The authors speculate that buflomedil may provoke coronary steal. It should be noted though that all 4 patients also received oral calcium antagonists for hypertension, coronary disease or both. However, caution is recommended when buflomedil is used intravenously since almost all patients with critical leg ischemia have overt or silent ischemic heart disease as well. The benefit/risk balance may easily shift to the wrong side.

Cinnarizine *(SED-11, 391)*
Flunarizine *(SED-11, 391; SEDA-12, 170; SEDA-13, 169)*

The adverse reactions observed with these two related substances with antihistamine properties and calcium-blocking activity are usually mild in clinical trials. *Sedation, fatigue, drowsiness* and *weight gain* were the most frequent complaints in two recent large clinical trials in which almost 2000 patients received 10 mg of flunarizine as prophylaxis of migraine for 4 and 6 months, respectively (2[r], 3[r]). In the largest trial, *depression* was verified in 3 patients (0.2%), one of whom had been in a depressive state before entering the study (2[r]).

Earlier reports of parkinsonism, tardive dyskinesia and depression (SEDA-11, 179; SEDA-12, 170) induced by the two piperazine derivatives provoked several new publications from Spain and Italy, two countries which appear to have a high consumption of the two drugs (4[c]–7[c]). Over 100 new cases of *extrapyramidal symptoms* and/or *depression* are described. Not all are elderly and the unwanted effects can occur with the recommended daily dosage. The symptoms disappeared in virtually all patients within 1 month of stopping the drug. From the available data, it is difficult to estimate the true incidence of these neurological and psychiatric side effects of flunarizine and cinnarizine, but physicians who prescribe one of the two drugs should be aware that they can occur.

Ergotamine *(see also Chapter 14)*

Ergot poisoning from food has almost disappeared, but the therapeutic use of ergot alkaloids remains responsible for occasional reports of severe *vasospasm*. In one study of 1500 consecutive cases of acute ischemia admitted to a vascular unit 4 were due to ergotamine intoxication (8[r]). Arterial spasm can be due to an ergotamine overdose, but some patients develop an exaggerated response to a normal therapeutic dose. Patients with hyperthyroidism, acute infections, shock, and pregnant women appear particularly vulnerable.

In recent years, ergotamine has been added

Side Effects of Drugs Annual 14
M.N.G. Dukes and L. Beeley, editors

to low-dose heparin to improve the prophylactic effect on deep vein thrombosis. The use of this combination, however, may occasionally result in leg ischemia due to arterial spasm, especially in patients with pre-existing obstructive arterial disease. The risk of vasospasm may also outweigh the potential benefit of the combination over heparin alone in trauma patients (9[c]).

Ergotamine taken for migraine can induce spasm in the visceral and coronary arteries as well. This can lead to a clinical picture of acute myocardial infarction as recently reported in 2 middle-aged women (10[c]). In both, protracted coronary spasm due to ergotamine administered for supposed migraine was considered responsible. Ultimately, the left ventricular ejection fraction returned to normal in both patients, suggesting that myocardial ischemia rather than necrosis had occurred.

Nicotinic acid and derivatives *(SED-11, 393)*

Nicotinic acid and some of its derivatives not only are potent vasodilators but also exhibit a cholesterol-lowering effect. β-Pyridylcarbinol, the alcohol corresponding to nicotinic acid, is completely absorbed from the gastrointestinal tract and oxidized to nicotinic acid by alcohol dehydrogenase of the liver. Large doses of nicotinic acid (>4 g/d) are known to induce liver injury with prominent cholestasis, hepatocellular disarray and nodule formation by fibrous tissue on liver biopsy, so-called niacin hepatitis. Two new cases of *hepatic lesions* following long-term treatment with a lower dose of β-pyridylcarbinol (1.5 g/d) have now been published (11[c]). Mild elevations of liver enzymes led to the discovery on ultrasound examination of a large tumor-like mass in the gallbladder region in one patient and of nodular changes in the whole liver resembling metastatic lesions in the other patient. A liver biopsy in the second patient revealed moderate enlargement of the portal fields with histiocytic and lymphocytic infiltration and formation of collagen septa in the parenchyma. The changes regressed markedly after discontinuation of the drug in both patients.

Despite the vasodilating properties of nicotinic acid, a patient with dystrophia myotonica experienced acute severe hand ischemia following a self-administered injection of nicotinic acid into the ulnar artery (12[c]). He had crushed up several tablets of nicotinic acid into tap water and attempted intravenous injection into the forearm but erronously punctured the ulnar artery. Endothelial damage, vasospasm and secondary thromboembolic vessel occlusion may have resulted from the acidic drug itself or from the cornstarch or talcum powder fillers used in oral preparations.

Pentoxifylline *(SED-11, 393; SEDA-12, 171; SEDA-13, 170)*

Because of its hemorheological properties, pentoxifylline is being evaluated in the acute phase of ischemic cerebrovascular disorders. A recent multicenter, double-blind, randomized and placebo-controlled trial tested the efficacy and safety of the drug in 297 adult patients with ischemic stroke. Pentoxifylline was administered intravenously in a continuous infusion for 3 days (16 mg/kg/d, maximum 1200 mg/d) followed by 400 mg t.i.d. by mouth for up to 4 weeks. Neurological deficit scores did not differ between groups throughout the study, except for the first few days when a few parameters were better in the pentoxifylline group, but the clinical benefits were small and not sustained. The frequency of severe effects was comparable between the two treatment groups: as expected from previous experience in peripheral vascular disease, the most frequently reported effect that could probably be related to treatment was some *gastrointestinal discomfort* (13[r]).

Suloctidil

Suloctidil was withdrawn from the Belgian market in 1985 because of reported *hepatotoxicity* (SEDA-11, 181). New cases of drug-induced hepatocellular damage continue to be published. A sharp rise in liver enzymes was observed during the 7th week of treatment (400 mg t.i.d.) in a patient who participated in a double-blind trial of suloctidil in Alzheimer's disease (14[c]). A needle biopsy of the liver demonstrated focal necrosis of hepatocytes, mild hyperplasia of Kupffer cells and other features suggestive of mild acute hepatitis. The drug was discontinued and the liver enzymes returned promptly to normal levels.

REFERENCES

1. Romano M, Spinelli A, Muzio L et al (1988) Insufficienza coronarica acuta grave in corso di terapia per via endovenosa con buflomedil cloridrato. *Minerva Cardioangiol., 36*, 451.
2. Martinez-Lage JM (1988) Flunarizine (Sibelium) in the prophylasis of migraine: an open, long-term, multicenter trial. *Cephalalgia, 8, Suppl. 8*, 15.
3. Lücking CH, Oestreich W, Schmidt R, Soyka D (1988) Flunarizine vs. propranolol in the prophylaxis of migraine: two double blind comparative studies in more than 400 patients. *Cephalalgia, 8, Suppl. 8*, 21.
4. Capella D, Laporte JR, Castel JM et al (1987) Parkinsonism, tremor, and depression induced by cinnarizine and flunarizine. *Br. Med. J. 297*, 722.
5. Lugaresi A, Montagna P, Galassi R, Lugaressi E (1988) Extrapyramidal syndrome and depression induced by flunarizine. *Eur. Neurol., 28*, 208.
6. Moretti A, Lucantoni C (1988) Flunarine-induced parkinsonism: clinical report. *It. J. Neurol. Sci., 12*, 295.
7. Brignolio F, Coppo F (1988) Valuzione clinica di 12 casi di M. di Parkinson iatrogeno indotto da terapia prolungata con flunarizina. *Gaz. Med. It. Arch. Sci. Med., 147*, 237.
8. Adebe Vallina EJ, Polvornos MF, Estevan Solano JM et al (1988) Isquemias agudas producidas por ergotamina: analisis de cuatro cavos. *Angiologia, 3*, 100.
9. Schackford SR, Davis JW (1988) Refractory vasospasm occurring in a trauma patient receiving dihydroergotamine and heparin. *Crit. Care Med., 16*, 909.
10. Slob J, Burgersdijk C, Ruiter JH (1988) Ergotamine; van hoofdpijn naar hartpijn. *Ned. Tijdschr. Geneeskd., 132*, 927.
11. Kello C, Zoller W, Wolfram G, Zollner N (1988) Unusual but reversible hepatic lesions following long-term treatment with pyridylcarbinol for familial hypercholesterolemia. *Klin. Wochenschr., 66*, 647.
12. Dyson A, Henderson AM (1987) Continuous axillary brachial plexus blockade following intra-arterial injection of nicotinic acid. *Anaesth. Intens. Care, 15*, 462.
13. Hsu CY, Norris JW, Hogan EL (1988) Pentoxifylline in acute non hemorrhagic stroke: a randomized, placebo-controlled, double-blind trial. *Stroke, 19*, 716.
14. Shung MW, Komorowski RA, Varma RR (1988) Suloctidil-induced hepatotoxicity. *Gastroenterology, 95*, 490.

Janice A. Steiner

21 Antihypertensive drugs

The last 2 years, judging from the review articles published, seem to have been something of a watershed. Much has been written (1[R]–3[R]) about the failure of the successful treatment of hypertension to prevent myocardial infarct, assumed to be due to the negative effect of drugs on serum lipid profiles. This certainly contrasts with attitudes perhaps 20 years ago when the prevention of stroke, malignant hypertension and renal failure was hailed as a medical victory. It also presumably reflects a changing population in which, in developed countries at least, control of hypertension is widespread.

At the same time, much attention has been paid to issues of well-being (4[R]) in treated and untreated hypertensive populations compared with the population at large. Where symptoms do occur, it has been difficult on many occasions to differentiate between the disease process and its treatment or some other unrelated, perhaps psychological, disturbance. Take, for example, the vexed question of sexual dysfunction in hypertension. The Hypertension Detection and Follow-up Program (HDFP) (5[R]) suggests that the commonest cause of change of therapy in men was sexual dysfunction. There is little conclusive evidence, however, that treated and untreated hypertensives differ in this regard. The authors of the HDFP point out that since compliance is regarded as more important than any specific drug regimen, treatment changes are made frequently as a first approach to the problem. Reviewing the situation, Bansal (6[R]) draws similar conclusions and implies that although theoretically there are many causes, be they psychogenic, hormonal, vascular or drug-related, none has been conclusively shown to be of overall importance. Perhaps in the subtle and multifactorial syndromes now facing us conclusive general proof of causation is not possible as indeed is the case for essential hypertension itself.

Side Effects of Drugs Annual 14
M.N.G. Dukes and L. Beeley, editors

Solez et al (7[R]) report briefly their review of 2 large databases containing information on antihypertensive treatment in renal transplant patients. Two β-adrenoceptor antagonists (propranolol and metoprolol) seem to have had a deleterious effect on late graft function while nifedipine appears to have improved it. Much substantial information such as the demography of the patient groups, duration of treatment, level of hypertension and etiology of the renal failure is missing, making the paper difficult to evaluate.

Stumpf (8[R]) has recently provided an overview of the management of hypertensive crisis. There does not appear to be any inherent difference between the use of antihypertensive agents in hypertensive crisis and less severe states. The point is well taken, however, that sudden lowering of blood pressure in a crisis may cause hypoperfusion of many organs including the brain, heart and kidneys. Special care should be taken whatever the agent used.

Wurzelman et al (9[R]) reviewed a case-controlled cohort of 487 subjects aged between 75 and 85 years for the effect of β-adrenoceptor antagonists and α-methyldopa on mental performance measured by a battery of subjective tests. Beta-blockers were without apparent effect. Patients taking methyldopa did worse than controls overall, although they only reached statistical significance in one test. Unfortunately, more modern antihypertensive agents were not included in this study.

ANGIOTENSIN CONVERTING-ENZYME (ACE) INHIBITORS *(SED-11, 403; SEDA-12, 172; SEDA-13, 173)*

The major step forward for ACE inhibitors has been in the field of cardiac failure rather than hypertension. Captopril has been accepted by the FDA as a treatment for hypertension and the CONSENSUS Trial has shown the improvement in mortality brought about by the use of enalapril in patients with severe heart failure. Adverse events in patients with heart failure do not differ qualitatively from those in hypertensives (10[R]). Hypotension remains the main cause for concern although, if the starting dose of ACE inhibitor is low enough, this problem should be avoided. Patients in heart failure may also be prone to deteriorating renal function and hyperpotassemia when given ACE inhibitors. These effects are reversible and are frequently avoided by using sufficiently low doses of drug; this is especially true for those ACE inhibitors whose main excretory route is via the kidney.

The renal effects of ACE inhibitors have been extensively reviewed (11[R]). The authors include interesting evidence that, far from injuring the kidney as previously postulated, captopril may prevent deterioration in renal function in patients with renal parenchymatous disease. Even in some instances of renovascular hypertension ACE inhibitors are of positive benefit.

Meanwhile, there is an appreciation that ACE inhibitors appear to have no long-term effects on serum lipids, do not cause hypokalemia, and improve quality of life by comparison with other standard therapies for hypertension (12[R]). This has led to calls for the use of ACE inhibitors as first-line therapy in a stepped-care approach to treatment (13[R]).

The general spectrum of ACE inhibitor side effects has been succinctly reviewed by Gavras and Gavras (14[R]) and by Weber (15[R]). A review of the use of ACE inhibitors in blacks concludes that the side effects profile is no different from that seen in Caucasians (16[R]).

Captopril *(SED-11, 403; SEDA-12, 172; SEDA-13, 174)*

Cardiovascular Four children are reported who had renal artery stenosis secondary to Takayasu's arteritis. When given captopril 0.5 mg/kg 3 out of 4 showed dramatic deterioration in renal function demonstrated by ^{99m}Tc-DTPA renograms. No further details are given (17[C]). Another 11-year-old child received captopril 50 mg t.d.s. following renal transplantation. After several days her creatinine level rose abruptly and then oscillated only to settle when captopril was stopped. The authors felt that this was due to a minor degree of *renal artery stenosis* which, in itself, was clinically insignificant (18[C]).

Nervous system Thirty-one male patients have been studied for *taste acuity* and plasma and urinary *zinc* concentrations (19[C]). Eleven were taking high doses of captopril (266 ± 34 mg/d), 6 had started captopril within the last 6 months (104 ± 40 mg/d) and 14 served as controls. The long-term group had significantly higher taste detection thresholds, lower zinc plasma concentrations and higher urinary zinc excretion than controls. The short-term group were found only to have higher taste thresholds in some modalities. It is difficult to be sure whether this relates more to dose or duration of treatment or to other co-medications such as diuretics. From this study it is also not clear whether there is any direct relationship between the taste abnormalities and the changes in zinc metabolism.

Respiratory *Cough* is a well-known side effect. If it is necessary to maintain captopril therapy, bupivacaine has been shown to afford temporary relief in a patient aged 73 with congestive cardiac failure (20[C]).

Metabolic A 34-year-old woman with severe hypertension and impaired renal function (creatinine clearance 40 ml/min) was treated with captopril 200 mg daily in addition to methyldopa and furosemide (21[C]). After 2 weeks the patient's serum potassium rose from 4.7 to 5.8 mEq/l and a normal anion gap metabolic acidosis was found. This resolved when captopril was stopped and recurred on rechallenge with captopril without any co-medications. The hyperkalemic acidosis was accompanied by a fall in plasma aldosterone and a rise in plasma renin activity and was reversed by the administration of fludrocortisone. Renal function remained constant throughout. The authors postulate that the acidosis may have been secondary to inappropriate urinary bicarbonate excretion and the *hyperkalemia* secondary to captopril-induced hypoaldosteronism.

Ten further patients with a similar syndrome are presented (22[C]). All were treated with unspecified ACE inhibitors and had renal insufficiency. Six had an associated metabolic acidosis. All were given heparin and became hyperkalemic, even though on ACE inhibitors alone they were normokalemic. It was postulated that the interaction between heparin and ACE inhibitors caused the hyperkalemia.

Urinary system In contrast to the hopeful reports of the beneficial effects of ACE inhibitors in renal parenchymal disease (11[R]) other reports suggest that this is not always the case. Ten patients with various glomerulopathies were given captopril 37.5 mg daily. In one *renal function* deteriorated quickly. In the other 9 proteinuria increased. This change was reversible (23[C]). In a 64-year-old man with diabetic nephropathy and renal artery stenosis, captopril caused a deterioration in renal function. It is not clear which renal pathology was the cause of this (24[C]).

Nine premature infants were treated with captopril 0.3 mg/kg for hypertension secondary to renal arterial or parenchymal disease (25[C]). Blood pressure proved difficult to control in this group with hypotension resistant to volume expansion and accompanied by oliguria occurring in 4 infants. In 3 other cases seizures secondary to hypotension occurred.

Skin and appendages Two further cases of *pemphigus* are described, one in a 51-year-old man taking 200 mg daily (26[C]) and the other in a 64-year-old woman with rheumatoid arthritis taking 37.5 mg daily (27[C]). Both cases were reversible when captopril was stopped. A 64-year-old woman was given captopril 75 mg daily and developed an *eczema* on light-exposed areas (28[C]). Subsequently she took a single 25 mg dose of captopril. This was followed by acute urticaria which resolved. The rash continued, becoming lichenified. Tests for porphyria and ANF titers were negative. Although captopril may have had a part to play in the etiology of this rash, the evidence is suggestive rather than conclusive. However, a mechanism has been proposed. Immune histological study of dermal filtrates from two chronic pemphigus and one lichenoid syndrome related to captopril showed the presence of a CD8 (T-suppressor) infiltrate (29[C]). The authors suggest that a T-cell cytotoxic reaction occurs in the epidermis which may be induced by a captopril-induced modification of keratinocytic antigens.

Endocrine A 34-year-old man with systemic lupus erythematosus was treated with captopril 75 mg daily for hypertension (30[C]). He also received prednisolone and cyclophosphamide. After 7 months of treatment, he developed painful left-sided *gynecomastia*. No hormonal or hepatic abnormalities were found. The symptoms and signs resolved when captopril was stopped.

Hematological An interesting in vitro study has been performed examining the cause of captopril-related *suppression of granulocytopoiesis* (31[C]). The results suggest that the active thiol group on the captopril molecule can interact with copper to generate hydrogen peroxide which may be toxic to neutrophil progenitor cells.

Enalapril *(SED-11, 405; SEDA-12, 174; SEDA-13, 176)*

Respiratory Five further cases of *cough* are reported (32[C]). Very few patient details are given, although the authors draw attention to the nocturnal nature of the complaint. They also point out that it may only occur after many months of treatment.

Gastrointestinal Enalapril (dose unspecified) was given to 4 very old patients in a clinical trial. All of these developed *abdominal pain* which was interpreted by the authors as mesenteric ischemia secondary to hypotension (33[C]). However, further details are not given.

A 60-year-old man was started on enalapril 5 mg daily. After the first dose he noted abdominal discomfort. After the second dose, persistent abdominal pain developed. Admitted to hospital, he was found to have a clinical and laboratory picture consistent with *acute pancreatitis*. This resolved and has not recurred. The authors believe it to be related to enalapril (34[C]).

Urinary system In 3 patients with severe heart failure high-dose enalapril caused severe hypotension with reversible *renal insufficiency* (35[C]). The cause for this seems to have been co-medication with diuretics in 2 patients and severe diarrhea in the 3rd. This last patient also became severely hyperkalemic (serum potassium 9.1 mmol/l) when co-medicated with spironolactone and potassium supplements. A similar case is described in a 72-year-old bronchitic patient also receiving enalapril and diuretics (36[C]).

Two further elderly patients are described who took enalapril and developed renal insufficiency (37[C]). Both were said to have small kidneys on ultrasound. It is difficult to know whether this implies bilateral renal artery stenosis as the authors suggest or bilateral chronic pyelonephritis since in one patient there was a definite history of analgesic abuse.

A 57-year-old diabetic patient, with normal renal function is described who was prescribed enalapril (dose not given). Eight months later his creatinine had risen 5-fold. This returned to normal when enalapril was stopped. Although his IVP was normal, a renal angiogram revealed a left *renal arterial stenosis* (24[C]).

The outcome of a large prescription event monitoring study has been published (38[C]). The case notes of 75 out of 913 patients were reviewed in detail because of a clinically significant *rise in creatinine* concentration associated with enalapril use. It was thought that enalapril might have contributed to the death of 10 of these patients. Factors which contributed to the majority of cases seemed to be heart failure (7/10), diuretics (9/10) and hyperkalemia (all). Three patients had severe diarrhea before developing renal failure. In all cases enalapril was withdrawn but without clinical improvement.

Hematological A 38-year-old man with end-stage renal failure received a living-related donor transplant (39[C]). After this, he became mildly polycythemic. At this stage he was treated with enalapril for hypertension. His creatinine concentration rose, but this was attributed to a mild episode of rejection. Meanwhile his hemoglobin concentration fell. Eventually, he was admitted to hospital after a severe diarrheal episode, hypokalemic and with a low hemoglobin and white cell count. Bone marrow biopsy revealed suppression. The *anemia* resolved when enalapril was stopped. The authors point out, however, that since the patient was also taking azathioprine at the time, it was not possible to attribute the bone marrow suppression to one drug or the other.

Hypersensitivity A review of data collected from complete adverse event recording in 3 studies of about 12 000 patients each suggests that *angioedema* occurs in about 1/3000 patients in the first week. After this the rate is about 1/42 000. Overall the incidence is about 0.1% of all patients treated. Most cases were mild and resolved when medication was discontinued (40[R]).

Lisinopril *(SEDA-12, 175; SEDA-13, 178)*

A number of large patient trials and evaluation of data from combined trials have been written up. Seven-hundred-and-fifty older (55 years or more) and 724 young (under 55 years) patients taking lisinopril alone were examined for their pattern of adverse events (41[R]). There were no substantial differences between the two age groups. The most frequent adverse events were *headache, dizziness, cough, diarrhea, nausea, fatigue* and *upper respiratory symptoms*. These occurred in 6% of patients or less. Symptomatic first-dose *hypotension* occurred in 0.7% of older patients and 1.5% of younger patients. Elevations of *serum creatinine* and *urea* were noted in 2.3% of patients or less.

This experience is borne out by a smaller study examining 97 older patients and 710 younger patients recruited to 4 multicenter trials (42[R]). Major differences between the two groups were not found. The most frequent adverse events were headache, cough, *rash*, fatigue, nausea, diarrhea and dizziness. These occurred in 8.3% of patients (headache in the older group) or less.

In a group of 130 patients with congestive heart failure most adverse events occurred with the same frequency in patients taking lisinopril or placebo (43[C]). Only dizziness and headache occurred more frequently with lisinopril.

In another study of 55 patients with heart failure, taking lisinopril 2.5–10 mg daily, the main most frequent adverse events were diarrhea, *asthenia*, fatigue, dizziness and *dyspnea*. Various other *gastrointestinal* complaints, headaches, rash and cough were also noted. Clinically significant rises in *blood urea nitrogen* and creatinine occurred in 26 and 21% of the patients, respectively (45[C]).

When given to 26 patients with hypertension and renal impairment, lisinopril was generally well tolerated (45[C]). One patient was withdrawn because of nausea and vomiting secondary to *reflex esophagitis*. A 2nd developed *angioneurotic edema*. Interestingly, this was treated with antihistamines and the patient was able to continue lisinopril. A 3rd patient reported a metallic taste in the mouth which resolved spontaneously. Other symptoms reported were mild and non-specific.

Cilazapril *(SEDA-12, 175)*

Thirty patients received cilazapril 2.5 or 5 mg, with or without hydrochlorothiazide (46[C]). Eleven developed a dry *cough* which could have started anywhere between 1 week and 13 months after starting cilazapril. These patients were investigated for other causes of cough, but none was found. This incidence of cough looks high by comparison with other ACE inhibitors. Publication of further data in a greater number of patients will doubtless set this problem into a wider perspective.

DRUGS ACTING ON THE SYMPATHETIC NERVOUS SYSTEM *(SED-11, 405; SEDA-12, 175; SEDA-13, 179)*

DRUGS INTERFERING WITH NEURO-TRANSMITTERS (SEDA-12, 176; SEDA-13, 179)

Methyldopa *(SED-11, 405; SEDA-12, 176; SEDA-13, 179)*

Cardiovascular A 22-year-old primigravida, 26 weeks pregnant, was admitted to hospital for treatment of hypertension, presumably pre-eclamptic in origin (47[C]). She was treated with atenolol and methyldopa without success and delivery was accordingly induced. Post partum she was well controlled with atenolol and methyldopa, so the latter was suspended. Her blood pressure immediately rose to 210/170 mmHg, she became drowsy and had 2 grand mal convulsions and her optic disc margins were blurred. A CT scan was normal, apart from an appearance consistent with cerebral edema. Her blood pressure was once more controlled, first with nitroprusside and then with methyldopa and atenolol. A few days later, she was successfully weaned off all antihypertensive agents and has remained normotensive. The authors have suggested that she suffered *rebound hypertension* as a result of methyldopa withdrawal in the presence of atenolol. While this may be so, one is also tempted to wonder how much the pre-eclampsia, if this is the right diagnosis, may have contributed to the severity of her response.

Gastrointestinal A 63-year-old woman was given methyldopa 250 mg bd. Two weeks later she experienced diarrhea, vomiting, undulating fever, chills and headaches. On examination, she was mildly pyrexic and had generalized abdominal tenderness. Extensive testing revealed only air scattered through the gastrointestinal tract, an eosinophilia and a mild elevation of alkaline phosphatase. Her methyldopa, as it so happened, was withheld because of transient hypotension and she promptly recovered. Rechallenge led to a recurrence of the symptoms (48[C]).

In another case a 64-year-old woman was admitted to hospital with a 3-month history of malaise, weakness and dyspepsia. She had been treated with methyldopa 500 mg daily for 5 years. She was pale and mildly jaundiced. Her hemoglobin was 8.1 g/100 ml and her reticulocyte count was 35.5%. Her direct antiglobulin test was positive. At gastroscopy, gastric biopsies were taken which revealed the presence of *chronic atrophic gastritis* in the antrum. Her blood was found to contain antiparietal cell antibodies. All symptoms and signs normalized when methyldopa was withdrawn (49[C]).

Hematological A 75-year-old man was treated with methyldopa 500 mg daily. Three months later he was found to have a hemoglobin of 6.2 g/100 ml. There was no evidence of hemolysis or Coombs positivity. Other formed elements in the blood and bone marrow were unaffected, but erythroid precursors were absent. In vitro tests suggested that methyldopa suppressed these erythoid percursors directly. The patient recovered rapidly once methyldopa was withdrawn (50[C]).

A 70-year-old woman who had been taking methyldopa and glibenclamide was admitted to hospital for treatment of a stroke. She was also found to have a platelet count of 40–45000/mm^3. Her antinuclear antibody was positive 1:640, but other titers were normal. When methyldopa was stopped her platelet count rose to normal and her antinuclear antibody titer fell (51[C]).

Reserpine

A 51-year-old hypertensive man was treated with reserpine 0.25 mg daily on which he did well clinically. When his cerebral blood flow was estimated using a xenon inhalation method, it was said to be lower than normal. This returned to normal when the drug was withdrawn (52[C]).

PRESYNAPTIC α-ADRENOCEPTOR AGONISTS (SED-11, 408; SEDA-12, 175; SEDA-13, 179)

Clonidine *(SED-11, 408; SEDA-12, 175; SEDA-13, 179)*

A 57-year-old black male was switched abruptly from oral clonidine 0.3 mg b.d. on which he was well controlled to transdermal clonidine. Six days later he was found to be severely hypertensive. Reinstatement or oral clonidine controlled his blood pressure. Whether this represents a true rebound or a return to his previous hypertensive state is a little difficult to evaluate from the information given (53[C]).

Tolerance to long-term transdermal clonidine was assessed in 23 patients (54[C]). Ten were obliged to give up transdermal therapy because of skin reactions. In 5 of these who consented to be tested further, this seemed to be due to a direct *allergic reaction* to clonidine itself.

Guanabenz *(SED-11, 410)*

An 87-year-old woman was admitted for investigation of syncopal episodes. She was being treated with digoxin 0.125 mg daily, indometacin, potassium chloride, chlorpropamide, furosemide and guanabenz 8 mg daily. Her ECG showed a bradycardia of 46 bpm and first-degree heart block. Serum digoxin and thyroid function tests were unremarkable. Challenge with guanabenz markedly prolonged the PR interval (840 ms) and subsequently paroxysmal second-degree heart block and Wenckebach phenomenon were noted with ventricular rates less than 40. Electrophysiological studies in the presence of guanabenz increased the sinus cycle length by 50% and sinus node recovery time by 42%. AV block occurred proximal to the His bundle and His-ventricular conduction time was prolonged by 42%. The authors suggest that guanabenz may have unmasked a latent sick sinus syndrome (55[C]).

POSTSYNAPTIC α-ADRENOCEPTOR ANTAGONISTS (SED-11, 407; SEDA-12, 177; SEDA-13, 179)

Alfuzosin

Alfuzosin was given to 12 hypertensive patients for 28 days. The only adverse events noted were complaints of *palpitations* (56[C]).

Prazosin *(SED-11, 407; SEDA-12, 177; SEDA-13, 179)*

Four patients suffering from narcolepsy are briefly described, all of whom were taking prazosin. All improved when prazosin was withdrawn. Two worsened on rechallenge with prazosin (57[C]).

The Australian Drug Reaction Committee reported its experience with prazosin as a cause of *urinary incontinence* between 1978 and 1986. There were 56 documented reports in all of which the symptom was cured by withdrawal of the drug. The daily dose was 0.5–15 mg/d (58[C]).

DIRECT VASODILATORS *(SED-11, 398; SEDA-12, 178; SEDA-13, 180)*

Diazoxide *(SED-11, 401)*

A neonate was treated with diazoxide 6 mg/kg/d for hypoglycemia. After 3 weeks *hypertrichosis* was noted on most parts of his body. This regressed slowly when the drug was stopped (59[C]).

Dihydralazine

Three elderly patients are described all of whom were given dihydralazine for their hypertension (60[C]). All developed *hepatic necrosis* which was fatal.

Hydralazine *(SED-11, 398; SEDA-12, 178; SEDA-13, 180)*

A 73-year-old woman was treated for hypertension with a beta-blocker to which hydralazine 25 mg b.d. was added. She then developed arthritis, a low-grade fever, a papular rash on her legs, a right pleural rub and anemia with an ESR of 70 mm/h. In hospital, she developed hoarseness and acute stridor which was found to be due to bilateral vocal cord palsies which led to a respiratory arrest. This was treated with a tracheotomy, steroids and withdrawal of hydralazine and has not recurred. Her antinuclear factor titer was 1/10, 240 for both IgM and IgG (61[C]).

A 60-year-old man who was a slow acetylator was treated with hydralazine 50 mg t.d.s. for 4 years (62[C]). This was stopped after he developed arthralgia. He subsequently presented with a dry mouth and eye discomfort. Parotid salivary flow was found to be diminished as was lacrimal flow. His antinuclear factor was positive (1/1000). He was treated symptomatically and the syndrome resolved spontaneously.

Minoxidil *(SED-11, 400; SEDA-12, 178)*

A 54-year-old man presented with a fungating lesion on the left arm. Incidentally he was noted to have an extensive weeping erythematous *rash* which had started as papules on the right foot about $2^1/_2$ months earlier. He was being treated with metoprolol, nifedipine, furosemide and minoxidil. His serum sodium was 127 mEq/l. Minoxidil and metoprolol were stopped and he was treated with diphenhydramine, fluocinolone acetate and occlusive dressings. The rash resolved over the next 3 days. The patient was inadvertently re-exposed to minoxidil for 2 doses and the rash recurred. Antinuclear and anti-DNA antibody titers remained normal throughout (63[C]).

POTASSIUM CHANNEL ACTIVATORS

Pinacidil *(SEDA-12, 179)*

Pinacidil is a powerful vasodilator. In an overview of its clinical pharmacology, the main side effects were said to be characteristic of this class of compounds. Dose-related *edema, tachycardia, palpitations, headache, hypertrichosis* and transient *T-wave ECG changes* were noted which seemed to have had no clinical sequelae (64[R]).

In a pharmacokinetic study carried out in 8 healthy volunteers (66[c]) 6 complained of *headache*. Other symptoms included *tiredness* (4 cases), palpitations (2 cases) *diarrhea* (1 case) and *vomiting* (1 case).

In a study comparing pinacidil 12.5–75 mg b.d. and prazosin ($n = 197$ and 204, respectively), substantial adverse reaction rates were obtained. Tachycardia occurred in 15–20% of both groups and palpitation in 13–15% of both groups. Edema occurred in 38.2% of patients taking pinacidil (prazosin 22.3%). *Postural hypotension* occurred in 4.7% of patients taking pinacidil and *asthenia* in 20.2%. Clearly pinacidil needs to be used carefully if it is to be successful (66[C]).

REFERENCES

1. Weinberger MH (1988) Cardiovascular risk factors and antihypertensive therapy. *Am. J. Med., 84, Suppl. 4A*, 24.
2. Stark RM (1988) The atherogenic risk of antihypertensive therapy. *Am. J. Med., 84, Suppl. 1B*, 86.
3. Howes LG, Louis WJ (1988) Effects of antihypertensive drugs on cardiovascular risk factors. *Clin. Exp. Pharmacol. Physiol., 15*, 199.
4. Bulpitt CJ, Fletcher AE (1988) Importance of well-being to hypertensive patients. *Am. J. Med., 84, Suppl. 1B*, 40.
5. Curb JD, Schneider K, Taylor JO et al (1988) Antihypertensive drug side effects in the hypertension detection and follow up program. *Hypertension, 11, Suppl. II*, II-51.
6. Bansal S (1988) Sexual dysfunction in hypertensive men: a critical review of the literature. *Hypertension, 12*, 1.
7. Solez K, Racusen LC, Keown PA et al (1988) The influence of antihypertensive drug therapy on renal transplant function and outcome. *Transplant. Proc., 20*, 618.
8. Stumpf JL (1988) Drug therapy of hypertensive crises. *Clin. Pharm., 7*, 582.
9. Wurzelman J, Frishman WH, Aronson M et al (1987) Neuropsychological effects of antihypertensive drugs. *Cardiol. Clin., 5*, 689.
10. Ryden L (1988) When and how to use angiotensin-converting enzyme inhibition in congestive heart failure. *Am. J. Cardiol., 62*, 75A.
11. Gans ROB, Hoorntje SJ, Donker AJM (1988) Renal effects of angiotensin-I converting enzyme inhibitors. *Neth. J. Med., 32*, 247.
12. Schoenberger JA (1988) Emerging benefits of angiotensin converting enzyme inhibitors versus other antihypertensive agents. *Am. J. Med., 84, Suppl. 4A*, 30.
13. Brunner HR, Waeber B, Nussberger J (1987)

Treatment of hypertension with ACE inhibitors as first step: pharmacologic and clinical considerations. *J. Cardiovasc. Pharmacol., 10, Suppl. 7*, S36.
14. Gavras H, Gavras I (1988) Angiotensin converting enzyme inhibitors: properties and side effects. *Hypertension, 11, Suppl. II*, II-37.
15. Weber MA (1988) Safety issues during antihypertensive treatment with angiotensin converting enzyme inhibitors. *Am. J. Med., 84, Suppl. 4A*, 16.
16. Shulman NB (1988) Treatment of hypertension in black patients with angiotensin-converting enzyme inhibitors. *J. Natl. Med. Assoc., 80*, 265.
17. Saieh C, Amaral H, Morales B (1988) Effect of captopril in Takayasu's arteritis. *Pediatr. Nephrol., 2*, 375.
18. Ogborn MR, Crocker JFS (1988) Captopril and transplant renal artery stenosis. *Nephron, 48*, 333.
19. Abu-Hamdan DK, Desai H, Sondheimer J et al (1988) Taste acuity and zinc metabolism in captopril-treated hypertensive male patients. *Am. J. Hypertens., 1*, 303S.
20. Brown RC, Turton CWG (1988) Cough and angiotensin converting enzyme inhibition. *Br. Med. J., 296*, 1741.
21. Sakemi T, Ohchi N, Sanai T et al (1988) Captopril-induced metabolic acidosis with hyperkalemia. *Am. J. Nephrol., 8*, 245.
22. Durand D, Ader J-L, Rey J-P et al (1988) Inducing hyperkalemia by converting enzyme inhibitors and heparin. *Kidney Int., 34, Suppl. 25*, S-196.
23. Traindl O, Pohanka E, Kovarik J (1988) Progression of chronic renal failure. *Lancet, 2*, 962.
24. Webster J, Murchison LE, Robb OJ (1988) Angiotensin converting enzyme inhibitors may cause renal impairment in diabetes mellitus. *Scott. Med. J., 33*, 247.
25. Tack ED, Perlman JM (1988) Renal failure in sick hypertensive premature infants receiving captopril therapy. *J. Paediatr., 112*, 805.
26. Dashore A, Choudhary SD (1987) Captopril induced pemphigus vulgaris. *Indian J. Dermatol. Venereol. Leprol., 53*, 293.
27. Blanken R, Doeglas MG, De Jong MCJM (1988) Pemphigus-like eruption induced by d-penicillamine and captopril in the same patient. *Acta Derm. Venereol. (Stockh.), 68*, 456.
28. Mauduit G, Granier F, Antoniotti O, Thivolet J (1988) Photosensibilisation après traitment au captopril. *Ann. Dermatol. Vénéréol., 115*, 167.
29. Bretin N, Dreno B, Bureau B, Litoux P (1988) Immunohistological study of captopril-induced late cutaneous eruptions. *Dermatologica, 177*, 11.
30. Markusse HM, Meyboom RHB (1988) Gynaecomastia associated with captopril. *Br. Med. J., 296*, 1262.
31. Hammond WP, Miller JE, Starkebaum G et al (1988) Suppression of in vitro granulocytopoiesis by captopril and penicillamine. *Exp. Haematol., 16*, 674.
32. De Groote P, Millaire A, Aisenfarb JC et al (1988) Toux et inhibiteurs de l'enzyme de conversion de l'angiotensine. *Ann. Cardiol. Angiol., 37*, 251.
33. O'Neill CJA, Bowes SG, Sullens CM et al (1988) Evaluation of the safety of enalapril in the treatment of heart failure in the very old. *Eur. J. Clin. Pharmacol., 35*, 143.
34. Tilkemeier P, Thompson PD (1988) Acute pancreatitis possibly related to enalapril. *N. Engl. J. Med., 318*, 1275.
35. Wieland T, Stäubli M (1988) Schwerwiegende Komplikationen unter Enalapril-Therapie wegen Herzinsuffizienz. *Schweiz. Med. Wochenschr., 118*, 1789.
36. Corsi A, Tasso A, Corsi G (1988) Insufficienza renale acuta de enalapril: considerazioni a proposito di un caso di osservazione personale. *Gaz. Med. Ital., 147*, 193.
37. O'Donnell D (1988) Renal failure due to enalapril and captopril in bilateral renal artery stenosis: greater awareness needed. *Med. J. Austr., 148*, 525.
38. Speirs CJ, Dollery CT, Inman WHW et al (1988) Postmarketing surveillance of enalapril. II. Investigation of the potential role of enalapril in deaths with renal failure. *Br. Med. J., 297*, 830.
39. Loftus WK, Levine F, Mathew TH (1988) Enalapril and anaemia. *Med. J. Austr., 148*, 209.
40. Slater EE, Merrill DD, Guess HA et al (1988) Clinical profile of angioedema associated with angiotensin converting-enzyme inhibition. *J. Am. Med. Assoc., 260*, 967.
41. Rush JE, Lyle PA (1988) Safety and tolerability of lisinopril in older hypertensive patients. *Am. J. Med., 85, Suppl. 3B*, 55.
42. Gomez HJ, Smith SG, Moncloa F (1988) Efficacy and safety of lisinopril in older patients with essential hypertension. *Am. J. Med., 85, Suppl. 3B*, 35.
43. Lewis GRJ (1988) Lisinopril versus placebo in older congestive heart failure patients. *Am. J. Med., 85, Suppl. 3B*, 48.
44. Uretsky BF, Shaver JA, Liang C-S et al (1988) Modulation of hemodynamic effects with a converting enzyme inhibitor: acute hemodynamic dose–response relationship of a new angiotensin converting enzyme inhibitor, lisinopril, with observations on long-term clinical, functional, and biochemical responses. *Am. Heart J., 116*, 480.
45. Donohoe JF, Kelly J, Laher MS, Doyle GD (1988) Lisinopril in the treatment of hypertensive patients with renal impairment. *Am. J. Med., 85, Suppl. 3B*, 31.
46. Lernhardt GB, Zeigler MG (1988) Cough caused by cilazapril. *Am. J. Med. Sci., 296*, 119.
47. Al-Ruhaimi MN, Muscat-Baron JM (1988) Rebound hypertension after sudden methyldopa withdrawal. *Emirates Med. J., 6*, 180.
48. Young BA, Girotti MJ (1988) Methyldopa hy-

persensitivity can mimic acute toxic enterocolitis. *Can. J. Surg.*, *31*, 165.
49. Giardina MG, Matarazzo M, Varriale A, Cacciatore L (1988) Concurrent autoimmune haemolytic anaemia and chronic atrophic gastritis in a patient under methyldopa treatment. *Ital. J. Gastroenterol.*, *20*, 151.
50. Itoh K, Wong P, Asai T et al (1988) Pure red cell aplasia induced by alpha methyldopa. *Am. J. Med.*, *84*, 1088.
51. Pai RG, Pai SM (1988) Methyldopa induced reversible immune thrombocytopenia. *Am. J. Med.*, *85*, 123.
52. Nobili F, Marenco S, Rodriguez G et al (1988) Cerebral blood flow recovery after reserpine withdrawal. *Ital. J. Neurol. Sci.*, *9*, 403.
53. Stewart M, Burris JF (1988) Rebound hypertension during initiation of transdermal clonidine. *Drug Intell. Clin. Pharm.*, *22*, 573.
54. Horning JR, Zawada ET, Simmons JL et al (1988) Efficacy and safety of two-year therapy with transdermal clonidine for essential hypertension. *Chest*, *93*, 941.
55. La Russo P, Jessup SA, Rogers FJ, Rogers JC (1988) Sinoatrial and atrioventricular dysfunction associated with the use of guanabenz acetate. *Can. J. Cardiol.*, *4*, 146.
56. Leto di Priolo S, Priore P, Cocco G et al (1988) Dose–titration study of alfuzosin, a new alpha$_1$-adrenoceptor blocker, in essential hypertension. *Eur. J. Clin. Pharmacol.*, *35*, 25.
57. Guilleminault C, Mignot E, Aldrich M et al (1988) Prazosin contraindicated in patients with narcolepsy. *Lancet*, *2*, 511.
58. Mathew TH, McEwen J, Rohan A (1988) Urinary incontinence secondary to prazosin. *Med. J. Austr.*, *148*, 305.
59. Prigent F, Gantzer A, Romain O et al (1988) Hypertrichose diffuse acquise au cours d'un traitement par diazoxide chez un nouveau-né. *Ann. Dermatol. Vénéréol.*, *115*, 191.
60. Machnik G, Bergert A, Justus J et al (1988) Arzneimittelhepatitis nach Dihydralazin mit tödlichem Verlauf. *Zentralbl. Allg. Pathol. Pathol. Anat.*, *134*, 167.
61. Chong WK, Dewhurst AG, Dathan JRE (1988) Acute laryngeal stridor with respiratory arrest in drug induced systemic lupus erythematosus. *Br. Med. J.*, *297*, 660.
62. Darwaza A, Lamey PJ, Connell JMC (1988) Hydrallazine induced Sjögren's syndrome. *Int. J. Oral Maxillofac. Surg.*, *17*, 92.
63. Ackerman BH, Townsend ME, Golden W, Bryan AB (1988) Pruritic rash with actinic keratosis and impending exfoliation, in a patient with hypertension managed with minoxidil. *Drug Intell. Clin. Pharm.*, *22*, 702.
64. Goldberg MR (1988) Clinical pharmacology of pinacidil, a prototype for drugs that affect potassium channels. *J. Cardiovasc. Pharmacol.*, *12, Suppl. 2*, S41.
65. McBurney A, Henry JA, Ward JW (1988) Accumulation of pinacidil *N*-oxide during chronic treatment with pinacidil. *Eur. J. Clin. Pharmacol.*, *35*, 93.
66. Goldberg MR, Sushak CS, Rockhold FW, Thompson WL (1988) Vasodilator monotherapy in the treatment of hypertension: comparative efficacy and safety of pinacidil, a potassium channel opener, and prazosin. *Clin. Pharmacol. Ther.*, *44*, 78.

Gordon T. McInnes

22 Diuretic drugs

GENERAL

Although no substantial new evidence has become available in the last year, the failure of diuretics to reduce cardiac morbidity and mortality in long-term trials in hypertension continues to fuel speculation that their metabolic effects may be detrimental (1[r], 2[R], 3[r], 4[R]–6[R]). Despite the lack of adequate support (SEDA-13, 184), links are postulated between disturbances of potassium and magnesium metabolism, ventricular ectopy and sudden death particularly in those with ECG abnormalities (3[r], 5[R], 6[R]), and between changes in lipids, uric acid and carbohydrate handling and enhanced development and progression of coronary heart disease (1[r], 3[r], 4[R]–6[R]). It is argued that the metabolic effects of diuretics may offset, negate or even reverse the benefit offered by successful blood pressure control (4[R]). The lack of a primary protective effect of other forms of antihypertensive therapy with dissimilar metabolic consequences is conveniently ignored (SEDA-11, 194). These authors also emphasize the probably exaggerated symptomatic side effects of the thiazide diuretics (SEDA-11, 197). Warnings are gradually becoming more muted, but there remains a note of caution about the use of diuretics as monotherapy (1[r], 3[r], 5[R]).

As emphasized previously (SED-11, 421; SEDA-13, 184), there is no good evidence that diuretic-induced hypokalemia or magnesium loss leads to significant arrhythmias in uncomplicated hypertensive patients (2[R], 7[r]). None of the long-term clinical trials has demonstrated an increase of serum cholesterol with diuretics although the lipid-lowering effects of diet may be blunted (7[r]). It is impossible to be definitive about whether the metabolic effects are detrimental and, if so, to what extent (8[r]). The long-term benefits of antihypertensive treatment with diuretics probably override potential negative metabolic effects (9[C]) and these drugs should not be abandoned unless more definitive outcome data demonstrate that other agents are clearly superior (8[r]). Since no new large-scale outcome studies will be reported in the near future, this is a reasonable position. However, to minimize biochemical changes doses should be kept as low as compatible with the desired antihypertensive effect (2[R], 7[r], 8[r]).

METABOLIC EFFECTS

Potassium metabolism *(SED-11, 421; SEDA-13, 184)* Walters and Barnes (10[C]) surveyed 1243 plasma samples from general practitioners and found potassium concentrations less than 3.6 mmol/l in 14% (3.0 mmol/l or less in 2.4%). Diuretics were being taken by 54% of those with low plasma potassium concentrations usually (62%) for the treatment of hypertension. In two surveys of attenders at blood pressure clinics (11[C], 12[Cr]), hypokalemia was more common in female and black patients. For black females, the odds ratios were 1.8 compared to white females, 10.8 compared to black males and 29.5 compared to white males (11[C]). There was no correlation between hypokalemia and symptoms (12[Cr]) or ventricular ectopy (12[Cr], 13[C]) even in those with ECG abnormalities prior to therapy (SEDA-13, 184).

As discussed previously (SEDA-9, 205), prior treatment with a thiazide or furosemide potentiates the hypokalemic effects of inhaled salbutamol or infused adrenaline (14[C], 15[C]); spironolactone has no such effect (15[C]). Although in elderly diuretic-treated patients with heart failure, concomitant β-adrenoceptor agonists did not significantly influence mean plasma potassium, withdrawals due to hypokalemia were more common in those taking β-adrenoceptor agonists (16[C]). The clinical significance of these findings is uncertain, but the risk of diuretic-induced hypokalemia appears to be increased during chronic β-adrenoceptor

Side Effects of Drugs Annual 14
M.N.G. Dukes and L. Beeley, editors

stimulation and the severity of hypokalemia during short-term rises in plasma adrenaline (such as after myocardial infarction) may be enchanced by chronic diuretic treatment.

The effect of diuretics on plasma potassium concentration is dose-related (12[C], 17[C], 18[C]), but blood pressure reduction is not closely related to dose (13[C], 17[C], 18[C]). Comparing cyclopenthiazide 125 and 500 μg daily, McVeigh et al (17[C]) observed similar antihypertensive effects but a much lesser hypokalemic effect (0.2 vs. 0.6 mmol/l) at the lower dose. Ziegler et al (18[C]) found no difference in blood pressure at daily doses, between 6.25 and 50 mg daily of hydrochlorothiazide. Chlortalidone 50 mg every 2nd day adequately controlled blood pressure in 62.5% patients with mild to moderate hypertension, but fall in plasma potassium was modest and no patient developed levels less than 3.0 mmol/l (13[C]). Thus, low-dose thiazide diuretic treatment regimens are effective and have only minor effects on potassium metabolism.

Potassium-sparing agents are effective in preventing or correcting thiazide-induced hypokalemia (9[C], 16[C]) and spironolactone-containing preparations appear to be the most satisfactory in maintaining plasma potassium concentrations (16[C]). However, during long-term therapy, potassium levels may not be maintained (16[C], 19[c]). In a comparison of amiloride, spironolactone and triamterene in combination with equivalent thiazide doses in elderly patients with heart failure (16[C]), plasma potassium concentrations fell progressively over 3 years. The eventual fall (0.5 mmol/l) was similar to that seen with a thiazide alone (SEDA-11, 193). Although the efficacy of amiloride may decline in the long-term (SEDA-11, 194), it is unclear to what extent the reported changes (16[C]) may reflect fluctuations in cardiac function.

Potassium supplements have little influence on serum potassium concentrations (SEDA-9, 206; SEDA-10, 187; SEDA-11, 195; SEDA-12, 182), but there continues to be speculation that such treatment may enhance the antihypertensive effect of thiazides (SEDA-10, 186). In an uncontrolled study of 24 black hypertensive patients taking bendrofluazide 10 mg daily, 48 mmol potassium chloride (Slow K) daily resulted in a significant fall in blood pressure (20[C]). The reduction was attributed to a decrease in intracellular sodium concentration, but the unsatisfactory study design precludes any valid conclusions. There remains no support for the use of potassium supplements in diuretic-treated patients.

Hyperkalemia is a much more serious complication than diuretic-induced hypokalemia (SEDA-9, 206). Although hyperkalemia is rare in elderly outpatients treated with diuretics and potassium-sparing agents (16[C]), a prospective study of hospital patients revealed a high incidence of serum potassium concentrations of at least 5.5 mmol/l especially in elderly patients treated with potassium supplements and potassium sparers in the presence of moderate renal impairment (21[Cr]). Durakovic et al (22[C]) and Rado (23[Cr]) have each reported extreme hyperkalemia in an elderly male with impaired renal function treated with a potassium sparer (amiloride + potassium chloride and spironolactone, respectively). These cases illustrate the risks of potassium-sparing agents and potassium salts in the elderly. Such agents should not be prescribed in combination to outpatients and should be used with caution in the face of significant impairment of renal function which can be difficult to assess in the elderly (SEDA-9, 206).

Magnesium metabolism *(SED-11, 422; SEDA-13, 185)* Reviewing the role of magnesium in hypertension, Wester and Dyckner (24[R]) reach several controversial conclusions: diuretic-induced electrolyte disturbances can interfere with the efficacy of antihypertensive drugs; extracellular and intracellular electrolyte disturbances are not corrected by potassium supplements alone but are improved when magnesium supplements are added; double correction probably restores antihypertensive responsiveness to diuretics better than provision of potassium alone; correction of diuretic-induced electrolyte disturbances by magnesium supplements may also prevent arrhythmias due to diuretic-induced magnesium depletion. The inadequacy of their database has been criticised previously (SEDA-10, 187; SEDA-13, 185). In well-conducted studies, repeated doses of thiazides, furosemide and spironolactone have no effect on plasma magnesium concentrations (14[C], 15[C], 17[C]). Thus, it remains uncertain that diuretics cause any important perturbation of magnesium metabolism.

Severe hyponatremia *(SED-11, 42; SEDA-12, 183; SEDA-13, 186)* Combined treatment with a thiazide diuretic and amiloride causes a modest mean reduction in serum sodium concentration (19[c]), but severe hyponatremia continues to be seen. Friedman et al (25[Cr]) compared 11 elderly patients with hyponatremia (serum sodium less than 130 mmol/l) after hydrochlorothiazide 50 mg + amiloride 5 mg (Moduretic) with 11 elderly patients previously treated uneventfully and 10 healthy volunteers. Each was challenged with a single dose of Moduretic. The previously hyponatremic patients responded with falls in serum sodium and osmolality significantly greater than in control subjects while body weight increased in susceptible patients and decreased in the others. No differences between the groups were seen in urine sodium, potassium or osmolality, free water clearance or circulating antidiuretic hormone (ADH). The authors conclude that polydipsia as reflected by increased body weight may play a major role in the development of severe hyponatremia, and that a single dose challenge may be predictive. It is doubtful whether the control groups were sufficient to allow such conclusions and Sonneblink et al (26[C]) have presented anecdotal evidence that inappropriate ADH activity induced by thiazides causes dilution of serum sodium concentrations. The mechanism underlying this problem remains unresolved.

Central pontine myelinolysis (CPM) has been reported in patients dying after diuretic-induced hyponatremia (SEDA-11, 195; SEDA-13, 186). Despite lack of evidence, the notion that uncorrected hyponatremia itself can lead to CPM persists (SEDA-11, 195). In a comprehensive review, Laureno and Karp (27[R]) conclude that CPM occurs in diuretic-induced hyponatremia only if there is rapid correction and that it is induced neither by hyponatremia nor overcorrection. Hyponatremia causes a generalized metabolic encephalopathy, usually if serum sodium drops precipitously to levels less than 125 mmol/l, but no specific neuropathological lesion is seen. It is usually reversible if sodium deficiency is corrected, but how rapid a rise in serum sodium is safe? In the absence of convulsions, conservative measures (discontinuation of diuretic and water restriction) suffices. If the patient convulses, hypertonic saline should be administered very slowly to allow an increase in serum sodium of no more than 12 mmol/l in the first 24 hours and thereafter even more slowly. Marked interindividual variability in response necessitates frequent monitoring.

Serum lipids *(SED-11, 420; SEDA-12, 183; SEDA-13, 186)* Although several authors appear convinced of the atherogenic influence of diuretics on serum lipids (1[r], 3[r], 4[R]–6[R]), the evidence for a major impact on these biochemical variables remains unconvincing. In a double-blind, placebo-controlled, randomized study of 3 doses of cyclopenthiazide (50–500 μg daily) for 8 weeks, McVeigh et al (28[Cr]) detected no changes in indices of lipid metabolism. Likewise, Salvadeo et al (19[c]) reported that hydrochlorothiazide 25 mg daily for 12 months induced no significant changes in serum cholesterol or triglycerides. Williams et al (29[C]) found no consistent influence of angiotensin converting-enzyme (ACE) inhibitors on lipid responses to hydrochlorothiazide. Indeed, changes after the thiazide showed considerable variability. This study demonstrated many of the confounding factors in evaluating drug effects on lipids: age, baseline fluctuation, small population size and the phenomenon at regression to the mean. In their study of the effects of thiazides, potassium-sparing diuretics and spironolactone, Jeunemaitre et al (9[C]) found that variability in serum cholesterol concentrations during treatment was mainly due to regression to the mean. Reports of diuretic-induced changes in serum lipids and any extrapolation to the pathogenesis of arteriosclerosis must be interpreted cautiously.

Glucose tolerance *(SED-11, 419; SEDA-12, 183; SEDA-13, 187)* Despite the known hyperglycemic tendency of thiazides, the Working Group on Hypertension in Diabetes (30[r]) recommends a thiazide-based, stepped-care approach to drug treatment. However, Kaplan et al (31[r]) and Bell (32[r]) suggest that diuretic use should be limited and other therapeutic regimens adopted especially if there is concomitant hypercholesterolemia.

The hyperglycemic response to diuretics is dose-related and low doses reduce blood pressure with little if any alteration in carbohydrate metabolism in the short term (13[C], 18[C], 19[C], 28[Cr]). In a large study of patients treated with low doses of spironolactone, or thiazides in combination with amiloride or triamterene over 20 months (9[C]), only non-significant changes in fasting blood sugar were observed, suggesting that reduction in blood pressure can be achieved without alteration of carbohydrate metabolism even in the long-term. Furthermore, as with cholesterol, changes in blood sugar were mainly due to regression to the mean: increases were seen only in those with low initial values. Thus concerns about the risk to those with hyperglycemia and hypercholesterolemia before treatment may have been exaggerated.

The hyperglycemic action of diuretics may be attributable to the effect of hypokalemia (SEDA-9, 206; SEDA-10, 191; SEDA-12, 183) or a direct effect of the diuretic on insulin-producing cells in the islets of Langerhans (32[r]). Potassium-sparing diuretics may correct hyperglycemia by virtue of their action on potassium metabolism. Some support for this came from the study of Jeunemaitre et al (9[C]) who observed a significantly different blood sugar response (a rise) in those where plasma potassium fell compared to (a fall) in those where plasma potassium increased.

There has been speculation that bumetanide may differ from furosemide in its lack of effect on carbohydrate metabolism (SEDA-9, 209). In mice, bumetanide causes acute and transient hyperglycemia possibly due to reduction in capacity to secrete insulin (33). Thus, bumetanide appears to differ little from furosemide in this respect. These findings require confirmation in man in direct comparison with furosemide at therapeutically equivalent doses.

Hyperuricemia and gout *(SED-11, 420)* In a survey of serum uric acid concentrations in an elderly rural population in Finland (34[C]), hyperuricemia was linked strongly to diuretic use. Compared to a similar survey 11 years earlier, the incidence was increased and this change was attributed to widespread use of diuretics during the intervening period.

Although a dose–response relation has been questioned (SEDA-13, 187), recent well-conducted studies have demonstrated that diuretic-induced changes in serum uric acid are dose-related (17[C], 18[C]). In low-dose regimens, as currently recommended, alterations are minor (13[C], 17[C], 18[C], 19[c]) and the risk of gout would appear to be slight.

Calcium metabolism *(SED-11, 422)* Thiazide treatment might prevent osteoporosis and bone fracture by inducing a positive calcium balance (SEDA-9, 207) although this postulate has been disputed (SEDA-11, 197). In a population-based case-control study of 905 Saskatchewan residents over 65 years (35[Cr]), relative risk of hip fracture dropped from 1.2 for less than 2 years use to 0.5 with prolonged use of 6 years or more when compared with a random sample of 5137 age- and sex-matched controls not taking drugs known to affect bone mass. If it is confirmed that diuretics can retard age-related bone loss, the clinical and public health consequences will be of considerable significance because of the serious physical, social and economic cost of hip and other osteoporotic fractures and the lack of proven therapy for osteoporosis in the elderly.

SPECIAL PROBLEMS

Skin reactions Furosemide has been associated with allergic vasculitis and bullous hemorrhagic eruptions (SED-11, 427). Lin (36[Cr]) describes an unusual presentation of furosemide-associated hypersensitivity angiitis.

A diffuse purpuric maculopapular eruption developed acutely over trunk, arms and legs of a 75-year-old man. It diminished gradually when furosemide was discontinued only to recur with fever and malaise when the drug was reintroduced. Histology revealed a leukocytoclastic angiitis. Other findings included tongue ulceration; anemia, leukocytosis and thrombocytopenia; elevated serum creatinine; proteinuria and hematuria; direct Coombs' test positive, immune complexes and cold agglutinins present and antinuclear antibody titers elevated. Thus, the patient had multisystem manifestations—mucocutaneous, hematological and renal—suggestive of systemic lupus erythematosus. There was gradual recovery on high-dose steroids although antinuclear antibody titers remained elevated for 5 months.

Furosemide must be added to the list of drugs which can cause a lupus-like syndrome.

Diuretics in premature infants *(SEDA-8, 219; SEDA-9, 208; SEDA-10, 194)* Guignard and Gouyon (37[R]) have reviewed the adverse effects of diuretics on the immature kidney. Unwanted reactions to furosemide including hypercalciuria, nephrocalcinosis, secondary hyperparathyroidism and bone disease are usually seen when the drug is administered chronically or in large doses. Renal calcification is seen after at least 2 mg/kg/d for at least 12 days and is worse if there is concomitant urinary tract infection. Partial dissolution of renal calcification and reduced urine calcium excretion appear to follow subsequent administration of a thiazide.

Kenney et al (38[C]) reported nephrocalcinosis in 3 very-low-birth-weight infants treated with furosemide for bronchopulmonary dysplasia. Renal function remained normal in all three. The ultrasound findings of diffuse medullary hyper-echogenicity appear to be specific for nephrocalcinosis and the authors recommend that all low-birth-weight babies treated with furosemide should undergo regular renal ultrasound examination. A clinical report by Fischer et al (39[C]) suggests that exposure to etacrynic acid in utero can result in polyhydramnios, massive diuresis after birth and nephrocalcinosis.

A retrospective examination of the clinical course of 17 preterm infants with chronic lung disease who received loop diuretics and developed nephrocalcinosis (40[CR]) indicated that calcification was associated with both furosemide treatment and the presence of multiple risk factors including alkaline urine and low urine output. In 9 children followed up for a mean of 21.3 months, calcification improved in 5 (total resolution in 4), renal length was normal in 17 of 18 kidneys, but renal function remained abnormal in 4 patients. Compared to control patients, hypercalciuria followed the administration of furosemide, hydrochlorothiazide and spironolactone to 30 low-birth-weight infants (41[CR]). It appears that a large intake of sodium can override the normal tendency of thiazides to promote calcium reabsorption in the distal tubules. Although neither study was prospective nor randomized, these findings suggest that renal function may be compromised after furosemide use in some infants and that thiazides too may increase the risk of nephrocalcinosis in premature infants. Further research is needed.

The above findings are the more disturbing in view of a prospective, randomized, blinded evaluation of the early prophylactic use of furosemide (2 mg/kg/d for 2 days) in 69 newborn infants with severe respiratory distress syndrome (42[C]) in which such treatment was of no benefit on any measure of pulmonary function. Furthermore, it led to more rapid postnatal weight loss, higher pulse rate, a greater sympathomimetic drug requirement and no expansion of plasma volume between 48 and 96 hours of age. Therefore, furosemide appears to produce undesirable volume depletion and exposes the infant to the risk of nephrocalcinosis without advantage.

In vitro, at concentrations likely to be achieved clinically in neonates, bumetanide significantly reduced binding of bilirubin to albumin from critically ill neonates and increased unbound bilirubin (43). Like furosemide, bumetanide seems to be a potent displacer of bilirubin and should be used with caution in jandiced neonates to avoid the risk of kernicterus.

Diuretics in the elderly Because of their high prescription rate, diuretics are the commonest cause of adverse drug reaction in this age group (44[r]). However, in reviewing the results of long-term studies of diuretic use in elderly hypertensives. Applegate (8[r]) observed that overall toxicity rates were acceptable and side effects appear no more common than in younger subjects. Although he urges caution especially in patients who develop metabolic complications, the use of low doses and aggressive treatment of hypokalemia, there remains insufficient negative evidence to proscribe diuretic use in the elderly.

Diuretics in ascites A thoughtful editorial has examined the use of diuretics in the management of hepatic ascites (45[c]). Electrolyte imbalance is seen in 20–80% of diuretic-treated patients while renal impairment and hepatic encephalopathy are also common. In patients with peripheral edema, which acts as a reserve compartment from which the intravascular compartment can be replenished, changes in plasma volume are slight and renal impairment is relatively uncommon. However, in patients without peripheral edema, plasma volume may fall by up to 24%, renal impairment is more likely and electrolyte abnormalities are also common.

Surreptitious diuretic abuse (*SED-11, 418*) A retrospective study (46[C]) of 31 patients presenting with hypokalemia of indeterminate origin and normal blood pressure over a 10-year period revealed 5 cases of pseudo-Bartter's syndrome due to diuretic ingestion (furosemide, chlortalidone, hydrochlorothiazide, clopamide and xipamide alone or in combination). In all cases, diagnosis by measurement of diuretic concentration in urine was delayed. Challenge with diuretic may provoke the syndrome while withdrawal leads to body weight increases and disappearance of metabolic alkalosis. These maneuvers may facilitate diagnosis.

Pancreatitis *(SED-11, 427)* Stenvinkel and Alvestrand (47[CR]) report a patient in whom pancreatitis was induced by both furosemide and bumetanide. The mechanism is unknown: possibilities include a direct toxic effect, diuretic-induced stimulation of pancreatic secretion or ischemia due to impaired pancreatic blood flow secondary to extracellular volume contraction. The similarity of the responses to two distinct agents suggests that the reaction depends on pharmacological properties rather than chemical structure.

Loop diuretics after envenomation Karnad et al (48[C]) present 5 patients with pulmonary edema secondary to severe envenomation following scorpion stings. Intravenous diuretic therapy was associated with resolution of pulmomary edema, but shock with low central venous pressure supervened rapidly. Diuretics should be used cautiously in such patients. If hypotension develops, afterload reduction with an ACE inhibitor together with fluid replacement appears to readily correct the hemodynamic disturbance.

Other topics Santos-Luna et al (49[C]) describe a further case of hydrochlorothiazide-induced *interstitial pneumonitis* presenting as pulmonary edema (SED-11, 419; SEDA-12, 183; SEDA-13, 188). The first reported incident precipitated by chlorothiazide (50[C]) suggests that this syndrome may occur with any drug of the thiazide group. Bailey (51[R]) and Sica and Gehr (52[R]) review *nephropathy* associated with potassium-sparing diuretics (SED-11, 429, 431). Although the overall incidence of nephrotoxicity is quite low, elderly patients and those with prior renal dysfunction are at particular risk. Special care is necessary in these circumstances.

DRUG INTERACTIONS

Ketanserin–diuretics The Ketanserin Trial Group (53[Cr]) report a large study involving 3899 patients with intermittent claudication randomized to ketanserin or placebo. During the trial, it became apparent that a harmful interaction between ketanserin and potassium-losing diuretics had resulted in an excess of deaths, forcing the withdrawal of patients receiving both drugs. The authors place the blame for the interaction firmly on diuretic-induced ventricular ectopy on the basis of largely discredited analyses of long-term studies in hypertension (SEDA-9, 203). However, there is a real risk of serious arrhythmia and sudden death if drugs such as ketanserin which prolong the QT interval are administered to patients with diuretic-induced hypokalemia (SEDA-9, 205). Combination therapy with potassium-losing diuretics and drugs of this type should be prescribed only with extreme caution; even mild hypokalemia must be avoided.

Non-steroidal anti-inflammatory drugs–diuretics *(SED-11, 423; SEDA-10, 193; SEDA-11, 198)*

Two reviews (51[R], 52[R]) have considered the interaction between non-steroidal anti-inflammatory drugs (NSAIDs) and potassium-sparing diuretics. Both types of drugs can cause nephrotoxicity and, in combination, the effects appear to be additive. This is a particular problem in the elderly where serum creatinine may be in the normal range even in the face of marked renal impairment. The availability of over-the-counter NSAIDs has increased the importance of this interaction. Plasma potassium and renal function should be monitored closely.

NSAIDs tend to offset the antihypertensive action of diuretics. No such interaction between ibuprofen and bendroflumethiazide was seen in the study of Davies et al (54[C]). However, this small study had serious design flaws and the data presented cannot exclude a clinically relevant interaction. More work is required.

SPECIFIC DRUGS

Furosemide *(SED-11, 425)*

The hemodynamic effects of furosemide may not always be favorable (SEDA-11, 199). In patients after myocardial infarction but without evidence of left ventricular failure (55[C]) single doses of furosemide 20 and 40 mg reduced pulmonary artery pressure within 1 hour. Administration of 40 mg every 8 hours for 24 hours produced a sustained reduction associated with temporary reduction in cardiac index, prolonged reduction in stroke volume, increased heart rate and systemic vascular resistance. Thus, after uncomplicated myocardial infarction, the hemodynamic benefit of furosemide may be limited. Whether loop diuretics have any role in this circumstance is uncertain.

Hydrochlorothiazide

Kavi and Mengel (56[C]) present findings in a patient with an acute debilitating myalgic syndrome and chills attributed to hydrochlorothiazide.

A 57-year-old black male with hypertension treated with hydrochlorothiazide for 1 year was admitted with diffuse myalgia and chills of some weeks' duration. He developed soreness of muscles whenever he ingested the drug and was afraid to take it regularly. Physical examination and all investigations were negative. On discontinuation, he became pain free only to relapse 3–4 h after a single 50 mg dose.

This patient clearly associated hydrochlorothiazide with symptoms and the anecdotal, subjective nature of the findings cast doubt on a causal relationship.

Indapamide *(SED-11, 424)*

Indapamide is structurally related to thiazides but is claimed to have additional properties in the management of hypertension. Two large but uncontrolled observational studies (57[C], 58[C]) indicate that indapamide is well tolerated. However, metabolic changes were similar to those expected with conventional diuretics. Therefore, these findings provide no convincing evidence of an advantage of indapamide over low doses of thiazide.

Spironolactone *(SED-11, 429; SEDA-13, 189)*

Four studies have reported adverse reactions in 116 patients (one male) treated with spironolactone for hirsutism or acne (59[c], 60[C], 61[C], 62[c]). The major side effects were related to antiandrogenic mechanisms: *menstrual disturbances*, and *breast enlargement or tenderness*. Although up to 80% of patients developed such problems usually early in the course of treatment, withdrawals were uncommon. Concomitant use of an oral contraceptive led to a lower incidence of menstrual abnormalities (61[C]). The frequency of side effects was dose-related and they were less often seen at doses of 100 mg daily than at higher doses (60[c]). In the only double-blind, adequately controlled trail (62[c]), menorrhagia was equally frequent after spironolactone 100 mg and placebo, and in some active treated patients, menstrual periods were more regular. However, no objective benefit in hair growth was seen.

Other adverse reactions included *urticaria, scalp alopecia* (60[C]) and *chloasma*, a previously unreported complication in 2 patients during prolonged treatment with 200 mg daily (61[C]).

A 35-year-old female with both acne and hirsutism complained of increasing patchy pigmentation on the cheeks, forehead and chin after 8 weeks treatment. Therapy was continued and hyperpigmentation persisted. A 30-year-old female treated for acne for 12 months noticed pigmentation on the forehead and around the eyes while on holiday in Spain. Spironolactone was stopped and the pigmentation gradually faded. Neither had a history of oral contraceptive use, previous pigmentation or recent pregnancy.

In a retrospective analysis of 699 men treated with spironolactone at a large blood pressure clinic (63[C]) 91 developed *gynecomastia*. This side effect was reversible and dose-related, being uncommon at doses less than 100 mg daily.

Although there are limitations in the interpretation of these data, spironolactone appears to cause few symptomatic side effects including those likely to be related to antiandrogenic mechanisms, if used at low doses.

REFERENCES

1. Challenor VF, Waller DG, (1988) Drugs for hypertension. II. Diuretics. *Cardiol. Pract., 6,* 32.
2. Hannedouche T, Delgado A (1988) Hypokaliémie, hypomagnésémie et arythmies ventriculaires au cours du traitement diurétique de l'hypertension artérielle. *Arch. Mal. Coeur Vaiss., 81,* 819.
3. Saunders E (1988) Drug treatment considerations for the hypertensive black patient. *J. Fam. Pract., 6,* 659.
4. Stark RM (1988) The atherogenic risk of antihypertensive therapy. *Am. J. Med., 84, Suppl. 1B,* 86.
5. Weinberger MH (1988) Diuretics and their side effects: dilemma in the treatment of hypotension. *Hypertension, 11, Suppl. II,* II-16.
6. Weinberger MH (1988) Cardiovascular risk factors and antihypertensive therapy. *Am. J. Med., 84, Suppl. 4A,* 24.
7. Moser M (1988) Less severe hypertension — where and how it should be treated. *Compr. Ther., 14,* 11.
8. Applegate WB (1989) Hypertension in elderly patients. *Ann. Intern. Med., 110,* 901.
9. Jeunemaitre X, Charru A, Chatellier G et al (1988) Long-term metabolic effects of spironolactone and thiazides combined with potassium-sparing agents for treatment of essential hypertension. *Am. J. Cardiol., 62,* 1072.
10. Walters EG, Barnes IC (1988) A survey of hypokalaemia in patients of general practitioners. *Br. J. Clin. Pract., 42,* 192.
11. Bloomfield RL, Wilson DJ, Buckalew VM (1986) The incidence of diuretic-induced hypokalaemia in two distinct clinical settings. *J. Clin. Hypertens., 4,* 331.
12. Waite WW, Wade WE, Cobb HH (1988) Effect of diuretic regimens on serum potassium. *Can. J. Hosp. Pharm., 41,* 243.
13. Plavnik FL, Ribeiro AB, Maranhão MFC et al (1988) Chortalidona em baixas dóses no tratamento da hipertensão arterial leve e moderada: analise de eficacia frequencia de hipocalemia e disturbios do ritmo cardiaco. *Arqu. Bras. Cardiol., 50,* 135.
14. Lipworth BJ, McDevitt DG, Balfour DJK, Struthers AD (1989) Prior treatment with diuretics augments the hypokalaemic and electrocardiographic effects of inhaled salbutamol in man. *Clin. Sci., 76, Suppl. 20,* 30P.
15. Whyte KF, Whitesmith R, Reid JL (1988) The effect of diuretic therapy on adrenaline-induced hypokalaemia and hypomagnesaemia. *Eur. J. Clin. Pharmacol., 34,* 333.
16. Sawyer U, Gabriel R (1988) Progressive hypokalaemia in elderly patients taking three thiazide potassium-sparing diuretic combinations for thirty-six months. *Postgrad. Med. J., 64,* 434.
17. McVeigh G, Galloway D, Johnston D (1988) The case for low dose diuretics in hypertension: comparison of low and conventional doses of cyclopenthiazide. *Br. Med. J., 297,* 95.
18. Ziegler MG, Lernhardt E, Solt-Buzsaki V (1988) Dose response to hydrochlorothiazide in hypertensives receiving a calcium channel blocker. *Clin. Exp. Hypertens. (A), A10,* 791.
19. Salvadeo A, Villa G, Segagni S et al (1988) Validità della associazione fissa atenololo/idrocloratiazide /amiloride (100/25/2.5 mg) nella terapia dell'ipertensione arteriosa essenziale. *Minerva Cardioangiol., 36,* 109.
20. Forrester TE, Grell GAC (1988) Changes in red cell sodium content and blood pressure levels with potassium supplementation in black hypertensive patients. *West Indian Med. J., 37,* 92.
21. Borra S, Shaker R, Kleinfeld M (1988) Hyperkalaemia in an adult hospital population. *Mt. Sinai J. Med., 55,* 226.
22. Durakovic Z, Sinalcelj A, Durakovic S (1988) Malignant ventricular arrhythmia due to hyperkalaemia in an elderly patient. *Rom. J. Gerontol. Geriatr., 9,* 57.
23. Rado JP (1988) Successful treatment of hyperkalemic quadriplegia associated with spironolactone. *Int. J. Clin. Pharmacol. Ther. Toxicol., 26,* 339.
24. Wester P-O, Dyckner (1987) Magnesium and hypertension. *J. Am. Coll. Nutr., 6,* 321.
25. Friedman E, Shadel M, Halkin H, Farfel Z (1989) Thiazide-induced hyponatraemia: reproducibility by single dose rechallenge and an analysis of pathogenesis. *Ann. Intern. Med., 110,* 24.
26. Sonneblink M, Algur N, Rosin A (1989) Thiazide-induced hyponatraemia and vasopressin release. *Ann. Intern. Med., 110,* 751.
27. Laureno R, Karp BI (1988) Pontine and extrapontine myelinolysis following rapid correction of hyponatraemia. *Lancet, 1,* 1439.
28. McVeigh GE, Dulie EB, Ravenscroft A et al (1989) Low and conventional dose cyclopenthiazide on glucose and lipid metabolism in mild hypertension. *Br. J. Clin. Pharmacol., 77,* 523.
29. Williams LL, Lopez LM, Thorman AD et al (1988) Plasma lipid profiles and antihypertensive agents: effects of lisinopril, enalapril, nitrendipine, hydralazine, and hydrochlorothiazide. *Drug Intell. Clin. Pharm., 22,* 546.
30. Members of the Working Group on Hypertension in Diabetes (1987) Statement on hypertension in diabetes. *Diabetes Care, 10,* 764.
31. Kaplan NN, Rosenstock J, Raskin P (1987) A differing view of treatment of hypertension in patients with diabetes mellitus. *Arch. Intern. Med., 147,* 1160.
32. Bell DSM (1989) Hypertension in the person with diabetes. *Am. J. Med. Sci., 297,* 228.
33. Sandstrom P-E (1988) Evidence for diabetogen-

ic action of bumetanide in mice. *Eur. J. Pharmacol., 150*, 35.

34. Takala J, Anttila S, Gref CG, Isomaki H (1988) Diuretics and hyperuricaemia in the elderly. *Scand. J. Rheumatol., 17*, 155.

35. Ray WA, Griffin MR, Downey W, Melton LJ (1989) Long-term use of thiazide diuretics and risk of hip fracture. *Lancet, 1*, 687.

36. Lin RY (1988) Unusual autoimmune manifestations in furosemide-associated hypersensititivty angiitis. *NY St. J. Med., 88*, 439.

37. Guignard J-P, Gouyon JB (1988) Adverse effects of drugs on the immature kidney. *Biol. Neonate, 53*, 243.

38. Kenney IJ, Aiken CG, Lenney W (1988) Furosemide-induced nephrocalcinosis in very low birth weight infants. *Pediatr. Radiol., 18*, 323.

39. Fischer AF, Parker BR, Stevenson DK (1988) Nephrolithiasis following in utero diuretic exposure: an unusual case. *Pediatrics, 81*, 712.

40. Ezzedeen F, Adelmann RD, Ahlfors CE (1988) Renal calcification in preterm infants: pathophysiology and long-term sequelae. *J. Pediatr., 113*, 532.

41. Atkinson SA, Shah JK, McGee C, Steele BT (1988) Mineral excretion in premature infants receiving various diuretic therapies. *J. Pediatr., 113*, 540.

42. Green TP, Johnson DE, Bass JL et al (1988) Prophylactic furosemide in severe respiratory distress syndrome: blinded prospective study. *J. Pediatr., 12*, 605.

43. Walker PC, Shankaran S (1988) The bilirubin-displacing capacity of bumetanide in critically ill neonates. *Dev. Pharmacol. Ther., 11*, 265.

44. Nolan L, O'Malley K (1989) Adverse drug reactions in the elderly. *Br. J. Hosp. Med., 41*, 446.

45. Anonymous (1988) Diuretics or paracentesis for ascites? *Lancet, 2*, 775.

46. Kunz-Kostomanolakis M, Walb D, Abdelhamid S et al (1988) Bartter-Syndrom oder Pseudo-Bartter-Syndrom durch verborgenen Diuretikaabusus: eine retrospective klinische Studie bei 10 Patienten. *Nieren- u. Hochdruckkr., 17*, S287.

47. Stenvinkel P, Alvestrand A (1988) Loop diuretic-indiced pancreatitis with rechallenge in a patient with malignant hypertension and renal insufficiency. *Acta Med. Scand., 224*, 89.

48. Karnad DR, Deo AM, Apre N et al (1989) Captopril for correcting diuretic induced hypotension in pulmonary oedema after scorpion sting. *Br. Med. J., 298*, 1430.

49. Santos-Luna F, Entrenas Costa LM, Munoy Cabrera L, Costano Pavedano A (1988) Edema pulmonar tras la ingestión de hidrochorotiacida. *Arch. Bronconeumol., 24*, 104.

50. Bowden FJ (1989) Non-cardiogenic pulmonary oedema after ingestion of chlorothiazide. *Br. Med. J., 298*, 605.

51. Bailey RR (1988) Adverse renal reactions to non-steroidal anti-inflammatory drugs and potassium-sparing diurectics. *Adverse Drug React. Bull., 131*, 492.

52. Sica DA, Gehr TWB (1989) Triamterene and the kidney. *Nephron, 51*, 454.

53. Prevention of Atherosclerotic Complications with Ketanserin Trial Group (1989) Prevention of atherosclerotic complications: controlled trial of ketanserin. *Br. Med. J., 298*, 424.

54. Davies JG, Rawlins DC, Busson M (1988) Effect of ibuprofen on blood pressure control by propranolol and bendrofluazide. *J. Int. Med. Res., 16*, 173.

55. Larsen FF (1988) Haemodynamic effects of high or low doses of furosemide in acute myocardial infarction. *Eur. Heart J., 9*, 125.

56. Kavi NG, Mengel CE (1988) Hydrochlorothiazide and myalgias. *Ann. Intern. Med., 109*, 84.

57. Leonetti G, Rappelli G, Salvetti A, Scapellato L (1988) Tolerability and well-being with indapamide in the treatment of mild-moderate hypertension: an Italian multicenter study. *Am. J. Med., 84, Suppl. 1B*, 59.

58. Werning C, Weitz T, Ludwig B (1988) Assessment of indapamide in elderly hypertensive patients with special emphasis on well-being. *Am. J. Med., 84, Suppl. 1B*, 104.

59. Azizlerli G, Ozarmagam G, Taklifi B et al (1988) Aknede spironolactone ile tedavi. *Deri Hast. Frengi Ars., 22*, 125.

60. Helfer EL, Miller JL, Rose LI (1988) Side-effects of spironolactone therapy in the hirsute woman. *J. Clin. Endocrinol. Metab., 66*, 208.

61. Hughes BR, Cunliffe WJ (1988) Tolerance of spironolactone. *Br. J. Dermatol., 118*, 687.

62. McLellan AR, Rentoul J, MacKie R, McInnes GT (1989) Lack of effect of spironolactone on hair shaft diameter in hirsute females. *Postgrad. Med. J., 65*, 459.

63. Jeunemaitre X, Chatellier G, Kreft-Jais C et al (1987) Efficacy and tolerance of spironolactone in essential hypertension. *Am. J. Cardiol., 60*, 820.

P.L.C.M. van Riel

23 Metals

Aluminium *(SED-11, 437; SEDA-12, 185; SEDA-13, 191)*

An excellent review article about aluminium toxicity in children was published by Freundlich in 1988 (1[R]). The patients who are at risk, the most important clinical manifestations of aluminium toxicity in prematures and infants and the prevention and treatment with deferoxamine are discussed.

Endocrine metabolic In a study of 12 children with chronic renal failure, the effect of two phosphate binders (aluminium hydroxide and calcium carbonate) on bone turnover and 1,25-dihydroxycholecalciferol were compared (2[C]). Both phosphate binders, in addition to mild dietary phosphorus restriction and small doses of vitamin D supplement, effectively suppressed the secondary hyperparathyroidism. However, in both treatment groups a mild mineralization defect present before treatment worsened, with a decrease in mineral appositional rate and increase in mineralization lag time. In spite of this it is suggested that the observed mineralization defect is due to aluminium toxicity. An argument for this may be the raised serum aluminium level in both groups due to treatment with aluminium hydroxide before this study began. Since calcium carbonate appeared to be as effective as aluminium hydroxide one should give preference to the less toxic calcium carbonate for the treatment of hyperphosphatemia.

Liver Besides effects on the central nervous system and bones aluminium may also affect the liver in which organ it is also accumulated.

A study in rats sought to determine whether chronic intravenous administration of aluminium could produce hepatic or biliary dysfunction (3[c]). Aluminium caused a dose- and time-dependent elevation of the total serum bile acid concentration and a decrease of the bile flow. On account of these findings it seems possible that aluminium has a role in the pathogenesis of parenteral nutrition-induced hepatobiliary dysfunction.

Skin and appendages A patient was described with persistent itchy, eczematous and slightly pigmented lesions at the sites of previous injections of DTP triple vaccine (5[c]). Aluminium hypersensitivity was suggested and confirmed by patch testing.

Miscellaneous Recently a causal association between aluminium and *Alzheimer's disease* has been suggested (4[R]). However, due to the many limitations of the study design, this association is still a matter of dispute. A prospective study is needed to give a decisive answer.

Bismuth *(SED-11, 439) (see also Chapter 38)*

Bismuth has been used in the treatment of dyspepsia for decades. Having fallen out of favor in the 1970s because of reports of encephalopathy it is regaining popularity in recent years because of the proven efficacy of the colloidal bismuth in the treatment of gastrointestinal ulcer disease, especially since it is known to have an effect on *Campylobacter pylori*. In a review article the pharmacokinetics-dynamics and toxicity of the bismuth salts have been discussed (6[R]). In Chapter 38 of this Volume some speculation as to the long-term safety of the preparations currently in use is discussed.

Gold *(SED-11, 443; SEDA-12, 186; SEDA-13, 191)*

Gold has evolved from an elixer of life which could cure all known diseases to a scientifically proven efficaceous drug in the treatment of a few diseases, notably rheumatoid arthritis and

Side Effects of Drugs Annual 14
M.N.G. Dukes and L. Beeley, editors

psoriatic arthritis (7[R]). Several review articles on the use of gold in the treatment of rheumatoid arthritis have been published (8[R], 9[R], 10[R]). In a double blind study of 26 weeks' duration 40 patients with rheumatoid arthritis were randomly treated with weekly intramuscular injections of either 10 mg methotrexate or sodium aurothiomalate (11[CR]). Methotrexate turned out to be as effective as sodium aurothiomalate; however, significantly more patients in the gold group had to be withdrawn from the study due to adverse reactions (7 vs. 2 patients).

It has been suggested that the concentration of 'free' gold might be a useful parameter for monitoring patients during chrysotherapy (12). A method has been described which makes it possible to obtain reliable measures of free gold concentrations (13[CR]). In the retrospective study which used the method, 6 out of the 7 patients with a higher free-to-total serum gold ratio turned out to have developed an adverse reaction. Prospective studies are needed to show whether the correlation indeed does exist.

Immune system *(SED-11, 447; SEDA-12, 186; SEDA-13, 191)* 151 white and 14 black rheumatoid arthritis patients treated with gold were studied to throw light on the relationship between HLA antigens and adverse reactions (14[CR]). Gold-induced dermatitis and stomatitis occurred with similar frequency among black and white patients; no association was found between HIA antigens and this adverse reaction. This study confirms the association between HLA-DR3 and gold-induced thrombocytopenia and proteinuria in whites. In addition a reduced frequency of HLA-DR7 was found among dermatitis patients in both racial groups suggesting a weak protective effect of this antigen. Due to the small number of black patients included in this study no conclusions could be reached with respect to the more uncommon adverse reactions such as thrombocytopenia and proteinuria.

Respiratory *(SED-11, 445; SEDA-12, 186)* Another case of bronchiolitis obliterans during chrysotherapy has been described (15[Cr]).

A 49-year-old woman with a severe seropositive rheumatoid arthritis was treated with naproxen 500 mg b.i.d., pulse methylprednisolone and gold sodiumthiomalate. After 2 months she experienced insidious onset of dyspnea on exertion and scant dry cough without upper respiratory symptoms. On examination, temperature was 38°C, cardiac and pulmonary examinations were normal. On chest radiograph soft nodular densities in both lung fields and faint air bronchogram were seen. A complete blood count was normal except for 5% eosinophilia. Naproxen and gold were discontinued. However, the respiratory symptoms persisted and the chest X-ray 1 week later showed progression. Pulmonary function test revealed no obstruction and a slightly decreased diffusion capacity. Bronchoscopy was normal and transbronchial biopsy was non-diagnostic. Bronchopulmonary lavage demonstrated an increased total cell count with a predominant increase in the percentage lymphocytes. Three weeks after the onset of respiratory symptoms an open lung biopsy was performed. A bronchiolitis obliterans with small bronchioles occluded by inflammatory cells, their walls thickened by granulation tissue, was found. In addition aberrations consistent with interstitial fibrosis were found. The patient was treated with methylprednisolone and cyclophosphamide and could be discharged after a 4-month hospital stay. The results of the bronchoalveolar lavage, namely an increase in the total cell count as well as an increase in the percentage lymphocytes, make it very likely that the bronchiolitis obliterans was due to a gold adverse reaction. Whether the interstitial fibrosis was part of the adverse reaction or just a coincidence remains uncertain.

Liver *(SED-11, 446)* Another case of hepatitis with onset 3 weeks after the start of aurothiomalate treatment was published (16[c]). No alternative causes for the hepatitis were found. Five weeks after discontinuation of the gold therapy the hepatitis had resolved completely.

Urinary *(SED-11, 446; SEDA-12, 187; SEDA-13, 192)* In an editorial on gold nephropathy attention has been paid to clinical features, the various histopathological lesions, pathogenetic mechanisms and the management of this adverse reaction (17[R]).

Renal damage by gold, presenting as proteinuria or microscopic hematuria, accounts for about 10% of all adverse reactions to gold treatment. Gold nephropathy occurs in 70% of the patients within the first year of treatment. It runs a benign course, usually resolving within 2 years after discontinuation of gold treatment without obvious damage to renal function. In 70% of the patients renal biopsy shows a membranous glomerulonephritis. As a pathogenetic mechanism it has been suggested that gold causes renal tubular damage, just as do such other heavy metals as lead, bismuth and mercury. This leads to release of renal tubular epithelial (RTE) cells. The RTE cells act as an autoantigen which induces the formation of RTE antigen-antibody immune complexes, and these localize in the glomerular subepithelial space, leading to membranous glomerulonephritis. Other renal lesions found in patients with gold nephropathy, and probably due to different pathogenetic mechanisms comprise mesangial glomerulonephritis, minimal change nephropathy and tubulointerstitial disease. In the majority of the cases withdrawal of gold treatment is the only measure needed and there is certainly no need for corticosteroids or immunosuppressive drugs.

In 20 rheumatoid arthritis patients, 10 treated with sodium aurothiomalate and the others with D-penicillamine, the effects of these medications on renal function and arachidonic acid metabolism were studied (18[Cr]). No influence of aurothiomalate treatment could be detected on *N*-acetyl-*β*-glucosaminidase activity or on the *β*-2-microglobulin concentrations in serum and urine, which are sensitive indicators of glomerular and tubular damage respectively. Nor did aurothiomalate treatment affect renal prostanoid excretion.

Miscellaneous *(SED-11, 447)* Recently a case of *lupus erythematosus* perhaps induced by gold has been described (19[Cr]).

A 12-year-old patient with a seronegative juvenile chronic arthritis after 10 months of gold sodium thiomalate treatment developed pericarditis and high titers of antinuclear antibodies as well as antibodies to native double-stranded DNA. After withdrawal of the gold medication the clinical symptoms disappeared and the titers of autoantibodies decreased to normal levels. However, in addition to withdrawal of the gold treatment the patient was also treated with high-dose corticosteroids and azathioprine, which makes drug induction of the lupus less likely.

A rheumatoid arthritis patient was described who had been on long-term intramuscular gold therapy and whose mammogram showed a nodule resembling an intramammary lymph node with microcalcifications (20[Cr]). A biopsy of the lesion was performed; histopathology showed a normal breast parenchyma without microcalcifications and an intramammary lymph node was indeed found. In the lymph node granular-dense black particles were found which by means of X-ray microanalysis were shown to be *gold particles*.

A patient was described who after 4 injections of aurothiomalate developed a diffuse *urticarial skin eruption* and *interstitial lung disease* (21[c]). Despite intensive supportive treatment and high doses of corticosteroids the patient died after 7 days. At autopsy nonbacterial thrombotic endocarditis of the mitral valve was found, supposed to be due to gold-induced immune complex depositions.

A patient with *panhypogammaglobulinemia* detected after he had been treated with a cumulative dose of 1020 mg aurothiomalate was described (22[CR]). Although no data as to the immunoglobulin levels were available prior to the start of the gold therapy, the panhypogammaglobulinemia was thought to have developed during the gold treatment as the patient started to complain of recurrent upper respiratory tract infections, a herpes zoster infection and a pneumococcal pneumonia shortly after the gold treatment was begun.

Use in children A retrospective study of the treatment of juvenile chronic arthritis with slow-acting antirheumatic drugs (gold, penicillamine, antimalarials, and sulfasalazine) and a review of the literature on this subject has been published (23[CR]). Due to lack of sufficient placebo-controlled and comparative studies, definite conclusions as to the efficacy of the different drugs cannot be made. However, gold appears to be one of the most efficacious of these drugs. More general agreement does exist with respect to toxicity. Discontinuation occurred most frequently with gold (21%) and least frequently with antimalarials (7%).

Auranofin *(SED-11, 448; SEDA-12, 189; SEDA-13, 194)*

In an open multicenter study 90 rheumatoid arthritis patients were treated with auranofin 6 mg daily for one year (24[Cr]). Over 35% of the patients developed adverse reactions, mainly between months 3 and 6 of the treatment; 50% of them had to be withdrawn from the investigation. The reported side effects were in order of decreasing frequency: gastrointestinal, skin and hematological in nature. Efficacy was more pronounced in the patient group with a disease duration of less than 2 years.

In a 24-month double-blind placebo-controlled trial the effect of early initiation of auranofin therapy in 138 patients with early rheumatoid arthritis was evaluated (25[CR]).

After 2 years 52% of the patients in the auranofin group were still on the original drug, 25% had been withdrawn due to side effects and 19% due to lack of efficacy. In the placebo-treated group 37% of the patients were still taking the original 'drug'. Patients in both treatment groups withdrawn due to lack of effect or side effects were treated, on an intention-to-treat policy, with D-penicillamine or hydroxychloroquine. At the end of the study period patients in the auranofin group had improved more than in the placebo group with respect to several clinical variables as well as in such outcome measurements as radiological progression. The authors concluded that early initiation of auranofin treatment compared to delayed initiation of second-line treatment in early rheumatoid arthritis modifies the course of the disease after 2 years as expressed by a lesser degree of radiological damage.

Gastrointestinal symptoms, mainly diarrhea and loose stools, are the most frequent adverse reactions of auranofin therapy.

137 rheumatoid arthritis patients treated with auranofin were prospectively followed with the aim to acquire more information, by means of a questionnaire, on this adverse reaction in long term treatment (26[Cr]). The definition of diarrhea used in this study was: 'any report of diarrhea, loose, runny, soft or semi-formed stools'. 101 patients (74%) reported at least 1 episode of diarrhea, usually within 1 month after the start of treatment. The prevalence diminished from 30–40% in the first 6 months of therapy to about 20% for patients treated for 1 year and 10% for those treated for more than 18 months. Only 8% of the patients had to be withdrawn due to this adverse reduction. The diarrhea usually responded well to temporary dose reduction and/or antidiarrheal medication.

Seventeen patients with pemphigus vulgaris were treated with 6 mg auranofin daily; 15 of them were also treated with a lower than usual dose of methylprednisolone: 45 mg daily (27[CR]). Clinical remission was observed in 14 patients. Mild side effects were seen in 2 patients. It is possible that adding auranofin to the corticosteroid treatment in pemphigus vulgaris has a corticosteroid-saving effect with minor adverse reactions.

Iron *(SED-11, 451; SEDA-12, 190; SEDA-13, 195)*

The administration of iron dextran intramuscularly or by intravenous infusion is frequently (in up to 30% of cases) accompanied by adverse reactions. These are divided into acute reactions (such as anaphylaxis and headache), delayed reactions (such as arthralgia, myalgia, fever and nausea) and local reactions including pain and skin staining at the site of injection and phlebitis.

A patient has been presented who experienced adverse reactions to an intravenous infusion (50 mg/d) of iron dextran, but tolerated without any problems a low dose of iron dextran (2 mg/d) in total parenteral nutrition (28[cr]). These authors also reviewed the literature on parenteral iron suppletion and found that iron dextran supplemented total parenteral nutrition up to doses of 100 mg/d was not associated with adverse reactions. This is probably due to the smaller iron dose used and the much longer administration period which is customary when iron is given to support total parenteral nutrition.

Experience with total dose intravenous infusion of iron dextran in a prospective study of 87 patients with anemia has been described (29[CR]).

Two patients developed anaphylactoid reactions shortly after the test dose of 1500 mg elemental iron. In 37 patients (42%) mild delayed adverse reactions (myalgia, arthralgia and fever) developed within 24 hours after infusion. In most instances these symptoms resolved soon after administration of a non-steroidal anti-inflammatory drug. Delayed reactions occurred in 4 patients. Pretreatment with aspirin, diphenhydramine or steroids did not appear to influence the incidence of delayed adverse reactions.

A patient was described with *local necrosis and ulceration* secondary to massive doses of intramuscularly-administered iron dextran (350 injections over a period of 5 years) (30[C]). Pathological examination revealed dense fibrosis, ulceration and massive accumulation of iron in the dermis.

Four patients with *erythropoietic protoporphyria* have been published in whom oral iron produced clinical and biochemical deterioration (31[Cr]). As some patients with this disease do improve on oral iron suppletion, this observation suggests that there are at least 2 different subgroups of patients with erythropoietic protoporphyria distinguished by their response to oral iron.

The toxicity of acute iron overload has been studied in an animal model (32). It was hypothesized that the toxicity of acute iron overload might be due primarily to hepatocellular damage, particularly of the mitochondrial membrane, resulting in lactic acidosis and probably also in cardiac toxicity.

Silver *(SED-11, 456)*

A report on a patient who developed a *ureteral stenosis* after retrograde intrapelvic instillation of silver nitrate and a review of the literature on this therapy has been published (33[CR]). Silver nitrate administered by retrograde injection in the ureter is being used in the treatment of essential hematuria although there is some controversy concerning its efficacy. The supposed mechanism of action is cauterization. Complications are minor (transient flank pain and nausea) provided the silver nitrate has been installed in the right place (i.e. not intravesically or retroperitoneally) and in the right dosage (0.125 – 1% silver nitrate). The patient described in the case-report had been treated with 2.5% silver nitrate.

Zinc *(SED-11, 456; SEDA-12, 191)*

Many people today regularly take a variety of vitamins and other non-prescribed supplements to maintain health and to prevent or treat disease. Recently a patient was reported who, after taking pharmacological doses of zinc to prevent prostatitis, developed *copper deficiency anemia* and *neutropenia* (34[C]).

A 44-year-old man developed fatigue and a sore throat. A blood count was obtained that revealed neutropenia and anemia. There was no alcohol abuse and the patient denied exposure to toxins. He was taking L-lysine 2 g/d to control genital herpes. He was also taking non-prescribed vitamin E, A, B complex, folic acid and pyridoxine. In addition he had used 200–300 mg zinc gluconate as a single daily dose for at least 2 years. Physical examination was normal except for pallor. Laboratory studies showed a total white blood cell count of 2000/μl, with 6% segmented neutrophils, 78% lymphocytes, 7% monocytes, 7% eosinophils, hemoglobin 9.0 g/dl hematocrit 25.7%, mean corpuscular volume 100, reticulocyte count 0.2% and platelet count 352 000/μl. Bone marrow morphology showed prominent cytoplasmic vacuoles in eary myeloid and erythroid forms. There were numerous ringed sideroblasts. Serum zinc was 262 μg/dl (normal 50–160), serum copper 15 μg/dl (normal 70–155), ceruloplasmin 2 μg/dl (normal 15–50), serum iron 32 μg/dl, and total iron binding capacity 212 μg/dl. Lead level was within the normal range. The patient discontinued all the nutritional supplements except pyridoxine and folic acid. Within 4 weeks the peripheral blood values returned to normal and a repeat examination of the bone marrow after 7 weeks as well as serum levels of zinc, copper and ceruloplasmin showed a return to normal.

Ingestion of large quantities of zinc leads to induction of the synthesis of the protein metallothionein in the mucosal cells. Because zinc bound to metallothionein is not absorbed in the intestine, zinc absorption is regulated by the induction of this protein. However, the metallothionein protein has a stronger affinity for copper than for zinc, resulting in copper depletion. It is the copper deficiency which causes anemia and neutropenia. The mechanism of the neutropenia is unknown; the anemia is thought to be due to reduced mobilization of iron from liver stores and impaired mitochondrial iron metabolism.

The induction of decreased copper absorption by prolonged oral zinc administration is used in the treatment of Wilson's disease (35[C]). Recently a case of successful treatment of Wilson's disease with oral zinc sulphate 600 mg daily in a patient having serious adverse reactions to D-penicillamine was reported (36[Cr]).

REFERENCES

1. Freundlich M (1988) The spectrum of aluminum toxicity in pediatrics. *Int. J. Pediatr. 3*, 41.
2. Turner C, Compston J, Mak RH et al (1988) Bone turnover and 1,25-dihydroxycholecalciferol during treatment with phosphate binders. *Kidney Int., 33*, 989.
3. Klein GL, Heyman MB, Lee TC et al (1988) Aluminum-associated hepatobiliary dysfunction in rats:

relationships to dosage and duration of exposure. *Pediatr. Res.*, 23, 275.
4. Martyn C, Osmond C, Edwardson JA et al (1989) Geographical relation between Alzheimer's disease and aluminium in drinking water. *Lancet, 1*, 59.
5. Cox NH, Moss C (1988) Cutaneous reactions to aluminium in vaccines: an avoidable problem. *Lancet, 2*, 43.
6. Borsch G (1988) Übersicht. Alte und neue Magentherapie mit Wismutsalzen. Pharmakokinetik, Pharmakodynamik, Toxizität. *Med. Klin., 83*, 605.
7. Hillson RM (1988) Gold, frankincense and myrrh. *J. R. Soc. Med., 81*, 542.
8. Davis P (1988) Gold therapy in the treatment of rheumatoid arthritis. *Can. Fam. Physician, 34*, 445.
9. Grasedyck K (1988) Wirkweise und Sicherheit der parenteralen Goldtherapie. *Aktuel. Rheumatol., 13*, 157.
10. Rau R (1988) Goldtherapie in der Praxis des niedergelassenen Arztes. *Akt. Rheumatol., 13*, 214.
11. Suarez-Almazor ME, Fitzgerald A, Grace M et al (1988) A randomized controlled trial of parenteral methotrexate compared with sodium aurothiomalate (Myochrysine) in the treatment of rheumatoid arthritis. *J. Rheumatol., 15*, 753.
12. Pedersen MP (1986) Binding of sodium aurothiomalate to human serum albumin in vitro at physiological conditions. *Ann. Rheum. Dis., 45*, 712.
13. Heath MJ (1988) Measurement of 'free' gold in patients receiving disodium aurothiomalate and the association of high free to total gold levels with toxicity. *Ann. Rheum. Dis., 47*, 18.
14. Fraser PA, Stern SH, Coblyn JS et al (1988) Immunogenetics and racial determinants of gold toxicity in rheumatoid arthritis. *J. Natl. Med. Assoc., 80*, 162.
15. Fort JG, Scovern H, Abruzzo JL (1988) Intravenous cyclophosphamide and methylprednisolone for the treatment of bronchiolitis obliterans and interstitial fibrosis associated with chrysotherapy. *J. Rheumatol., 15*, 850.
16. Tebib J, Colson F, Noel E et al. (1988) Un nouveau cas d'hépatite aurique au cours du traitement d'une polyarthrite rhumatoïde. *Rev. Rhum., 55*, 705.
17. Hall CL (1988) Gold nephropathy. *Nephron, 50*, 265.
18. Seppala E, Lehtinen K, Isomaki H et al (1988) Effects of long-term aurothiomalate and D-penicillamine treatments on renal function and urinary excretion of prostanoids in patients with rheumatoid arthritis. *Int. J. Clin. Invest., 3*, 149.
19. Korholz D, Nurnberger W, Gobel U et al (1988) Gold-induzierter systemischer Lupus erythematodes. *Monatsschr. Kinderheilkd., 136*, 644.
20. Bolen JW, Shaw de Paredes E, Carter T (1988) Mammographic determination of gold deposits simulating malignant calcifications in an intramammary lymph node. *Breast Dis., 1*, 105.
21. Kollef MH, Irvine T, Cragun WH (1988) Nonbacterial thrombotic endocarditis associated with gold-induced pulmonary disease. *Ann. Intern. Med., 106*, 903.
22. Pearson SL, Stewart IC, Kellett RJ (1988) Panhypogammaglobulinaemia caused by gold therapy. *Scot. Med. J., 33*, 343.
23. Grondin C, Malleson P, Petty RE (1988) Slow-acting antirheumatic drugs in chronic arthritis of childhood. *Semin. Arthritis Rheum., 18*, 38.
24. Klein G, Schwann H, Thumb N et al (1988) Klinische Wirksamkeit und Verträglichkeit von Auranofin bei Patienten mit chronischer Polyarthritis. Ergebnisse einer multizentrischen Langzeitstudie. *Z. Rheumatol., 47*, 342.
25. Borg G, Allander E, Lund B et al (1988) Auranofin improves outcome in early rheumatoid arthritis. Results from a 2-year, double blind, placebo controlled study. *J. Rheumatol., 15*, 1747.
26. Wallin BA, McCafferty JP, Fox MJ et al (1988) Incidence and management of diarrhea during long term auranofin therapy. *J. Rheumatol., 15*, 1755.
27. Magnin PH, Spillman DH, Oxilia MR (1988) Aureoterapía oral en el penfigo. *Rev. Argent. Dermatol., 69*, 184.
28. Porter KA, Blackburn GL, Bristian BR (1988) Safety of iron dextran in total parenteral nutrition: a case report. *J. Am. Coll. Nutr., 7*, 107.
29. Auerbach M, Witt D, Toler W et al (1988) Clinical use of the total dose intravenous infusion of iron dextran. *J. Lab. Clin. Med., 111*, 566.
30. Fuller JD, Williams HJ, McRory TI (1988) Necrotic bilateral buttocks ulcerations occurring after multiple intramuscular iron dextran injections. *Arch. Dermatol., 124*, 1722.
31. Milligan A, Graham-Brown RAC, Sarkany I et al (1988) Erythropoietic protoporphyria exacerbated by oral iron therapy. *Br. J. Dermatol., 119*, 63.
32. Rosenmund A, Brand B, Werner Straub P (1988) Hyperlactataemia, hyperkalaemia and heart block in acute iron overload: the fatal role of the hepatic iron-incorporation rate in rats on ferric citrate infusions. *Eur. J. Clin. Invest., 18*, 69.
33. Vijan SR, Keating MA, Althausen AF (1988) Ureteral stenosis after silver nitrate instillation in the treatment of essential hematuria. *J. Urol., 139*, 1015.
34. Simon SR, Branda RF, Tindle BH et al (1988) Copper deficiency and sideroblastic anemia associated with zinc ingestion. *Am. J. Hematol., 28*, 181.
35. Hoogenraad TU, Van der Hamer CJ, Van Hattum J (1984) Effective treatment of Wilson's disease with oral zinc sulphate: two case reports. *Br. Med. J. 289*, 273.
36. Kaur U, Bambery P, Bhushnurmath SR et al (1988) Successful long term oral zinc in florid Wilson's disease: a case report. *Trop. Geogr. Med., 40*, 161.

R.H.B. Meyboom and I.A. Jaffe

24 Metal antagonists

Originally, this chapter discussed a small number of very specialized and medically unrelated drugs; most of the information concerned penicillamine and mainly on its role as a 'slow acting' antirheumatic drug. In the past 15 years penicillamine has proved to be one of the most interesting drugs in the field of adverse reactions and has become a welcome tool in experimental research into the molecular basis of immune resistance and its regulation. In the past few years also the medical applications for other 'chelators' such as deferoxamine have proliferated (and now experimentally also include rheumatoid arthritis), whereas improved and more effective methods of administration (self-administration of deferoxamine by subcutaneous injection by the patient is now possible) (1^{C}) have made the drug more attractive. New iron chelators that can be taken by mouth have been introduced for experimental use in man, e.g. pyridoxal isonicotinoyl hydrazone (PIH) and α-ketohydroxypyridine (2^{CR}), drugs that may be expected to appear in future Annuals.

Because of their capacity to influence cellular enzymatic processes and the flow of peroxides through their affinity for trace metals, 'metal antagonists' are now a major object of promising research in molecular biology and pathophysiology as well as in clinical medicine, and are becoming a group of drugs that really deserve a separate chapter. Furthermore, the diversity and severity of the adverse reactions already recognized leave no doubt that the benefits from these drugs will not be achieved without risks.

Penicillamine *(SED-11, 461; SEDA-12, 194; SEDA-13, 198)*

General The history of the use of penicillamine in man has recently been reviewed by Miehlke (3^{R}). In the management of rheumatoid arthritis there has been a tendency towards more aggressive and earlier therapeutic intervention with slow-acting antirheumatic drugs such as penicillamine, presumably reflecting an attempt to improve the ultimate outcome of the disease (4^{R}). This development may not be without problems, however, since adverse reactions and loss of effect frequently cause the premature cessation of such drugs.

A large multicentre study lasting 7 years collected information on 5124 Japanese patients receiving penicillamine for rheumatoid arthritis (5^{cr}). The mean initial daily dose was 175 mg and the maintenance dose after 3 months was about 200 mg/d. Of these patients 28.1% experienced one or more side effects. *Skin reactions* were most frequent with an incidence of 14.6%. *Loss of taste* and *gastrointestinal symptoms* were frequent only at an early stage of the treatment. *Agranulocytosis* and *aplastic anemia* each occurred in 3 patients. Interestingly, serious *nephropathy* was rarely observed (4 cases of nephrosis), which is in accordance with previous preliminary information and may reflect the rare occurrence of the HLA antigens B8 and DR3 in Japanese people (see 'Risk situations, genetic factors' and also SEDA-8, 235, Ref. 7). Valuable reviews of cystinuria and its treatment have updated our knowledge of the use of penicillamine in this condition (6^{CR}, 7^{R}). In a series of 38 patients early *rashes*, often associated with mild *pyrexia*, were frequent (about 25%) but did not necessitate withdrawal (6^{c}). Severe *proteinuria* developed in 4 subjects and was associated wih a *nephrotic syndrome* in 2; with the exception of transient *thrombocytopenia*, blood dyscrasias did not occur. Of interest is the observation of Horoupian and coworkers that despite the dramatic beneficial effect of penicillamine on the neuropsychiatric manifestations of Wilson's disease, the drug does not seem to cause a significant decrease in the cerebral copper content or to produce a regression or healing of the neuropathological le-

(Biomedical Division)
Side Effects of Drugs Annual 14
M.N.G. Dukes and L. Beeley, editors

sions to degrees that are commensurate with the clinical improvement (8[CR]).

Respiratory A review of *obliterating bronchiolitis* (OB) has again referred to the diversity of this condition (SEDA-8, 236; 9[R]). In his commentary on this issue, Camus underlined that OB as encountered in patients with rheumatoid arthritis is probably a distinct entity which is different from OB in association with chronic pulmonary disease (10[R]). Rheumatoid-arthritis-associated OB is notable for its severity and irreversibility, leaving the patient in a seriously disabled and life-threatening state. There seems to be a predominance of OB in patients receiving penicillamine, but it has also occurred without penicillamine (SEDA-8, 236; 10[R]). An increased prevalence of the histocompatibility antigen DR4 may indicate an association between the pathogenesis of OB and rheumatoid arthritis (11[C]). Also if OB is essentially a complication of rheumatoid disease, it might be possible that penicillamine acts in one way or another as a facilitating factor (10).

The case has been described of a patient who repeatedly had *rhinitis* and *bronchospasm* after occupational exposure to penicillamine (12[C]). This patient had a history of allergy with bronchospasm to cats and to guar gum, but the mechanism of the reactions to penicillamine could not be elucidated.

Nervous system Commencing penicillamine in patients with Wilson's disease can initially cause neurological deterioration (SED-11, 462; see also 'Risk situations').

One of the interesting aspects of penicillamine-induced *autoimmune reactions* is whether or not they differ from idiopathic autoimmune diseases. In 19 patients with penicillamine-associated *myasthenia gravis*, antigenic specificities of circulating acetylcholine receptor antibodies were assessed with monoclonal antibodies and compared with those in patients with idiopathic myasthenia (13[CR]). The results showed that the AChR antibody patterns of penicillamine and idiopathic myasthenia are very similar with a predominance of antibodies to the extracellular surface of the α-subunit. However, there appear to be interesting differences in the genetic findings, as has already been discussed in earlier volumes (SEDA-8, 235). On the basis of 2 original and 45 literature cases, Paladini and colleagues provided further evidence that myasthenic reactions to penicillamine can occur in a special genetic subgroup of patients (14[CR]). The prevalence of HLA antigens DR1 and Bw35 is increased in these patients, whereas that of the antigens DR3 (which is associated with idiopathic myasthenia) and DR4 (which is increased in rheumatoid arthritis) is decreased.

Hematological In previous volumes, several reports have been reviewed describing *thrombotic thrombocytopenic purpura* (TTP, Moschcowitz syndrome) in connection with penicillamine (SED-11, 463). A review from the Netherlands of 12 patients with TTP has provided valuable information on this rare disease (15[C]). In one (fatal) case out of this series of 12, the condition was suspected to be induced by penicillamine. The authors concluded that TTP is a syndrome of diverse etiology and is probably caused by different pathogenic mechanisms, and they emphasized that the syndrome is variable and often incomplete and should therefore be considered in any patient presenting with thrombocytopenia or hemolytic anemia.

The mechanisms underlying drug-induced *granulocytopenia* are poorly understood. In experiments with bone marrow, Hammond and colleagues demonstrated that penicillamine (and also captopril but not enalapril) in the presence of copper caused inhibition of granulocyte/macrophage colony formation (16). Catalase reversed the inhibition of colony formation. The findings indicated that drugs with a reactive thiol group can interact with copper to generate H_2O_2, which can be toxic to neutrophilic progenitor cells and suggested a novel hematotoxic mechanism. Variations in sensitivity between individuals might be a complex function of drug levels, trace metal concentrations, endogenous free thiol concentrations and the presence of intact oxidant scavenging systems.

In a trial with 39 patients with primary sclerosing cholangitis, 3 cases of *hemolysis* were listed as 'possible drug related side effects' but no details were given (17[c]).

Gastrointestinal For the development of an oroantral fistula in suspected connection with penicillamine, see 'Risk situations'.

Urinary system In their study of 84 children with low-level lead poisoning, Shannon and coworkers provided the first report on *urinary incontinence* as a suspected side effect of penicillamine (18[c]). For three of these children treated with penicillamine, the parents spontaneously reported the onset or worsening of urinary incontinence, improving or resolving once treatment was terminated. In contrast, there were no unsolicited reports of enuresis in the control group. Unfortunately no more details were given and the issue remains unclear.

Apart from a moderate increase of urinary PGE_2 excretion, no biochemical evidence was found of impairment of renal function in a 2-year follow-up study of 10 patients taking penicillamine for rheumatoid arthritis (19[c]). Emery and Panayi have re-emphasized the potential importance of their finding of a strong association between impaired sulfoxidation ability and the risk of *nephropathy* with penicillamine (and also gold) (20). The mechanism for this association remains speculative, but may relate to altered metabolism of the thiol moiety in these drugs (see also 'Immune system' and 'Risk factors'). The risk of toxicity for patients possessing either HLA-DR 3 or poor sulfoxidation appears to be increased 25-fold as compared with those possessing neither. If these tests could be simplified, they would be a valuable tool for identifying patients at risk (20[R]).

In a series of 38 cystinuria patients, Stephens divided *proteinuria* into 3 groups: mild (less than 1 g/24 h), which was apparently related to urinary tract infection or stone and not to penicillamine, moderate (1–5 g/24 h) and severe (6[cr]). Moderate proteinuria appeared to be associated with penicillamine, but usually remained at a similar level despite continuation of penicillamine and did not seem to cause clinical harm. Severe proteinuria (11–19 g/24 h) developed in 4 of 38 patients and was associated with a *nephrotic syndrome* in two. In all 4 patients proteinuria recovered over a period of several months after stopping penicillamine. Interestingly in one of the patients with nephrosis penicillamine was later on restarted without recurrence of proteinuria. The author concluded that penicillamine may be continued in cystinuric patients so long as proteinuria does not exceed 5 g/24 h. The continuation of penicillamine without progression of proteinuria has also been documented in patients with rheumatoid arthritis and low doses of penicillamine have been well tolerated in patients with previous penicillamine nephropathy (21[CR]). Yet the advice of Hall and Tighe with regard to its use in rheumatoid arthritis is much more restrictive, since alternative medicines are usually available (21). In an autopsy study in the Netherlands rheumatoid arthritis was found surprisingly to be associated with renal pathology (22[CR]). *Membranous glomerulopathy* (8 cases in 132 autopsies) was observed only in patients who had received penicillamine or gold; this association was not statistically significant, however, because of the large proportion of patients treated with these drugs. In an etiological study in France of 82 consecutive patients with membranous glomerulonephritis, the disease was found to be secondary to other factors in 17 patients (23). Interestingly medicines were thought to be a likely cause in 5 of these 17 patients, and penicillamine in 3 subjects. In a series of 122 patients in East Germany, receiving penicillamine for Wilson's disease, serious adverse reactions were found in 14 patients, with nephropathy in 10 of them (24[cr]). In a large multicentre study in Japan, on the other hand, involving 5124 patients receiving penicillamine for rheumatoid arthritis, only 4 cases of nephrosis were observed (5[cr]). This finding is of special interest since the HLA antigens B8 and DR3, which were identified as a risk factor for penicillamine nephropathy in several studies (SEDA-11, 212), is known to be rare in Japanese people (SEDA-8, 235).

Skin and appendages In persons receiving long-term treatment with high doses of penicillamine (e.g. for Wilson's disease or cystinuria), characteristic *hemorrhagic skin lesions* may develop as a result of faulty collagen and elastin production (SED-11, 465; 25[CR]). Ultrastructural examination reveals alterations of collagen and elastin fibers. In histological, immunochemical and ultrastructural studies in one such patient, Goldstein and co-workers also found multiple *lymphangiectases* with blood vessel to lymphatic anastomosis within the lesions, a finding not previously reported (26[C]).

A *yellow nail syndrome*-like condition has occasionally been reported in the past in association with penicillamine (SEDA-9, 223). Recently the complete syndrome (dystrophy of the nails, lymphedema, pleural effusion and bronchial involvement) has been described in 2 patients as a suspected adverse reaction to penicillamine (27[CR]).

Three further cases of penicillamine-induced *pemphigus foliaceus* have been reported. One case was interesting in that a prodromal rash had occurred 3 years earlier and that the eruption persisted up to 4.5 years after stopping penicillamine (28[C]). In another patient the eruption started as annular and geographic lesions, mimicking *erythema annulare* (29[C]). Although a variety of drugs have occasionally been reported to cause pemphigus, there is in the literature no other single drug so strongly associated with pemphigus as penicillamine (SEDA-12, 195; 30[R]).

Special senses *Disturbance of taste,* although a characteristic and well-known side effect of penicillamine in adult patients, has not been reported in children (SED-10, 221). In a recent study of 84 children receiving penicillamine for lead poisoning, again no taste alterations were documented (31[c]).

Genital system Penicillamine-induced *breast enlargement* has previously been observed in female and occasionally male patients (SEDA-11, 214). A very comprehensive case-report described a further female patient with massive enlargement of the breasts, apparently induced by penicillamine (32[CR]). Her breasts were tender and grew progressively larger during each menstrual period. Endocrine evaluation was unremarkable and the breast enlargement resolved with danazol therapy. The condition resembles the pubertal form of massive breast enlargement. Histological examination mainly shows increased fibrous tissue. Regression of breast size with danazol treatment is often sufficient to avoid surgical treatment. Breast biopsy prior to endocrine therapy is advised, to rule out inflammatory carcinoma of the breast.

Muskuloskeletal See 'Nervous system' for *myasthenia gravis* as an adverse reaction to penicillamine.

Immune system and autoimmune reactions Several experimental studies have contributed to the unraveling of the complex effects of penicillamine and, in addition, illustrate the value value of drugs for the progress of the study of autoimmunity (33–38). Penicillamine presumably produces autoimmune reactions by inhibiting (in synergism with copper or ceruloplasmin and via the production of H_2O_2): (a) the proliferation of T-lymphocytes and the activity of helper T-cells in supporting the generation of antibody-forming cells (33); (b) endothelial cell proliferation and neovascularization (34); (c) fibroblast proliferation (35); and (d) clearance of circulating immune complexes by the complement system (36[CR], 37[R]).

In systemic *lupus erythematosus* (SLE) and in *membranous glomerulopathy,* the deposition of immune complexes is a characteristic feature and the handling of immune complexes by the complement system has been shown to be impaired in SLE patients. Penicillamine presumably inhibits the clearance of immune complexes by reacting with the carbonyl group of the exposed thiol ester in C4b. The reaction with C4 also inhibits activation of C3, the central component in the complement pathway. The inhibition by penicillamine of the complement cascade probably contributes to both the therapeutic anti-inflammatory action of the drug (through control of the generation of anaphylatoxins) and the development of side effects such as SLE and nephropathy (36, 37). While studying the effects of penicillamine on the immune system in rheumatoid arthritis patients, a fall in rheumatoid factor was observed which corresponded with the clinical improvement (38[CR]). In this study no changes were found in natural killer cell activity and in the numbers of T4, T8 and HLA-DR positive lymphocytes.

As a new autoimmune phenomenon induced by penicillamine, *anti-centromere antibodies* were detected in 6 patients (39[C], 40[c]). Although anti-centromere antibodies are usually a marker for serious autoimmune diseases, in all 6 cases the phenomenon was not associated with clinical symptoms and disappeared after stopping penicillamine. In these patients other abnormal antibodies were not found (e.g. no anti-DNA, antimitochondrial, anti-smooth muscle, or antibodies to intermediate filaments). In an assay using penicillamine attached to inert microspheres, evidence for antibodies against penicillamine was more frequently in patients with various adverse reactions to the drug than in patients without adverse reactions (41[cr], 42[CR]).

The clinical meaning of this finding needs further exploration, however.

Multisystem reactions The striking ability of penicillamine to elicit different serious adverse reactions simultaneously (SEDA-13, 201), was recently observed in a patient who developed both *pemphigus* and *nephrosis* (*minimal change nephropathy*) (43[C]).

Risk situations, genetic factors The results of HLA assessments in 95 Greek patients treated with penicillamine or gold for rheumatoid arthritis were in accordance with earlier findings in that the B8 antigen was more frequent in patients with *nephropathy* whereas *skin reactions* were more common in the presence of DRw6 (44[cr]). As Emery and Panayi have pointed out, two parameters have been found to be especially associated with an increased risk of adverse reactions to penicillamine, especially nephropathy: the sulfoxidation capacity and the histocompatibility antigen DR3 (see ‘Urinary’) (20). This finding is compatible with the view of Sim and colleagues that genetic determinants (the complement system is related to the histocompatibility antigens) and metabolic factors may contribute to an impaired handling of circulating immune complexes and to the subsequent development of autoimmune reactions such as SLE and immune complex glomerulonephritis (36, 37). A possible mechanism for this association is discussed under ‘Urinary’. The presence of antibodies to Ro(SSA) cellular antigen, seems to be another risk factor for adverse reactions to penicillamine. In a comparative study of patients with rheumatoid arthritis, Skopouli and colleagues concluded that anti-Ro(SSA) antibodies seem to characterize a distinct group of RA patients who are almost exclusively female, express more activated B-cell function, have a high prevalence of features of Sjögren’s syndrome and commonly develop adverse reactions to penicillamine, i.e. in 72% as compared with 27% patients without Ro(SSA) (45[CR]).

It has been known for a long time that commencing penicillamine in patients with Wilson’s disease may initially cause *neurological deterioration* (SED-11, 462; 46[R]). It is uncertain, however, if this results from alterations of copper distribution at submolecular, subcellular, transcellular or transorgan levels, or whether it results from some other property of penicillamine (e.g. its capacity to donate sulfhydryl groups). Pall and co-workers have pointed out that it seems likely that the initial damage is caused by copper decompartmentalization and suggested that pretreatment with lipid-soluble antioxidants such as vitamin E might be useful (46[R]).

In the past it was thought that penicillamine might, because of its effects on collagen synthesis, disturb normal *wound healing*. Experience in 217 operations in 150 patients did not disclose such effects and suggested that it is unnecessary to stop penicillamine before surgery (47[CR]). Another case observation, on the other hand, supports the view that penicillamine may, at least in some cases, interfere with wound healing: removal of an impacted maxillary third molar in a patient with Wilson’s disease treated with penicillamine was followed by the development of an *oroantral fistula*, presumably as a result of impaired collagen synthesis (48[C]).

Use in children Shannon and colleagues collected information on 84 children receiving penicillamine for low-level lead poisoning (31[C]): 28 subjects experienced side effects, leading to premature discontinuation of treatment in 8, the most common cause being a skin rash. *Thrombocytopenia* and *leukopenia* were frequent, but mostly mild and transient. Interestingly taste alterations were not recorded, which is in accordance with previous studies (SED-10, 221).

Second-generation effects A review of the literature on the use of penicillamine during pregnancy (49[R]) is in accordance with the view expressed in SED-11 (p. 469). Whereas the benefit of penicillamine outweighs the risk in patients with Wilson’s disease and probably cystinuria, a small number of reports of malformations (especially of cutis laxa) is reason to stop the drug during pregnancy in patients with rheumatoid arthritis.

Miscellaneous In a study in patients with scleroderma penicillamine was found to have a normalizing effect on collagen metabolism, via a decrease in β-galactosidase activity (50[C]). Penicillamine was found to cause a spurious variant of *α-antitrypsin*, which may be the cause of diagnostic errors (51[C]).

RELATED DRUGS

Pyritinol *(SED-11, 469)*

As has been pointed out earlier, the side effects of pyritinol and penicillamine appear to be very similar (SED-11, 469). The first report has now been published of *autoimmune hypoglycemia*, with demonstrated anti-insulin antibodies, probably induced by puritinol (52[C]). This syndrome has previously been described in connection with other thiol compounds, i.e. penicillamine, methimazol and tiopronin (SED-11, 214; 52[R]).

Tiopronin (mercaptopropionylglycine) *(SED-11, 469; SEDA-12, 197; SEDA-13, 202)*

Further to a series of patients with cystinuria referred to in SEDA-13 (p. 202), Sigaud and colleagues have presented experiences with tiopronin in 69 rheumatoid arthritis patients (53[Cr]), again showing a pattern of side effects resembling that of penicillamine, with *rashes, ageusia, stomatitis, proteinuria, thrombocytopenia and leukopenia.* Of special interest in this series was a patient who first had pemphigus in association with penicillamine and later on had a relapse when tiopronin was taken (53[c]). In another patient the development of *obstructive bronchiolitis* was thought to be secondary to tiopronin (first report; 53[c]). Amor and colleagues, in their review of the use of tiopronin in rheumatoid arthritis, also emphasised the similarity of the side effects to those of penicillamine: *stomatitis, rashes, lichenoid eruption, alopecia, ageusia, fever, proteinuria, thrombocytopenia, cholestatic hepatitis and polymyositis* can all occur (54[cr]). Most of their material appears to have been used in a publication 2 years earlier (SEDA-11, 215, Ref. 51). The introduction of the name 'acadione' for tiopronin (54), may increase the already existing confusion with regard to the identity of this drug.

One further case of tiopronin-associated *pemphigus* has recently been described, the total number of published cases now amounting to 7 (55[cR]). A report, probably the first, of *myasthenia gravis* in association with tiopronin underlines the similarity between the patterns of adverse reactions to penicillamine and tiopronin (56[C]).

A study of 2 cases in Japan (where tiopronin seems to be widely used, e.g. for liver dysfunction, allergic disorders, cataract and cystinuria) documents the occurrence of a *lichenoid skin eruption* and *alopecia* in association with tiopronin (57[C]). Other Japanese reports concerned *drug fever*, with and without a *rash*, in which hypersensitivity to tiopronin was demonstrated by eczematous reactions to a patch test (58[C]), and a patient with both *toxic epidermal necrolysis* and *cholestatic hepatitis* suspected in connection with tiopronin (this patient was also taking other drugs, including rescinnamine and nicomol) (59[C]).

OTHER METAL ANTAGONISTS

Deferoxamine *(SED-11, 470; SEDA-12, 197; SEDA-13, 202)*

Pharmacokinetics Information about the pharmacokinetics and metabolism of deferoxamine has been limited, so it is useful to have the studies of Kruck et al (60[CR]). Deferoxamine is rapidly converted into two metabolites, both of which are capable of binding iron and/or aluminium. As the parent molecule decreases, the metabolites increase and reach a maximum concentration at 2 h. As the amount of metal-free deferoxamine decreases, the rate of metabolite generation decreases and elimination of the metal-deferoxamine complexes by the kidney becomes the controlling factor. Preliminary data indicate marked differences in metabolite formation and elimination kinetics in different individuals and there are indications that metabolite pharmacokinetics may be related to the occurrence of side effects (60). A study in patients on continuous ambulatory peritoneal dialysis, showed an easy exchange of deferoxamine between plasma and the peritoneal fluid (61[C]). Peritoneal administration of deferoxamine cannot be recommended, however, because the addition of deferoxamine to the dialysis fluid could increase the risk of infection (see also 'Opportunistic infections'). Another study, in 8 children with thalassemia, emphasized the delay in obtaining a deferoxamine plus ferrioxamine plateau in plasma, the important interindividual variations and the slow decrease of the drug after finishing the infusion (62). Intravenous administration of 1 g deferoxamine to an anephric patient led to marked increases in the fecal elimination of aluminium and iron; dialysate removal of these metals also increased but to a lesser extent (63[C]). Apparently the biliary/fecal route of excretion may contribute significantly to deferoxamine-induced losses of aluminium and iron in dialysis patients.

Opportunistic infections Since the Special Review in SEDA-11 (p. 215), reports are accumulating of *opportunistic infections* with *Yersinia enterocolitica* and a variety of other micro-organisms with otherwise low virulence, in association with deferoxamine use and iron overload (SEDA-13, 203). In the period covered in this Annual, reports have included infections with *Yersinia, Pneumocystis carinii, Cunninghamella bertholletiae, Rhizopus oryzae* and *Rhizopus microsporus* (mucormycosis) occurring in association with deferoxamine in adults and in children. It should be added, however, that iron overload is already in itself associated with an increased risk of serious infections and that the role of deferoxamine remains difficult to establish (63a[CR]).

Sepsis with *Yersinia enterocolitica* developed 4 days after a single infusion of deferoxamine (60 mg/kg) in a 51-year-old patient with long-standing iron overload and renal failure (64[CR]). In such patients *Yersinia* infection should be suspected even in the absence of digestive symptoms. Also in a 26-year-old woman with thalassaemia major, splenectomy and hemosiderosis, *Y. enterocolitica* septicemia developed in temporal association with deferoxamine (65[C]). Interestingly this patient later on had a relapse of *Yersinia* sepsis when deferoxamine administration was resumed, necessitating permanent discontinuation of this drug. Another situation in which *Yersinia* sepsis can occur is when deferoxamine is used in children with acute iron poisoning. In view of the severity of this condition, Hadjiminas recommends the prophylactic use of antibiotics whenever deferoxamine is administered to children from areas with a high incidence of yersiniosis (66[R]). Pneumonia occurring during treatment with high doses of deferoxamine (2–2.5 g by continuous infusion) in a patient with thalassemia major was found to be due to *Pneumocystis carinii* (67[CR]). The authors postulate that high doses of deferoxamine and low levels of circulating iron may have led to an excess of free deferoxamine, which in turn may have caused lymphocyte inhibion and a decreased immune response. Several new reports of fatal cases of mucormycosis underline the danger of acquiring disseminated fungal infection in patients receiving deferoxamine (86–70). Mucormycosis, which can present clinically as rhinocerebral, pulmonary, gastrointestinal, cutaneous or widely disseminated infection, is otherwise rare and mainly restricted to patients with uncontrolled diabetes mellitus, hematological malignancies or organ transplantation (68[CR]). The patient described by Johnson and co-workers had cerebral mucormycosis with bilateral cavernous sinus and carotid artery thrombosis (69[CR]). The report emphasizes the limitations of neuroimaging techniques in establishing the diagnosis of both cerebral mycormycosis and cavernous sinus thrombosis. In another patient mucormycosis started with a vasculitis-like skin lesion (70[CR]). Also in a patient with a fatal invasive pulmo-arterial *Rhizopus oryzae* infection in association with the use of deferoxamine, the disorder had started with a skin lesion resembling infarction of cutaneous tissue (71[CR]). In another case-report fatal mucormycosis peritonitis and septicemia developed in a 17-year-old boy in probable association with deferoxamine and ambulatory peritoneal dialysis (72[CR]).

Although *Cunninghamella bertholletiae* is an ubiquitous soil saprophyte, infections with this organism have so far only very rarely been documented. A recent report describing fatal disseminated *C. bertholletiae* infection suggests that iron overload and deferoxamine treatment may increase the pathogenicity of this species too. Perhaps deferoxamine decreases host resistance by depleting the pool of iron available to the macrophage cytotoxic system (73[CR]). Only members of the Mucoraceae and *C. bertholletiae* are known to produce the characteristic angio-invasive pulmonary and rhinocerebral syndromes. Boelaert and colleagues reviewed 24 published cases up to January 1989 of rhizopus infections in dialysis patients, of which 21 were fatal (74[R]). At least 21 of the 24 patients received deferoxamine; there was evidence of iron overload in 6 and no evidence in 12. The authors emphasize that, because of the increasing use of deferoxamine in dialysis, there is an urgent need to identify the predisposing factors and they announce the establishment of an international registry of cases of mucormycosis developing during long-term dialysis (Dr. J.R. Boelaert, Algemeen Ziekenhuis Sint Jan, B-8000 Brugge, Belgium).

Nervous system and special senses Important news with regard to deferoxamine is the suggestion that its use may precipitate progressive dialysis *dementia*. In 5 out of a series of 35 patients with chronic renal failure and aluminium osteopathy, the administration of standard doses of deferoxamine was complicated by the development of *mental disturbances* (confusion, agitation, abnormal behavior, myoclonus), diagnosed as dialysis dementia (75[CR]). In 3 patients the condition had a fatal course. Concomitant parathyroid hypofunction may have placed these patients at increased risk for aluminium toxicity. Also other evidence indicates that aluminium is more neurotoxic than was previously thought (76) and the exacerbation of neurological symptoms when deferoxamine is started is reminiscent of similar experiences with penicillamine in Wilson's disease (see Penicillamine, 'Nervous system').

Evidence of *auditory neurotoxicity* (SED-11, 470) was present in 13 (causing deafness in 5) of 50 patients receiving long-term deferoxamine chelation for thalassemia (77[CR]). All patients showed improvement of hearing when deferoxamine was substituted with calcium diethylene triamine penta-acetic acid (Ca-DPTA). Also in an audiometric screening study of 153 children with β-thalassemia, sensorineural hearing loss was detected in 38% of the subjects (78[CR]). The observations that hearing loss was greater in younger patients, appeared to be correlated with the mean and peak deferoxamine doses and was higher in subjects with lower iron load, were arguments in favor of deferoxamine as the cause. Masala and colleagues, on the other hand, did not report an increased frequency of hearing loss in subjects receiving deferoxamine, perhaps reflecting the use of lower doses of the drug (79[CR]). With regard to *ocular toxicity* (SED-11, 470), a recent case-report was alarming in that irreversible *visual loss* occurred after a single small dose (40 mg/kg) of deferoxamine (80[CR]). Pall and co-workers described reversible ocular toxicity in 2 out of 3 patients receiving deferoxamine for rheumatoid arthritis (81[CR]). Both had abnormal electro-oculograms; one also had visual failure. The authors suggest that because of low iron stores in rheumatoid patients deferoxamine may chelate copper, which in turn may cause retinal damage. In the case of a 4-year-old child with refractory leukemia, acute retinal damage with impairment of visual acuity and color vision developed after the administration of high doses of deferoxamine (82[C]). A detailed study of 3 patients with optic neuropathies while undergoing chronic hemodialysis, obviously associated with deferoxamine in one, underscored the heterogeneity of optic nerve disease in patients with uremia (82a[CR]).

Skin and appendages An edematous, erythematous and itching *rash* of the legs developed in a 62-year-old woman within 48 h after the infusion of deferoxamine (83[c]).

Metabolic In an experimental study of its influence on peroxidase-catalyzed reactions, deferoxamine was shown to have multiple effects on the formation and activity of phagocyte-derived oxidants (84). Deferoxamine does not seem to react with or to remove heme iron (84). In another study deferoxamine was found to protect the red cell membrane against iron-induced oxidative stress (85). Deferoxamine was shown to inhibit in vitro the iron-containing enzymes cyclo-oxygenase and lipoxygenase and human platelet aggregation; hence the drug may perhaps be effective in atherosclerosis and inflammatory joint disease (86). Iron plays an important role in oxygen-radical-induced genetic damage and deferoxamine has been shown to have a protective effect in this respect (87).

Interference with diagnostic routines Experiences in a patient with a cerebral hemorrhage showed that chelation of gallium by deferoxamine may interfere with the diagnostic value of a ^{67}Ga scan (88[C]).

Edetate *(SED-11, 471; SEDA-13, 203)*

Edetate-dependent *pseudothrombocytopenia* (ED-PTP) is a rare but misleading phenomenon, the recognition of which is important in order to avoid expensive and potentially harmful procedures. In a study involving 33 623 hospital admissions, ED-PTP was found in 23 subjects; the prevalence rate of 0.07% is in accordance with previous studies (89[CR]). As a case-report of Hoyt and Durie shows, similar antibodies may occur that are edetate-independent (90[C]). The great practical importance of a proper diagnosis of ED-PTP was illustrated in a report of a patient in whom ED-PTP was mistaken for heparin-induced thrombocytopenia (91[C]).

There has been some discussion that edetate, as a reagent red cell diluent, may on rare occasions cause *inhibition of anti-A1 (of the ABO system) antibodies*, but the case has not yet been settled (92[C], 93[R]).

Urea-EDTA

Urea-EDTA (with methylhexyl ether) was used without side effects for the dissolution of calcified gallbladder stones in 2 patients (94[c]).

REFERENCES

1. Van Deursen CTBM, Goey SH, Fickers MMF (1988) Maintenance treatment with desferrioxamine via subcutaneous injections in a patient with HbE thalassaemia. *Neth. J. Med., 33,* 178.
2. Fucharoen S, Rowley PT, Paul NW et al (1988) (Eds.) *Thalassemia: Pathophysiology and Management. Birth Defects: Original Article Series, Vol. 23, No. 5B.* Alan R. Liss, New York.
3. Miehlke K. (1988) D-Penicillamin – ein Rückblick. *Z. Rheumatol., 47, Suppl. 1,* 3.
4. Spector TD, Thompson PW, Evans SJW, Scott DL (1988) Are slow-acting antirheumatic drugs being given earlier in rheumatoid arthritis? *Br. J. Rheumatol., 27,* 498.
5. Kashiwazaki S (1988) Current status of D-penicillamine therapy in Japan. *Z. Rheumatol., 47, Suppl. 1,* 38.
6. Stephens AD (1988) Cystinuria and its treatment: 25 years experience at St. Bartholomew's Hospital. *J. Inherit. Metab. Dis., 12,* 197.
7. Jaeger P (1989) Cystinuria: pathophysiology and treatment. *Adv. Nephrol., 18,* 107.
8. Horoupain DS, Sternlieb I, Scheinberg IH (1988) Neuropathological findings in penicillamine-treated patients with Wilson's disease. *Clin. Neuropathol., 7,* 62.
9. Bignon J, Jaubert F, Laurent P (1987) Les bronchiolites obstructives. *Rev. Mal. Respir., 4,* 199.
10. Camus Ph (1988) A propos des bronchiolites oblitérantes. *Rev. Mal. Respir., 5,* 193.
11. Sweatman MC, Markwick JR, Charles PJ et al (1986) Histocompatibility antigens in adult obliterative bronchiolitis with or without rheumatoid arthritis. *Dis. Markers, 4,* 19.
12. Lagier F, Cartier A, Dolovich J, Malo J.-L (1989) Occupational asthma in a pharmaceutical worker exposed to penicillamine. *Thorax, 44,* 157.
13. Tzartos SJ, Morel E, Efthimiadis A et al (1988) Fine antigenic specificities of antibodies in sera from patients with D-penicillamine-induced myasthenia gravis. *Clin Exp. Immunol., 74,* 80.
14. Paladini G, Mazzanti G, Mysco G et al (1988) La sindrome miastenica indotta da D-penicillamina nell'artite reumatoide: caratteri clinici e genetic. *Reumatismo, 40,* 139.
15. Holdrinet RSG, Namdar Z, Haanen C (1988) Thrombotic thrombocytopenic purpura: clinical course and response to therapy in twelve patients. *Neth. J. Med. 33,* 113.
16. Hammond WP, Miller JE, Starkebaum G et al (1988) Suppression of in vitro granulocytopoiesis by captopril and penicillamine. *Exp. Hematol., 16,* 674.
17. Larusso NF, Wiesner RH, Ludwig J et al (1988) Prospective trial of penicillamine in primary sclerosing cholangitis. *Gastroenterology, 95,* 1036.
18. Shannon M, Graef J, Lovejoy FH (1988) Efficacy and toxicity of D-penicillamine in low-level lead poisoning. *J. Pediatr., 112,* 799.
19. Seppälä E, Lehtinen K, Isomäki H et al (1988) Effect of long-term aurothiomalate and D-penicillamine treatments on renal function and urinary excretion of prostanoids in patients with rheumatoid arthritis. *Int. J. Clin. Pharmacol. Res., 8,* 149.
20. Emery P, Panayi G (1988) Penicillamine nephropathy. *Br. Med. J., 296,* 1538.
21. Hall CL, Tighe R (1989) The effect of continuing penicillamine and gold treatment on the course of penicillamine and gold nephropathy. *Br. J. Rheumatol., 28,* 53.
22. Boers M, Croonen AM, Dijkmans BAC et al (1987) Renal findings in rheumatoid arthritis: clinical aspects of 132 autopsies. *Ann. Rheum. Dis., 46,* 658.
23. Cahen R, François B, Trolliet P et al (1989) Aetiology of membraneous glomerulonephritis: a prospective study of 82 adult patients. *Nephrol. Dial. Transplant., 4,* 172.
24. Bachman H, Löszner J, Biesold D et al (1988) Aktuelle Erfahrungen und Probleme mit der Langzeitbetreuung von Patienten mit Wilsonscher Erkrankung in der DDR. *Z. Ärztl. Fortbild., 82,* 297.
25. Pasquali Ronchetti I, Quaglino D, Baccarani Contri M et al (1989) Dermal alterations in patients with Wilson's disease treated with D-penicillamine. *J. Submicrosc. Cytol. Pathol., 21,* 131.
26. Goldstein JB, Scott McNutt N, Hambrick GW, Hsu A (1989) Penicillamine dermatopathy with lymphangiectases. *Arch. Dermatol., 125,* 92.
27. Dubost JJ, Fraysse P, Ristori JM, Rampon S (1988) Syndrome des ongles jaunes avec dilatation des bronches après traitement d'une polyarthrite

rhumatoïde par la D-pénicillamine. *Sem. Hôp., 64,* 1548.

28. Buckly C, Barry C, Woods R et al (1988) Penicillamine induced pemphigus – a report of 2 cases. *Ir. J. Med. Sci., 157,* 267.
29. Aydemir EH, Isçimen A, Aksoy F (1988) D-Penisilamin'e bagli eritem anuler benzeri pemfigus. *Deri Hast. Frengi Ars., 22,* 247.
30. Civatte J (1989) Durch Medikamente induzierte Pemphigus-Erkrankungen. *Dermatol. Monatsschr., 175,* 1.
31. Shannon M, Graef J, Lovejoy FH (1988) Efficacy and toxicity of D-penicillamine in low-level lead poisoning. *J. Pediatr., 112,* 799.
32. Craig HR (1988) Penicillamine induced mammary hyperplasia: report of a case and review of the literature. *J. Rheumatol., 15,* 1294.
33. Lipsky PE (1988) Suggested mode of action of D-penicillamine as an immunosuppressive agent in rheumatoid arthritis. *Z. Rheumatol., 47, Suppl. 1,* 6.
34. Matsubara T, Saura R, Hirohata K, Ziff M (1989) Inhibition of human endothelial cell proliferation in vitro and neovascularization in vivo by D-penicillamine. *J. Clin. Invest., 83,* 158.
35. Matsubara T, Hirohata K (1988) Suppression of human fibroblast proliferation by D-penicillamine and copper sulfate in vitro. *Arthritis Rheum., 31,* 964.
36. Sim E, Dodds AW, Goldin A (1989) Inhibition of the covalent binding reaction of complement component C4 by penicillamine, an anti-rheumatic agent. *Biochem. J., 259,* 415.
37. Sim E (1989) Drug-induced immune-complex disease. *Complement Inflammation, 6,* 119.
38. Thoen J, Helgetveit K, Førre Ø et al (1988) Effects of piroxicam and D-penicillamine on T lymphocyte subpopulations, natural killer cells and rheumatoid factor production in rheumatoid arthritis. *Scand. J. Rheumatol., 17,* 91.
39. Haberhauer G, Bröll H (1989) Drug-induced anticentromere antibody? *Z. Rheumatol., 48,* 99.
40. Haberhauer G (1989) D-Penicillamine (DPA)-induced anticentromere antibody (ACA). *Int. J. Rheum. Connect. Tissue Dis., 7,* 332.
41. Storch WB (1988) Clinical significance of penicillamine antibodies. *Lancet, 2,* 214.
42. Storch W, Keitel W (1988) Antikörper gegen D-Penicillamin bei Patienten met chronischer Polyarthritis – diagnostische Hilfe unerwünschter und ungenügender Arzneimittelwirkung? *Z. Rheumatol., 47, Suppl. 1,* 44.
43. Savill JS, Chia Y, Pusey CD (1988) Minimal change nephropathy and pemphigus vulgaris associated with penicillamine treatment of rheumatoid arthritis. *Clin. Nephrol., 29,* 267.
44. Pachoula-Papasteriades C, Boki K, Varla-Leftherioti M et al (1986) HLA-A, -B and -DR antigens in relation to gold and D-penicillamine toxicity in Greek patients with RA. *Dis. Markers, 4,* 35.
45. Skopouli FN, Andonopoulos AP, Moutsopoulos HM (1988) Clinical implications of the presence of anti-Ro (SSA) antibodies in patients with rheumatoid arthritis. *J. Autoimmunity, 3,* 381.
46. Pall HS, Williams AC, Blake DR (1989) Deterioration of Wilson's disease following the start of penicillamine therapy. *Arch. Neurol., 46,* 359.
47. Zacher J, Spath S, Wessinghage D, Waertel G (1988) Basistherapie der chronisch-entzündlichen Gelenkerkrankungen met D-Penicillamin und Wundheilungsstörungen bei rheumaorthopädischen Eingriffen. *Z. Rheumatol., 47, Suppl. 1,* 41.
48. Greene MW, King RC, Alley RS (1988) Management of an oroantral fistula in a patient with Wilson's disease: case report and review of the literature. *Oral Surg. Oral Med. Oral Pathol., 66,* 293.
49. Miehle W (1988) Aktuelles zu D-Penicillamin und Schwangerschaft. *Z. Rheumatol., 47, Suppl. 1,* 20.
50. Schulze E, Herrmann K, Haustein U-F et al (1988) Einfluss von Penicillin und D-Penicillamin auf die Beta-galactosidaseaktivität bei Patienten met progressiver Sklerodermie. *Dermatol. Monatsschr., 174,* 661.
51. Whitehouse DB, Lovegrove JU, Hopkinson DA (1959) Variation in alpha-1-antitrypsin phenotypers associated with penicillamine therapy. *Clin. Chim. Acta, 179,* 109.
52. Faguer de Moustier B, Burgard M, Boitard C et al (1988) Syndrome hypoglycémique auto-immun induit par le pyritinol. *Diabète Métab., 14,* 423.
53. Sigaud M, Maugars Y, Maisonneuve H, Prost A (1988) Tiopronine dans 69 cas de polyarthrite rhumatoïde traités antérieurement par la D-pénicillamine. *Rev. Rhum. 55,* 467.
54. Amor B, Mery C, De Gery A (1988) L'acadione, un nouveau traitement de fond de la polyarthrite rhumatoïde. *Rev. Rhum., 55,* 462.
55. Meunier J, Krause E, Guillot B et al (1988) Pemphigus induit par l'alphamercaptopropionylglycine. *Presse Méd., 17,* 647.
56. Menkes CJ, Job-Deslander C, Bauer-Vinassac D et al (1988) Myasthénie induite par la tiopronine au cours du traitement de la polyarthrite rhumatoïde. *Presse Méd., 17,* 1156.
57. Kawabe Y, Mizuno N, Yoshikawa K, Matsumoto Y (1988) Lichenoid eruption due to mercaptoprionylglycine. *J. Dermatol., 15,* 434.
58. Komura A, Tamaki (1988) Clinical analysis of drug allergy due to tiopronin. *Skin Res., 30, Suppl. 4,* 197.
59. Matsueda K, Matsuoka Y, Mizuno M et al (1988) A case of drug-induced toxic epidermal necrolysis complicated with severe liver injury. *Acta Hepat. Jpn., 29,* 949.
60. Kruck TPA, Teichert-Kuliszewska K, Fisher E, Kalow W (1988) High-performance liquid chromatographic analysis of desferrioxamine, pharmacokinetic and metabolic studies. *J. Chromatogr., 433,* 207.
61. Allain P, Chaleil D, Mauras Y et al (1988) Pharmacokinetics of desferrioxamine and of its iron

and aluminum chelates in patients on peritoneal dialysis. *Clin. Chim. Acta, 173,* 313.
62. Llados i Vallory EA, Girot R, Lenoir G et al (1989) Studies of variations of subcutaneously infused desferrioxamine and iron movements in thalassaemia children. *Eur. J. Pediatr., 148,* 503.
63. McCarthy JT, Kurtz SB, Mussman GV (1987) Deferoxamine-enhanced fecal losses of aluminum and iron in a patient undergoing continuous ambulatory peritoneal dialysis. *Am. J. Med., 82,* 367.
63a. Tielemans C, Lenclud C (1988) Respective role of haemosiderosis and desferrioxamine therapy in the risk from infection of haemodialysed patients. *Q. J. Med., 255,* 573.
64. Hoen B, Renoult E, Jonon B, Kessler M (1988) Septicemia due to *Yersinia enterocolitica* in a long-term hemodialysis patient after a single desferrioxamine administration. *Nephron, 50,* 378.
65. Masters AP, Hopkinson RB (1988) *Yersinia enterocolitica* septicaemia. *Intens. Care Med., 14,* 585.
66. Hadjiminas JM (1988) Yersiniosis in acutely iron-loaded children treated with desferrioxamine. *J. Antimicrob. Chemother., 21,* 680.
67. Kouides PA, Slapak CA, Rosenwasser LJ, Miller KB (1988) *Pneumocystis carinii* pneumonia as a complication of desferrioxamine therapy. *Br. J. Haematol., 70,* 383.
68. Boelaert JR, Van Roost GF, Vergauwe PL et al (1988) The role of desferrioxamine in dialysis-associated mucormycosis: report of three cases and review of the literature. *Clin. Nephrol., 29,* 261.
69. Johnson EV, Kline LB, Julian BA, Garcia JH (1988) Bilateral cavernous sinus thrombosis due to mucormycosis. *Arch. Ophthalmol., 106,* 1089.
70. Sombolos K, Kalekou H, Barboutis K, Tzarou V (1988) Fatal phycomycosis in a hemodialyzed patient receiving deferoxamine. *Nephron, 49,* 169.
71. Sane A, Manzi S, Perfect J et al (1989) Deferoxamine treatment as a risk factor for zygomycete infection. *J. Infect. Dis., 159,* 151.
72. Nakamura M, Weil WB, Kaufman DB (1989) Fatal fungal peritonitis in an adolescent on continuous ambulatory peritoneal dialysis: association with deferoxamine. *Pediatr. Nephrol., 3,* 80.
73. Rex JH, Ginsberg AM, Fries LF et al (1988) *Cunninghamella bertholletiae* infection associated with deferoxamine therapy. *Rev. Infect. Dis., 10,* 1187.
74. Boelaert JR, Fenves AZ, Coburn JW (1989) Mucormycosis among patients on dialysis. *N. Engl. J. Med., 321,* 190.
75. Sherrard DJ, Walker JV, Boykin JL (1988) Precipitation of dialysis dementia by deferoxamine treatment of aluminum-related bone disease. *Am. J. Kidney Dis., 12,* 126.
76. Altmann P, Dhanesha U, Hamon C et al (1989) Disturbance of cerebral function by aluminium in haemodialysis patients without overt aluminium toxicity. *Lancet, 2,* 7.
77. Wonke B, Hoofbrand AV, Aldouri M et al (1989) Reversal of desferrioxamine induced auditory neurotoxicity during treatment with Ca-DPTA. *Arch. Dis. Child., 64,* 77.
78. Albera R, Pia F, Morra B et al (1988) Hearing loss and desferrioxamine in homozygous beta-thalassemia. *Audiology, 27,* 207.
79. Masala W, Meloni F, Gallisai D et al (1988) Can deferoxamine be considered an ototoxic drug? *Scand. Audiol., Suppl. 30,* 237.
80. Bene C, Manzler A, Bene D, Kranias G (1989) Irreversible ocular toxicity from single 'challenge' dose of deferoxamine. *Clin. Nephrol., 31,* 45.
81. Pall H, Blake DR, Winyard P et al (1989) Ocular toxicity of desferrioxamine – an example of copper promoted auto-oxidative damage? *Br. J. Ophthalmol., 73,* 42.
82. Kaplinsky C, Stark B, Goshen Y et al (1988) Deferoxamine (desferal)-induced ocular toxicity. *Pediatr. Hematol. Oncol., 5,* 1293.
82a. Hamed LM, Winward KE, Glaser JS, Schatz NJ (1989) Optic neuropathy in uremia. *Am. J. Ophthalmol., 108,* 30.
83. Venencie P-Y, Rain B, Blanc A, Tertian G (1988) Toxidermie à la déféroxamine (Desféral). *Ann. Dermatol. Venereol., 115,* 1174.
84. Klebanoff SJ, Waltersdorph AM (1988) Inhibition of peroxidase-catalyzed reactions by deferoxamine. *Arch. Biochem. Biophys., 264,* 600.
85. Rice-Evans C, Baysal E, Kontoghiorghes GJ et al (1985) Oxidative effects of iron on erythrocytes. *Free Radicals Res. Commun., 1,* 55.
86. Barradas MA, Jeremy JY, Kontoghioghes GJ et al (1989) Iron chelators inhibit human platelet aggregation, thromboxane A2 synthesis and lipoxygenase activity. *FEBS Lett., 245,* 105.
87. Weitberg AB, Corvese D (1989) Hydroxy- and hydroperoxy-6,8,11,14-eicosatetraenoic acids induce DNA strand breaks in human lymphocytes. *Carcinogenesis, 10,* 1029.
88. Baker DL, Manno CS (1988) Rapid excretion of gallium-67 isotope in an iron-overloaded patient receiving high-dose intravenous deferoxamine. *Am. J. Hematol., 29,* 230.
89. Vicari A, Banfi G, Bonini PA (1988) EDTA-dependent pseudothrombocytopaenia: a 12-month epidemiological study. *Scand. J. Clin. Lab. Invest., 48,* 537.
90. Hoyt RH, Durie BGM (1989) Pseudothrombocytopenia induced by a monoclonal IgM Kappa platelet agglutinin. *Am. J. Hematol., 31,* 50.
91. Perrier JF, Nace L, Mariot J et al (1988) Pseudothrombopénie en présence d'EDTA évoquant une thrombopénie à l'héparine. *Réanim. Soins Intens. Méd. Urg., 4,* 313.
92. Tedrow HE, Zeigler ZR (1988) Evidence of anti-A1 inhibited by EDTA. *Transfusion, 28,* 177.
93. Judd WJ, Barnes BA (1989) EDTA-saline and ABO system antibodies. *Transfusion, 29,* 84.
94. Swobodnik W, Baumgaertel H, Janowitz P et al (1988) Dissolution of calcified gallbladder stones by treatment with methylhexyl ether and urea-EDTA. *Lancet, 2,* 216.

G. Reybrouck

25 Antiseptic drugs and disinfectants

ALCOHOLS *(SED-11, 474; SEDA-12, 201)*

Benzyl alcohol *(SED-11, 475; SEDA-12, 201)*

In 1982 the FDA recommended that bacteriostatic saline and water (i.e. containing benzyl alcohol as a preservative) should not be used as intravascular flush solutions nor as diluents for medications in newborn infants.

Jardine and Rogers (1^{Cr}) reviewed the hospital and autopsy records of infants admitted to a nursery during the prior 18 months in whom fluids containing benzyl alcohol were used as flush solutions to clear intravascular lines (218 patients) and compared them with those of neonati admitted during the following 18 months (232 patients). Exposure to benzyl alcohol was significantly associated with the development of *kernicterus* (15 patients out of 49 exposed to benzyl alcohol, no cases after benzyl alcohol were withdrawn) and *intraventricular hemorrhage*. Withdrawal of benzyl alcohol from clinical use had no demonstrable effect on mortality.

The toxicity of benzyl alcohol in neonates is mainly related to an excessive body burden relative to weight, but the load of benzoic acid, the metabolite of benzyl alcohol, may exceed the capacity of the immature liver or kidney for detoxification, especially in pre-term newborns (2^{C}).

ALDEHYDES *(SED-11, 476; SEDA-12, 202)*

Formaldehyde *(SED-11, 476; SEDA-12, 202)*

Side Effects of Drugs Annual 14
M.N.G. Dukes and L. Beeley, editors

Donahue and Frank (3^{R}) identified in an extensive search of the literature 235 cases of intractable hemorrhagic cystitis treated with *intravesical* formalin (37% formaldehyde solution) (SEDA-9, 225).

Increasing concentration of formalin slightly improved the effectiveness of therapy: the 10%, 5% and 1% formalin solutions had complete response rates of 83%, 78% and 71%, respectively. The average duration of complete response before recurrence of bleeding was 3 to 4 months. The recurrence rate showed a gradual decrease with higher concentrations of formalin. Minor complications (mild or transient problems not requiring surgical intervention) included fever, tachycardia, transient or minor elevations of blood urea nitrogen or creatinine, mild hydronephrosis, grades I and II vesicoureteral reflux, frequency, urgency, incontinence, suprapubic pain or a decrease in bladder capacity not requiring urinary diversion. These minor complications appeared to be related directly to the concentration of formalin used: 10% formalin had a 2-fold increase in minor complication rate compared to 5% formalin and a 5-fold increase compared to 1% formalin. Major complications were defined as those requiring surgical intervention, resulting in the loss of renal function or inducing damage to the supravesical urinary tracts (stricture formation). They included anuria, acute tubular necrosis, papillary necrosis, ureteral or retroperitoneal fibrosis, ureterovesical or ureteropelvic junction obstruction, severe hydronephrosis, grades III and IV vesicoureteral reflux, any vesical fistula or a decrease in bladder capacity requiring urinary diversion. Major complications occurred in all treatment groups, including those treated with 1% formalin. The higher rate observed with 10% formalin was not significantly different from that with 5% or 1% formalin. The mortality rates were 2.2% for the 5% formalin groups and 5.7% for the 10%, but they are not significantly different.

A 10% formalin solution resulted in a higher 'complete and favorable response' rate, a lower 'recurrence rate', equal 'major complication and mortality' rates and a 3-fold higher 'minor complication' rate than 5% formalin in patients whose hemorrhagic cystitis was due to radiotherapy for bladder tumor. In contrast, 5% formalin was more effective than the 10% solution in treating patients with intractable hematuria due to unresectable bladder tumors or cyclophosphamide cystitis.

Glutaraldehyde *(SED-11, 478; SEDA-12, 202)*

Jonas et al (4[C]) observed a unique form of *colitis* during endoscopy of the lower gastrointestinal tract in 21 patients. They were found to have discrete or confluent white plaques adherent to the colonic mucosa, mild to severe erythema of the surrounding mucosa, and variable amounts of foamy liquid upon withdrawal of the endoscope. Some patients developed rectal bleeding, tenesmus, and increased frequency of stools, lasting up to 12 days. The authors believe that these cases were due to chemical exposure to residual endoscope cleaning solution in the air-water channel. Most cases occurred where hydrogen peroxide was used for endoscope cleaning (before disinfection with 2% glutaraldehyde was introduced): there are many similarities with reported cases of colitis caused by enemas containing hydrogen peroxide. One case, however, was encountered after hydrogen peroxide was no longer used. This raises the possibility that glutaraldehyde may have been the responsible agent causing a chemical colitis similar to that induced by hydrogen peroxide.

CHLORHEXIDINE *(SED-11, 480; SEDA-12, 202; SEDA-13, 206)*

Chlorhexidine gluconate (CHX) is widely used over the world as a medical disinfectant and it is generally safe. Care should be taken during preoperative preparation of the facial skin to keep CHX out of the eye (5[c]). If CHX is accidentally introduced into the eye, it should be flushed copiously with sterile saline solution or water. Even then epithelial defects of the cornea and *corneal opacification* can develop.

Allergic adverse reactions to CHX such as contact dermatitis, contact urticaria and photosensitive dermatitis are relatively rare. Okano et al (6[Cr]) described 6 patients who developed life-threatening *anaphylactic reactions* (generalized *urticaria, dyspnea, shock*) after the use of 0.5% or 1% (in one case 0.05%) CHX. Using intradermal, scratch and epicutaneous tests, CHX was confirmed as the causative agent of the hypersensitivity. The authors also summarize previous information on adverse reactions to CHX reported to the Japanese Ministry of Welfare from 1967 to 1984: the records included 22 cases with a fall in blood pressure, 13 with dyspnea, 9 with anaphylactic shock, 4 with cyanosis; 19 cases showed erythema, 11 urticaria, 9 pruritus, 7 facial wheals. In 1984 the Japanese Ministry of Welfare recommended that the use of CHX on mucous membranes be prohibited because of the evidence that this application can provoke anaphylactic shock. Application of CHX to wound surfaces appears to be safe, but it should be used at the lowest bactericidal concentration (0.05%).

ETHYLENE OXIDE *(SED-11, 479; SEDA-12, 202)*

Watschinger et al (7[C]) evaluated the presence of antibodies against ethylene oxide (EO) which is used for sterilization of dialysers. By means of a radio-allergo-sorbent-test (RAST) only 2 out of 52 hemodialysis patients were found to exhibit EO antibodies. There was, however, no significant correlation between these EO antibodies (2/52) and eosinophilia (11/52), IgE elevation (8/52) or symptoms of hypersensitivity (20/52) during the 624 dialyses performed in these patients. The reasons for these findings may be thorough rinsing and sufficiently long storage time of the dialysers.

IODOPHORS *(SED-11, 487; SEDA-12, 203; SEDA-13, 207)*

Povidone-iodine *(SED-11, 487; SEDA-12, 203; SEDA-13, 207)*

It is generally accepted that povidone-iodine (polyvinyl-pyrrolodine-iodine, PVP-I) is relatively non-toxic and non-irritating to tissues. It has been advocated for local application to prevent wound sepsis following surgery, and although a significant reduction in wound infection has been observed by some workers, Eggert and Baumann (8[c]) found in a study of 91 appendectomized patients an increase of the postoperative *wound infection* rate from 8% to 26% after the intraoperative application of 2% PVP-I (10–20 ml instilled in the wound before the opening and after the closing of the peritoneum). Tissue toxicity was found to outweigh bactericidal effect. Another side effect is the development of polyvinylpyrrolidone *thesaurismosis* in the vicinity of postoperative fistulae, irrigated for an extended period by diluted PVP-I (9[C]).

Skin disinfection with PVP-I in obstetrics results in iodide overload of the mother due to cutaneous absorption of iodine. Iodide readily crosses the placenta and is actively concentrated in the mammary gland. Consequently, newborn infants born to mothers who have undergone an epidural anesthesia or a cesarean section requiring disinfection with PVP-I are exposed to iodine overload, especially if breastfed. Infants born to exposed mothers had a shift of thyroid-stimulating hormone towards high values on the 5th day of life (10[C]). This shift is much more important in the case of breast-feeding: there is a 25- to 30-fold increase in the recall rate at screening for congenital hypothyroidism in the breast-fed infants, whereas in bottle-fed infants the recall rate was barely modified. The use of PVP-I in mothers at deliverly unnecessarily increases the recall rate and consequently the cost of the screening and the stress on families. It can result in a mild and transient *Wolff-Chaikoff effect* in the infant (11[c]). It must be remembered that the premature infant is at higher risk for developing PVP-I-induced hypothyroidism, and that an infant with omphalocele is particularly susceptible, because the area for absorption is large and composed of easily permeable membranes (12[Cr]).

Even in adults absorption of iodine occurs, especially if the skin barrier is no longer intact. Rath et al (13[Cr]) reported 2 burn patients with apparently normal thyroid glands who developed *hyperthyroidism* after topical treatment with PVP-I, whereas about 150 other patients have been treated without any complications.

In a 34-year-old male with an 80% body surface area (BSA) burn, 1% PVP-I ointment was applied on an area of 36% BSA for 6 weeks. PVP-I was first applied on the burn eschar and after necrectomy on granulation tissue without any coverage by skin or skin substitutes; closed treatment of the burn wounds was used and PVP-I was applied once a day. The patient developed clinical signs of hyperthyroidism, i.e. agitation, tachycardia and no increase in weight in spite of adequate nutritional support. The effective thyroxine ratio (ETR) was 1.29 (normal range 0.87–1.12) and the total thyroxine (T4) 13.5 μg/dl (normal 4.3–13.3 μg/dl); the total triiodothyronine (T3) was within the normal range. Subsequent determinations of ETR and T4 1 week after the end of the PVP-I application and during treatment with methimazole revealed normal values.

Campistol et al (14[Cr]) described a patient with a suppurative mediastinitis treated with continuous PVP-I irrigation who developed an acute *oliguric renal failure*.

A 63-year-old woman developed mediastinitis 12 days after a triple coronary artery bypass graft with saphenous vein. A closed system of continuous mediastinal irrigation with 0.1% PVP-I at a rate of 10 l a day was instituted; 12 days after the re-exploration, a recurrence of the purulent discharge was observed, and the infected sternum was removed, leaving the wound packet with sterile gauze impregnated with PVP-I. About 4 weeks after this 3rd operation, the patient began to develop progressive decrease of urinary output (<300 ml/24 h) with concomitant increase of creatinine to 5.4 mg/dl (at the time of the last intervention still 1.1 mg/dl) and blood urea nitrogen (BUN) to 118 mg/dl (previously 25 mg/dl). There was no proteinuria and the sediment was normal. The patient began an effective diuresis 40 hours after the treatment was started (furosemide 500 mg/24 h and saline solutions) and the PVP-I application was discontinued, and creatinine and BUN decreased to normal levels. Unfortunately serum iodine concentration could not be determined.

It must be remembered that aqueous solutions of PVP-I, like many other disinfectants and antiseptics (SEDA-9, 228), can be contaminated by *Pseudomonas* sp., usually *P. cepacia* or *P. aeruginosa*, and that these solutions can cause infections or pseudoinfections (15[c]).

PARABENS *(SED-11, 484)*

Parabens (4-hydroxybenzoic acid alkyl esters) are the most widely used preservatives in topical medicaments and cosmetics. They are certainly present in some thousands of preparations (16[c]). Their sensitization potential is low; about 1% of eczema patients react to a paraben mixture in patch tests. This frequency is confirmed once more in a study of 8020 consecutive patients of a dermatological clinic (17[Cr]): 76 patients showed positive patch tests to the paraben mixture; retesting with the individual esters showed a positive reaction to methylparaben in 25 cases, ethylparaben in 23, propylparaben in 21, butylparaben in 30 and benzylparaben in 12 patients.

PEROXIDES *(SEDA-12, 203)*

Hydrogen peroxide *(SEDA-11, 221; SEDA-12, 203)*

Hydrogen peroxide solution has been shown to be active against the human immunodeficiency virus and therefore has been recommended as a disinfectant for tonometer tips, other ophthalmic instruments and trial contact lenses (18).

Pogrebniak and Sugar (19[c]) described the case of a circular *corneal epithelial defect* caused by the contact with a tonometer; the tip had been left soaking in a 3% hydrogen peroxide solution, but the solution had evaporated overnight, and the tonometer tip had not been rinsed prior to use. The usual 3% solution, however, seemed to be safe and drops of 3% hydrogen peroxide caused no reaction when placed directly on the cornea of rabbits, nor did the tonometer tips taken directly from fresh 3% hydrogen peroxide without rinsing. Nevertheless, the tips taken from a solution that had evaporated overnight caused the same marked reaction as in the patient. The reason why the tip became toxic is unclear. It is advisable to rinse ophthalmic instruments before use in order to dilute or remove potential toxins.

QUATERNARY AMMONIUM COMPOUNDS *(SED-11, 489)*

Benzalkonium chloride *(SED-11, 489)*

Paradoxical *bronchoconstriction* may occur following inhalation of nebulizer solutions in which benzalkonium chloride is present as a preservative. When ipratropium bromide nebulizer solution alone was administered, bronchodilation occurred in subjects who had previously developed marked bronchoconstriction with the ipratropium bromide solution containing benzalkonium chloride. Miszkiel et al (20[C]) demonstrated that the initial bronchoconstrictor effect of benzalkonium chloride is due, in part, to histamine release. The bulk of the adverse effect, however, relates to a different, as yet unrecognized mechanism.

Cetrimide *(SED-11, 490)*

A dilute antiseptic solution containing 0.05% chlorhexidine and 1% cetrimide was accidentally fed, in place of sterile water, to 5 normal breast-fed babies, 4 born on the previous day and one 6 days before (21[Cr]). They developed *caustic burns* of the lips, mouth and tongue within minutes and became fretful and restless. The baby most severely affected became severely ill due to acute *pulmonary edema* associated with prominent oral frothing. There was no evidence of any CNS depression or excitation, nor of hepatotoxicity or nephrotoxicity. It is likely that the symptoms were mainly due to the caustic nature of 1% cetrimide and that the dose ingested was negligible. All survived without sequelae.

OTHER ANTISEPTICS

Mahaur et al (22[C]) studied the prevalence of contact sensitivity to antiseptics and topical antibiotics in 200 individuals, including 127 apparently normal persons and 73 patients with non-eczematous minor dermatoses. None of them showed a positive patch test to Savlon (0.1% chlorhexidine, 0.5% cetrimide); 1 individual in the normal group and 1 patient in the 'minor-dermatoses' group reacted to Dettol (4.8% chloroxylenol, 9% terpineol), the same numbers to 1% mercurochrome, and 1 patient in the dermatoses group to Piodin and to Betadine (both PVP-I; it could not be deduced whether it was the same patient). The most frequent sensitizing substance in the battery, apart from the antibiotics, was benzoic acid (5 cases in the normal group and 8 in the minor-dermatoses group; 6.5% of the individuals tested): this is a fairly high frequency.

REFERENCES

1. Jardine DS, Rogers K (1989) Relationship of benzyl alcohol to kernicterus, intraventricular hemorrhage, and mortality in preterm infants. *Pediatrics, 83*, 153.
2. LeBel M, Ferron L, Masson M et al (1988) Benzyl alcohol metabolism and elimination in neonates. *Dev. Pharmacol. Ther., 11*, 347.
3. Donahue LA, Frank IN (1989) Intravesical formalin for hemorrhagic cystitis: analysis of therapy. *J. Urol., 141*, 809.
4. Jonas G, Mahoney A, Murray J, Gertler S (1988) Chemical colitis due to endoscope cleaning solutions: a mimic of pseudomembranous colitis. *Gastroenterology, 95*, 1403.
5. Tabor E, Bostwick DC, Evans CC (1989) Corneal damage due to eye contact with chlorhexidine gluconate. *J. Am. Med. Assoc., 261*, 557.
6. Okano M, Nomura M, Hata S et al (1989) Anaphylactic symptoms due to chlorhexidine gluconate. *Arch. Dermatol., 125*, 50.
7. Watschinger BH, Graf H, Kovarik J et al (1988) Äthylenoxidinduzierte Antikörper und Hypersensitivitätsreaktionen während Hämodialyse. *Wien. Med. Wochenschr., 138*, 110.
8. Eggert A, Baumann M (1988) Der Effekt von intraoperativer lokaler Polyvinylpyrrolidon-Jod-Applikation auf das Wundinfektionsrisiko nach Appendektomie. *Zentralbl. Chir., 113*, 391.
9. Balaton AJ, Vaury P, Vuong PN et al (1988) Fistules digestives persistantes: une forme inhabituelle de thésaurismose à la polyvinylpyrrolidone. *Arch. Anat. Cytol. Pathol., 36*, 23.
10. Chanoine JP, Boulvain M, Bourdoux P et al (1988) Increased recall rate at screening for congenital hypothyroidism in breast fed infants born to iodine overloaded mothers. *Arch. Dis. Child., 63*, 1207.
11. Clemens PC, Neumann RSJ (1989) The Wolff-Chaikoff effect: hypothyroidism due to iodine application. *Arch. Dermatol., 125*, 705.
12. Cosman BC, Schullinger JN, Bell JJ, Regan JA (1988) Hypothyroidism caused by topical povidone-iodine in a newborn with omphalocele. *J. Pediatr. Surg., 23*, 356.
13. Rath Th, Meissl G, Weissel M (1988) Induction of hyperthyroidism in burn patients treated topically with povidone-iodine. *Burns, 14*, 320.
14. Campistol JM, Abad C, Nogué S, Bertrán A (1988) Acute renal failure in a patient treated by continuous povidone-iodine mediastinal irrigation. *J. Cardiovasc. Surg., 29*, 410.
15. Centers for Disease Control (1989) Contaminated povidone-iodine solution – Texas. *Morbid. Mortal. Wkly Rep., 38*, 133.
16. Wilden I, Jorde W (1988) Farb- und Konservierungsstoffe als Auslöser (pseudo)-allergischer Reaktionen. *Allergologie, 11*, 321.
17. Menné T, Hjorth N (1988) Routine patch testing with paraben esters. *Contact Derm., 19*, 189.
18. Recommendations for preventing possible transmission of human T-lymphotropic virus type III/lymphadenopathy-associated virus from tears. *Morbid. Mortal. Wkly Rep., 34*, 533.
19. Pogrebniak AE, Sugar A (1988) Corneal toxicity from hydrogen peroxide-soaked tonometer tips. *Arch. Ophthalmol., 106*, 1505.
20. Miszkiel KA, Beasley R, Rafferty P, Holgate ST (1988) The contribution of histamine release to bronchoconstriction provoked by inhaled benzalkonium chloride in asthma. *Br. J. Clin. Pharmacol., 25*, 157.
21. Mucklow ES (1988) Accidental feeding of a dilute antiseptic solution (chlorhexidine 0.05% with cetrimide 1%) of five babies. *Hum. Toxicol., 7*, 567.
22. Mahaur BS, Sharma VK, Kumar B, Kaur S (1987) Prevalence of contact hypersensitivity to common antiseptics, antibacterials and antifungals in normal persons. *Indian J. Dermatol., Venereol. Leprol., 53*, 269.

T. Midtvedt

26 Penicillins, cephalosporins and tetracyclines

Go back for decision
All affairs
(The Qur'an, 35:4)

℞ The importance of post-marketing surveillance

Pivampicillin and carnitine deficiency *Pivampicillin has now been on the market for more than 15 years, and pivmecillinam for more than 5 years. These pivaloyl-oximethyl-esterified antibiotics are hydrolyzed in the body, and pivalic acid, formaldehyde and the β-lactam antibiotic in question are formed. Until recently, pivalic acid has been regarded as a harmless acid, rapidly excreted in the urine. However, there is no natural source of pivalic acid and, as has often happened before, a 'man-made' compound turns out to have biological effects which were neither anticipated nor at the time it was developed. The need for further investigations in patients receiving pivalic acid-containing antibiotics was underlined in a recent volume in this series (SEDA-12, 209). It has now been shown that short-term administration of pivampicillin and pivmecillinam – in the recommended doses – invariably results in a significant decrease of the serum carnitine concentration and an increase in the excretion of acylcarnitine in urine (1[c]). These changes were found to persist for more than 10 days after cessation of therapy. In 7 girls on long-term treatment with a mixture of pivampicillin and pivmecillinam the mean serum carnitine concentration fell to 15% (range 7–27%) or pre-treatment values. Muscle carnitine concentrations in 2 girls treated with the antibiotics for 22 and 30 months were only 10% of the mean reference value.*

The serum and muscle carnitine concentrations described here fall within the range encountered in patients with carnitine deficiencies of other etiologies in which life-threatening metabolic crises have been reported (2[c], 3[c]). However, it should be added that the degree of carnitine depletion at which symptoms arise is not known. Since the symptomatology of carnitine deficiency is vague, we need to watch out for adverse effects of these drugs, particularly during long-term treatment.

Several forms of carnitine deficiency have been described. In the present connection, primary or hereditary carnitine deficiency can be left out of consideration. Secondary carnitine deficiency, defined as an abnormally low concentration of carnitine in the serum and tissues, occurs in some forms of organic acidurias (2[c], 3[c]), in patients with the Fanconi syndrome (4[c]), in preterm infants (5[c]) and in some patients on chronic dialysis (3[c]). It seems most appropriate to compare the metabolic situation in pivampicillin- or pivmecillinam-treated patients with that in organic acidurias in which carnitine deficiency is caused by excretion of abnormal carnitine esters. In short-term treated patients, pivaloylcarnitine was the main metabolite in the urine, the quantities encountered representing about 35% recovery of the ingested pivalic acid.

Obviously, as the investigators concerned remark, 'it seems prudent to avoid the use of drugs that give rise to pivalic acid if there is a good alternative' (1[C]). However, the main lesson is far more serious. Pivampicillin had been on the market for some 20 years before it was found that carnitine metabolism was markedly influenced, and that the effect indeed occurred in all the patients so far investigated. Such a finding really underlines the necessity for better follow-up after new drugs have entered the market. The same

Side Effects of Drugs Annual 14
M.N.G. Dukes and L. Beeley, editors

lesson was learned as regards cephalosporins and their effect on vitamin K. Latamoxef had been on the market for a considerable time before it became obvious that bleeding disorders occurred in a high frequency, and cefoperazone had been extensively investigated world-wide before these complications were discovered (SEDA-12, 210).

The time has come to improve things – and there may be several ways of approaching this. The key word should be more co-operation and not more regulations. In his presidential address to the Infectious Disease Society of America, Dr. Baude proposed a 'joint venture' between the pharmaceutical industry and the academic infectious disease community and outlined the essentials of a 'nationwide institute for research and development' to promote research on antimicrobial drugs (6[R]). Unfortunately, the proposal has never been carried out.

An initiative taken by the World Health Organization in association with the National Institutes of Health in the United States, to evaluate various aspects of the world-wide usage of antibiotics was effectively thwarted by the pharmaceutical industry (SEDA 11, 222; SEDA-12, 206); the work seems to have stopped entirely once the various task force groups had completed their reports (7[r], 8[r], 10[r]-12[r]). Individual pharmaceutical companies as well as the pharmaceutical industry as a whole should surely accept their responsibility for encouraging the proper use of antimicrobial drugs. Instead of sending an increasing number of drug-prescribing doctors to the exotic places, where company-sponsored meetings are so often held nowadays, the pharmaceutical industry should put the money involved into research and development – including an extension of work on drugs already on the market. Of one thing I am certain: the industry cannot continue to behave in its present way until the cows come home.

In the case of pivalic acid it seems relatively easy to tell the pharmaceutical companies what has to be done. They should start by making it entirely clear to all doctors that, in every individual so far investigated, pivalic acid is excreted together with carnitine. Concomitantly, they should start investigations in patient groups supposedly at high risk for the development of carnitine deficiency. Until the results of these investigations are available, pivalic-acid-containing antibiotics should not be given to these groups. Adequate alternatives are of course at hand. Another thing of which I am certain: If the companies ignore the message about carnitine depletion in patients receiving pivampicillin or pivmecillinam and something happens in a patient at risk, they deserve to be the object of derision. Stupidity has always had its own price.

Immediate hypersensitivity reactions and cross-reactions to β-lactam antibiotics *(SEDA-13, 214)*

The first death from penicillin anaphylaxis was reported shortly after benzylpenicillin had been generally introduced. Since then, an overwhelming number of reports of hypersensitivity have appeared, described a variety of reactions to penicillins as well as to the newer classes of β-lactam antibiotics in clinical use, i.e. cephalosporins, monobactams and carbapenems. The following is by no means an attempt to review the present situation in its entirety; instead it will focus on the incidence of immediate hypersensitivity cross-reactions.

Almost everybody who receives a penicillin will develop specific IgG and IgM antibodies. These antibodies may cause so-called Type II and III reactions. Whether a reaction occurs or not depends upon the quality and quantity of antibody and the amount of antigen (drug) present in the patient. Because the specific factors involved in this course of events have not been determined, it is difficult to predict these reactions prospectively. The same holds true for Type IV reactions, i.e. contact dermatitis or delayed hypersensitivity, to penicillins.

Immediate hypersensitivity reactions to drugs are mediated by IgE antibodies. The reactions include IgE-dependent activation of mast cells and basophils with rapid release of vasoactive and bronchoactive mediators such as histamine, prostaglandins (D_2), leukotrienes (C_4) and platelet-activating factor, which together produce urticaria, laryngeal edema, bronchoconstriction and hypotension.

The incidence of such immediate reactions seems to be about 0.05%, with a mortality of 0.0002%, in all patients receiving penicillin (13[R]). The widespread use of penicillins has endowed a substantial number of subjects with the label 'allergic to penicillin'. However, it is only the risk of an anaphylactic reaction, insofar as *this can be predicted that comprises a major contradiction. Confirmation of IgE-related sensitization to penicillins may be obtained by standard skin-prick testing with a derivative of the so-called major determinant (benzylpenicillin polylysine) and the minor determinants including benzylpenicillin itself (13[R], 14[R], 15[r]). Only about 10% of patients with a history of 'penicillin allergy' have positive skin test results (13[R]). There seem to be very few false-negative results. One group quotes that 'we have yet to see a patient with a negative skin test develop an IgE-mediated penicillin reaction, and have done more than 1000 tests during the past ten years' (14[R]). Such data make the interpretation of an adequately performed skin test fairly straight-forward. The presence of a positive test means that a patient is at great risk of immediate hypersensitivity reactions whereas negative tests strongly predict a lack of any immediate hypersensitivity reaction.*

Shortly after cephalosporins had been introduced into clinical use, reports of anaphylaxis began to appear (16[c]). The chemical structure of cephalosporins and penicillins is similar, and the question of possible cross-reactions between these two groups of β-lactam antibiotics was soon brought forward. Initially, it was assumed that cephalosporins would have to be given with great care to patients with a history of penicillin allergy. However, it was soon realized that these first cephalosporins contained trace amounts of penicillin (17[c]). It is conceivable that early studies of cephalosporin and penicillin allergy may, because of such penicillin contamination have overestimated the degree of cross-reactivity.

An accurate determination of cephalosporin allergy awaits the definition of the haptenic determinants actually involved in the production of cephalosporin allergy. At present, there are no reliable test reagents. A positive or negative cefalotin skin test seems to provide little assistance in taking clinical decisions as to the choice of an antibiotic choice (14[R], 15[r]). After 25 years in clinical use, the most important risk factor to be considered in prescribing a cephalosporin is still a history of penicillin or cephalosporin allergy, and clinicians are well-advised to rely primarily upon their own common sense (18[c]).

The cross-reactivity of cephalosporins with penicillins has been studied in many animal systems. In a recent review, it was argued that these data suggest less cross-reactivity among cephalosporin derivatives than among penicillin derivatives, and that the data also indicate that the 'degree of cross-reactivity between cephalosporin derivatives is much greater than the degree of cross-reactivity between cephalosporins and penicillins' (14[R]). For humans, however, no exact figures can be given. At present, it must be accepted that the true incidence of clinical cross-reactivity between cephalosporins and penicillins awaits more accurate determination.

The monobactams contain only a monocyclic ring structure in contrast to the bicyclic ring contained in penicillins and cephalosporins. The prototype monobactam is aztreonam and this drug was originally judged 'to be a safe drug in patients allergic to penicillins or cephalosporins' (SEDA-10, 236). In a more recent report, 26 patients with IgE antibodies to penicillin determinants were treated with therapeutic doses of aztreonam (14[R]). No patient had a clinical reaction, none developed IgE antibodies to aztreonam detectable by solid-phase radio-immunoassay, and there was no rise in the levels of pre-existing antipenicillin antibodies. These data and further in vivo evidence of the lack of immune cross-reactivity between aztreonam and the penicillins. At least in experimental animals, anti-aztreonam antibodies are directed at the side-chain of the monobactam moiety. The new cephalosporin ceftazidime however has a side-chain identical to that of aztreonam. The possibility therefore exists that an individual allergic to aztreonam may react to ceftazidime, and vice versa. Furthermore, if monobactams with side-chains similar to that of a penicillin should be introduced, their safety in patients who are allergic to penicillins will have to be questioned.

Carbapenems, like penicillins, have a bicyclic nucleus comprising of β-lactam with an associated 5-member ring. The prototype is imipenem. In most of the initial clinical trials, patients with a history of serious β-lactam allergy were excluded (SEDA-10, 237), and the question about cross-reaction could not be adequately answered. Recently, imipenem determinants analogous to the penicillin determinants, have been synthesized and then tested, in a dose-dependent manner, in patients with and without IgG-dependent reactions to penicillin (14[R]). The results clearly show a high degree of immune cross-reactivity, justifying the conclusion that 'any patient who shows an IgE-mediated response to one or more of the penicillin determinants should be given im-

ipenem only under close observation and with the same degree of caution as if the patients were to receive penicillin' (14[R]).

Desensitization to β-lactams It is generally accepted that 'patients who had a strong history of penicillin anaphylaxis and who need penicillin for an overwhelming bacterial infection should be desensitised' (13[R]). However, the mechanism(s) responsible for the induction of clinical tolerance in such patients are not well-understood. The leading hypothesis is that the tolerance is induced by desensitization of IgE-laden blood basophils and tissue mast cells by low levels of circulating drug allergen (19[C], 20[C]). This hypothesis has been strongly challenged by some recent findings in a penicillin-allergic patient who required therapy with β-lactam antibiotics for osteomyelitis of the sternum (21[C]). After desensitization with increasing parenteral doses of penicillin G, the patient tolerated, without signs of allergic reactions, intravenous piperacillin. Concurrently, a long series of immunological studies were undertaken to investigate humoral and cellular changes accompanying desensitization process. Serum penicilloyl IgG and IgE antibodies did not change significantly during induction of clinical tolerance to the drug. The patient's previously positive immediate skin reaction to penicilloyl polylysine (PPL) converted to negative. Non-specific releasability of skin mast cells as determined using the polymyxin B skin test was unchanged. In contrast, in vitro blood basophil activation, by both specific antigen (penicilloyl-human albumin) and a non-specific IgE-dependent stimulus (anti-IgE) remained strong after the desensitization procedure and during some weeks of high-dose piperacillin therapy. A monovalent penicilloyl hapten inhibited penicilloyl-albumin-induced basophil histamine release, whereas the patient's own serum, obtained during piperacillin treatment, did not. Moreover, while the patient was receiving piperacillin, his serum was able to trigger histamine from passively sensitized basophils of a donor not allergic to penicillin, suggesting the presence of a sufficient amount of complete multivalent antigen to initiate release and/or desensitization. The presence of high concentrations of penicilloylated serum proteins in the patient's treatment serum was confirmed by immunoassay.

Basophil histamine release could, nevertheless, be elicited from the patient's whole blood sample taken during piperacillin treatment by adding penicilloyl-human albumin in vitro.

Taken together, these data clearly demonstrate that clinical tolerance (desensitization) to haptenic drugs such as penicillin is more complicated than was previously believed. The authors advance the suggestion that 'the conditions for cellular desensitization in mast cells and basophils may be fundamentally different in vivo. This could be due to different biochemical processes in the two cell types or to the protective effect of some serum factor that is not operating in the microenvironment of the skin mast cell.' Obviously, there is a need for further investigations in this important area of clinical immunology.

Neurotoxicity of β-lactam antibiotics The neurotoxic effect of benzylpenicillin was established as early as 1945 when the first case of myoclonic twitching following intravenous administration of the drug was reported (22[c]). Experimental studies confirmed the neurotoxicity of benzylpenicillin after intracisternal administration or application to the cerebral cortex of cats, monkeys and man (23[c]–25[c]). The first reports on benzylpenicillin neurotoxicity following intravenous administration appeared in the mid-1960s (26[C]–28[C]). Since then, reports of severe neurotoxic side effects of benzylpenicillin have continued to appear, mostly in patients with impaired renal function and patients undergoing open heart surgery with pulmonary bypass.

Several experimental studies have been undertaken to investigate the neurotoxic effects of other penicillin derivatives. In general, the results show that they all have neurotoxic effects, but that, with the possible exception of nafcillin, they are considerably less potent than benzylpenicillin (29[c]).

It became apparent at an early stage that the cephalosporins may also show neurotoxic manifestations after both intravenous and intrathecal administration (30[c]–32[c]). The neurotoxicity of cephalosporins was recently summarized in a report describing neurotoxic symptoms in 3 patients following intraventricular injection of cefazolin (33[C]). In general, the cephalosporins are looked upon as being less neurotoxic than benzylpenicillin.

This is in sharp contrast to the findings with imipenem. Seizures are observed in approximately 1% of the patients receiving imipenem (34[R]). In a retrospective study, covering 1754 patients treated with imipenem in phase III dose-ranging studies in the United States, a series of risk factors (CNS disorders, renal function, amount of drug received, and suchlike) were evaluated (35[R]). It was recommended that patients with certain diseases of the CNS should be treated with antibiotics other than imipenem unless the benefit clearly outweighs the risk of seizure. Patients with renal impairment clearly require dosage modification.

Although extensively studied, the pathogenesis of neurotoxic reactions to β-lactam antibiotics is still not clarified. It is generally held that the reactions result from alterations in synaptic transmission. At least for the penicillins, a possible mechanism may be excitation of the CNS neurons by a blockade of the synaptic activity of the inhibitory neurotransmitter, γ-aminobutyric acid (GABA), possibly at the GABA-receptor level (36[c]). Additionally, it has been found that various penicillins may bind to the benzodiazepine receptor in the brain (37[c]). The authors found a very good correlation between the affinity for the various penicillin derivatives for this receptor and their neurotoxicity, and they suggested that besides antagonism at the GABA receptor, antagonistic properties at the benzodiazepine receptor could be involved in the neurotoxicity of penicillins.

Obviously, there is a need for further research and new experimental models in order to clarify the relative neurotoxicity of the various groups of β-lactam antibiotics. A Swedish group has shown an electroencephalographic (EEG) model in rabbits to be a suitable and reproducible method for such comparative work (38[c]–42[c]). Defining neurotoxicity as epileptogenic EEG activity, they found that the mean doses of benzylpenicillin and imipenem precipitating such activity were 486 and 86 mg/kg respectively (41[c]). The neurotoxicity was related more closely to the antibiotic concentrations in the brain tissue fluid than to those in the cerebrospinal fluid. Utilizing the same EEG model in rats, the group has more recently demonstrated a pharmacokinetic interaction between benzylpenicillin and thiopental (42[c]). The most probable site of this interaction was claimed to be the organic acid transport system, which both drugs seem to use as a common transport system out of the CNS. In fact, the neurotoxic effects of penicillin (and most probably those of other β-lactam antibiotics as well) in patients undergoing surgery may be due to an interaction with the anesthetic drug used.

Regardless of the method employed, investigations of neurotoxicity in animals are time-consuming and expensive. In a recent study the effects of benzylpenicillin, cefuroxime, ceftazidime, ceftriaxone, amikacin and chloramphenicol on growth and differentiation of rat brain-cell cultures were followed (43[c]). Drug concentrations were chosen so as to represent peak values attained in the ventricular cerebrospinal fluid during intravenous therapy and their 5- and 10-times multiples that correspond to the concentration range reached by intraventricular antibiotic administration. Amikacin, cefuroxime and ceftazidime inhibited DNA synthesis and cerebral sulfate transferase activity at concentrations corresponding to the peak cerebrospinal fluid values attained by intraventricular therapy in patients.

Direct extrapolation of these in vitro results to the in vivo situation and to other species is obviously unrealistic. However, the method could represent an important screening method in the early assessment for neurotoxicity of newer antimicrobial agents. It might also be reasonable to 'suggest' that the clinical use of antimicrobial agents that produce significant inhibition of cell growth and differentiation in this brain cell culture model implies close monitoring for potential neurotoxicity, especially during intraventricular administration (43[c]).

Passage of penicillins in milk and possible consequences The increased permeability of penicillins into the CSF in patients with meningitis as a result of greater permeability is well known. To investigate whether comparable kinetic alterations occur when other organs are affected, the milk excretion of penicillin V (Pen V) was studied from both breasts in 12 patients with mastitis and in 4 healthy volunteers (44[C]). Maximum milk concentrations of Pen V in the 12 patients were significantly higher in mastitic than in non-mastitic breasts. The latter concentrations were significantly higher than those in breast milk from healthy controls. This suggests that in human subjects unlike in cows (45[c]), unilateral mastitis may have general pathophysiological implications. The mechanisms underlying these bilateral alterations are, however, not known.

The average infant dose of Pen V ingested during the first day of therapy was estimated to be 0.06, 0.05 and 0.04 mg/kg, respectively, if nursing from mastitic, non-mastitic and control breast milk. Although the penicillin dose ingested by the baby was very low, 3 out of 12 infants had looser fecal evacuations during maternal therapy. Additionally, one had a rash on the buttocks on the last day. Unfortunately, 'no controls of these observations were available' (44[C]). According to the authors, their findings justified 'breast-feeding during maternal penicillin treatment, unless the infant is hypersensitive to penicillin'.

In another study, the same group have reported milk concentrations in 6 mothers treated with pivampicillin for puerperal infections during the postpartum days 1–8 in the maternity ward (46[C]). However, only one of the patients had mastitis, and no controls were included. It was found that the breast-fed infants received less than 0.4% of the dose/kg given to the mother. Unfortunately, no further information was given about the babies, and any possible influence of pivampicillin upon carnitine metabolism (see earlier in this Chapter) was not studied. Bearing in mind these very recent findings concerning the pivalic acid part of the pivampicillin, it may be somewhat premature to conclude, as these investigators do, that 'breast-feeding during maternal treatment with pivampicillin... would appear to be safe, unless the infant is already hypersensitive to penicillins' (46[C]).

In sucklings, immediate hypersensitivity reactions to β-lactam antibiotics must be extremely rare. Their own production of IgE is negligible, and passive transfer of IgE through milk implies that the mother herself is allergic to penicillin, and therefore unlikely to receive it. In addition, it has to be stressed that a diagnosis of hypersensitivity to penicillin cannot be established without thorough investigation. In a recent study, a total of 298 children, 1–5 years old, with a history of penicillin allergy in connection with prior penicillin treatment, were investigated using a radioallergosorbent test, the skin prick test, and oral challenge with Pen V (47[C]). Skin prick tests were negative in all patients. In one patient, the radio-allergosorbent test indicated a high titer and this patient was the only one in whom no oral challenge was performed. Of the remaining 297 children who were given Pen V as a challenge, 30 showed clinical reactions, mainly with symptoms such as exanthema with pruritus or urticaria. No serious reactions or anaphylaxis were seen.

Clavulanic acid — another 'helper compound' with its own problem?

In order to resist breakdown by bacterial β-lactamases various β-lactam antibiotics can be given together with enzyme inhibitors (48[c]). Clavulanic acid was the first β-lactamase inhibitor to be marketed more than 10 years ago and, so far, few serious adverse reactions, specific for clavulanic acid have been described (49[R]). A few cases of *jaundice*, with an uncertain relationship to the drug, were reported (50[c], 51[c]). More recently the link with cholestasis seems to have become more firmly established in the light of a well-documented case-report (52[C]).

A 66-year-old man was treated with amoxicillin and clavulanic acid (500/125 mg t.i.d.) for exacerbation of chronic obstructive pulmonary disease. He received two 7-day-courses with an interval of 3 weeks, and 10 days later became icteric. Extrahepatic and viral causes were excluded. A diagnostic laparotomy showed no signs of obstruction and a liver biopsy showed centrilobular cholestasis. The patient had an uneventful recovery and, at that time, no causal relationship between the intake of clavulanic acid and jaundice was suspected. Eighteen months later, however, the patient was again treated with amoxicillin/clavulanic acid for 4 days, after which the drug was discontinued because of dyspepsia; 5 days later he became jaundiced. He remained icteric for several days. At control 3 months later, all liver function tests were normal. It may be noted that the patient had received 6 courses of amoxicillin therapy (as well as 2 courses of cefaclor and 4 courses of doxycycline therapy) without any sign of jaundice.

There seems to be no reason to disagree with the author's statement that 'clavulanic acid seems to be the most likely cause of cholestasis in this patient'.

TETRACYCLINES *(SED-11, 521; SEDA-12, 212; SEDA-13, 215)*

Tetracyclines and staining of the teeth Tooth discoloration associated with the use of tetracycline in children was first described in 1956 (53[C]), 8 years after the introduction of this group of antibiotics. Two theories have been advanced to explain this discoloration, the one being chelation of the mineral portion of the tooth and the other the formation of a metal-organic matrix combination of the tetracycline complex. The severity of the discoloration depends on 3 factors; namely the time (age) and duration of administration (54[R], 55[R]), the type of tetracycline administered (56[R]–58[R]) and the dosage (56[R]–58[R]). Anterior deciduous teeth are susceptible to tetracycline discoloration from 4 months in utero to 9 months postpartum and anterior permanent teeth are susceptible from 3–5 months postpartum onwards to the age of 7 years (58[R]). It may be safe to use tetracyclines after the age of about 7 years, by which time the permanent teeth are 90% mineralized, but the generally recognized age after which usage is more generally recognized as safe is 12 years (59[R]).

Although this discoloration has been known for decades, tetracyclines in syrup form are still available for prescription to young children. In an investigation in Great Britain it was found that in 1982 approximately 15% of children aged between 3 and 5 years had received a tetracycline at some time during the first 3 years of their life (60[R]).

Most investigators have found that most of the tetracyclines reside in the dentine, with only minimal amounts in the enamel (58[R], 61[R]). Consequently, only temporary bleaching effects have been found following the use of externally applied oxidizing agents (vital bleaching). More recently, various clinical case-reports (62[C]–64[C]) and an animal study (65[c]) have shown the effectiveness of bleaching tetracycline-stained teeth by intentional pulp devitalization followed by internal application of oxidizing agents directly to the dentin via the pulp chamber (walking bleaching). However, this is a somewhat drastic procedure, at least if it has to be carried out in all 12 anterior teeth.

In a recent investigation it was found that irradiation with short-wave ultraviolet light (200–300 nm) had a bleaching effect on the dentine of tetracycline-stained rat incisors within a 24-hour exposure time (66[R]). The effect appeared to be more than a surface phenomenon.

There are of course many problems to be addressed before this mode of treatment can be considered for use in patients with tetracycline-stained teeth. However, there is at least a faint glimmer of hope for them. In the meantime, the use of tetracyclines in children should be strictly limited and wherever possible entirely avoided.

Tetracyclines, topical use and contact hypersensitivity Ever since they were introduced into medicine some decades ago, the tetracyclines have been used topically. In general, they have been looked upon as safe drugs, giving rise to very few side effects. There are no reports of systemic illness following the use of topical tetracyclines, nor has staining of the teeth been reported (59[R]). Allergic contact sensitivity has also been thought to be a rare event, but this last statement has recently been challenged (67[C]). Two hundred individuals including 127 apparently normal persons and 73 patients with non-eczematous minor dermatoses were patch-tested with 26 commercially available topical antimicrobial preparations. Sensitivity to oxytetracycline was found in 3 and 2 persons in the 2 groups, respectively, placing oxytetracycline among the 4 most common sensitizers.

The authors stress that the spectrum of topical drugs causing hypersensitivity is likely to vary from time to time, depending upon prescribing trends, availability and the frequency of use at any given time. It is essential that studies be conducted regularly at different places to get some idea of the prevalent sensitivity for any given drug.

Tetracycline hydrochloride, delivered in a vehicle containing *n*-decylmethylsulfoxide to enhance the penetration of the tetracycline into the skin, is now in use in several countries for the long-term treatment of acne vulgaris (68[C]). It would seem wise to investigate the risk of contact hypersensitivity to tetracycline following this modification of the topical approach.

Last, but not least: the safety of subsequent systemic therapy with tetracyclines in patients with contact hypersensitivity to these drugs has not been established.

Minocycline *(SED-11, 528; SEDA-12, 213; SEDA-13, 217)*

Pigmentation Reports dealing with this colorful side effect of minocycline therapy continue to appear. The pigmentation can occur in several places in the body, and here just two locations will be commented upon briefly.

A black thyroid, found at operation or at autopsy, can be confusing, and surgeons and pathologists need to be aware of the phenomenon. Findings in and the mechanisms underlying a 'black thyroid gland' are discussed in 2 recent reports (69[c], 70[c]).

The second location, and one in which the pigmentation can be diagnostically misleading, is the nail. Ever since Sir Jonathan Hutchinson wrote a short report in the *British Medical Journal* (71[r]), more than 100 years ago, a periungual hyperpigmentation together with a pigmented streak or other pigmented lesion of the nail ('Hutchinson's sign') has been considered pathognomonic for subungual melanoma. A 33-year-old woman who developed Hutchinson's sign in her right 4th toenail was initially regarded as a case of minocycline hyperpigmentation (72[C]). Two biopsies however revealed the presence of a melanoma. Her daily intake of 100 mg minocycline was stopped. Five years later, the pigmentation could still be seen, although it had faded somewhat.

Thus, Hutchinson's sign is probably not pathognomonic for melanoma and should not, by itself, be the basis for aggressive management until the patient has been asked about intake of minocycline.

REFERENCES

1. Holme E, Jacobson C-E, Nordin I et al (1989) Carnitine deficiency induced by pivampicillin and pivmecillinam therapy. *Lancet, 1*, 469.
2. Stanley CA (1987) New genetic defects in mitochondrial fatty acid oxidation and carnitine deficiency. *Adv. Pediatr., 34*, 59.
3. Engel AG (1987) Carnitine deficiency syndromes and lipid storage myopathies. In: Engel AG, Blanker BQ (Eds.), *Mycology, Basic and Clinical*, p. 1663. McGraw-Hill, New York.
4. Bernardini I, Rizzo WB, Dalakas M et al (1985) Plasma and muscle free carnitine deficiency due to renal Fanconi syndrome. *J. Clin. Invest., 75*, 1124.
5. Shenai JP, Borum PR (1984) Tissue carnitine of newborn infants. *Pediatr. Res., 18*, 679.
6. Braude AI (1984) A joint venture. *J. Infect. Dis., 149*, 295.
7. Col NF, O'Connor RW (1987) Estimating worldwide current antibiotic usage: Report of Task Force 1. *Rev. Infect. Dis., 9*, 232.
8. O'Brien ThF et al (1987) Resistance of bacteria to antibacterial agents: Reports of Task Force 2. *Rev. Infect. Dis., 9*, 244.
9. Simon HJ, Folb PI, Rocha H (1987) Policies, laws and regulation pertaining to antibiotics: Report of Task Force 3. *Rev. Infect. Dis., 9*, 261.
10. Kunin CM, Lipton HL, Tupasi T et al (1987) Social behavioral, and practical factors affecting antibiotic use worldwide: Report of Task Force 4. *Rev. Infect. Dis., 9*, 270.
11. Avorn J, Harvey K, Soumerai SB (1987) Information and education as determinants of antibiotic use. Report of Task Force 5. *Rev. Infect. Dis., 9*, 286.
12. Liss RH, Batchelor FR (1987) Economic evaluations of antibiotic use and resistance — a perspective: Report of Task Force 6. *Rev. Infect. Dis., 9*, 297.
13. Holgate ST (1988) Penicillin allergy: how to diagnose and when to treat. *Br. Med. J. 296*, 1213.
14. Saxon A, Beall GN, Rohr AS et al (1988) Immediate hypersensitivity reactions to beta-lactam antibiotics. *Urology, Suppl. 31*, 14.
15. Penicillin allergy. In: Medical Letter (ISSN 0026-732X).
16. Kabins SA, Eisenstein B, Cohen S (1965) Anaphylactoid reaction to an initial dose of sodium cephalotin. *J. Am. Med. Assoc., 193*, 165.
17. Pedersen-Bjergaard J (1967) Cephalothin in the treatment of penicillin-sensitive patients. *Acta Allergol., 22*, 299.
18. Parker WA, Martin ME, Reid MJ (1988) Cephalosporins and the penicillin-allergic patients *N. Engl. J. Med., 319*, 520.
19. Sullivan TJ (1982) Antigen-specific desensitization of patients allergic to penicillin. *J. Allergy Clin. Immunol., 69*, 500.
20. Naclerio R, Mizrahi EA, Adkinson NF Jr (1983) Immunologic observations during desensitization and maintenance of clinical tolerance to penicillin. *J. Allergy Clin. Immunol., 71*, 294.
21. Plenkowski MM, Kazmier WJ, Adkinson NF (1988) Basophil histamine release remains unaffected by clinical desensitization to penicillin. *J. Allergy Clin. Immunol., 82*, 171.
22. Johnson HC, Walker AE (1945) Intraventricular penicillin. A note of warning. *J. Am. Med. Assoc., 127*, 217.

23. Walker AE, Johnson HC (1945) Convulsive factor in commercial penicillin. *Arch. Surg., 50,* 69.
24. Walker AE, Johnson HC, Kollros JJ (1945) Penicillin convulsions. The convulsive effect of penicillin applied to the cerebral cortex of monkey and man. *Surg. Gynecol. Obstet., 81,* 692.
25. Borkowski WJ, Forster FM (1948) Convulsant effects of penicillin on the cerebral cortex. *J. Neuropathol. Exp. Neurol., 6,* 201.
26. Weinstein L, Lerner PL, Chew WH (1964) Clinical and bacteriologic studies of the effect of 'massive' dose of penicillin G on infections caused by gram-negative bacilli. *N. Engl. J. Med., 271,* 525.
27. New PS, Wells CE (1965) Cerebral toxicity associated with massive intravenous penicillin therapy. *Neurology, 15,* 1053.
28. Olstone MB, Nelson E (1966) Central nervous system manifestations of penicillin toxicity in man. *Neurology, 16,* 693.
29. Brozanski BS, Scher MS, Albright AL (1988) Intraventricular afcillin-induced seizures in a neonate. *Pediatr. Neurol., 4,* 188.
30. Yoshioka H, Nambu H, Fujita H et al (1975) Convulsion following intrathecal cephaloridine. *Infection, 3,* 123.
31. Yost RL, Lee DJ, O'Leavy JP (1977) Convulsions associated with sodium cefazolin: a case report. *Am. Surg., 43,* 417.
32. Wu M-J, Narsete TA, Hussey JL et al (1978) Cephalotin neurotoxicity in renal failure (letter). *Ann. Intern. Med., 89,* 429.
33. Manzella JP, Paul RL, Butler IL (1988) CNS toxicity associated with intraventricular injection of cefazolin. Report of three cases. *J. Neurosurg., 68,* 970.
34. Lipman B, Neu HC (1988) Imipenem: a new carbapenem antibiotic. *Med. Clin. North Am., 72,* 567.
35. Calandra G, Lydick E, Carrigan J et al (1988) Factors predisposing to seizures in seriously infected patients receiving antibiotics: experience with imipenem/cilastatin. *Am. J. Med., 84,* 911.
36. Macdonald RL, Barker JL (1978) Specific antagonism of GABA-mediated postsynaptic inhibition in cultured mammalian spinal cord neurons: a common mode of convulsant action. *Neurology, 28,* 325.
37. Antoniadis A, Muller WE, Wollert U (1980) Benzodiazepine receptor interactions may be involved in the neurotoxicity of various penicillin derivatives. *Ann. Neurol., 8,* 71.
38. Schliamser SE, Bolander H, Kourtopoulos H et al (1988) Neurotoxicity of benzylpenicillin: correlation to concentrations in serum, cerebrospinal fluid and brain tissue fluid in rabbits, *J. Antimicrob. Chemother., 21,* 365.
39. Schliamser SE, Bolander H, Kourtopoulos H et al (1988) Neurotoxicity of benzylpenicillin in experimental *Escherichia coli* meningitis. *J. Antimicrob. Chemother., 22,* 251.
40. Schliamser SE, Bolander H, Broholm KA et al (1989) Neurotoxicity of benzylpenicillin in experimental renal failure and *Enterobacter cloacae* meningitis. *J. Antimicrob. Chemother., 24,* 515.
41. Schliamser SE, Broholm KA, Liljedahl AL et al (1988) Comparative neurotoxicity of benzylpenicillin, imipenem/cilastatin and FCE 22101, a new injectible penem. *J. Antimicrob. Chemother., 22,* 687.
42. Schliamser SE, Karlsson K, Larsson JE et al (1989) Interaction between benzylpenicillin and thiopental in the central nervous system of the male rat. *Pharmacol. Toxicol., 64,* 222.
43. Schaad UB, Guenin K, Steffen C et al (1988) Effects of antimicrobial agents used for therapy of CNS infections on dissociated brain cell cultures. *Pediatr. Res., 24,* 367.
44. Matheson M, Samseth M, Løberg R et al (1988) Milk transfer of phenoxymethylpenicillin during puerperal mastitis. *Br. J. Clin. Pharmacol., 25,* 33.
45. Ziv G (1980) Practical pharmacokinetic aspects of mastitis therapy—1: Parenteral treatment. *Vet. Med., 75,* 277.
46. Matheson I, Samseth M, Sande HA (1988) Ampicillin in breast milk during puerperal infections. *Eur. J. Clin. Pharmacol., 34,* 657.
47. Graff-Lonnevig V, Hedlin G, Lindfors A (1988) Penicillin allergy—a rare paediatric condition? *Arch. Dis. Child., 63,* 1342.
48. Fink AL (1985) The molecular basis of β-lactamase catalysis and inhibition, *Pharm. Res., 2,* 55.
49. Watson ID, Stewart MJ, Platt DJ (1988) Clinical pharmacokinetics of enzyme inhibitors in antimicrobial chemotherapy. *Clin. Pharmacokin., 15,* 133.
50. Mehtar S, Ball AP (1985) Intravenous augmentin in bacteraemia and severe invasive polymicrobial sepsis. *J. Antimicrob. Chemother., 15,* 765.
51. Anyanwu CH, Umeh BUO (1988) A clinical evaluation of clavulanate-potentiated amoxycillin in the management of moderate to severe respiratory tract infections, *J. Int. Med. Res., 16,* 210.
52. Van den Broek JWG, Buennemeyer BLM, Stricker BH CH (1988) Cholestatische hepatitis door de combinatie amoxicilline en clavulaanzuur (Augmentin). *Ned. Tijdschr. Geneeskd., 132,* 1495.
53. Schwachman H, Schuster A (1956) The tetracyclines applied pharmacology. *Pediatr. Clin. North Am., 3,* 295.
54. Swallow JN (1964) Discoloration of primary dentition after maternal tetracycline ingestion in pregnancy. *Lancet, 2,* 611.
55. Genet MT (1970) Effects of administration of tetracycline in pregnancy on the primary dentition of the offspring. *J. Oral Med., 25,* 75.
56. Wehman J, Porteous JR (1963) Tetracycline staining of teeth: a report of clinical material. *J. Dent. Res., 42,* 1111.

57. Grossman ER, Walcheck A, Freeman H (1971) Tetracycline and permanent teeth: the relation between dose and tooth color. *Paediatrics, 47*, 567.
58. Moffitt JM, Cooley RO, Olsen NH et al (1974) Prediction of tetracycline-induced tooth discoloration. *J. Am. Dent. Assoc., 88*, 547.
59. Wright AL, Colver GB (1988) Tetracyclines—how safe are they? *Clin. Exp. Dermatol., 13*, 57.
60. Kinirons MJ (1983) Reduction in evidence in children's teeth of the use of tetracyclines. *Br. Med. J., 287*, 1515.
61. Bennett IC, Law DB (1965) Incorporation of tetracycline in developing dog enamel and dentin. *J. Dent. Res., 44*, 788.
62. Takamizu M, Momoi Y, Furuya K et al (1980) Bleaching teeth discolored by tetracycline therapy. *Dent. Surv., 56*, 17.
63. Abou-Rass M (1982) The elimination of tetracycline discoloration by intentional endodontics and internal bleaching, *J. Endod., 8*, 101.
64. Fields J (1982) Intracoronal bleaching of tetracycline-stained teeth: a case report. *J Endod., 8*, 512.
65. Walton RE, O'Dell NL, Lake FT et al (1983) Internal bleaching of tetracycline stained teeth in dogs. *J. Endod., 9*, 416.
66. Lin LC, Pitts DL, Burgess Jr LW (1988) An investigation into the feasibility of photobleaching tetracycline-stained teeth. *J. Endod., 14*, 293.
67. Mahaur BS, Sharma VK, Kumar B et al (1987) Prevalence of contact hypersensitivity to common antiseptics, antibacterials and antifungals in normal persons. *Indian J. Dermatol. Venereol. Leprol., 53*, 269.
68. Budden MG (1988) Topical and oral tetracycline in the treatment of acne vulgaris. *Practitioner, 232*, 669.
69. Hanzlick R, Wilson R (1988) Minocycline-related black thyroid. *Am. J. Forensic Med. Pathol., 9*, 201.
70. Suzuki K, Yamamoto K, Adachi S et al (1988) A clinicopathological study of black thyroid in the elderly. *Chemotherapy, 36*, 563.
71. Hutchinson J (1986) Melanosis often not black: melanotic whitlow. *Br. Med. J., 1*, 491.
72. Mooney, E., Bennett RG (1988) Periungual hyperpigmentation mimicking Hutchinson's sign associated with minocycline administration. *J. Dermatol. Surg. Oncol., 14*, 1011.

T. Midtvedt

27 Miscellaneous antibiotics

Wilmaaaaaaaa!
(F. Flintstone)

MACROLIDES *(SED-11, 557; SEDA-12, 218; SEDA-13, 221)*

New and old macrolides, interactions and cytochrome P-450

The class of macrolide antibiotics can be divided into 2 main subgroups depending on the number of atoms within the macrolide ring. Erythromycin, which is a 14-membered macrolide, is the derivative most in use world-wide. Oleandomycin and troleandomycin (TAO) both also have a 14-membered nucleus, whereas josamycin, kitasamycin, midecamycin, spiramycin and tylosin all have a 16-membered nucleus. The number of new derivatives is steadily increasing. Substances likely to enter regular clinical practice in the foreseeable future may include azithromycin, clarithromycin, dirithromycin, flurithromycin, miokamycin, rokitamycin and roxithromycin. Their chemical structures and antimicrobial activities have recently been summarized and commented upon (1[R]–3[R]).

Their hepatic metabolism will be as important as their antimicrobial properties. The macrolides are extensively oxidized in the liver by a multienzymatic system, the terminal oxidase of which is cytochrome P-450. In the liver, this system is composed of different isoenzymes. To date, at least 21 different cytochromes P-450 have been purified from rat liver, each one having its own characteristic structure, substrate binding affinities and differential responses to drug or other xenobiotics (4[R]). Because each cytochrome appears to reflect expression of a unique gene, a standard nomenclature has been proposed based on dividing the P-450 genes into families and subfamilies, according to nucleotide sequence homology (5[R]). Functionally, it is worth noting that no xenobiotic or drug will induce all cytochrome isoenzymes, but only one or several of them. The system can also be inhibited by various mechanisms. The fact that several nitrosoalkanes have the undesirable property of forming stable complexes with cytochrome P-450 is of clinical importance. Erythromycin and more especially TAO, but not josamycin, midecamycin or spiramycin, form such nitroso-alkanes in vivo (SEDA-10, 242).

It is well-known that the macrolides can interact with a large variety of drugs which also are metabolized via the cytochrome P-450 system. The clinical occurrence of such interactions is often difficult to predict, and single-dose kinetic studies are, in fact, of little value.

In theory, it should be possible, by choosing an appropriate substrate, to estimate the amounts of the various cytochrome P-450 isoenzymes or subclasses in the liver using a breath test. In a recent study, the utility of this approach was shown very elegantly (6[C]). The major glucocorticosteroid-inducible cytochrome P-450 is within the P-450IIIA gene family (5[R]), present in the liver of rats (P-450p) and man (HLp). Since HLp and P-450p are enzymes that catalyze and, in most instances, limit the rate of erythromycin N-demethylation in liver microsomes prepared from their respective species (7[c]), the authors reasoned that the rate of production of breath $^{14}CO_2$ after injection of a test dose of N-methyl[^{14}C]-erythromycin should provide a convenient and selective measure of the catalytic activity of these cytochromes in vivo. Erythromycin was supposed to be an ideal substrate for a breath test because demethylation appears to be a major metabolic pathway (8[r]). Furthermore, N-desmethyl erythromycin is excreted in bile and does not appear to undergo a second demethylation

Side Effects of Drugs Annual 14
M.N.G. Dukes and L. Beeley, editors

(9^r). The authors also reasoned that because in man HLp is known to be induced by glucocorticosteroid (7^c, 10^c), and is inhibited by TAO (7^c) (probably by formation of nitroso-alkanes), these treatments should provide a means of validating the breath test as an HLp-specific assay in man.

The authors hit the jackpot, as subsequent work showed:

In rats, the rate of demethylation correlated well with erythromycin N-demethylase activity (r=0.90) and the concentrations of immunoreactive P-450p protein (r=0.70) and holocytochromes P-450p, determined in the liver microsomes prepared from each rat. Thereafter, N-methyl[^{14}C]erythromycin was administered to 30 patients and there was a 6-fold interindividual variation in breath $^{14}CO_2$ seemingly unrelated to medications, smoking status or age. However, in female patients the average breath test values were twice as high as in male patients ($P<0.01$). Breath $^{14}CO_2$ production rose significantly in patients retested after treatment with the P-450IIIA inducers dexamethasone or rifampicin, and was significantly decreased after treatment with TAO.

Obviously, the erythromycin breath test should provide a means of determining genetic and environmental factors involved in HLp regulation. The test could have fairly immediate clinical implications since recent experiments suggest that HLp (or a closely related cytochrome P-450) (11^c) may play a major role in the metabolism of such commonly used drugs as quinidine (12^C), nifedipine (13^C) and ciclosporin A (14^C). The test may also be used to evaluate whether the new macrolides show inhibitory activity to that exerted by TAO.

In future, this (and similar tests) will allow us to evaluate the patient's own P-450 enzymatic profile, thereby giving us a rationale to tailor the best drug—or combination of drugs—to a particular patient. The present trial-and-error-evaluations of interactions via the cytochrome P-450 system could then be considered as being as primaeval as Fred Flintstone.

Erythromycin *(SED-11, 557; SEDA-12, 218)*

Erythromycin and ototoxicity Reports of ototoxic effects of erythromycin therapy continue to appear and the 2 reports below describe typical cases.

A 73-year-old woman was admitted to hospital for pneumonia, and treatment was started with intravenous erythromycin lactobionate, 500 mg q.i.d. (15^C). After 48 hours of therapy, the patient began to complain of a decrease in hearing. Erythromycin therapy was stopped 5 days later, after the patient had received a total of 14 g. An audiogram performed 3 days after the therapy was withdrawn revealed moderate to severe bilateral sensorineural hearing loss. Another audiogram, taken approximately 6 months later, showed no significant improvement.

Another woman, 78 years of age, received intravenous erythromycin lactobionate 1000 mg q.i.d. for her pneumonia (16^C). After 2 days of therapy she developed a sudden neurosensorial hearing loss, which receded when the drug was discontinued.

The pharmacological and electrophysiological dynamics of these changes are still unknown. A recent review reported that when erythromycin was infused intravenously in anesthetized guinea-pigs at a rate of 125 mg/kg/h, 'the initial effect was an increase in the latency of the 4th peak of the auditory brainstem evoked response' (17^C). These effects were subsequently followed by similar changes in the 3rd and 2nd waves. When drug administration was discontinued, all changed values returned to control values. No changes were found in the alternating current cochlear potential or compound action potential thresholds. If the CNS does represent the site of the ototoxic effect of erythromycin, it would suggest that there is some drug-induced change in the CNS that results in the ototoxic effect. Indeed, other CNS effects of erythromycin, such as psychiatric disturbances, might prove to be caused by the same mechanism. So far, however, this is no more but speculation.

Ototoxicity may be more commonly encountered in females than in males (18^C). As commented upon elsewhere in this chapter, there may be a sex-dependent difference in the hepatic metabolism of erythromycin (6^C). In the present state of knowledge, high-dose therapy should be given with the greatest care to elderly patients as well as to patients with impaired hepatic or renal function.

Erythromycin and psychiatric complications There are a few reports in which erythromycin therapy has been associated with complications such as *confusion, paranoia, visual hallucinations, fear, lack of control* and *nightmares*

(19[c], 20[R], 21[R], 22[C], 22[R]). The onset of these suspected psychiatric side effects has been within 12–48 hours of starting therapy with conventional doses of erythromycin. When the drug was stopped, the symptoms resolved quickly within a few days. In 2 patients, the psychiatric disturbances were accompanied by hearing loss (22[C]). In another 2 patients, receiving a second exposure to erythromycin, the psychiatric complications recurred (21[R]). In addition to the published cases, one may note that the Committee on Safety of Medicines in the U.K. had up to 1988 received 21 reports on psychiatric disturbances associated with erythromycin (20[R]). Sex distribution in these 21 cases was not stated. In the published cases, there is a female dominance.

It seems reasonable to assume that such complications are under-reported. The 2 main areas of erythromycin therapy are pediatric infections and sexually-transmitted diseases (STD). It is, of course, not easy to determine whether nightmares in a child with fever are caused by the drug given. Correspondingly, drug-related nightmares do not immediately spring to mind in a woman with STD.

The mechanisms behind these reactions are unknown.

CHLORAMPHENICOL *(SED-11, 543; SEDA-12, 218; SEDA-13, 221)*

Hepatotoxicity A 1988 'Guide to Drug Dosage in Hepatic Disease' covers more than 60 different drugs, of which more than 20 are anti-infective agents (23[R]). Chloramphenicol is claimed to be the drug of which clearance is most markedly affected in liver disease. It is quite simply stated that the drug should be avoided in such patients.

Problems in pediatric practice The 'gray baby syndrome', occurring in neonates who have been exposed to chloramphenicol, is thought to be caused by a combination of inadequate hepatic conjugation (due to inadequate glucuronyl transferase activity) and decreased glomerular filtration at that age group – particularly since the phenomenon can also occur in older children if these same two functions are impaired (SEDA-8, 258). In most countries, therefore, so-called recommended dosage schedules have been established (25[R]). The value of such recommendations has recently been challenged (26[C]).

In 252 neonates, infants and children, from 45 hospitals, all of whom were receiving chloramphenicol, samples of serum and cerebrospinal fluid were assayed for chloramphenicol and the treatment regimens were analyzed: 41 of the patients were less than 1 week of age, 112 were 1–4 weeks old, and the remainder was more than 1 months of age. Less than 50% of neonates and 25% of infants received the recommended dose of chloramphenicol. In older children, however, the recommended dose was generally given. Of 39 neonates who received the recommended dose intravenously, only 16 (40%) had serum concentrations within the therapeutic range (15–25 mg/l). Altogether, 31% of neonates and infants had potentially toxic serum concentrations. Twelve neonates and infants (5.5%) suffered toxic side effects and 4 of them died. A further 8 babies accidentally received a 2- to 10-fold overdose and in 3 others an overdose was assumed following assay. No overdoses of toxic effects were reported in children over 1 year of age. Eight patients with impaired renal function had elevated serum levels and 3 showed toxic symptoms.

Interestingly, peak chloramphenicol serum concentrations were significantly higher in infants who were also receiving penicillin (means 23 vs 14; $P<0.02$), even though these patients received a significantly lower dose of chloramphenicol ($P<0.01$) than those receiving monotherapy (48 mg/kg/d vs 71 mg/kg/d). The authors 'were unable to account for the higher serum chloramphenicol concentrations among infants who also received penicillin'.

Taken together, the above data clearly indicate that even when a recommended dosage regimen for chloramphenicol is followed, serum from all patients under approximately 1 year of age should be assayed every 48–72 hours. That seems to be the only way to ensure that safe and effective levels are maintained.

AMINOGLYCOSIDES *(SED-11, 546; SEDA-12, 220; SEDA-13, 223)*

Aminoglycosides and ototoxicity

The first report of clinical efficacy of the very first aminoglycoside antibiotic, streptomycin, also described the problem of hearing loss resulting from use of the drug (25[c]). Since then, the fact that this group of antibiotics can produce ototoxicity is overwhelmingly well-established in man as well as in experimental animals. The number of reports is very high, as are the numbers of reviews on this topic. A recent 'review of reviews' commented upon 28 such papers; all but one appeared during the last 10 years (28[R]). However, despite the vast amount of knowledge that has accumulated as to the ototoxicity of these drugs, the true incidence of hearing loss resulting from aminoglycoside use in humans remains controversial. As in modes of fashion, the question whether one aminoglycoside is more likely than another to result in ototoxicity is in dispute. In addition, the basic mechanisms underlying the ototoxicity are also questioned. These 3 main questions are discussed below.

The question of the incidence of ototoxicity originates from the discrepancy between clinical observations, in which very few patients receiving these drugs actually complain of developing a hearing loss, and the reported incidence of ototoxicity of up to 41% in studies in which auditory thresholds were obtained (29[C]). According to Brummett and Fox (28[R]), there are 2 main reasons for this discrepancy. The first relates to the fact that aminoglycosides give high-frequency hearing losses well before they affect the speech frequency range in which they can be detected by the patient. To understand speech, we rely greatly on our hearing at lower frequencies, from 0.3–3 kHz, which are affected only with very extensive aminoglycoside damage. Therefore, patients are most unlikely to complain about any loss of hearing, even if asked, until considerable damage has been done (30[C], 31[C]). In cases in which the only damage occurs at frequencies above 8 kHz, it will often not be detected since many audiometers only test frequencies at 8 kHz and below. Furthermore, patients who have a hearing loss from 4–8 kHz may have difficulty in understanding speech, especially in a noisy working environment. Thus, a hearing loss recognized by the patient weeks after he has left hospital and any association with the aminoglycoside treatment, that he received weeks previously is difficult to establish.

The second reason for the discrepancy between the clinical and experimental incidences of aminoglycoside-antibiotic-induced ototoxicity has to do with the established criteria for ototoxicity. Brummet and Fox (28[R]) give references to many reports lacking information about the criteria used to determine whether ototoxic changes had occurred, to reports considering ototoxicity as a 15-dB or more increase in the auditory threshold at any 2 frequencies, to reports considering a change of 15 dB or greater at any threshold to represent ototoxicity, and to some reports using combinations of the criteria given above. The problem of not having a universally agreed-upon standard for the definition of drug-induced ototoxicity has been underlined by several authors (28[R], 30[C]).

At present, most of the studies now reported seem to accept a 15-dB change in threshold at any frequency as a meaningful change sufficient to representing ototoxicity. The reason for this is that it is standard procedure to use 5-dB steps in sound intensity when obtaining auditory thresholds. Experimental error allows a ±5-dB discrepancy between audiograms, and a 15-dB change is thus the smallest change to exceed the inherent error of the method.

However, this standard can be questioned. It has been shown (in healthy subjects) that changes of 17–20 dB at some frequencies must occur before statistical significance reaches the 5% confidence level between repeat audiograms (32[C]). By contrast, it is possible, in sick people, that even greater changes do not represent a meaningful or significant alteration. Of 27 hospitalized patients who did not receive any known ototoxic drug, 15 had a change in the threshold between 20 and 35 dB at one or more frequencies during their stay in hospital (33[C]).

Thus, if it is true that sick patients receiving no ototoxic drugs can have day-to-day auditory changes exceeding the most commonly established criteria for ototoxicity, all assumptions about the incidence of ototoxicity must be looked at very critically. In comparative studies of the incidence of ototoxicity of different aminoglycosides, it is very often assumed that non-drug-related changes are the same in the different treatment groups, thereby justifying a comparison. In many of these studies, the sample sizes are very small and it is indeed possible that some samples are biased because of some unrecognized variable. Until more data can be presented, non-randomized comparative studies seem to be of rather little – if any – value. At present, it does not seem justified to claim that any one of the commonly-used aminoglycosides is more or less ototoxic than any other.

However, this lack of data should not mislead us into ignoring the real risk of ototoxic changes in patients receiving aminoglycosides. The classical example, published 20 years ago, is still valid (29[C]). In that instance a patient, suffering from Gram-negative bacteria infection, received a single injection of 1 g kanamycin, and two hours later the patient was given a single 50-mg intravenous dose of etacrynic acid. Thirty minutes after the etacrynic acid, he began to complain of difficulties in hearing. No more of either drug was given, and when he was well enough to have his hearing tested he was found to have a 60–70 dB loss at all frequencies.

The last question to be discussed is that of the basic mechanisms underlying the ototoxic effects of aminoglycosides. Early studies of aminoglycoside distribution in cochlear fluids resulted in the misconception that a plasma threshold existed for entry of the drugs into the inner ear and that accumulation in the inner-ear fluid was the primary determinant in the development of ototoxicity. It was suggested that below certain threshold concentrations the aminoglycosides were excluded from the perilymph and that they were transferred into the inner ear only at high peak serum levels. Early findings and postulates were recently critically reviewed in 1988 by Hentley and Schacht (34[R]) and, to quote their summary, 'the literature is replete with studies attempting to correlate aminoglycoside levels in inner-ear and whole tissues with selective toxicity. It is abundantly clear that aminoglycoside toxicity does not necessarily correlate with plasma perilymph or whole-tissue levels of these drugs; at these levels the 'concentration = toxicity' approach is inadequate in explaining the mechanisms by which these important chemotherapeutic agents exert their toxic actions'. These same authors present on their own a multistep molecular hypothesis of aminoglycoside ototoxicity. The initial action is thought to involve binding of the aminoglycoside to the outer plasma membrane of the cell, as an acute effect of electrophysiological processes such as the cochlear microphonic response. These effects are reversible and probably antagonized by the divalent cations calcium, zinc and magnesium (35[r], 36[R]). The next step may be energy-dependent uptake into the cell; here the aminoglycosides will interfere with a number of essential intracellular processes and cause disruption of membrane integrity and function. Aminoglycosides seem to inhibit the polyphosphoinositide second messenger system and other intracellular reactions regulated by the polyphosphoinositides (SEDA-11, 235). In addition, the aminoglycosides may in several ways compete with the polyamines for uptake and binding (37[R]), and they may inhibit cochlear ornithine decarboxylase, i.e. the enzyme catalyzing the initial reaction in polyamine synthesis (38[R]). As has been pointed out (34[R]), this could result in inhibition of cellular repair mechanisms which might be initiated by the cell following the damage caused by the aminoglycosides. Such an inhibition would prevent recovery of the cell and represent a final biochemical insult leading to cellular death.

Pending the final answers to these very complicated biochemical questions, one must remain as alert as ever for possible ototoxic effects whenever aminoglycosides are given.

Several questions concerning hearing loss in pre-term infants were recently addressed (39[C]). The perinatal histories of 16 pre-term infants who had a confirmed moderate-to-profound sensorineural deficit were compared with the histories of infants in 2 other groups. The first group, which was selected to identify the 'at-risk' infants for screening purposes, consisted of 226 surviving pre-term infants from the same intensive care unit. The second group comprised 16 pre-term infants with normal hearing who were matched to infants with hearing deficits according to gestational age, birthweight percentile and sex. All but 1 of the infants with a hearing deficit were tested during the postnatal period and 'identified correctly by persistently-elevated brainstem auditory-evoked response threshold'. Concerning the aminoglycosides, it was found that the mean duration of therapy in infants with hearing loss was significantly longer than in those with normal hearing (15 days vs 8 days). The authors recommend that early identification of pre-term infants with a hearing deficit should be achieved by recording brainstem auditory-evoked responses just before discharge from the intensive care unit.

The findings above may also fit into an old theory, first proposed by Dayal et al in 1974 (40[C]), that aminoglycoside antibiotics can have their ototoxic potential exacerbated by excessively loud sounds. Their major concern was in fact that the use of aminoglycosides in premature infants who are kept in isolators may be dangerous because of the possibility of such an interaction. Many such isolators are fairly noisy. Experimentally, these investigators reported a slightly increased loss of cochlear hair cells in guinea-pigs exposed to kanamycin and incubator noise as compared to those of animals exposed to kanamycin alone or to incubator-noise alone. Several investigators have tried to confirm these data – with varying results. However, as recently summarized (41[R]), 'when all of the data are considered as a whole, it is apparent that when doses of the aminoglycoside antibiotics sufficiently large as to produce some cochlear hair loss alone, are combined with sound intensities that will produce some cochlear hair cell loss alone, an exaggerated damage results that is greater than the additive effects of the 2 agents.'

Brummett (41[R]) cites several sources of noise in a hospital. Measuring the intensity of sound that some patients listen to on their Walkman-type radios or tape players, he found intensities as high as 115 dB. Such intense sound may enhance aminoglycoside-induced auditory damage. He advocated that in the absence of any contradictory evidence, it would be prudent to keep patients who are receiving aminoglycosides in as quiet an environment as possible.

Finally, one must realize that more than two risk factors may sometimes be present.

When the ear is exposed to loud sounds, the tensor tympani and stapedius muscles contract, thereby impairing the transfer of sounds from the middle ear to the cochlea. As Brummett (41[R]) has remarked, we have a long list of drugs such as tranquillizers, sedatives, muscle relaxants – and ethyl alcohol – that could interfere with the ability of the middle ear muscles to function properly, and thereby have an additive effect on the toxicity caused by aminoglycosides and sounds. In short: an aminoglycoside, a Walkman and a beer – and nothing you will hear!

MISCELLANEOUS REPORTS/AGENTS

Vancomycin *(SED-11, 561; SEDA-12, 222)*

Vancomycin and endotoxin Previously it has been shown that endotoxin potentiates the nephrotoxic effect of aminoglycosides (SEDA-8, 259). It has now been found that the same holds true for vancomycin – at least in rats (42[c]).

A single injection of vancomycin was given to rats which were infused intravenously with saline (control) or endotoxin. Injection of endotoxin was associated with a significant increase in the half-life of vancomycin, an increase in the area under the serum concentration curve of vancomycin and a higher accumulation of vancomycin in the renal cortex and medulla. The results indicate that endotoxin modifies the renal handling of vancomycin.

Previously, endotoxin has been shown to increase the negative charge of biological membranes formed from different phospholipids (43[R]). The possibility therefore exists that binding between positively-charged vancomycin and negatively-charged phospholipids in tubular cell membranes may have been enhanced by endotoxin. Whatever the mechanism, the increase in vancomycin levels within the renal parenchyma might be associated with a higher incidence of nephrotoxicity. Although vancomycin primarily acts upon Gram-positive, non-endotoxin-forming organisms, it is often used in combination with an aminoglycoside or a β-lactam antibiotic in patients with infections of unknown or mixed etiology. Endotoxin will then be liberated in the blood of these patients, and the nephrotoxic property of vancomycin might thus be potentiated. Research along these lines seems clinically relevant.

Teicoplanin *(SED-11, 561; SEDA-13, 226)*

The spectrum of adverse effects following teicoplanin therapy is becoming increasingly like that of vancomycin. More cases of *ototoxicity* are now reported.

A female patient (age not given), who received a total dose of 3000 mg teicoplanin over 7 days, demonstrated normal audiograms before therapy and on day 6, but abnormal audiograms on days 12 and 22 (44[C]). The findings were described as '20–30-dB decrease in auditory threshold over the high frequency range in both ears'. During therapy, the teicoplanin concentrations in serum never exceeded 10 mg/l.

Another case of vestibular damage has been reported in a patient after 59 days of intravenous teicoplanin therapy (45[c]). This patient also received gentamicin concomitantly. The serum concentrations of teicoplanin and gentamicin were not reported. Two cases of hearing loss were recently reported (46[c]), and 1 of them was described in some detail.

A 68-year-old female was treated with teicoplanin (8.9 mg/kg/day/i.v.) for 41 days. She had normal audiograms when treatment was instituted and developed a 50- to 60-dB decrease in high frequency (2000–8000 Hz) auditory threshold, recognized at the end of the treatment period. This side effect persisted 2 years later.

Experimental studies in the rat revealed dose-dependent *nephrotoxicity* following administration of teicoplanin (47[R]). No significant differences were observed in the comparative nephrotoxicity of vancomycin and teicoplanin at a 10:1 dose ratio. So far, however, only a few cases of teicoplanin-associated renal impairment have been described (48[C], 49[c]).

Given by the intramuscular route, teicoplanin may cause symptoms of *local pain* which can be avoided if the drug is given in a 1% lidocaine solution (44[C]). Other reported adverse effects include a *transient rise in serum aminotransferase, drug fever, neutropenia, skin rash, bronchospasm, eosinophilia* and *thrombophlebitis.* Relevant references are given in 2 recent reviews (50[R], 51[R]).

Evidence of *cross-sensitivity* between teicoplanin and *vancomycin* is still controversial. One patient has been reported to exhibit cross-sensitivity between vancomycin and teicoplanin, with rash and other symptoms of an allergic reaction to vancomycin, also occurring when the patient subsequently received teicoplanin (52[c]). However, others suggest that patients may be successfully treated with teicoplanin despite vancomycin allergy (53[c]).

Last but not least: few—if any—reactions resembling the vancomycin *'red-neck'* or *'red-man'* syndrome have so far been reported (50[R]). That might turn out to be the only difference in the side-effect spectra of teicoplanin and vancomycin.

Fusidic acid *(SED-11, 560; SEDA-13, 226)*

Granulocytopenia Granulocytopenia during treatment of severe infections can be due to the infection itself or may be a side effect of the drug(s) used. In fact, there are reports describing the occurrence of this side effect in connection with usage of nearly all groups of antimicrobial drugs, and fusidic acid can now line up with the others (54[C]).

An 18-year-old man was admitted with osteomyelitis and arthritis caused by *Staphylococcus aureus.* Surgical drainage and intravenous flucloxacillin and fusidic acid (dose not given) were successful. However, a routine blood count after 4 days revealed severe neutropenia (0.1×10^9/l). All drugs were stopped and the neutrophil count rose promptly. Although the patient had received 12 different drugs, including anesthetics, the flucloxacillin was judged to be the most likely cause. Because he still required antistaphylococcal drugs he was started on oral fusidic acid and erythromycin. However, the neutropenia recurred immediately. Consequently, the fusidic acid was stopped, and the neutrophil count rose immediately. Later he was treated with flucloxacillin and erythromycin without adverse effects.

According to the authors, the files of the U.K. Committee on Safety of Medicines contain 13 cases in which fusidic acid was one of several drugs taken by patients demonstrating granulocytopenia. They claim that 'the clinical and laboratory features point to a direct toxic or hapten-antibody mechanism'. Whatever the mechanism(s) might be, it now seems well-proven that fusidic cid can cause granulocytopenia.

REFERENCES

1. Kirst HA, Sides GD (1989) New directions for macrolide antibiotics: structural modifications and in vitro activity. Minireviews. *Antimicrob. Agents Chemother., 33,* 1413.
2. Hardy DJ, Hanson CW, Hensey DM et al (1988) Susceptibility of *Campylobacter pylori* to macrolides and fluoroquinolones. *J. Antimicrob. Chemother., 22,* 631.
3. Hardy DJ, Hensey DM, Beyer JM (1988) Comparative in vitro activities of new 14-, 15- and 16-membered macrolides. *Antimicrob. Agents Chemother., 32,* 1710.
4. Black SD, Coon MJ (1986) Comparative structures of P-450 cytochromes. In: Ortiz de Montellano PR (Ed), *Cytochrome P-450: Structure, Metabolism and Biochemistry,* p. 161. Plenum, New York.
5. Nebert DW, Adesnik M, Coon MJ et al (1987) The P450 gene superfamily: recommended nomenclature. *DNA, 6,* 1.
6. Watkins PB, Murray SA, Winkelman LG et al

(1989) Erythromycin breath test as an assay of glucocorticoid-inducible liver cytochromes P-450. *J. Clin. Invest.*, *83*, 688.
7. Watkins PB, Wrighton SA, Maurel P et al (1985) Identification of an inducible form of cytochrome P-450 in human liver. *Proc. Natl. Acad. Sci. USA*, *82*, 6310.
8. Lee CC, Anderson RC, Chen KK (1956) The excretory products of *N*-methyl-^{14}C-erythromycin in rats. *J. Pharmacol. Exp. Ther.*, *117*, 274.
9. Mao JC, Tardew PL (1965) Demethylation of erythromycin by rabbit tissues in vitro. *Biochem. Pharmacol.*, *14*, 1049.
10. Molowa DT, Schuetz EG, Wrighton SA et al (1986) Complete cDNA sequence of a cytochrome P-450 inducible by glucocorticoids in human liver. *Proc. Natl. Acad. Sci. USA*, *83*, 5311.
11. Beaune PH, Umbenhauer DR, Bork RW et al (1986) Isolation and sequence determination of a cDNA clone related to human cytochrome P-450 nifedipine oxidase. *Proc. Natl. Acad. Sci. USA*, *83*, 8064.
12. Guengerich FP, Muller-Enoch D, Blair IA (1986) Oxidation of quinidine by human liver cytochrome P-450. *Mol. Pharmacol.*, *30*, 287.
13. Guengerich FP, Martin MV, Beaunne PH (1986) Characterization of rat and human liver microsomal cytochrome P-450 forms involved in nifedipine oxidation, a prototype for genetic polymorphism in oxidative drug metabolism. *J. Biol. Chem.*, *261*, 5051.
14. Kronbach T, Fischer V, Meyer RA (1988) Cyclosporine metabolism in human liver: identification of a cytochrome P-450III gene family as the major cyclosporine-metabolizing enzyme explains interactions of cyclosporine with other drugs. *Clin. Pharmacol. Ther.*, *43*, 630.
15. Dylewski J (1988) Irreversible sensorineural hearing loss due to erythromycin. *Can. Med. Assoc. J.*, *139*, 230.
16. Marti DJ, Mutio L, Alonso A et al (1988) Hipoacusia neurosensorial reversible secundaria a erithromicina. *An. ORL Iber.-Am.*, *15*, 429.
17. Brummett RE, Fox KE (1989) Minireviews. Vancomycin- and erythromycin-induced hearing loss in humans. *Antimicrob. Agents Chemother.*, *33*, 791.
18. Haydon RC, Thelin JW, Davis WE (1984) Erythromycin ototoxicity: analysis and conclusions based on 22 case reports. *Otolaryngol. Head Neck Surg.*, *92*, 678.
19. Black RJ, Dawson TAJ (1988) Erythromycin and nightmares. *Br. Med. J.*, *296*, 1070.
20. Murdoch J (1988) Psychiatric complications of erythromycin and clindamycin. *Can. J. Hosp. Pharm.*, *41*, 277.
21. Cohen IJ, Weitz R (1981) Psychiatric complications with erythromycin. *Drug Intell. Clin. Pharm.*, *15*, 388.
22. Umstead GS, Neumann KH (1986) Ototoxicity and acute psychotic reaction in cancer patients with hepatic dysfunction. *Arch. Intern. Med.*, *146*, 897.
23. Williams NR (1988) Erythromycin: a case of nightmares. *Br. Med. J.*, *296*, 214.
24. Bass NM, Williams RL (1988) Guide to drug dosage in hepatic disease. *Clin. Pharmacokin.*, *15*, 396.
25. British Medical Association and the Pharmaceutical Society of Great Britain (1984) British National Formulary Number 9.
26. Mulhall A, Berry DJ, DeLouvois J (1988) Chloramphenicol in paediatrics: current prescribing practice and the need to monitor. *Eur. J. Pediatr.*, *147*, 574.
27. Hinshaw HC, Feldman WH (1945) Streptomycin in treatment of clinical tuberculosis: a preliminary report. *Proc. Staff Meet. Mayo Clin.*, *20*, 313.
28. Brummett RE, Fox KE (1989) Aminoglycoside-induced hearing loss in humans. *Antimicrob. Agents Chemother.*, *33*, 797.
29. Sataloff J, Wagner S, Menduke H (1964) Kanamycin ototoxicity in healthy men. *Arch. Otolaryngol.*, *80*, 413.
30. Katz J, White TP (1982) Introduction to the handicap of hearing impairment in the adult: auditory impairment versus hearing handicap. In: Hull RH (Ed) *Rehabilitative Audiology*. Grune and Stratton, New York, p. 13.
31. Newby HA, Popelka GR (1985) *Audiology, 5th ed.* Prentice-Hall Inc., Englewood Cliffs, 360.
32. Bryan ME (1976) Industrial audiometry. In: Stephens SDG (Ed) *Disorders of Auditory Function II*. New York, Academic Press Inc. p. 77.
33. Davey PG, Jabeen FJ, Harpur ES et al (1983) A controlled study of the reability of pure tone audiometry for the detection of gentamicin auditory toxicity. *J. Laryngol. Otol.*, *97*, 27.
34. Hentley III CM, Schacht J (1988) Pharmacokinetics of aminoglycoside antibiotics in blood, inner-ear fluids and tissues and their relationship to ototoxicity. *Audiology*, *27*, 137.
35. Pasternak CA, Mahadevan D (1988) Novel role of extracellular calcium and zinc: protection against membrane damage induced by cytotoxic agents. *Ind. J. Biochem. Biophys.*, *25*, 1.
36. Günther T, Rebentisch E, Vormann J et al (1988) Enhanced ototoxicity of gentamicin and salicylate caused by Mg deficiency and Zn deficiency. *Biol. Trace Element Res.*, *16*, 43.
37. Williams SE, Smith DE, Schacht J (1987) Characteristics of gentamicin uptake in the isolated crista ampullaris of the inner ear of the guinea pig. *Biochem. Pharmacol.*, *36*, 89.
38. Henley CM, Gerhardt H-J, Schacht J (1987) Inhibition of inner ear ornithine decarboxylase by neomycin in vitro. *Brain Res. Bull.*, *19*, 695.
39. Pettigrew AG, Edwards DA, Henderson-Smart

DJ (1988) Perinatal risk factors in preterm infants with moderate-to-profound hearing deficits. *Med. J. Aust., 148*, 174.
40. Dayal VS, Smith EL, McCain G (1974) Cochlear and vestibular gentamicin toxicity. *Arch. Otolaryngol., 100*, 338.
41. Brummett RE (1988) Insults of hearing (interactions) Review article. *Pharmindex ACPE 1. D. No.: 679–405, 11.*
42. Ngeleka M, Auclair P, Tardif D et al (1989) Intrarenal distribution of vancomycin in endotoxic rats. *Antimicrob. Agents Chemother., 33*, 1575.
43. Onji T, Liu MS (1989) Changes in surface charge density on liposomes induced by *E. coli* endotoxin. *Biochim. Biophys. Acta, 558*, 320.
44. Bibler MR, Frame PT, Hagler DN et al (1987) Clinical evaluation of efficacy, pharmacokinetics, and safety of teicoplanin for serious gram-positive infections. *Antimicrob. Agents Chemother., 31*, 207.
45. Williams AH, Gruneberg RN, Webster A, Ridgway GL (1986) Teicoplanin in the treatment of infections caused by Gram-positive organisms. *J. Hosp. Infect., Suppl. A*, 101.
46. Leport C, Perronne C, Massip P et al (1989) Evaluation of teicoplanin for treatment of endocarditis caused by Gram-positive cocci in 20 patients. *Antimicrob. Agents Chemother., 33*, 871.
47. Marre E, Schulz E, Graefe H, Sack K (1987) Teicoplanin: renal tolerance and pharmacokinetics in rats. *J. Antimicrob. Chemother., 20*, 697.
48. Smith SR, Cheesbrough J, Spearing R, Davies JM (1989) Randomized prospective study comparing vancomycin with teicoplanin in the treatment of infections associated with Hickman catheters. *Antimicrob. Agents Chemother., 33*, 1193.
49. Van Laethem Y, Kermans P, De Wit S, Glumeck N (1987) Clinical and biological experience with teicoplanin at various dosages in severe *S. aureus* methicillin-resistant septicemia. Abstract presented at: 15th International Congress on Chemotherapy, Istanbul, 1987.
50. Babul N, Pasko M (1988) Teicoplanin: a new glycopeptide antibiotic complex. *Drug. Intell. Clin. Pharm., 22*, 218.
51. Pryka RD, Rodvold KA, Rotschafer JC (1988) Drug Reviews. Teicoplanin: An investigational glycopeptide antibiotic. *Clin. Pharm., 7*, 647.
52. McElrath MJ, Goldberg D, Neu HC (1986) Allergic cross-reactivity of teicoplanin and vancomycin (Letter to Editor), *Lancet, 1*, 47.
53. Schlemmer B, Falkman H, Boudjada A et al (1988) Teicoplanin for patients allergic to vancomycin. *N. Engl. J. Med., 318*, 1127.
54. Revell P, Nicholson F, Pearson TC (1988) Granulocytopenia due to fusidic acid. *Lancet, 2*, 454.

A.V. Astakhova and V.K. Lepakhin

28 Antifungal drugs

Amphotericin B *(SED-11, 568; SEDA-12, 226; SEDA-13, 230)*

℞ *Management of amphotericin B nephrotoxicity*

During the year under consideration a number of new papers on the management of nephrotoxicity induced by amphotericin B have been published, including a major review (1[R]).

Sodium loading appears to have a beneficial effect on amphotericin B nephrotoxicity in humans. Sodium can be delivered in the form of ticarcillin or by a normal saline or bicarbonate infusion. The amount of sodium in a daily dose of ticarcillin approximately equals the sodium content in 500–1000 ml of normal saline. Since volume depletion is a risk factor for amphotericin B nephrotoxicity, normal fluid volume should be maintained. Prophylactic administration of 500–1000 ml of normal saline per day should be considered if the patient's cardiovascular status allows. Observations by Stein et al (2[C]) confirm the hypothesis that sodium can prevent renal dysfunction in patients receiving amphotericin B therapy; their investigation was conducted on leukemic patients.

Since ticarcillin at doses of 18 g/d represents the administration of a considerable salt load (93.6 mmol/d), these authors hypothesized that leukemic patients receiving both ticarcillin and amphotericin B might be protected by this serendipitous administration of saline. They therefore reviewed an extensive series of their patients receiving empiric amphotericin B therapy with respect to administration of ticarcillin and with respect to the total intake of intravenous sodium. By means of univariant and multivariant analysis they identified factors associated with an increased risk of renal failure during amphotericin B therapy. Nephrotoxicity was found to have developed in 12 patients (19%) receiving amphotericin B and aminoglycosides (creatinine value ⩾ 2.0 mg/100 ml). Patients with nephrotoxicity tended to be older than patients without; sex and total amphotericin B dose were not correlated with nephrotoxicity. In this series, among patients receiving ticarcillin at ⩾ 18 mg/d, the incidence of nephrotoxicity was 1:30 (3.3%). A multivariate analysis showed that this protective effect of ticarcillin was not dependent on the fact that patients receiving ticarcillin were less likely to receive vancomycin. There were insufficient patients receiving sodium in the absence of ticarcillin to study the effect of sodium alone. Time to renal failure was the dependent variable; age, baseline serum creatinine, vancomycin administrtion; adequacy of ticarcillin administration and adequacy of total sodium administration were the independent variables. Only age and inadequacy of ticarcillin dosage were significantly related to development of nephrotoxicity.

It may thus be considered established that administration of sodium in one form or another is helpful; its use in the form of saline should be considered if the patient's cardiovascular status allows. Other therapeutic maneuvers, such as infusion of mannitol, saralasin or theophylline, are of no proven benefit in human amphotericin B nephrotoxicity. Wherever possible the administration of other nephrotoxins such as gentamicin or ciclosporin should be avoided, since these drugs may potentiate the renal toxic effects of amphotericin B (1[R]).

In Raymond's opinion (1[R]) management strategies must also be directed at detecting and countering specific nephrotoxic effects of amphotericin B. Tubular defects can easily be detected (by urinalysis, serum chemistry and arterial blood gas analysis) and dealt with by the clinician. Azotemia is a more difficult problem. Blood urea nitrogen and creatinine levels may rise days to months after the initiation of therapy. In

Side Effects of Drugs Annual 14
M.N.G. Dukes and L. Beeley, editors

many cases a rapid reduction of azotemia may be achieved by discontinuing amphotericin B for 1–3 days and then resuming the drug with a 25–50% reduction in the daily dose. Alternative methods include reducing the daily dose by 50% or switching to an every-other-day schedule, with or without a drug hiatus. If the azotemia diminishes or stabilizes, amphotericin B is continued. If renal function continues to deteriorate, the status of the patient's fungal infection must be re-evaluated. If the infection is still life-threatening, amphotericin should be continued at the same or a higher daily dose, and preparations should be made for hemodialysis or peritoneal dialysis. If the fungal infection has improved but the azotemia has worsened, therapy should be continued at the current daily dose or at a reduced dose with careful clinical observation. Transient dialysis may be required and is at all events preferable to a fatal outcome. Amphotericin B probably should not be discontinued for more than 3 days in the presence of a fungal infection which is believed to be life-threatening. Little or no dosage adjustment is required in chronically azotemic, anephric or dialysis patients. Nephrotoxicity is in such cases not a concern (or not a primary one) and to date no investigators have demonstrated a clinically significant difference in the serum amphotericin B levels of uremic and non-uremic patients.

The clinical usefulness of amphotericin B is thus often complicated by nephrotoxicity, though it is usually reversible where amphotericin B can be and is withdrawn. In Raymond's view, to which one must subscribe, the patient's chance of survival should be compromised to save the kidneys. If, despite prophylactic and therapeutic measures, renal function continues to deteriorate, and the fungal infection is considered life-threatening, amphotericin B should be continued and preparations for dialysis made.

Amphotericin B and systemic candida infections in the very young As a result of their rapidly increasing incidence, acquired systemic candida infections have become a significant problem in neonates and pre-term infants. A paper by Bottineau (3[r]) has provided an overview of this problem.

These infections are severe, both because they develop in infants with significant risk factors (gestational age of e.g. 30 weeks, birthweight perhaps 1250 g, intensive care, antibiotic therapy, intravascular catheters), and because they may remain clinically latent. Clinical features include a broad spectrum of manifestations but are all non-specific; the diagnosis should therefore be routinely considered. Many organs may be involved, particularly the digestive tract (90%), kidney (48%), lung (26%) and central nervous system (20–60%). Diagnosis is urgent and rests mainly upon the routine performance of mycological studies using special media in all infants with risk factors or undergoing unexplained clinical deterioration. *Candida albicans* appears to be responsible for some 90% of the cases. Curative treatment should be instituted promptly. This treatment is today almost exclusively medical and centers around an intravenous infusion of the amphotericin B/flucytosine combination or oral ketoconazole.

The experience of Loke et al (4[cr]) confirms the point of view that when systemic candidiasis and pneumonia are recognized early, effective and safe treatment can be achieved with favorable short- and long-term outcome. They themselves observed 22 pre-term infants with systemic candidiasis. All except 1 were of very low birthweight. Fifteen infants had positive cultures of blood, cerebrospinal fluid or urine, and 7 had candida pneumonia only. The diagnosis was made after death in 2 infants. In the remaining 20 infants, treatment was initiated between 5 and 97 days of age, with a median delay of 4 days after the first positive cultures were taken. The standard treatment protocol for systemic candidiasis consisted of amphotericin for 4 weeks and flucytosine for 6 weeks. Amphotericin was given in a once-daily dose of 0.1 mg/kg/d, increasing by 0.1 mg/kg/d to a maximum of 0.5 mg/kg/d (3 infants) and 0.3 mg/kg/d (27 infants). 5-Flucytosine (5-FC) was given as a slow infusion over 1 hour in a total daily dose of 100 mg/kg in 4 divided doses. However, amphotericin was sometimes withheld because of azotemia.

Five (25%) infants developed complications which could be related to the treatment, namely *hypertension, azotemia, thrombocytopenia* or *cholestasis*. The authors conclude that the main objective in the management of systemic candidiasis and pneumonia in pre-term infants must be prevention. A number of prophylactic measures, such as the application of povidone-iodine ointment to site of possible infection or even twice-daily administration of antifungal agents, have been proposed and employed. Oral administration of such agents as nystatin is also being used to limit the overgrowth of candida in the gut, thus reducing the risk of systemic invasion. As neither toxicity nor resistance to nystatin has been reported, its use may be considered justified. However, the efficacy of such prophylactic measures has yet to be proven.

Neonatal pediatricians should have a high index of suspicion for systemic candida infections and pneumonia in very-low-birthweight infants, who may acquire such infections either antenatally or postnatally. Loke et al. (4[cr]) recommend that antifungal therapy be initiated with the first positive blood, urine or cerebrospinal fluid culture in clinically ill infants and when respiratory deterioration occurs in infants with positive tracheal aspirate culture. They also recommend a combined therapeutic regimen of amphotericin and 5-FC as described in this study.

Pharmacokinetics and adverse effects of amphotericin B in infants and children Despite more than 3 decades of clinical use of amphotericin B only a little information exists on its pharmacokinetics and safety in infants and children. Pediatric dose recommendations have been derived by extrapolation from adult experience without verification of their appropriateness in achieving effective and safe antifungal concentrations in this age group. For this reason a study by Korel et al (5[C]) is of special interest; its goal was to determine the range of dosages needed to achieve antifungal serum concentrations in the pediatric age group.

The kinetics and safety of amphotericin B were studied in 13 infants and children (aged from 3 weeks to 18 years) treated with the drug for proven (n = 11) or suspected (n = 2) fungal infections. The dose on the first day was 0.5 mg/kg, followed in most patients by double this daily dose for the rest of the treatment period. The drug was infused over 4–6 hours. During the first day, serum concentrations were above the target therapeutic level of 0.3 μg/ml in all patients at 2 and 6 hours from the start of the infusion, in 12 of 13 patients at 12 hours, but in only 6 of 13 patients at 24 hours. On the third day, all concentrations were > 0.3 μg/ml throughout the 24-hour period and in 12 of 13 patients they were in excess of 0.5 μg/ml. The same kinetic profile prevailed on days 7–10 of therapy, with a tendency for concentrations to increase. Elimination half-life was 9.93 ± 1.6 hours, clearance rate was 25 ± 5 ml/kg/h and distribution volume was 378 ± 25 ml/kg. The half-life inversely correlated with the patient's age. Pharmacokinetic values calculated during the first day were no different from those calculated on day 3. Significant differences in hemoglobin, platelets and serum potassium concentration were recorded along with significant increases in serum creatinine, urea and aspartate transaminase values. Changes in laboratory values associated with amphotericin B therapy in these children are summarized in Table 1.

Four children experienced adverse clinical events associated with amphotericin B infusions. One child had *generalized pain*, necessitating the use of a narcotic analgesic; 1 had *flushing, chills and high fever*

Table 1. *Changes in laboratory values associated with amphotericin B treatment*

Test (units)	Before amphotericin B treatment	During amphotericin B treatment	Significance*
Hb (gm/l)	105.5 ± 4.1	0.5 ± 5.2	$P < 0.01^{+}$
K (mmol/l)	3.81 ± 0.18	3.14 ± 0.26	$P < 0.025$
Urea (mmol/l)	2.83 ± 0.4	9.8 ± 2.8	$P < 0.025$
Ca (mmol/l)	2.17 ± 0.04	1.8 ± 0.3	n.s.
Mg (mmol/l)	1.08 ± 0.27	0.85 ± 0.19	n.s.
Creatinine (mmol/l)	33 ± 2.1	69.6 ± 16.3	$P < 0.05$
Alkaline phosphatase (IU/mm^3)	170 ± 59	349 ± 120	n.s.
AST (IU/mm^3)	30 ± 7.3	45 ± 9.8	$P < 0.05$

AST = Aspartate transaminase; Hb = hemoglobin; n.s. = not significant. Values are mean + SEM.
*Paired t-test.
$^{+}$12 of 13 patients required erythrocyte and platelet transfusions during amphotericin B treatment.

temporally associated with the administration of the drug and favorably responding to diphenhydramine and prednisone; a 3rd patient developed *urticaria* and a 4th had *nausea and vomiting*.

The above study indicates that the current practice of monitoring amphotericin B therapy according to the degree of nephrotoxicity is not adequate in the young, because in most children the serum concentrations are likely to exceed the needed antifungal concentrations with a dose of 0.5 mg/kg. Although in some children the dose will have to be increased to 1 mg/kg, the continuous increase in concentrations which occurs (because of slow equilibration) may allow a gradual decrease in dose later on. The study points to the need to individualize amphotericin B in children by using therapeutic drug monitoring. This will allow reduction in toxicity to be achieved while ensuring effective fungicidal levels. Serum concentrations of amphotericin B should be measured during days 2 and 3 of therapy both at the peak level (end of infusion) and through level (before the next dose). Repeated measurements after 7–10 days of continuous therapy will detect possible drug accumulation and in many cases should render it possible to decrease the daily dose in the interests of safety without undermining the treatment.

Miscellaneous problems *Influence of the infusion rate on reactions* The influence of the infusion rate of amphotericin B on the incidence of adverse reactions has hitherto received only sparse attention. Cleary et al (6[C]) have now performed a controlled cross-over study of 2-hour versus 45-minute infusions of amphotericin B in patients in order to assess the incidence of infusion-related reactions at these different infusion rates.

Seventeen bone-marrow-transplant recipients in whom amphotericin B was to be initiated for known or suspected fungal infections were recruited. After standardized premedication with hydrocortisone, diphenhydramine and acetaminophen) patients received 8 daily infusions of amphotericin B (0.5 mg/kg/d, concentration 0.25 mg/ml). The rate was assigned using a randomized, cross-over pair design. The axillary temperature, occurrence of chills and the meperidine dose required to resolve the chills was monitored for each infusion. For the first pair of infusions, fever (defined as an increase of body temperature by 1°C) occurred frequently, namely in 12 of 17 (70.5%) and in 13 of 17 patients (76.4%), with a mean rise of 1.6°C (range 1.1–3.7°C) and 1.7°C (1.1–3.5°C) for the 45-minute and 2-hour infusions respectively. Meperidine requirements for rapid and slow infusions were similar as well ($P = 0.12$). These data suggest that, for patients free of pre-existing renal and cardiac disease, rapid amphotericin B infusions are well-tolerated and produce adverse reactions (fever and chills) similar in nature and severity to slower infusions.

Shivering A paper by Rutledge et al (7[R]) reviews within a nursing context what is known about shivering associated with amphotericin B therapy. This common and distressing reaction reflects the drug's inherent pyrogenicity and thus resembled febrile shivering. The loss of heat has both metabolic and psychological consequences. It is important for the nurse to recognize and report the phenomenon, and measures need to be taken to restore lost heat, alongside the use of drugs to suppress the fever and thus the shivering. Table 2 provides a summary of the assessment parameters for this adverse reaction.

Treatment of paracoccidioidomycosis Köhler et al (9[C]) have reported on a 49-year-old patient who developed paracoccidioidomycosis after working in a gold mine in South America. The patient suffered from cheilitis, stomatitis, laryngitis and bilateral pneumonia. There was also evidence of cerebral granuloma. The diagnosis was confirmed by culture and serological methods. *Paracoccidioides brasiliensis* grows slowly and more than a month may elapse (in this case 6 weeks) before typical yeast-like forms with multiple buds appear in culture; in cases where there is no typical clinical picture this may complicate the making of a diagnosis. The patient was treated with amphotericin B and sulfamethoxazole/trimethoprim and a clinical response to therapy was observed. However, treatment had to be stopped because of severe side effects *(allergic exanthema, increase of creatinine levels, phlebitis at the site of infusion)*. Ketoconazole was less effective, but further clinical improvement was achieved on itraconazole without untoward side effects.

Interactions Goren et al (8[CR]) prospectively studied the effect of amphotericin B therapy on *aminoglycoside (amikacin and gentamicin) clearance* in 20 consecutive child patients dur-

Table 2. *Amphotericin B-associated shivering (7^R)*

Levels of shivering	Symptoms	Assessment	Suggested nursing approaches
Prevention	None	Temperature (oral) Blood pressure Pulse Respiration	Prevention of dehydration Increasing room temperature and making extra covers and clothes available for patient before infusion Administration of premedication. The following may be helpful: – Acetaminophen p.o. 4–6 h before infusion; repeated 30 min before diphenhydramine p.o., 30 min before infusion – Hydrocortisone mixed with infusion – Meperidine p.o. 30 min before infusion – No bathing of patient during amphotericin infusion.
Level 1	Sense of coldness Tenseness masseter	Temperature (axillary) Blood Pulse Respiration	Use of relaxation techniques Use of hypnosis if available
Level 2	'Chest quivering' Trunk involvement: neck and pectoral muscles		Administration of meperidine intravenously as required Provision of additional covers, if desired by patient
Level 3	Long muscle group involvement: arms and legs		Increasing room temperature Offering warm fluids if tolerated
Level 4	Total body involvement, teeth chattering		Suggesting isometric leg and arm movements to decrease tremors

ing the remission-induction phase of chemotherapy for acute myelocytic leukemia. Increases (≥ 50%) in the half-life for aminoglycoside excretion were not associated with antileukemic or aminoglycoside therapy alone but occurred in 12 of 17 children when amphotericin B was added to the antimicrobial regimen. Seven children had impaired aminoglycoside clearances without increases of ≥ 50% in serum creatinine; hence the resulting adjustments in aminoglycoside dosage would not have been made had the authors relied solely on serial measurements of serum creatinine. Evidence for increased excretion of the renal enzymes N-acetyl-β-D-glucosaminidase and alanine aminopeptidase during amphotericin B therapy suggested that damage to proximal tubular cells may contribute to the renal impairment that has been associated with the drug.

The toxicity that these authors observed with aminoglycoside and amphotericin therapy is consistent with reports of increased clinical nephrotoxicity when each agent is administered with other potentially nephrotoxic drugs. Their findings underscore the value of monitoring serum aminoglycoside concentrations in patients being treated simultaneously with drugs other than amphotericin B.

IMIDAZOLE DERIVATIVES *(SED-11, 572; SEDA-12, 228; SEDA-13, 232)*

Ketoconazole *(SED-11, 572; SEDA-12, 228; SEDA-13, 232)*

Endocrine effects Ketoconazole has been shown to interfere with several steps in adrenal steroidogenesis in a dose-related manner, but actual *adrenal insufficiency* among patients receiving ketoconazole has in the past been reported only once with sufficient documentation to prove its presence. A second case has now appeared from Best et al (10[C]).

The report describes a patient with symptomatic adrenal insufficiency shortly after daily therapy was started with 400 mg ketoconazole for pulmonary blastomycosis. Her pulmonary blastomycosis was cured with a 6-month course of ketoconazole, but endocrine evaluation revealed adrenal insufficiency and the patient required glcocorticoid replacement therapy for the next 2 years. In addition to symptoms of adrenal insufficiency and low cortisol levels this patient had electrolyte abnormalities (decreased serum sodium and increased serum potassium levels). she was also noted to have an increased γ-glutamyl transferase level of 62 IU/l and alkaline phosphatase level of 163 IU/l. 3 days after ketoconazole therapy was begun. All of the patient's liver enzyme values returned to normal once treatment with hydrocortisone was begun.

This case makes it clear that adrenal insufficiency can be induced even by low-dose treatment and can run a prolonged course. The authors consider that any patient treated with ketoconazole, and especially those receiving higher doses (e.g. more than 800 mg daily), should be monitored for possible adrenal corticosteroid deficiency; in those patients who appear to have borderline low adrenal function or lack of response to an ACTH infusion, replacement therapy should be given.

The endocrine effects of imidazole antimycotic agents have been studied more broadly in an in vitro model by Mason et al (11). They evaluated the ability of imidazoles to inhibit steroid aromatase activities in human placental and fetal liver material, and their effects on the progesterone 16α-, 17α- and 21-hydroxylases of human fetal adrenal. It was shown that ketoconazole is a most potent inhibitor of all these 3 human fetal adrenal progesterone hydroxylases, while clotrimazole and imazalil (enilkonazole) are the most potent inhibitors of progesterone 21-hydroxylase. These results are strongly supportive of the belief that imidazole drugs are selective inhibitors not only of steroid aromatase but also of other microsomal steroid hydroxylases. The authors believe that the results suggest the need for studying their effects on estrogen formation as well. Other modifications of these drugs may result in compounds that could prove to be selective inhibitors of other cytochrome P-450-dependent steroid hydroxylase enzymes.

Prophylaxis of fungal infections with ketoconazole König et al (12[C]) treated 147 women and 214 men (mean age 51.9 years) over a period of 42 months for neoplastic diseases with cytostatic chemotherapy; in order to prevent mycotic infection in these immunocompromized patients, ketoconazole was given in an oral dosage of 200 mg/d (the mean duration of prophylactic treatment being 5.8 months). Fungal infections were diagnosed in 28 patients (7.7%) and the serum concentration of candida antibodies was significantly elevated in 22 patients (5.9%). Chemoprophylaxis with ketoconazole had to be stopped in 8 cases (2.2%) because of extreme elevations of liver transaminases. In spite of these hepatic side effects, the prophylaxis was considered to have reduced the incidence of fungal infections below that which would otherwise have been expected.

Cross-sensitivity of the imidazoles The imidazoles, though widely prescribed, are infrequently implicated in allergic contact dermatitis and cross-sensitivity has only rarely been documented. Carmichael and Foulds (13[c]) have now for the first time observed cross-reactions between several imidazoles, including sulconazole. Cross-sensitivity between miconazole, econazole and sulconazole and the lack of cross-sensitivity with clotrimazole are readily understood if their structures are considered; those cross-reacting are all β-substituted 1-phenethyl imidazoles, whilst clotrimazole has an altogether different ring structure. The evidence from these authors adds substance to the previous theoretical warning given in data sheets that sulconazole is contraindicated in patients hypersensitive to imidazoles.

Fluconazole

Fluconazole represents a new alternative for the oral therapy of disseminated cryptococcosis and cryptococcal meningitis. This drug is a triazole derivative, related to the imidazole ketoconazole. The drug is water-soluble and very well absorbed after oral administration, with bioavailability approaching 90%. Fluconazole crosses the blood–brain barrier, so that cerebrospinal fluid concentrations reach more than 80% of those attained in serum. The long half-life of about 25 hours permits once-daily dosing, a practical consideration in optimalizing compliance during long-term therapy.

Sugar and Saunders (14[c]) conducted an open non-randomized trial of oral fluconazole as maintenance suppressive therapy of disseminated cryptococcosis in patients with AIDS. Twenty patients with AIDS, 19 of whom had cryptococcal meningitis, were studied. Patients were followed for up to 21 months. All patients received amphotericin B as primary therapy, from 20–257 days prior to entry. Fluconazole was given once daily in doses of 50–200 mg/d. The results demonstrate that fluconazole provides effective suppressive therapy for long periods of time and that it is well-tolerated by a population that typically exhibits increased adverse reactions to many medications. The most common side effects in this series concerned the gastrointestinal tract. *Nausea, vomiting* and/or *abdominal discomfort* occurred in 12 patients. *Elevated liver function test* results were observed in 5 patients. Because of concern as regards the possibility that fluconazole could be toxic to the liver, the drug was withheld in 3 cases, to be resumed after transaminase levels had stabilized or returned to normal; in all 3 cases fluconazole was resumed within 7–15 days without incident. Thrombocytopenia developed in 1 patient and resolved once fluconazole was discontinued.

This study demonstrates that many patients with AIDS and disseminated cryptococcosis can receive maintenance treatment with once-daily oral fluconazole for at least 6 months without evidence of culture-proven relapse of this otherwise fatal disorder. In the light of this initial experience with fluconazole, the authors believe that this drug represents a viable alternative to life-long suppressive therapy for disseminated cryptococcosis, especially cryptococcal meningitis, in patients with AIDS.

Hypersensitivity Kotani et al (15[c]) report on a patient with AIDS who on 2 occasions developed anaphylactoid reactions after taking flucytosine. After taking the tablets the patient suddenly developed a temperature of 38.9 °C, diffuse erythema, pruritis, conjunctival injection and abdominal pain. A few hours later the became edematous with tachycardia and hypotension demanding volume support. He recovered rapidly except for desquamation of the skin.

Candidiasis and cryptococcosis constitute major fungal infections in AIDS. These opportunistic infections can usually be controlled with appropriate use of antifungal agents such as amphotericin B, ketoconazole, flucytosine or miconazole. The development of anaphylaxis to flucytosine in this patient was unexpected because no such cases have been reported previously. The fact that anaphylaxis recurred on rechallenge with flucytosine seems to confirm the causal role of the drug. Clearly it should be used with caution in patients with AIDS.

KP-363

A skin safety (patch) test was performed in 36 healthy volunteers by Itoh (16[c]) using KP-363, a new antifungal benzylamine derivative. Test preparations were 0.6% and 0.1% creams and solution and the relevant vehicles used as a control. Reference preparations were econazole, bifonazole and tolciclate, the latter being tested as cream only. The results pointed to a less degree of irritation when using KP-363 as cream or solution, and there were also favorable results with bifonazole and tolciclate.

REFERENCES

1. Raymond JR (1988) amphotericin B nephrotoxicity. *Am. Fam. Physician, 38,* 199.
2. Stein S, Albridge K, Lemox RK et al (1988) Nephrotoxicity in leukemic patients receiving empirical amphotericin B and aminoglycosies. *South Med. J., 81,* 1095.
3. Bottineau MC, Roze JC, Mouzard A (1988) Candidoses néonatales systémiques. *Ann. Pédiatr., 35,* 235.
4. Loke HL, Verber I, Szymonowicz W (1988) Systemic candidiasis and pneumonia in preterm infants. *Aust. Paediatr. J., 24,* 138.

5. Koren G, Lau A, Klein J et al (1988) Pharmacokinetics and adverse effects of amphotericin B in infants and children. *J. Pediatr., 113,* 559.
6. Cleary JD, Weisdorf D, Fletcher CV (1988) Effect of infusion rate on amphotericin B-associated febrile reactions. *Drug Intell. Clin. Pharm., 22,* 769.
7. Rudledge DN, Holtzclaw BJ (1988) Amphotericin B-induced shivering in patients with cancer: a nursing approach. *Heart Lung, 17,* 432.
8. Goren MP, Viar MJ, Shenep JZ (1988) Monitoring serum aminoglycoside concentrations in children with amphotericin B nephrotoxicity. *Pediatr. Infect. Dis. J., 7,* 698.
9. Köhler C, Klotz M, Daus H et al (1988) Viszerale Paracoccidioidomykose bei einem Goldgräber aus Brasilien. *Mycoses, 31,* 395.
10. Best TR, Jenkins SK, Murphy FG et al (1987) Persistent adrenal insufficiency secondary to low-dose ketoconazole therapy. *Am. J. Med., 82,* 676.
11. Mason JI, Carr BR, Murry BA (1987) Imidazole antimycotics: selective inhibitors of steroid aromatization and progesterone hydroxylation. *Steroids, 50,* 179.
12. König HJ, Georgion A, Krapt P et al (1988) Mykoseprophylaxe mit Ketoconazol bei Tumorpatienten unter zytostatischer Therapie. *Mycoses, 31,* 324.
13. Carmichael AJ, Foulds IS (1988) Imidazole cross-sensitivity to sulconazole. *Contact Derm., 19,* 237.
14. Sugar AM, Saunders C (1988) Oral fluconazole as suppressive therapy of disseminated cryptococcosis in patients with acquired immunodeficiency syndrome. *Am. J. Med., 85,* 481.
15. Kotani S, Hirose S, Niiya K et al (1988) Anaphylaxis to flucytosine in a patient with AIDS. *J. Am. Med. Assoc., 260,* 3275.
16. Itoh M (1988) Skin safety study of KP-363, a new antifungal agent, in healthy volunteers. *Skin Res., 30,* 507.

I. Nir

29 Antiprotozoal drugs

ANTIMALARIAL DRUGS *(SED-11, 581; SEDA-12, 239; SEDA-13, 238)*

The present status of antimalarial drugs

Chemoprophylaxis *Malaria continues to be a high health risk not only for people living in affected areas but also for those from unaffected places when travelling to malaria-endemic zones. The appearance of drug-resistant strains of* ***Plasmodium falciparum*** *throughout much of the world has made chemoprophylaxis and chemotherapy of the disease increasingly difficult. Moreover, the serious adverse reactions experienced with many of the alternative antimalarials potentiate the risk of exposure to chemoprophylaxis, making the problem a much more difficult one. The risk of acquiring malaria, depending on circumstances and personal protective measures should definitely be weighed when considering an appropriate regimen for malaria chemoprophylaxis (1[R]). When decided upon, chemoprophylaxis should begin 1–2 weeks prior to travel to malaria areas and continue for about 4 weeks after departure from the same (1[R]). In addition to the degree of risk of acquiring malaria, previous responses by the same individual to antimalarial drugs should be taken into account. For travel to an area where chloroquine-resistant* ***P. falciparum*** *(CRPF) has not been reported, on the whole once-weekly use of chloroquine should be satisfactory. In largely CRPF-affected areas, Fansidar in addition to chloroquine should be considered (2[R], 3[R]). Fansidar, however, may cause severe cutaneous adverse reactions, erythema multiforme, Stevens-Johnson syndrome and toxic epidermal necrolysis. It is definitely contraindicated in persons with histories of sulfonamide intolerance. Mefloquine, another antimalarial, is highly effective against chloroquine and Fansidar-resistant* ***P. falciparum****. With prophylactic doses, the side effects observed were usually mild and self-limited gastrointestinal disturbances. The drug should not be taken together with cardiovascular drugs. Amodiaquine has been used as an alternative prophylactic in areas where CRPF is endemic. However, agranulocytosis has been associated with this drug and it can hardly be recommended. Maloprim (pyrimethamine + dapsone) is usually well-tolerated and could be useful together with chloroquine (300 mg/wk). Proguanil has been shown to be efficient in Kenya and should be taken daily in combination with weekly chloroquine. Other circumstances affecting the selection of appropriate malaria chemoprophylaxis which must be taken into account are pregnancy and breast-feeding. Malaria infection may be more severe in pregnant than non-pregnant women and the risk of adverse pregnancy outcome is increased. Chloroquine is considered a permissible prophylactic regimen. However, women who are pregnant, or likely to become so, should avoid travelling to CRPF areas as no chemoprophylactic regimen is completely effective or absolutely free from possible teratogenic effects. If entry into endemic malaria zones is unavoidable, prophylaxis must be taken since the danger of malaria itself outweighs the potential toxicity of the drugs used in its prevention. Very small amounts of antimalarial drugs are secreted in the milk of lactating women and the quantity of drug transferred is not thought to be harmful to the nursing infant but it is also insufficient to provide adequate protection against malaria.*

So far we have been considering mainly the ***P. falciparum*** *strain of malaria infection, but there are species other than that and they introduce additional problems. For instance,* ***P. vivax*** *and* ***P. ovale*** *have forms that can persist in the liver and cause relapses even several years after chemoprophylaxis has been discontinued. This may be prevented by taking primaquine during the last 2 weeks after exposure in the endemic area has ended, in addition to the usual prophylaxis*

(Biomedical Division)
Side Effects of Drugs Annual 14
M.N.G. Dukes and L. Beeley, editors

schedule. G6PD-deficient individuals should however be excluded from the use of primaquine.

Adverse reactions of antimalarials, particularly when used for prophylaxis over long periods, have been of increasing concern in recent years, and the situation has been rendered more difficult by the progressive spread of multiple drug resistance, notably involving ***P. falciparum.*** *There is no ideal non-toxic drug effective against all forms of malaria and reliance needs to be placed on the various antimalarials according to their qualities and the circumstances of prevention.*

Chemotherapy *The chemotherapy of malaria, especially when the disease is severe, requires much higher dosages than those applied in prophylaxis and its potential toxicity is thus increased. Chloroquine is the drug of choice for treating infections caused by all malarial species except chloroquine-resistant* ***P. falciparum.*** *It should be used in the oral form if possible. Parenteral use of chloroquine has been questioned because of its arrhythmogenic properties, while in children who had received chloroquine previously some deaths have occurred from inadvertent administration of the drug, possibly in overdosage (3[r]). Parenteral therapy should be reserved for severely ill patients, including those who are vomiting. Rapid intravenous administration of chloroquine (bolus i.v. infusion) is contraindicated (3[r]).*

The spread of chloroquine-resistant plasmodium forms in Africa, Asia and South America has led to increased use of alternative drugs, especially quinine, which has been shown to be satisfactorily effective. However, partial resistance to quinine has been reported from Burundi (4[C]) and resistance has been claimed to be already in existence in other areas, especially South East Asia. Quinine commonly causes a complex of symptoms in the form of headache, tinnitus, gastrointestinal and visual disturbances, arrhythmias and blood dyscrasias. The parasitological response to quinidine is comparable to that of quinine for the treatment of CRPF infections, but electrocardiographic effects have been associated with high plasma levels of quinidine. When in addition to CRPF the malaria is also quinine-resistant, mefloquine is the drug of choice. It has been found to be effective against certain chloroquine- and quinine-resistant strains of ***P. falciparum*** *in a single oral dose. Unfortunately, mefloquine resistance has already emerged and has even been found in areas where mefloquine has never been used. Another drug advocated for resistant forms of* ***P. falciparum*** *is pyrimethamine + sulfadoxine, which is usually administered together with mefloquine. Nausea and vomiting is a major problem, while neuropsychiatric disturbances and sinus bradycardia have also been documented with this combination. Qinghaosu has been found to be effective in vivo in the treatment of CRPF infections and especially useful in cerebral malaria (3[r]). Primaquine is the only drug in current use which has activity against the exoerythrocytic stages of infection and is thus able to achieve radical cure in* ***P. vivax*** *and* ***P. ovale*** *malaria. However, it has no effect on the asexual blood forms of the parasite at therapeutically used doses (2[r]). With proguanil, although active against asexual blood stages of the various species in human malaria, the clinical response is slow, limiting the usefulness of the drug in treatment of acute infections.*

Malaria remains a major health problem world-wide. Large-scale attempts to eradicate the vector have failed. Vaccines against the various stages of the parasite do not at present appear forthcoming. Despite the many potent drugs available, none seems to solve all current problems.

Chloroquine *(SED-11, 582; SEDA-12, 239; SEDA-13, 238)*

Interesting information regarding the use of chloroquine as an antimalarial has been obtained from recently published reports. Resistance to *P. falciparum* could be reversed in vitro by using the calcium-channel blocker verapamil (5[C]). This finding could bring new hope for chloroquine, a reliable, relatively non-toxic and non-teratogenic drug. A report from the Philippines notes that asexual parasitemia could be cleared in men with uncomplicated *P. falciparum* malaria, whereas 4 of the 5 isolates were found resistant in vitro to chloroquine (6[C]). No major differences were found in the pharmacokinetics of chloroquine between a group of Thai patients with *P. vivax* malaria and a matched group of healthy volunteers (7[C]).

Ocular toxicity A survey of detailed changes in the visual apparatus before and after chloroquine treatment of 30 subjects suffering from chronic discoid lupus erythematosus has been presented (8[C]). In addition, observations concerning examinations of 1500 patients receiving either chloroquine or hydroxychloroquine and ocular findings in 46 patients with irreversible bilateral early retinopathy seen for about 8 years have been reported. Patients presenting with normal color vision and relative paracentral scotomas appear not to deteriorate over short-term follow-up of 5 years. Retinopathy in patients presenting with less than 20/20 vision, abnormal color vision and positive fluorescein angiography may progress even if treatment with the medication is discontinued (9[C]). However, reassurance that there is no danger of developing retinopathy due to chloroquine if a maximal daily dose of not more than 6.5 mg/kg body wt. is adhered to, comes from West Germany (10[r]).

Convulsions Case-reports of tonic clonic convulsions following various prophylactic antimalarial drugs have been described in 2 young and 2 middle-aged women (11[C]). These occurred 3–4 weeks after commencing treatment with chloroquine with occasionally the addition of dapsone, Maloprim or Fansidar. All 4 patients responded to antiepileptic treatment and remained seizure-free; 3 of them had never had tonic clonic seizures before; 1 had experienced a tonic clonic seizure many years previously. None had further tonic clonic seizures after stopping antimalarials. When considering malaria prophylaxis, patients should be advised about the risk of antimalarial drugs provoking seizures.

Psoriasis Psoriatic erythrodermia and general pustular psoriasis developed in a 75-year-old man 2 weeks after beginning antimalarial treatment with chloroquine (12[C]). Some psoriasis vulgaris plaques persisted for 6 months after the acute exacerbation despite active treatment.

Pregnancy Eight women with systemic lupus erythematosus (SLE) had 14 pregnancies while receiving antimalarial drugs throughout the entire course of their pregnancies. Six normal full-term spontaneous deliveries resulted from these pregnancies with no congenital abnormalities. Fetal wastage is very high in subjects with SLE, especially during disease activity (13[C]). The author concludes that it is possible for women taking large amounts of chloroquine phosphate (500 mg/d) or hydroxychloroquine sulfate (200 mg/d) during pregnancy to produce normal live babies. The lupus activity remains one of the most important factors determining the outcome of pregnancies of women with the disease, and in patients with SLE who become pregnant while taking chloroquine or hydroxychloroquine, it may be more advantageous to continue antimalarial therapy than to discontinue it and run the risk of losing control of the disease process.

Quinine *(SED-11, 590; SEDA-12, 243; SEDA-13, 243)*

Pharmacokinetic aspects Much information on the pharmacokinetics of quinine (and quinidine) has been produced using healthy volunteers; some of it may be misleading since it seems likely that malaria infection alters many of the pharmacokinetic variables of these agents. Plasma quinine levels during malaria infection are higher than those encountered in healthy subjects given the same dose. However, although the total plasma concentration of quinine is increased during infection, the concentration of free drug may be little altered as a result of changes in plasma protein concentrations during infection. Above plasma concentrations of 15 μg/ml electrographic changes such as prolongation of the Q-T interval and widening of the QRS complex occur in quinine and quinidine therapy. T-wave flattening may also occur. Quinine crosses the placenta in relatively high concentrations in cord blood and also is excreted in breast milk. Data concerning its teratogenicity are scant, so it should therefore be avoided in the first trimester of pregnancy (2[R]).

To investigate the toxic potential of rapid intravenous quinine administration in severe malaria the pharmacokinetic properties were studied in 7 patients with cerebral malaria receiving low-dose quinine injection (4 mg/kg body wt.) followed 1 hour later by infusion of 16 mg/kg body wt. over 3 hours (14[C]). Plasma quinine concentrations closely followed a bi-exponential decline and volumes of distribution were significantly smaller than reported in healthy subjects, rendering intravenous injection of the standard therapeutic dose of 10 mg/kg over 10–20 min potentially toxic in severe malaria. The authors suggest quinine dihydrochloride 7.0 mg/kg over 30 min and a subsequent maintenance infusion over 4 hours to achieve a nontoxic therapeutic level.

Photosensitivity Quinine is commonly used to treat nocturnal cramps. Topical contact with quinine has been reported to cause both contact and photocontact allergy. Systemic treatment with quinine can result in an eczematous type of photosensitivity with increased erythemal sensitivity to UVA radiation or, in the case of lichen planus, in a photosensitive distribution. The action spectrum for 24-hour ultraviolet erythema has been determined in 3 elderly patients who presented with photosensitive eruptions after taking quinine sulfate for night cramps (15[C]). The report presents results of the action spectrum whilst taking and after discontinuing quinine sulfate and comparing the in vivo action spectra with the in vitro absorption spectrum of quinine.

Purpura Two weeks after he began taking a quinine-containing preparation against leg cramps, gingival bleeding and purpuric lesions occurred on the lower extremities of a 50-year-old man (16[C]). There was no hematuria, hematemesis or epistaxis and all biochemical and hematological tests were normal, except the platelet count which was 7000/mm^3. The case was diagnosed as quinine-induced thrombocytopenia, although idiopathic thrombocytopenic purpura could not be excluded. The patient responded rapidly and well to intravenous corticosteroids and immunoglobulins and returned to normal within 1 week.

Hypoglycemia The incidence of hypoglycemia and the effect of quinine on it was assessed in 46 patients with severe *P. falciparum* (17[C]). Plasma glucose and immunoreactive insulin were determined before and after quinine therapy. In 5 patients the initial plasma glucose level was in the hypoglycemic range, the lowest value being 12 mg/100 ml in a pregnant patient. Following quinine administration a significant fall in plasma glucose was recorded in most of the remaining patients but not to the hypoglycemic range. A good correlation was found between the glucose and insulin changes, the latter increasing accordingly. Patients with severe *P. falciparum* malaria, particularly those on quinine therapy, should be watched for hypoglycemia.

Amodiaquine *(SED-11, 587; SEDA-12, 241; SEDA-13, 238)*

In vitro dose-dependent inhibition of bone marrow proliferation was demonstrated in patients recovering from amodiaquine-induced agranulocytosis and using human liver microsomes. It was observed that amodiaquine readily forms a reactive derivative which could play a part in its toxicity (18[c]).

Halofantrine *(SEDA-12, 240; SEDA-13, 240)*

Halofantrine is highly effective against drug-resistant isolates of *P. falciparum*. Its curative effect was evaluated in a randomized double-blind trial comprising a group of 82 patients in Thailand infected with *P. falciparum* (19[C]). Halofantrine proved effective in 65% of 20 patients who received 1000 mg followed by an additional 500 mg 6 hours later, and in 88% of 60 patients who received 500 mg every 6 hours for 3 doses. The mean parasite clearance time ranged from 50–60 hours. The side effects in patients treated with halofantrine consisted of *nausea, vomiting, abdominal pain* and *diarrhea* (15–20% of patients) as well as single incidences of *neuromuscular spasms, jaundice, mouth ulcers* and *premature ventricular contractions*, and were not significantly different from those of patients treated with mefloquine in the same study. Halofantrine, therefore, appears to be of comparable efficacy to mefloquine in treating multidrug-resistant *P. falciparum* malaria.

Mefloquine *(SED-11, 587; SEDA-12, 241; SEDA-13, 241)*

In the aforementioned study (19[C]) mefloquine was curative in 88% of 25 patients given a single dose of 1000 mg and in 97% of 30 patients given a single oral dose of 1500 mg. Side effects consisted mainly of *nausea* and *diarrhea* with isolated cases of *arthralgia, jaundice, hemolysis* and *premature ventricular contraction* in the high-dose group.

Seizures Partial and general seizures appeared in a 38-year-old man after he had taken a first, and 1 week later a second, dose of 250 mg mefloquine. The seizures responded to clonazepam. The subject began having complex partial seizures when aged 15. Mefloquine may therefore aggravate (and perhaps even provoke) latent epilepsy, a point which should be taken into consideration when prescribing the drug to epileptic patients (20[C]).

Pyrimethamine *(SED-11, 588)*

Pyrimethamine therapy was instituted in a pregnant woman at the 26th week of gestation because of a toxoplasma infection (21[C]). Treatment was stopped at the 3rd day due to symptoms suggestive of a common cold. Next day ulcerative buccal lesions, purpurae and hematomas were evident. On day 10 following pyrimethamine treatment severe *pancytopenia* and *hypercellular bone marrow* were diagnosed. After appropriate treatment the patient became symptomless, had normal hematological values and delivered a mature healthy baby by cesarian section.

Another hematological adverse effect ascribed to pyrimethamine therapy of toxoplasmosis in a pregnant woman has been reported (22[C]). At 22 weeks of gestation a 32-year-old woman was treated with pyrimethamine. After a week she developed malaise, nausea, vomiting and epistaxis and an erythematous skin rash. Hematological values were 10000 platelets/mm^3, 600 leukocytes/mm^3 and 9.1% hemoglobin.

Pyrimethamine 25 mg + sulfadoxine 500 mg (Fansidar) *(SED-11, 589; SEDA-12, 242; SEDA-13, 241)*

Thrombocytopenia was observed in a 41-year-old man treated for toxoplasmosis with pyrimethamine (8 mg/kg/d) and sulfadiazine (100 mg/kg/d) (23[c]).

On day 10 his hematological values were: thrombocytes 70000/μl, leukocytes 2500/μl and hemoglobin 11g%; on day 16 they measured 6000/μl, 6700/μl and 8 g%, respectively. Treatment with pyrimethamine + sulfadiazine was stopped and the patient slowly recovered.

Pyrimethamine 25 mg + sulfadoxine 500 mg + mefloquine 250 mg (Fansimef) *(SED-11, 590; SEDA-13, 242)*

A randomized double-blind study in long-term malaria chemoprophylaxis was performed in Nigeria in 211 volunteer Austrian industrial workers and their families ranging in age from 9–60; 101 received Fansimef and 110 chloroquine for 3–18 months (24[C]). *Insomnia, palpitations, dizziness, nausea* and *headaches* appeared in 7 subjects on Fansimef and in 2 on chloroquine. A few minor complaints of *burning eyes* and *gastric pain* were also reported in both groups. At 3 months laboratory checks showed a transient significantly *increased serum glutamic oxalacetic transaminase and glutamyl transpeptidase*. Antibodies against blood stage parasites could be demonstrated at different stages of the study, indicating that these 2 antimalarials are not causal prophylactic agents.

Quinacrine (mepacrine) *(SED-11, 592; SEDA-13, 241)*

Contrary to chloroquine and hydroxychloroquine, which accumulate in the retinal pigment epithelium and, when taken in large doses, produce retinal damage, the 9-aminoacridine compound is non-toxic to the retina. Quinacrine does result in *yellow staining*, of the sclerae, skin, nails and salivary glands; the incidence is dose-related and reversible on discontinuation of the drug (2[R]).

DRUGS USED IN THE TREATMENT OF OTHER PROTOZOAL INFECTIONS *(SED-11, 593; SEDA-12, 244; SEDA-13, 243)*

Metronidazole *(SED-11, 595; SEDA-12, 244; SEDA-13, 243)*

Present status The diverse uses of metronidazole range from a protozoacide against amoebae, bactericide, potentiating agent in radiotherapy, as well as widespread application with increased dosages and duration of treatment for such maladies as Crohn's disease (25[R]). In patients with *chronic liver disease*, especially those who also have renal disease, the metronidazole half-life is prolonged, leading to drug accumulation and toxicity, making dosage reduction necessary. The common adverse reactions are *gastrointestinal*, in particular nausea, vomiting and a metallic taste in the mouth. Pseudomembranous colitis has occurred but only rarely. The most serious toxicity has been reported in the central nervous system. Rarely, usually with high doses or prolonged therapy, *convulsions, ataxia* and *confusion* may occur. Sensory *peripheral neuropathy* has also occasionally been noted. For many years there has been concern about the possible *teratogenicity* and *carcinogenicity* of metronidazole. The reduction products of metabolism are mutagenic in bacteria and cancers have occurred in animals after long-term metronidazole use. Extrapolation of these findings to humans has been difficult and there has been no evidence that metronidazole is either carcinogenic or teratogenic and the risk of cancer in patients receiving conventional short courses of metronidazole is negligible (25[R]). Beneficial effects were achieved by treatment of duodenal ulcer with metronidazole, which was very well-tolerated by the patients (26[C]).

Metronidazole (and tinidazole) were found activated within anaerobic trophozoites by partial enzymic reduction of the nitro-group to produce a toxic compound that alkylates DNA and blocks nucleic acid synthesis. Simultaneously drug intake into the amoeba is facilitated (27[r]).

Pneumonitis A case of pneumonitis believed by the reporting author to be the first case of metronidazole-induced lung disease has been described by Kristenson (28[c]).

A patient known to have a pollen allergy and who had been taking oral contraceptives for years, developed recurrent vaginitis. On the day after metronidazole treatment was started she developed high fever, cough, conjunctivitis and a generalized maculopapular exanthema. A chest X-ray showed pulmonary infiltrates and bilateral pleural effusion. Following stoppage of metronidazole and erythromycin treatment the patient recovered completely after 3 days and all tests were negative. A very similar event occurred in the same patient 5 months later when metronidazole was again initiated for vaginitis. After 2 days' treatment the metronidazole was stopped and the patient recovered completely within a few days.

Postpartum psychosis It is possible that metronizadole might precipitate a psychosis in very high-risk patients, as a case in 1988 suggests (29[C]).

A 44-year old Laotian woman with no previous affective symptoms or psychosis and no history of psychiatric disease in her family had a normal premature spontaneous vaginal delivery without complication or anesthesia. Because of *Entamoeba coli* cysts in her stool the patient was given oral metronidazole 750 mg 3 times a day. She was doing well and was discharged; the newborn remained in the nursery because of its prematurity. One week later the patient was admitted to a residential psychiatric treatment center, since, according to her family, she acted weirdly, talked nonsense, did not sleep and complained of abdominal and chest pain and nausea. In fact, nausea, vomiting and abdominal pain occurred on the same day and she was taken to the emergency room. Suspicion that the distress was being caused by metronidazole was raised and so the drug was stopped. The patient became much improved, but 3 days later developed auditory and visual hallucinations, refused any kind of food, did not sleep, wanted to commit suicide and was therefore admitted to the psychiatric unit. She was treated with haloperidol and after 1 month of hospitalization was free of any psychiatric symptoms and discharged.

It should be noted that this patient had previously experienced several spontaneous abortions, a premature delivery and deaths of children aged 1 and 6. The authors, McCahill and Braff (29[C]), tend to believe this to be rather a multifactorial case; that because of her postpartum status the patient was in a state of biological vulnerability and the high dose of metronidazole facilitated the expression of her atypical *psychosis*. They advocate careful consideration of each case before applying high doses of metronidazole during the puerperium.

Neuropathy Three cases of peripheral neuropathy due to metronidazole have been reported from Seoul, Korea, after long-term administration of metronidazole 134, 105 and 81.5 g, respectively. Clinical characteristics were distal sensory polyneuropathy without definite motor involvement. Electrophysiological studies suggest distal sensory axonal degeneration showing loss of sensory nerve potential over distal segment and normal motor nerve conduction studies, F-waves and H-reflexes. The severity of clinical and electrophysiological abnormalities were closely related to the total amounts of metronidazole administered (30[C]).

Neutropenia A 74-year-old Japanese woman treated for pseudo-membranous colitis with vancomycin and metronidazole developed neutropenia. It was not established whether metronidazole had been the cause (31[c]).

Effects on the breast-fed neonate Metronidazole and its metabolite hydroxymetronidazole concentrations were measured in breast milk and plasma of 12 breast-feeding mothers following multiple doses of metronidazole (400 mg 3 times daily) and in plasma of suckling infants; 35 infants were monitored for adverse reactions to maternal therapy and in addition 2 groups of infants whose mothers received either ampicillin or no drugs served as controls.

The mean milk to plasma ratio was 0.9 for metronidazole and 0.76 for hydroxymetronidazole, while the mean milk metronidazole concentration was 15.5 μg/ml and the mean milk hydroxymetronidazole concentration was 5.7 μg/ml. Infant plasma metronidazole ranged from 1.27–2.41 μg/ml. There was no significant increase in adverse reactions in the infants which could be attributed to maternal metronidazole therapy and the amount of the drug in the milk caused no serious reactions in the 35 suckling infants studied. In their report, Passmore et al (32[C]) conclude that metronidazole may be administered in doses of 3×400 mg daily to mothers wishing to breast-feed their infants.

OTHER COMPOUNDS

Difluoromethylornithine (DFM)

DFM has been recently proposed as an effective curative drug in various *Trypanosoma* species infections. A study has been performed in Belgium in 3 Africans from Zaire and 2 whites who had lived there, suffering from Gambian trypanosomiasis (early and late stages of the disease), using DFM by intravenous and oral routes of administration (33[C]). During 1–4 days parasites were cleared from the blood with a marked improvement of clinical symptoms. Loose stools in 3 patients and anemia and decreased auditory acuity in 1 occurred, but all side effects were transient and mild. DFM penetrated the CSF into the central nervous system. These preliminary results are encouraging.

Melarsoprol

From Kinshasa comes a report on 5 male and female young and middle-aged patients with trypanosomiasis treated with the arsenical preparation Melarsopol usually 3 mg/kg/d i.v. in 3 series of 4 injections. *Peripheral neuropathy* predominantly in the extremities developed within 2–5 weeks of commencing treatment, with muscular pain and abolition of osteo-tendinous reflexes (34[C]).

Praziquantel *(SED-11, 598; SEDA-13, 242)*

This drug is highly effective against the major species of schistosomes that infect man as well as in cerebral cysticercosis and pulmonary paragonimiasis. It can be administered orally and usually produces only mild transient side effects such as drowsiness, headache, nausea, backache and abdominal discomfort. The recommended dosage varies with the infecting species and lies between 40 and 75 mg/kg/d. Cysticercosis is treated with 15 mg/kg/d for 15 days (35[r]).

Hemiplegia An unusual case of severe hemiplegia resulting from a vasculitic infarct during the course of praziquantel therapy of neurocysticercosis is of much interest (36[C]).

The event occurred in a 48-year-old man with a 16-year history of tonic clonic seizures. He was given praziquantel 50 mg/kg/d in 2 divided doses and after each intake the patient became confused with a high fever of 39°C. After a break of 6 days a gradual dose increment was introduced starting with 5 mg/kg. On reaching 50 mg/kg confusion with high fever developed, the patient became aphasic and a right permanent hemiplegia evolved. Praziquantel was discontinued, but the patient remained severely incapacitated.

Woo et al (36[C]) who report the event believe it was probably precipitated by a massive inflammatory response due to the destruction of a large number of cysts.

Pentamidine *(SED-11, 598; SEDA-12, 244; SEDA-13, 243)*

Cardiovascular effects A case of *ventricular tachycardia* has been described in a 29-year-old man with acquired immunodeficiency syndrome (AIDS) who was also suffering from visceral leishmaniasis and receiving pentamidine isethionate 4 mg/kg/d i.m. for *Pneumocystis carinii* pneumonia (37[c]).

ECG changes including ventricular bigeminy, marked QT interval prolongation and T-wave inversion with episodes of non-sustained ventricular tachycardia, were recorded after 10 days of pentamidine treatment. The ECG recorded before commencing pentamidine therapy had been normal.

It should be noted that this is a potentially life-threatening complication of pentamidine treatment and may be particularly relevant to AIDS patients. The ECG changes may be preceded by dizziness (37[c]).

Hypoglycemia Hypoglycemia as a side effect of intravenous pentamidine administration is not uncommon, occurring in 10–30% of patients treated with the drug. It has been assumed that by delivering pentamidine by inhalation directly to the site of infection, the adverse effects may be reduced. A case of intermittent hypoglycemia in a 45-year-old homosexual man with *P. carinii* pneumonia following 5 days of treatment with a daily dose of 300 mg pentamidine inhaled over 30 min has been reported (38[c]). After a 9-day period of treatment the hypoglycemia resolved despite continued pentamidine therapy.

With regard to association of hypoglycemia with pentamidine administration in general, another incident in a 35-year-old homosexual with AIDS who was treated with pentamidine for *P. carinii* pneumonia has been reported from Madrid, Spain. The hypoglycemia was recorded on the 8th day of treatment with 240 mg/d (39[c]). To assess the risk factors associated with pentamidine treatment and hypoglycemia the Division of Parasitic Diseases of the Center for Infectious Diseases in Atlanta reviewed hospital charts of patients treated with pentamidine in New York City during 4 months in 1984 (40[C]). Out of 164 patients, 97% of whom had a diagnosis of AIDS, hypoglycemia occurred in 23 (14%). It is apparent that hypoglycemia was more likely to develop in patients who received pentamidine therapy of longer duration and in higher dosages and in those who had received pentamidine previously, as well as in subjects who experienced azotemia during treatment. Waskin et al (40[C]) conclude that this serious, potentially fatal reaction is particularly dangerous in those receiving prolonged or recurrent pentamidine therapy and should be evaluated carefully in all patients before it is prescribed.

Hyperglycemia In a study carried out in India, of 490 cases of kala-azar treated with pentamidine isethionate, 11 developed hyperglycemia which was reversed in 8 upon cessation of therapy but persisted in the other 3, indicating the development of diabetes mellitus (41[C]).

Use of inhalations Regarding the nebulized form of pentamidine application, it should be noted that other systemic side-effects such as hypoglycemia (see above) neutropenia have also been observed in patients with inhaled pentamidine (38[c]). A case of hypersensitivity to nebulized pentamidine was also described in a 35-year-old man with AIDS to whom 600 mg was applied weekly for *P. carinii* prophylaxis (42[C]).

This was well-tolerated until 3 days after the 17th dose, when he developed an urticarial rash. A week later the rash had almost completely cleared and he received the 18th dose of nebulized pentamidine. A high fever with general urticarial rash occurred 1 hour after the inhalation, suggesting that the rash was due to pentamidine although the patient had received in addition certain other medication.

Rashes and toxic epidermal necrolysis have been described with parenteral pentamidine. This patient was allergic to co-trimoxazole and had had hypotension during intravenous pentamidine therapy. Others (43[c]) had not found any ill effects from the use of nebulized pentamidine in 2 AIDS patients with *P. carinii* pneumonia who had a history of serious reactions to parenteral pentamidine.

Treatment of *P. carinii* pneumonia To update the status of pentamidine in treatment of *P. carinii* pneumonia, its relevant properties have been reviewed by Salamone and Cunha (44[R]). Interest in its use for this purpose has increased with the rising number of patients with AIDS who have *P. carinii* pneumonia. Approximately 50% of patients who receive the drug by the intravenous or intramuscular route experience some drug toxicity, i.e. local pain, sterile abscesses at the intramuscular injection site, hypoglycemia, hypotension and azotemia, while adverse effects after aerosol therapy include bronchial irritation but less systemic toxicity. Pentamidine has clearly emerged as a mainstay of therapy in the management of *P. carinii* pneumonitis in AIDS, but it must be realized that any adverse reactions which emerge may be persistent since the drug may be detectable in the urine for 6–8 weeks after the last dose.

Sodium stibogluconate *(SED-11, 599)*

A rational regimen of treatment of kala-azar with sodium stibogluconate has been evaluated in India (45[C]). In a randomized study of 371 patients with kala-azar sodium stibogluconate 20 mg/kg/d for 40 days was found to produce the best rate of cure (97% of 62 patients). One patient in this and 3 in other groups became unresponsive to antimony. The patients tolerated the longer duration of treatment safely and side effects were minor.

REFERENCES

1. Recommendations for the prevention of malaria in travelers (1988) Leads from the Morbidity and Weekly Report, Vol. 37, Center for Disease Control, Atlanta. *J. Am. Med. Assoc., 259,* 3390.
2. Wistanley PA, Breckenbridge AM (1987) Currently important antimalarial drugs. *Ann. Trop. Med. Parasitol., 81,* 619.
3. Krogstadt DJ, Herwaldt BL, Schlesinger PH (1988) Antimalarial agents: specific treatment regimens. *Antimicrob. Agents Chemother., 32,* 957.
4. Coosemans M, Laroche R, Buhetura S et al (1988) Réponse de *Plasmodium falciparum* à la quinine en milieu hospitalier dans un region à chloroquine-résistance. *Méd. Trop., 48,* 139.
5. Ryall JC (1987) Reversal of chloroquine resistance in Falciparum malaria. *Parasitol. Today, 3,* 256.
6. Watt G, Long GW, Padre LP et al (1988) Chloroquine and quinine: a randomized double-blind comparison of efficacy and side effects in the treatment of *Plasmodium falciparum* malaria in the Philippines. *Trans. R. Soc. Trop. Med. Hyg., 82,* 205.
7. Edwards G, Looareesuwan D, Davies AJ et al (1988) Pharmacokinetics of chloroquine in Thais: plasma red cell concentrations following an intravenous infusion of healthy subjects and patients with *Plasmodium vivax* malaria. *Br. J. Clin. Pharmacol., 25,* 477.
8. Rossi A, Rinaldi M, Vozza A et al (1988) Studio dell' apparato visivo in 30 suggetti con LED trattati con idrossichlorochina. *G. Ital. Dermatol. Venereol., 123,* 189.
9. Easterbrook M (1988) Ocular effects and safety of antimalarial agents. *Am. J. Med., 85,* 23.
10. Ochsendorf FR, Runne U (1988) Chloroquin-Retinopathie: vermeidbar durch Beachtung der maximalen Tagesdosis. *Hautarzt, 39,* 341.
11. Fish DR, Espir MLE (1988) Convulsions associated with prophylactic antimalarial drugs: implications for people with epilepsy. *Br. Med. J., 297,* 526.
12. Nicholas J-F, Mauduit G, Haond J et al (1988) Psoriasis grave induit par la chloroquine (Nivaquine). *Ann. Dermatol. Vénéréol., 15,* 289.
13. Parke AL (1988) Antimalarial drugs, systemic lupus erythematosus and pregnancy. *J. Rheumatol., 15,* 607.
14. Davis TME, White NJ, Looareesuwan S et al (1988) Quinine pharmacokinetics in cerebral malaria: predicted plasma concentrations after rapid intravenous loading using a two-compartment model. *Trans. R. Soc. Trop. Med. Hyg., 82,* 542.
15. Diffey BL, Farr PM, Adams SJ (1988) The action spectrum in quinine photosensitivity. *Br. J. Dermatol., 118,* 679.
16. Mitchell TR, Morrow JD, Morgan HJ (1988) Quinine purpura. *J. Tenn. Med. Assoc., 81,* 578.
17. Das BS, Satpathy SK, Mohanty D et al (1988) Hypoglycemia in severe falciparum malaria. *Trans. R. Soc. Trop. Med. Hyg., 82,* 197.
18. Maggs J, Killeringham N, Breckenridge A et al (1987) Antoxidative formation of chemically reactive intermediate from amodiaquine amyelotoxin and hepatotoxin in man. *Biochem. Pharmacol., 36,* 3365.
19. Boudreau EF, Pang LW, Dixon KE et al (1988) Malaria treatment efficacy of halofantrine (WR 171,669) in initial field trials in Thailand. *Bull. WHO, 66,* 227.
20. Jallon P (1988) Use of mefloquine in epileptic patients. *J. Neurol. Neurosurg. Psychiatry, 51,* 732.
21. Pajor A, Hintalan A, Lintner F (1988) Pyrimethamin (Tindurin) által okozott pancytopenia terhességben. *Magy. Noorv. Lapja, 51,* 147.
22. Reyes P, Paucar J, Navarro J et al (1987) Toxicidad hematologica por pirimetamina. *Rev. Sanid. Fuerzas Polic., 48,* 79.
23. Termínassían D, Reygagne P, Lecompte T et al (1988) Thrombopénie non carentielle survenue à l'occasion d'un traitement par sulfadiazine-pyriméthamine. *Med. Mal. Infect., 18,* 250.
24. Kollaritsch H, Stemberger H, Mailer H et al

(1988) Tolerability of long-term prophylaxis with combination mefloquine + sulfadoxine + pyrimethamine (Fansimef): results of a double-blind trial versus chloroquine in Nigeria. *Trans. R. Soc. Trop. Med. Hyg.*, *82*, 524.
25. Scully B (1988) Metronidazole. *Med. Clin. North Am.*, *72*, 613.
26. Feliu IL, Diaz MQ (1988) Ulcera duodenal ensayo terapeutico mediante la utilizaciòn de acetazolamide versus metronidazol. *Rev. Cubana Med.*, *27*, 20.
27. Knight R (1988) Amoebiasis. *Prescr. J.*, *28*, 103.
28. Kristenson M (1988) Pneumonitis caused by metronidazole. *J. Am. Med. Assoc.*, *260*, 184.
29. McCahill ME, Braff DL (1988) Atypical postpartum psychosis possibly associated with metronidazole therapy. *J. Fam. Pract.*, *27*, 323.
30. Sunwoo IN, Kim SM, Choi MS et al (1988) Metronidazole neuropathy; report of three cases. *J. Korean Med. Assoc.*, *31*, 561.
31. Chiba M, Itoh S, Tsurui N et al (1988) A case of non-antibiotic pseudomembranous colitis with vancomycin and of metronidazole-induced neutropenia. *J. Jpn. Soc. Coloproctol.*, *41*, 395.
32. Passmore CM, McElnay JC, Rainey EA et al (1988) Metronidazole excretion in human milk and its effect on the suckling neonate. *Br. J. Clin. Pharmacol.*, *26*, 45.
33. Taelman H, Schecter PJ, Marcelis L et al (1987) Difluoromethylornithine, an effective new treatment of Gambian trypanosomiasis. *Am. J. Med.*, *82*, 607.
34. Nkanga NG, Mutombo L, Kazadi K et al (1988) Neuropathies arsénicales après traitement de la trypanosomiase humaine au mélarsoprol. *Méd. Afr. Noire*, *35*, 73.
35. Ramos O (1988) Praziquantel for the treatment of parasitic infections. *Int. Pediatr.*, *3*, 38.
36. Woo E, Yu YI, Huang CY (1988) Cerebral infarct precipitated by praziquantel in neurocysticercosis – a cautionary note. *Trop. Geogr. Med.*, *40*, 143.
37. Pujol M, Carratala J, Mauri J et al (1988) Ventricular tachycardia due to pentamidine isethionate. *Am. J. Med.*, *84*, 980.
38. Karboski JA, Godley PJ (1988) Inhaled pentamidine and hypoglycemia. *Ann. Intern. Med.*, *108*, 490.
39. Estopinan V, Montilla P, Riobo P et al (198) Hipoglucemia y diabetes mellitus como complicaciones del tratamiento con pentamidina. A proposito de un caso. *Med. Clin. (Barc.)*, *90*, 675.
40. Waskin H, Stehr-Green JK, Kelmick CG (1988) Risk factors for hypoglycemia associated with pentamidine therapy for pneumocystis pneumonia. *J. Am. Med. Assoc.*, *260*, 345.
41. Prakash N, Sinha SP, Sinha AN (1988) Development of diabetes mellitus in kala-azar patients after treatment with pentamidine isethionate. *Indian J. Clin. Biochem.*, *3*, 83.
42. Leen CLS, Mandal BK (1988) Rash due to nebulised pentamidine. *Lancet*, *2*, 1250.
43. Havlichek D (1988) Aerosolised pentamidine therapy. *Ann. Intern. Med.*, *109*, 167.
44. Salamone FR, Cunha BA (1988) Update of pentamidine for the treatment of *Pneumocystis carinii* pneumonia. *Clin. Pharm.*, *7*, 501.
45. Thakur CP, Kumar M, Kumar P et al (1988) Rationalisation of regimens of treatment of kala-azar with sodium stibogluconate in India. A randomised study. *Br. Med. J.*, *296*, 1557.

J.E. Idänpään-Heikkilä and K. Aranko

30 Miscellaneous antibacterial and antiviral drugs

ANTIBACTERIAL DRUGS

Nitrofurantoin (*SED-11, 614; SEDA-12, 248; SEDA-13, 250*)

Nitrofurantoin-induced *cholestatic hepatitis* after repeated automedication was reported in a 41-year-old woman with alcoholic liver cirrhosis. She had taken nitrofurantoin because of symptoms of dysuria. Treatment with 40 mg prednisolone resulted in progressive improvement (1[C]). A cholestatic form of acute liver injury that remits rapidly after cessation of therapy is a typical but rare complication of the short-term use of nitrofurantoin. In prolonged therapy a syndrome closely simulating chronic active hepatitis or lupus-like syndrome has occasionally been found (SEDA-5, 285).

A 64-year-old woman developed a *chronic lung reaction* with interstitial fibrosis (2[C]). She had used 100 mg of nitrofurantoin daily for chronic urinary tract infections. After 5 months of therapy with corticosteroids the *X*-ray still revealed some fibrosis. Similar cases have previously been reported and described in detail in the literature (3[C]).

Sulfonamides and trimethoprim (*SED-11, 603; SEDA-12, 248; SEDA-13, 250*)

The critical discussion about the role of co-trimoxazole (SEDA-12, 248, SEDA-13, 250) in the treatment of ordinary infections continues (4[R], 5[r], 6[c], 7[c]). In an extensive overview (4[R]) Turnidge summarized the published data on emergence of resistance, adverse drug reactions, and comparative efficacy of co-trimoxazole. He also compared the Australian experience of adverse reactions to co-trimoxazole with that of amoxicillin. There were 2466 reports on co-trimoxazole (24 deaths) to the Adverse Drug Reaction Advisory Committee from 1972–1988. This compares with 1450 reports and 10 deaths for amoxicillin during the same period of time. When the numbers were corrected by consumption figures, there was a 2-fold higher incidence of reactions to co-trimoxazole than to amoxicillin. Though a number of valid indications exist, the author concluded that co-trimoxazole can be substituted in the majority of its common indications.

Bachrach and Svartz (8[R], 9[R]) summarized and discussed all adverse drug reactions to sulfasalazine detected in the early trials. The reported incidence of side effects in the 27 early trials (from 1949–1973) varied from 13–60% and the treatment was discontinued in 0–22% of the patients. In addition, the mechanism of toxicity was discussed with a review of the data on hematological effects and lung reactions.

Single dose and 10-day treatment regimens of co-trimoxazole for acute dysuria were compared in a double-blind, randomized and placebo-controlled trial (10[c]).

In this elegant trial 116 women were given trimethoprim 320 mg and sulfamethoxazole 1600 mg in a single dose and 125 women the combination of trimethoprim 160 mg + sulfamethoxazole 800 mg twice daily for 10 days. The overall adverse effect frequency was statistically significantly lower in the single-dose group (12%) than in the 10-day treatment group (25%), including *rashes* in 1% vs. 7%, and *yeast vaginitis* in 4% vs. 12%, respectively. However, there were no differences in the reports of *gastrointestinal upset* (8% vs. 7%, respectively).

Stein et al (11[c]) reported drug-related side effects in 26% of patients during 10-days' co-trimoxazole treatment compared to 44% in

(Biomedical Division)
Side Effects of Drugs Annual 14
M.N.G. Dukes and L. Beeley, editors

those randomized to receive an additional 32 days of co-trimoxazole for upper urinary tract infection. The difference in adverse drug reaction frequency reached a statistically significant level in the number of rashes (5% vs. 20%, respectively). The only case of *leukopenia* was reported from the 6-weeks' treatment group. In addition, the number of withdrawals due to adverse effects was significantly higher among patients randomized to 6-week (24%) than in the 10-day (3%) regimen. Rash was the most common cause of discontinuation and occurred in all cases after 10 days' therapy.

Renal Another reminder of the perils of prolonged sulfonamide administration is an occurrence of *allergic interstitial nephritis* in 4 women with frequent urinary tract infections (12[c]).

These 4 postmenopausal women (54–67 years) suffered from frequently recurring urinary tract infections and a progressive fall in glomerular filtration rate. They all had eosinophiluria and their creatinine clearance averaged 34 ml/min (range 11–47 ml/min) at the time sulfonamides were discontinued. In addition to prophylactic sulfonamide (or co-trimoxazole) therapy 1 woman had both hydrochlorothiazide and furosemide, and another unspecified diuretic. Unfortunately no further details of medication were given. However, all sulfonamide preparations were discontinued and creatinine clearance improved markedly within less than 1 month in 3 patients. In the 4th patient improvement was less rapid but significant. Corticosteroids were not used and it took from 3 weeks to 3 months before eosinophiles were no longer found in the urinary sediment. Renal biopsy was not performed, but the authors suspected in all these cases eosinophilic interstitial nephritis due to chronic sulfonamide therapy.

Skin and appendages In the FDA spontaneous report system there were 97 reports of Stevens-Johnson syndrome associated with co-trimoxazole from 1981–1985 (13[c]). This outweighs the respective number of ampicillin (2 reports), cefaclor (7 reports), and cefalexin (2 reports). Additional cases of Stevens-Johnson syndrome (14[c]) or toxic epidermal necrolysis (6[c], 15[c]) associated with sulfonamides were also reported in the current literature.

Respiratory In a recent case-report, rechallenge verified sulfapyridine to be the causative agent in a sulfasalazine-induced *pulmonary eosinophilia*. Treatment with olsalazine, a 5-aminosalicylic acid compound, was successfully introduced without recurrence of pulmonary symptoms (16[c]). Two other case-reports describe the typical clinical picture of a pulmonary eosinophilia and response to withdrawal of sulfasalazine (17[c], 18[c]). The significance of this association was, however, questioned. A case of self-limiting primary pulmonary eosinophilia in a young woman receiving continuous sulfasalazine was reported (19[c]).

Other adverse effects *Systemic lupus erythematosus* was encountered in 2 patients on sulfasalazine and causative relationship was postulated (20[c], 21[c]).

A severe allergic reaction to co-trimoxazole was accompanied by *corneal ring formation* in a 55-year-old man (22[c]). He had a diffuse erythematous maculopapular rash involving his entire body, temperature of 39.5 °C, myalgias and arthralgias. Furthermore, he complained of a foreign-body sensation in both eyes and slit-lamp examination revealed marginal corneal ring infiltrates in both eyes. The patient had significantly higher levels of sulfamethoxazole-specific IgG, IgE and IgM than the controls. Topical and systemic corticosteroids were given and both systemic and ocular manifestations disappeared within 4 weeks.

Sperm penetration assay was used to document a case of sulfasalazine-induced *infertility* in a 32-year-old-man with colitis ulcerosa (23[c]). Three months after discontinuation of sulfasalazine and initiation of treatment with 5-aminosalicylic acid enemas, sperm penetration assay returned to normal. Six months later the patient's wife became pregnant. This strongly suggests that sulfapyridine component was responsible for this well-established adverse effect of sulfasalazine therapy.

NALIDIXIC ACID AND CONGENERS *(SED-11, 617; SEDA-12,249; SEDA-13, 251)*

Fluoroquinolones *(SED-11, 618; SEDA-12, 250; SEDA-13, 251)*

A special review on the safety of fluoroquinolones was published in a previous volume of this series (SEDA-12, 250). Since then the clini-

Table 1. *Adverse reactions in 1540 patients treated with norfloxacin in clinical trials**

Neuropsychiatric	(%)	*Gastrointestinal*	(%)
Headache	1.8	Nausea	1.9
Dizziness	1.2	Abdominal pain	0.3
Insomnia	0.4	Dyspepsia	0.3
Somnolence	0.3	Constipation	0.3
Depression	0.3	Flatulence	0.3
Taste disturbance	0.2	Heartburn	0.3
Skin and allergic		*Abnormal laboratory tests*	
Erythema	0.2	Leukopenia	0.4
Pruritus	0.2	Eosinophilia	0.1
Rash	0.4	Elevations in liver function tests	0.1
Urticaria	0.1		

*Modified from Corrado et al (31).

cal use of fluoroquinolones has increased and additional safety information has become available.

Ciprofloxacin Acute renal failure developed in a 64-year-old woman 11 days after the start of ciprofloxacin treatment (750 mg orally twice a day) for pneumonia (24[C]). Her blood urea nitrogen was 79 mg/100 ml and serum creatinine 8.2 mg/100 ml. The percutaneous renal biopsy finding supported the diagnosis of an *allergic interstitial nephritis*. Ciprofloxacin was probably the cause of this renal complication.

A striking rise in serum creatinine level (up to 14.1 mg/100 ml) after 4 days of concomitant therapy with ciprofloxacin and ciclosporin was observed in a 58-year-old man who had undergone bipolar hip arthroplasty 34 months following a heterotopic cardiac transplantation (25[C]). The patient had received daily ciclosporin since transplantation without any complications. Ciprofloxacin was introduced because of wound infection. The creatinine levels normalized when ciprofloxacin was discontinued although ciclosporin was continued. Apparently ciprofloxacin and ciclosporin acted synergistically to produce *nephrotoxicity* which seems to occur in about 1% of patients receiving ciclosporin alone. Crystalluria was found in 1 of the 12 healthy volunteers who received a single 400-mg dose intravenously (30 min infusion) of ciprofloxacin (26[R]). Crystalluria was not observed in subjects receiving lower doses (200 or 300 mg) of ciprofloxacin.

The safety and efficacy of ciprofloxacin (500 mg orally twice daily) was studied in 25 elderly (mean age 70.4 years) patients (27[R]) who suffered from complicated urinary tract infections. Adverse reactions were seen in 7 patients (25%): *eosinophilia* (1), eosinophilia and *reduced leukocyte count* (1), *crystalluria* (1), *granular casts* (1), *elevation of serum creatinine and blood urea nitrogen levels* (1) and *nausea* (2 patients). None of these adverse reactions warranted discontinuation of the therapy.

Among 38 patients with osteomyelitis who received ciprofloxacin from 500–1500 mg twice daily, 9 patients developed adverse events as follows: *phototoxic reactions* (2 cases), *impaired color vision* (2 cases) and 1 each of *exanthema, abdominal pain, malaise, drug fever, peripheral neuropathy* and *eosinophilia* (28[R]).

Phlebitis occurred in 6 of 34 patients who received ciprofloxacin 200 or 300 mg i.v. twice daily (29[R]).

Enoxacin Intravenous enoxacin treatment (from 200–400 mg twice daily) caused *phlebitis* and *headache* in 3 of 8 patients and *paresthesia, dizziness, urticaria* and *disturbances of liver function tests* each in 1 of the 8 patients (30[R]).

Norfloxacin Corrado et al from the Merck Sharp and Dohme Research Laboratories at West Point reviewed the safety data that the producer has collected during developmental studies of norfloxacin. Both norfloxacin and nalidixic acid produced arthropathy with lameness in immature dogs whereas rabbits developed arthropathy without lameness. Because lameness was caused by erosion of the articular cartilage in some of the affected animals it seemed to be prudent to restrict the use of norfloxacin and fluoroquinolines in general to adults only (31[R]).

In early human trials with about 200 volunteers and patients on the relative safety of norfloxacin, erythromycin and placebo an almost similar number of adverse reactions was observed with each of the drugs. The material was not extensive enough for any final conclusions to be drawn about their relative safety. The clinical trials of efficacy and safety involved 1540 patients. The norfloxacin-associated adverse reactions of these trials are summarized in Table 1.

In a study conducted in 7 countries, 392 persons with acute diarrhea received either norfloxacin 400 mg twice daily, norfloxacin 400 mg 3 times a day or trimethoprim + sulfamethoxazole (160/800 mg) twice daily. Two patients (2%) of those receiving the lower dose of norfloxacin, 2 patients (3%) of those receiving trimethoprim + sulfamethoxazole and 3 patients (4%) of those receiving the higher dose of norfloxacin experienced transient adverse hematological (*leukopenia*) or blood chemistry reactions (*abnormal liver function tests*). Two patients receiving norfloxacin and 2 patients receiving trimethoprim + sulfamethoxazole developed *urticaria* (32[R]).

In 21 patients with complicated urinary tract infection norfloxacin was associated with *abdominal pain, diarrhea, insomnia, myalgia* and *scintillating scotoma* (33[R]). Similar observations were reported from 3 studies involving 485, 477 and 42 patients with urinary tract infections (34[c], 35[c], 34[R]–36[R]).

Ofloxacin The safety and efficacy of ofloxacin (400–800 mg twice daily) was studied in 553 elderly patients (over 65 years) suffering from different infections. Nineteen patients (3.4%) complained of adverse effects such as *gastric pain, nausea, vomiting, rash, erythema, itching, vertigo, glossitis* and *stomatitis* (37[R]). Three patients discontinued ofloxacin due to these symptoms. Four patients developed *abnormal liver and renal function tests*.

In pharmacokinetic studies of ofloxacin in healthy volunteers *insomnia* and *gastrointestinal disturbances* were the leading adverse effects (38[R]).

It is interesting if one considers preclinical animal studies which have shown arthropathy in young animals that 1 of 63 patients with pulmonary tuberculosis who were treated with ofloxacin (300–600 mg/d) for more than 3 months, suffered from *arthralgia* (39[R]). No further details were available about this case to make any final conclusions.

Perfloxacin Two cases of confusion, 1 with cerebellar dysfunction and the other with an extrapyramidal syndrome, were reported during treatment with perfloxacin (400 mg daily) (40[C]). In both cases (a 64- and a 67-year-old-woman) the *neurological symptoms* appeared shortly after the start of perfloxacin and the symptoms disappeared a few days after the withdrawal of the drug. Accumulation of perfloxacin or its metabolites might have been possible in both cases due to renal and hemodynamic problems.

Myoclonus, disorientation and *psychiatric disorder*, each in 1 patient, were reported among 46 patients who received perfloxacin (800 or 1200 mg daily) for treatment of nosocomial pulmonary infection. In addition, diffuse *non-bullous toxidermia* was noted in 4 patients (41[c]).

NY-198 (Lomefloxacin) Ny-198, a new quinolone derivative (pyridonecarboxylic acid derivative) has been studied in a number of small short-term clinical terms (from 1–14 days) in patients and healthy volunteers. *Edema of palpebrae, skin eruptions, photosensitivity dermatoses, headache, dizziness, sleeplessness, stomach ache, diarrhea, decrease in WBC, eosinophilia* and *abnormalities in liver function tests* were reported occasionally in these trials (42[R]).

ANTIVIRAL DRUGS *(SED-11, 620; SEDA-12, 251; SEDA-13, 253)*

Interferons *(SED-11, 623; SEDA-12, 251; SEDA-13, 253)*

After a decade of continuously increasing clinical use the adverse effect profile of interferons of various classes is well-established (SEDA-8, 284; SEDA-9, 261; SEDA-10, 262; SEDA-11, 262; SEDA-12, 251; SEDA-13,

253). They all share the characteristic pattern of interferon toxicity; however, β-interferons seem to be better tolerated than α-interferons and both show less frequent and important adverse effects than γ-interferons (SEDA-13, 254).

Crockett et al (43[CR]) have systematically described the side effects and toxicity of interferons in a series of 25 children (mean age 7.5 years). Natural α-interferon, α_{N1}-interferon, or α_{2b}-interferon (3–7 × 10^6 /m^2) were given in the treatment of recurrent respiratory papillomatosis for 26–263 weeks. In addition to other detailed data on adverse reactions, the preliminary findings suggest *growth retardation* during long-term interferon therapy and subsequent tendency to increased growth in height after cessation of treatment. In spite of the limitations of this retrospective observation in 9 out of 10 children, the apparent growth suppression of interferons warrants further studies. Another recent study of some special interest is a cross-over comparison of the efficacy and tolerability of β_{ser}-interferon (5 × 10^6 U daily) and γ-interferon (2 or 20 × 10^6 U daily) as well as their combination in the treatment of chronic hepatitis B (44[C]). The small sample size (7 patients) and the short treatment period (8 days) excludes any formal analysis of adverse effects, but *fever* occurred more frequently when higher doses of γ-interferon or the combination were administered. One patient receiving 20 × 10^6 U γ-interferon was withdrawn on the 3rd day due to *myalgia*. *Proteinuria* developed in 2 patients on the 8th day of treatment with a combination of β- and γ-interferons, suggesting additive toxicity. However, there was no additional bone-marrow toxicity with γ-interferon. Severe *headache* was reported by 1 subject during lower- and by 3 subjects during higher-dose treatment with γ-interferons alone. No additive or synergistic effects on the inhibition of hepatitis B virus, as monitored by measuring serum levels of viral DNA polymerase activity, were seen after administration of these 2 interferons. In an anecdotal report severe *influenza-like systemic side effects* were described when well-tolerated α-interferon treatment was changed to treatment with γ-interferon (45[c]).

Neutralizing antibodies Development of neutralizing antibodies against various interferons and patients' increased resistance to long-term interferon therapy have caused concern (46[c], 47[C], 48[c]). However, the main body of evidence has been reviewed, with some dispute concerning the antibody assay employed (49[R], 50[R]), in 2 scrutinies of the large clinical experience with both α_{2a}-interferon (49[R]) and α_{2b}-interferon (51[R]).

A statistically significant association between the development of neutralizing antibodies and clinical resistance against α_{2a}-interferon was shown in 51 patients with hairy-cell leukemia (47[c]). Neutralizing antibodies were present in 16 patients (31%) and 6 of them had various degrees of resistance to interferon. All other patients continued to respond after a minimum of 2 years of therapy. In agreement with previous findings (52[c], 53[c]), antibodies were specific and did not neutralize the interferon activity of purified natural α-interferon. In 2 other reports (46[c], 48[c]) a loss of responsiveness to α_{2b}-interferon was documented parallel to development of anti-interferon antibodies in 5 patients with leukemia and 2 patients with carcinoid tumor. Interestingly, natural, leukocyte-derived α-interferons restored the clinical efficacy in all but 1 patient. Wussow et al (53[c]) reported also that the initial influenza-like syndrome occurred after the first natural interferon injection with the exception of the 4th patient who did not respond.

α-Interferon *(SED-11, 623; SEDA-13, 253)* A case report of α_{2a}-interferon-related *cardiomyopathy* (54[c]) was a new adverse effect since the previous edition. α_{2a}-Interferon (3–6 × 10^6 U daily) was introduced for the treatment of renal cell carcinoma in a 62-year-old woman who subsequently experienced the rapid onset of congestive heart failure due to a dilated cardiomyopathy. The authors of the report conclude that the patient history, clinical findings, and results of postmortem examination were consistent with a drug-related cardiomyopathy. A new form of *neurotoxicity* was also described. The authors suggest a causal relationship between spastic diplegia and human leukocyte interferon therapy in a 2-year-old boy who had juvenile laryngeal papilloma (55[c]).

The high-dose therapy with α_{2a}-interferon proved to be poorly tolerated and the initial dose which was as low as 10 or 27–36 × 10^6 U had to be reduced due to side effects. These occurred in over one-third of patients with chronic hepatitis B infection (79[c]) or AIDS-related Kaposi's sarcoma (80[c]). In a clinical trial in immunosuppressed herpes zoster patients with daily doses of 36 or 68 × 10^6 U α_{2a}-interferon the higher dose caused frequent and severe adverse effects resulting in early termination of that arm of treatment (81[c]). A case of *paranoid schizophrenia* and 1 case of *mental confusion* with nightmares, both responding to reduction of dose or withdrawal, were encountered during high-dose therapy (79[c]).

γ-Interferon *(SED-11, 623; SEDA-13, 254)* Autoimmune side-effects of interferons have also been associated with recombinant γ-interferon (56[c]). Six of the 13 patients with rheumatoid arthritis responded to γ-interferon. During maintenance treatment for 2–8 months antinuclear antibodies were present in 3 patients. The presence of antinuclear antibodies was accompanied by a simultaneous clinical exacerbation of the disease activity. The first case of a severe renal toxicity associated with γ-interferon was reported in a 12-year-old boy with *acute renal failure* and *acute tubular necrosis* 19 days after treatment was started. The treatment was for acute lymphoblastic leukemia (57[c]). Renal function returned to normal after discontinuation of interferon therapy. The renal-biopsy findings were different from those described in a case of acute renal failure following α-interferon (SEDA-9, 263).

Aciclovir (acyclovir) *(SED-11, 621; SEDA-13, 254)*

Intravenous therapy with aciclovir in patients with hypovolemia or pre-existing impaired renal function may lead to renal damage (SEDA-7, 204; SEDA-8, 283, SEDA-11, 263). A *crystal nephropathy* may develop which occurs when the drug is concentrated in the renal tubules and collecting ducts in excess of its solubility. An additional case of acute transient renal failure has been reported in a patient who became dehydrated during aciclovir therapy (58[C]).

Aciclovir crystalluria might be an early diagnostically valuable sign of aciclovir crystal nephropathy.

Among 20 patients with herpes simplex or herpes zoster infections receiving aciclovir 10 mg/kg i.v. 3 times daily for 10 days one 28-year-old woman developed cloudy urine and heavy crystalluria on the 2nd day of treatment (59[C]). The crystals were fine, elongated and more or less rectangular. They were morphologically identical with crystals in the aciclovir infusion fluid when it was acidified to pH 5. The patient's serum creatinine did not increase but she was suspected of suffering from aciclovir crystal nephropathy. After administration of additional intravenous fluid the crystals disappeared in 2 days. The crystalluria was accompanied by tubular impairment as evidenced by increased urinary β_2-microglobulin excretion.

Neutropenia associated with oral aciclovir therapy was reported for the first time in a 32-year-old white man with AIDS (60[C]).

He was first treated for shigellosis with intravenous trimethoprim + sulfamethoxazole and developed neutropenia. One month later his WBC count was normal but because of perianal herpes simplex infection aciclovir treatment, 200 mg 4 times daily p.o. was instituted. On the 2nd day of treatment his WBC count fell to 1800 cells/mm^3 and remained in this range over the next 2 days. On day 5 of treatment aciclovir was discontinued and the patient's WBC count rose over the next 2 days to 4131 cells/mm^3. Because of fever, treatment with nafcillin, ticarcillin and gentamicin was started and oral aciclovir was also restarted. On the following day the patient's WBC count fell and on the 3rd treatment day was 1400/mm^3. Aciclovir and antibiotics were discontinued and the neutrophil count rose to 5580/mm^3.

Intravenous but not oral administration of aciclovir has been associated with neutropenia in earlier reports (SEDA-8, 283). The neutropenia in the present case was possibly immune-mediated and the patient had AIDS. AIDS patients may be at greater risk than other populations for drug-induced bone marrow toxicity.

Fluid retention and *peripheral edema* developed in 2 women who had received oral aciclovir 200 mg 5 times and 400 mg 5 times a day for herpes zoster infection (61[C]). Both patients had been on a diuretic due to heart insufficiency. Discontinuation of aciclovir and increase in the dose of diuretics resulted in healing within a few days.

Sixty-four patients with herpes zoster were entered into a randomized placebo-controlled trial of 5% aciclovir cream applied 5 times daily for 5 days. Twelve aciclovir and 10 placebo-treated patients experienced erythema or desquamation or both during the treatment (62[R]). The similar incidence of skin reactions in both groups suggested that they were related to the cream base rather than to aciclovir. The adverse reactions to aciclovir in topical therapy have been discussed previously (SEDA-9, 263).

Four extensive reviews were published in which the efficacy and safety of aciclovir alone or in combination with vidarabine were evaluated in the treatment of varicella zoster, herpes simplex and cytomegalovirus infections (63[r]–66[r]).

Burroughs Wellcome Company operated a program of pharmacoepidemiology from 1982–1987 in which the safety experience with aciclovir was monitored during the first 5 years of its clinical use (67[R]). It was estimated that aciclovir had been used in over 10 million courses of treatment in more than 40 countries that have given a sales licence to the drug. Wellcome and its worldwide affiliations collected adverse experiences which had been reported directly to the company by practitioners or other agents and through the published literature. Outside the United States a total of 274 reports involving 474 events had been received. Within the United States a total of 730 adverse experiences involving 469 patients had been reported. Aciclovir in oral formulations was associated most often with *rashes, nausea/vomiting, headache, pruritus, malaise/asthenia, abdominal pains, diarrhea, confusion, fever/flu syndrome, urticaria, leukopenia and liver function abnormalities*. Aciclovir injection was associated most often with *confusion, hallucinations, agitation/acute brain syndrome, rashes, creatinine increases, leukopenia, fever, liver function abnormalities, convulsions, kidney failure and reactions at the injection site*. These drug reactions come as no surprise if compared with the reports and publications which have been reviewed over the years in these Annuals (SEDA-8, 283; SEDA-9, 263; SEDA-10, 264; SEDA-11, 262).

Ganciclovir *(SEDA-13, 255)*

Ganciclovir is an acyclic nucleosodiguanine (also known as DHPG, BW-B759U, BIOLF-62 and 2-NDG); it has excellent activity against cytomegalovirus in vitro (68). The drug has been recommended for U.S. FDA approval by the agency's anti-infective drugs advisory committee in May 1989 for the treatment of sight-threatening cytomegalovirus infections in AIDS patients (69).

Twelve liver and 5 kidney transplant recipients received ganciclovir 7 mg/kg/d i.v. for cytomegalovirus infection. The patients also received bone marrow suppressant agents. Transient *neutropenia* occurred in 3 patients and transient *thrombocytopenia* in 1 patient (68[r]). In a similar trial with 9 liver and 3 kidney transplant recipients leukopenia occurred in 8 patients, but no adverse effects with regard to platelet counts or hemostasis were observed (70[c]). In 15 bone marrow transplant patients who were treated with ganciclovir reversible neutropenia developed in 8 patients after 10–19 days of treatment (71[r]).

Based on the data of over 3000 AIDS patients treated with ganciclovir for serious cytomegalovirus infection, Drew (72[R]) summarized the adverse reactions as follows. Neutropenia defined as an absolute neutrophil count $< 1000/mm^3$ occurred in nearly 25% of ganciclovir recipients; 16% of patients developed neutrophil counts $< 500/mm^3$. Neutropenia normally occurs early but may also occur later during therapy. *Leukopenia* is often reversible, but at least 5 patients are known to have had irreversible suppression. AIDS patients may have low WBC counts and the contribution of ganciclovir to leukopenia may not be entirely clear. The dosage should be reduced or discontinued (neutrophil counts $< 500/mm^3$); this may reverse the neutropenia.

Thrombocytopenia occurred in 9% of AIDS patients who received ganciclovir.

Adverse effects on the *CNS* occur in 17% of patients receiving ganciclovir. *Confusion* occurs in about 3% of the patients whereas 2% may experience *convulsions, dizziness, headache* and/or *thinking disorders*.

Some 15% have *gastrointestinal complaints*, nausea being the most frequent one (5%) followed by vomiting (4%), abnormal liver function tests (3%) and diarrhea (2%). In preclinical animal studies ganciclovir was found to be a potent inhibitor of spermatogenesis.

Sperm counts in humans have been performed only occasionally but follicle-stimulating hormone and luteinizing hormone increase in about 30% of the patients. Patients wishing to reproduce should use ganciclovir only for the strongest indications.

Studies are in progress to determine whether the combination of zidovudine and ganciclovir is more toxic than either agent alone.

Foscarnet sodium *(SED-11, 621)*

Foscarnet (phosphonoformic acid trisodium salt) is an antiviral drug with in vitro activity against human immunodeficiency virus (HIV) as well as against human herpesvirus. It reduces the proportion of positive HIV cultures compared with those before treatment in AIDS patients and it also reduces the ability to detect HIV antigen in serum during treatment. Five of 6 AIDS patients reported *diarrhea* during treatment with oral foscarnet (4000 mg every 6 hours for 3 days (73[r]). Sudden *nausea* and *vomiting* after the morning dose and slight *dizziness* were noted by 2 of the patients. Oral treatment was followed by intravenous infusion for 3 days and the daily dose was the same as that given orally. Two patients had *thrombophlebitis* during the intravenous treatment and 1 patient reported 'hangover'-like symptoms on the first day of intravenous administration.

Pentamidine *(SED-11, 598; SEDA-12, 244; SEDA-13, 243)*

Pentamidine has been used for *Pneumocystis carinii* pneumonia in patients with AIDS. Pentamidine has been available in the United States under an IND treatment protocol since February 1989. The U.S. FDA's anti-infective drugs advisory committee in May 1989 gave its approval for the use of pentamidine for primary as well as secondary prophylaxis against *P. carinii* pneumonia in HIV-infected patients (74).

Parenteral pentamidine may cause *pain, swelling* and *sterile abscesses* at the intramuscular injection site and occasionally also *hypotension* (75[r]). *Thrombophlebitis, urticaria, hypotension* and *hypoglycemia* (up to 62%) have been reported with intravenous administration (75). *Impaired renal function, elevated liver enzymes, neutropenia, thrombocytopenia, fever, hypocalcemia, hallucinations, arrhythmias* and *pancreatitis* are other adverse reactions attributed to pentamidine. The high frequency of adverse reactions with systemic use of pentamidine has led to the development of new formulations.

Aerosolized pentamidine was considered a useful formulation because of the intra-alveolar location of *P. carinii*. In addition, this means of administration may cause fewer systemic reactions. Corkery and Luce (75) reviewed the data collected during first 2 years with aerosolized pentamidine. Complications experienced by patients included *bronchospasm, fatigue, burning sensation in the back of the throat, mild hypoglycemia* and *unpleasant taste*.

Zidovudine (AZT) *(SEDA-13, 246)*

A review of the safety of zidovudine was published in the previous volume of this series. The main adverse reactions of zidovudine therapy in patients with AIDS are *hematological complications* including *macrocytic anemia* and *neutropenia*.

Lithium seems to help in reversing neutropenia induced by zidovudine (76[C]).

Five patients with AIDS developed zidovudine-induced neutropenia which required discontinuation of zidovudine therapy. Lithium dosage (lithium carbonate 600–1200 mg/d p.o.) was titrated to achieve serum concentrations of 0.6–1.2 mEq/l in each of the 5 cases. Initial responses in neutrophil counts allowed reinstitution of zidovudine therapy and in the majority of cases they were able to tolerate full or nearly full doses of zidovudine.

Further studies may be needed in order to determine the influence of lithium upon the prognosis of these patients.

Among 113 zidovudine-treated patients [80 with AIDS, 33 with AIDS-related complex, (ARC)], 8 (7 AIDS, 1 ARC) developed clinical and biochemical evidence of *myopathy* after 240–386 (mean 329) days on the treatment (77[r]). The myopathy was clinically subacute, developing insidiously over several weeks. Weakness in the upper legs and pain in the affected muscles were the major symptoms. Creatinine phosphokinase was raised in 6 of the 7 patients tested. The myopathy resolved on cessation of zidovudine but not on dose reduction.

Pseudomembranous colitis occurs usually in the presence of antibiotic exposure. A patient with AIDS who received zidovudine for 8 weeks and aciclovir for 12 weeks (for anogenital herpes simplex) but did not receive any antibiotics developed a classical *Clostridium difficile*-induced diarrhea (78[C]). The sigmoidoscopical finding was typical. Both zidovudine and aciclovir were discontinued and vancomycin treatment resulted in resolution of the diarrhea in 10 days. The weak antibacterial activity exerted by aciclovir and possibly also by zidovudine may alter the intestinal milieu of the colon, thus promoting endogenous or acquired clostridial growth. Even AIDS may alter the intestinal microflora.

REFERENCES

1. Pauwels W (1988) Cholestatische hepatitis door nitrofurantoine. *Tijdschr. Geneeskd., 44,* 841.
2. Valcke Y (1988) Pulmonale complicaties van nitrofurantoin. *Tijdschr. Geneeskd., 44,* 1379.
3. Sovijärvi ARA, Lemola M, Stenius B, Idänpään-Heikkilä J (1977) Nitrofurantoin induced acute subacute and chronic pulmonary reactions. A report of 66 cases. *Scand. J. Respir. Dis., 58,,* 41.
4. Turnidge J (1988) A reappraisal of co-trimoxazole. *Med. J. Aust., 148,* 296, Corrigendum (1989) *151,* 355.
5. Simon A, Carbon C (1988) Imidazoles and co-trimoxazole. *Rev. Prat., 38,* 1033.
6. Whittington RM (1989) Toxic epidermal necrolysis and co-trimoxazole. *Lancet, 2,* 574.
7. Carmichael AJ, Tan CY (1989) Fatal toxic epidermal necrolysis associated with co-trimoxazole. *Lancet, 2,* 808.
8. Bachrach WH (1988) Sulfasalazine. I. An historical perspective. *Am. J. Gastroenterol., 83,* 487.
9. Svartz N (1988) Sulfasalazine II. Some notes on the discovery and development of salazopyrin. *Am. J. Gastroenterol., 83,* 497.
10. Fihn SD, Johnson D, Roberts PL et al (1988) Trimethoprim–sulfamethoxazole for acute dysuria in women: a single-dose or 10-day course. *Ann. Intern. Med., 108,* 350.
11. Stein GE, Gurwith D, Gurwith M (1988) Randomized clinical trial of rifampin–trimethoprim and sulfamethoxazole–trimethoprim in the treatment of localized urinary tract infections. *Antimicrob. Agents Chemother. 32,* 802.
12. Privette M, Cade R, Peterson J, Mars D (1988) Prevention of recurrent urinary tract infections in postmenopausal women. *Nephron, 50,* 24.
13. Platt F, Dreis MW, Kennedy DL, Kuritsky JN (1988) Serum sickness-like reactions to amoxicillin, cefaclor, cephalexin, and trimethoprim–sulfamethoxazole. *J. Infect. Dis., 158,* 474.
14. Guerra R, Trevisanuto E, Corradin MT (1988) Un caso di sindrome di Lyell: contributo alla casistica. *Chron. Dermatol., 19,* 31.
15. Phillips-Howard PA, Behrens RH, Dunlop J (1989) Stevens-Johnson syndrome due to pyrimethamine/sulfadoxine during presumptive self-therapy of malaria. *Lancet, 2,* 803.
16. Scherpenissa J, Van der Valk, PDLPM, Van den Bosch JMM et al (1988) Olsalazine as an alternative therapy in a patient with sulfasalazine-induced eosinophilic pneumonia. *J. Clin. Gastroenterol., 10,* 218.
17. Klein HP, Rupp M, Thiele-Fischabach A (1988) Sulphasalazine-induced alveolitis. *Dtsch. Med. Wochenschr., 113,* 1239.
18. Jordan A, Cowan RE (1988) Reversible pulmonary disease and eosinophilia associated with sulphasalazine. *J. R. Soc. Med., 81,* 233.
19. Trewby PN, Connolly CK (1988) Reversible pulmonary disease and eosinophilia associated with sulphasalazine. *J. R. Soc. Med., 81,* 558.
20. Clementz GL, Dolin BJ (1988) Sulfasalazine-induced lupus erythematosus. *Am. J. Med., 84,* 535.
21. Capdevila JA, Ocana I, Ribera E et al (1988) Lupus eritematoso inducido por sulfasalazina. *An. Med. Intern. (Madrid), 5,* 363.
22. Gutt L, Feder JM, Feder RS et al (1988) Corneal ring formation after exposure to sulfamethoxazole. *Arch. Ophthalmol., 106,* 726.
23. Chatzinoff M, Guarino JM, Corson SL et al (1988) Sulfasalazine-induced abnormal sperm penetration assay reversed on changing to 5-aminosalicylic acid enemas. *Dig. Dis. Sci., 33,* 108.
24. Rippelmeyer DJ, Synhavsky A (1988) Ciprofloxacin and allergic interstitial nephritis. *Ann. Intern. Med., 109,* 170.
25. Avet CK, Krinsky D, Kirklin JK et al (1988) Synergistic nephrotoxicity due to ciprofloxacin and cyclosporine. *Am. J. Med., 85,* 452.
26. Torsteinsson SB, Bergan T, Rohwedder R (1988) Tolerance of intravenously administered ciprofloxacin. *Chemotherapy, 34,* 256.
27. Preheim LC, Cuevas TA, Roccaforte JS (1987) Oral ciprofloxacin in the treatment of elderly patients with complicated urinary tract infections. *Am. J. Med., 82, Suppl. 4A,* 285.
28. Karlman K, Bresky B, Carlsson L et al (1988) Therapy of acute and chronic Gram-negative osteomyelitis with ciprofloxacin. *J. Antimicrob. Chemother., 22,* 221.
29. Scully BE, Neu HC (1987) Treatment of serious infections with intravenous ciprofloxacin. *Am. J. Med., 82, Suppl. 4A,* 369.
30. Bailey RR, Walker RJ, Lynn KL (1988) Intravenous enoxacin for treatment of acute pyelonephritis. *Br. J. Clin. Pharmacol., 25,* 223.
31. Corrado ML, Struble WE, Peter C (1987) Norfloxacin: review of safety studies. *Am. J. Med., 82, Suppl. 6B,* 22.
32. Dupont HL, Corrado ML, Sabbaj J (1987) Use of norfloxacin in the treatment of acute diarrheal disease. *Am. J. Med., 82, Suppl. 6B,* 79.

33. Sheehan GJ, Harding GK, Haase DA (1988) Double-blind randomized comparison of 24 weeks of norfloxacin and 12 weeks of norfloxacin. *Antimicrob. Agents Chemother., 32,* 1292.
34. Schaeffer AJ (1987) Multiclinic study of norfloxacin for treatment of urinary tract infections. *Am. J. Med., 82,* 53.
35. Heseltine PNR, Corrado ML (1987) Compassionate use of norfloxacin, *Am. J. Med., 82,* 88.
36. Falck G (1988) Double-blind comparison of 3-day versus 7-day treatment with norfloxacin in symptomatic urinary tract infections. *Scand. J. Infect. Dis., 20,* 619.
37. Fostini R, Girelli M, Dalle VP (1988) Safety profile of ofloxacin in elderly patients. *Drugs Exp. Clin. Res., 14,* 393.
38. Leigh DA, Walsh B, Harris K et al (1988) Pharmacokinetics of ofloxacin and the effect on the faecal flora of healthy volunteers. *J. Antimicrob. Chemother., 22,* 115.
39. Matsumoto T, Ikeda N, Kanetsuna F (1988) Therapeutic effect of ofloxacin on intractable pulmonary tuberculosis. *Kekkaku, 63,* 37.
40. Lucket J-C, Tilly H, Lerebours G (1988) Neurological toxicity related to perfloxacin *J. Antimicrob. Chemother., 21,* 811.
41. Martin C, Gouin F, Fourrier F et al (1988) Perfloxacin in the treatment of nosocomial lower respiratory tract infections in intensive care patients. *J. Antimicrob. Chemother., 21,* 795.
42. Aoki T, Saito M, Shimizu N et al (1988) Clinical study on NY-198 in infectious enteritis. *Chemotherapy, 36,* 792.
43. Crockett DM, Luska RP, McCabe BF, Mixon JH (1987) Side effects and toxicity of interferon in the treatment of recurrent respiratory papillomatosis. *Ann. Otol. Rhinol. Laryngol., 96,* 601.
44. Bisset J, Eisenberg M, Gregory P et al (1988) Recombinant fibroblast interferon and immune interferon for treating hepatitis B virus infection: patients' tolerance and the effect on viral markers. *J. Infect. Dis., 157,* 1076.
45. Gross F, Ellinger K, Roussaki A et al (1988) Epidermodysplasia verruciformis in a patient with Hodgkin's disease: characterization of a new papillomavirus type and interferon treatment. *J. Invest. Dermatol., 91,* 43.
46. Von Wussow P, Freund M, Block B et al (1987) Clinical significance of anti-IFN-α antibody titres during interferon therapy. *Lancet, 2,* 635.
47. Steis RG, Smith JW, Urba WJ et al (1988) Resistance to recombinant interferon α_{2a} in hairy-cell leukemia associated with neutralizing anti-interferon antibodies. *N. Engl. J. Med., 318,* 1409.
48. Öberg K, Alm G, Magnusson A et al (1989) Treatment of malignant carcinoid tumors with recombinant interferon α_{2b}: development of neutralizing interferon antibodies and possible loss of antitumor activity. *J. Natl. Cancer Inst., 81,* 531.
49. Itri LM, Campion M, Dennin R et al (1987) Incidence and clinical significance of neutralizing antibodies in patients receiving recombinant interferon α_{2a} by intramuscular injection. *Cancer, 59,* 668.
50. Jacobs SJ, Sullivan LM, Salfi M et al (1988) Minimal antigenicity of Intron A in human recipients demonstrated by three analytical methods. *J. Biol. Response Modif., 7,* 447.
51. Spiegel RJ, Spicehandler JR, Jacobs SL, Oden EM (1988) Low incidence of serum neutralizing factors in patients receiving recombinant α_{2b} interferon (Intron A). *Am. J. Med., 80,* 223.
52. Eife R, Mertens R, Holtman H (1985) Development of anti-interferon (IFN) antibodies after long-term therapy with IFN-β. *Pediatr. Res., 19,* 1079.
53. Von Wussow P, Hartmann F, Freund M et al (1988) Leucocyte-derived interferon-α in patients with antibodies to recombinant IFN-α_{2b}. *Lancet, 1,* 882.
54. Cohen MC, Huberman MS, Nesto RW (1988) Recombinant α-2 interferon-related cardiomyopathy. *Am. J. Med., 85,* 549.
55. Vesikari T, Nuutila A, Cantell K (1988) Neurologic sequelae following interferon therapy of juvenile laryngeal papilloma. *Acta Paediatr. Scand., 77,* 619.
56. Seiz M, Kranke M, Kirchner H (1988) Induction of antinuclear antibodies in patients with rheumatoid arthritis receiving treatment with human recombinant interferon gamma. *Ann. Rheum. Dis., 47,* 642.
57. Ault BH, Stapleton FB, Gaber L et al (1988) Acute renal failure during therapy with recombinant human gamma interferon. *N. Engl. J. Med., 319,* 1397.
58. Dickins JRE, Smith JT, Graham SS (1988) Herpes zoster oticus: treatment with intravenous acyclovir. *Laryngoscope, 98,* 776.
59. Peterslund NA, Larsen ML, Mygid H (1988) Acyclovir crystalluria. *Scand. J. Infect. Dis., 20,* 225.
60. McPherson ML, Plaisance KI (1988) Neutropenia associated with oral acyclovir and multiple antibacterial agents. *Clin. Pharm., 7,* 398.
61. Hisler BA, Daneshwar SA, Aronson PJ et al (1988) Peripheral edema and oral acyclovir. *J. Am. Acad. Dermatol., 18,* 1142.
62. Mandal BK, Dunbar EM, Ellis ME et al (1988) A double-masked, placebo controlled trial of acyclovir cream. *J. Infect., 17,* 57.
63. Saral R (1988) Management of mucocutaneous herpes simplex virus infections. *Am. J. Med., 85,* 57.
64. Meyers JD (1988) Management of cytomegalovirus infection. *Am. J. Med., 85,* 102.
65. Balfour HH (1988) Varicella zoster virus infections in immunocompromised hosts. *Am. J. Med., 85,* 68.
66. Shepp DH, Dandliker PS, Meyers JD (1988) Current therapy of varicella zoster virus infection in

immunocompromised patients. *Am. J. Med., 85,* 96.
67. Tilson HH (1988) Monitoring the safety on antivirals. *Am. J. Med., 85,* 116.
68. Paya CV, Hermans PE, Smith TF et al (1988) Efficacy of ganciclovir in liver and kidney transplant recipients. *Transplantation, 46,* 229.
69. Anonymous (1989) Ganciclovir approval recommended in U.S. *Scrip, 1410,* 20.
70. Harbison MA, Girolami PC, Jenkins RL (1988) Ganciclovir therapy of severe cytomegalovirus infections in solid-organ transplant recipients. *Transplantation, 46,* 82.
71. Reed EC, Shepp DH, Dandliker PS et al (1988) Ganciclovir treatment of cytomegalovirus infection of the gastrointestinal tract after marrow transplantation. *Bone Marrow Transplant., 3,* 199.
72. Drew WL (1988) Cytomegalovirus infection in patient with AIDS. *J. Infect. Dis., 158,* 449.
73. Sjövall J, Karlsson A, Ogenstad S (1988) Pharmacokinetics and absorption of foscarnet after intravenous and oral administration. *Clin. Pharmacol. Ther., 44,* 65.
74. Anonymous (1989) Pentamidine cleared for U.S. approval. *Scrip, 1410,* 22.
75. Corkery KJ, Luce JM, Montgomery AB (1988) Aerosolized pentamidine for treatment and prophylaxis of *Pneumocystis carinii* pneumonia. *Respir., Care, 33,* 676.
76. Roberts DE, Berman SM, Nakasato S et al (1988) Effect of lithium carbonate on zodovudine-associated neutropenia in AIDS. *Am. J. Med., 85,* 428.
77. Herbert M, Fletcher T, Peddle B et al (1988) Zidovudine-associated myopathy. *Lancet, 3,* 689.
78. Colarian J (1988) *Clostridium difficile* colitis following antiviral therapy in the acquired immunodeficiency syndrome. *Am. J. med., 84,* 1081.
79. Lok ASF, Lai CL, Wu PC, Leung EKY (1988) Long-term follow-up in a randomized controlled trial of recombinant α_2-interferon in Chinese patients with chronic hepatitis B infection. *Lancet, 2,* 298.
80. De Wit R, Schattenkerk JKME, Boucher CAB et al (1988) Clinical and virological effects of high-dose recombinant interferon-α in disseminated AIDS-related Kaposi's sarcoma. *Lancet, 2,* 1214.
81. Winston DJ, Eron L, Ho M et al (Hoffmann-La Roche Herpes Zoster Study Group) (1988) Recombinant interferon α_{2a} for treatment of herpes zoster in immunosuppressed patients with cancer. *Am. J. Med., 85,* 147.

C.J. Ellis

31 Drugs used in tuberculosis and leprosy

DRUGS USED IN TUBERCULOSIS *(SED-11, 633; SEDA-12, 255; SEDA-13, 259)*

Combination therapy for tuberculosis *(SED-11, 633; SEDA-12, 255; SEDA-13, 259)*

In England and Wales, 9% of all patients notified as having pulmonary tuberculosis in 1983 suffered a toxic reaction to treatment necessitating a change in regime while in a further 4% some temporary modification was required (1[R]). All the patients had been started on a regime which included rifampicin and isoniazid, and, of the 64% who completed treatment as planned, 67% had initially received ethambutol, 12% ethambutol plus pyrazinamide and 7% pyrazinamide at the start. To quote the original analysis: 'In the opinion of the clinician in charge, hepatitis occurred in 41 patients, 28 with jaundice. Of the 219 patients who received isoniazid plus rifampicin with pyrazinamide initially (with or without ethambutol) 11 (5%) had hepatitis, 9 with jaundice, whereas for the 795 who received isoniazid plus rifampicin without pyrazinamide the corresponding figures were 24 (3%) and 16 (2%) ($P > 0.3$ for both comparisons). Eight patients, all receiving ethambutol, were suspected of having toxic ocular reactions, but in none was this confirmed at ophthalmological assessment. Four of the 32 patients with cutaneous reactions had a generalized hypersensitivity reaction.'

It should be pointed out that at the present day an increasing number of patients are receiving pyrazinamide as the sole addition to the rifampicin and isoniazid regime with fewer receiving ethambutol either as a third or a fourth drug.

Comparison of these data with those on 160 children treated for tuberculosis in Arkansas suggests that increasing age may make adverse reactions more likely in that only one of the children suffered toxicity (urticaria, jaundice and fever) necessitating a change of therapy (2[R]).

Antituberculous therapy reduces serum $25(OH)D_3$ concentrations and was found to abolish its normal summer increase in 27 patients studied in Wales (3[R]). All patients received rifampicin and isoniazid and, on completion of treatment, vitamin D levels rose rapidly to normal. Rifampicin acts by induction of an enzyme which promotes conversion of $25(OH)D_3$ to an inactive metabolite and isoniazid by inhibition of 25 and 1 hydroxylation. The authors point out the particular risk of osteomalacia in Asian women in northern winters and advise consideration of supplementing antituberculous therapy with oral vitamin D but emphasize the importance of monitoring serum calcium to avoid possible hypercalcemia.

Ethambutol *(SED-11, 639; SEDA-12, 256; SEDA-13, 260)*

The gradual abandonment of ethambutol which has followed the demonstration that it appears superfluous to the now favoured short course regime of rifampicin and isoniazid, with pyrazinamide for the first two months, is challenged by Campbell and Ormerod (4) who point out that the British Committee on Safety of Medicines received fewer reports of deaths from ethambutol than from the other 3 agents from 1963–1987. In the same period ethambutol was linked with only one death and with four cases of blindness. These authors are answered by Kahana (5) who points out that how-

Side Effects of Drugs Annual 14
M.N.G. Dukes and L. Beeley, editors

ever safe, ethambutol, which is mycobacteriostatic, contributes little or nothing to antituberculous regimes based on the other three drugs and furthermore, that deaths are likely to be rare if the offending agent is promptly withdrawn. A review of 13 patients with bilateral optic neuritis attributed to ethambutol from China (6[R]) mirrors earlier published reports but gives no denominator figures.

Isoniazid *(SED-11, 634; SEDA-12, 257; SEDA-13, 261)*

Immune system A *lupus-like syndrome* may be induced by isoniazid. Hwang et al (7[R]) report a prospective study on the effect of isoniazid on the induction of antinuclear antibodies (ANA). Ten of 50 patients (20%) developed ANA during treatment, but more exhibited features of the lupus-like syndrome. The authors consequently advise that the detection of ANA in such patients should be ignored or, to put it more practically, ANA should not be looked for in asymptomatic patients in the first place.

Nervous system Various psychiatric disturbances have been attributed to isoniazid including *anxiety*, *paranoia* and *schizophrenic features*. Slow-acetylators, the elderly and the alcoholic appear to be at most risk. A case of *mania* is described (8[c]), in an 18-year-old man with a normal personality hitherto. Normal behavior returned on stopping isoniazid with mania again supervening when it was re-introduced. On replacing isoniazid with pyrazinamide his behavior again returned to normal. This effect is presumed to result from the action of isoniazid on the GABA neurotransmitter system.

Rifampicin *(SED-11, 637; SEDA-12, 258; SEDA-13, 261)*

Cardiovascular A hitherto undescribed association of rifampicin with *deep venous thrombosis (DVT)* is reported from South Africa (9[R]). In a retrospective analysis of lower limb DVT proven by contrast venography, DVT complicated admission in 46 (3.4%) of 1366 adult patients treated in a tuberculosis hospital. Analysis of 7542 admissions during 1978-86 showed a relative risk of 4.74 in patients treated with regimes including rifampicin compared with others. DVT was significantly more common in winter months and usually occurred within 2 weeks of the start of treatment. The author points out that the use of warfarin in patients receiving rifampicin is frequently complicated by interaction so that large doses are often required. Abrupt cessation of rifampicin while continuing warfarin is hazardous.

Respiratory *Pulmonary fibrosis* developed in a 79-year-old man undergoing treatment for pulmonary tuberculosis (10[c]). The fibrosis appeared to improve when rifampicin, isoniazid and ethambutol were stopped and did not progress when the latter 2 were resumed. The patient's lymphocytes were not transformed by incubation with rifampicin and a non-immune toxic mechanism was therefore invoked.

Renal *Acute interstitial nephritis* and *acute tubular necrosis* are the most commonly reported effects of rifampicin on the kidney although hemoglobinuric renal failure, secondary to hemolysis, renal cortical necrosis and proliferative glomerulonephritis have also been described. Light chain proteinuria was found in 27 out of 38 tuberculous patients treated with rifampicin but did not appear to be of significance. Subsequently 5 patients have been separately reported in whom light chain deposition led to acute renal failure. One group of authors speculate (11[c]) that rifampicin interferes with reabsorption of normally filtered light chains since in their patients' light chain concentration in the serum was not increased.

Interactions Rifampicin is a potent enzyme-inducer resulting in a steady stream of reports of drug interactions. Enhancement of elimination of *nifedipine may* have been the explanation for the return of angina after the commencement of antituberculous therapy in a man whose symptoms had hitherto been controlled (12[c]). An added twist to the well-documented consequences of the acceleration of cortisol metabolism by rifampicin will probably become increasingly important as the AIDS epidemic progresses. Inadequate adrenal reserve is not uncommon in AIDS patients and rifampicin therapy may precipitate overt adrenal insufficiency. In one such case (13[c]), the baseline cortisol was normal in a patient with classical features of acute adrenal insufficiency but there was only minimal response to Synacthen. The patient's condition was unaltered by conventional doses of dexamethasone, the metabolism of which is more markedly accelerated by rifampicin than is that of other glucocorticoids. The authors state that in these circumstances 25 mg of dexamethasone daily may be required as replacement.

DRUGS USED IN LEPROSY *(SED-11, 643; SEDA-12, 258; SEDA-13, 262)*

In 1982 the WHO published a report on the chemotherapy of leprosy for control programme (14). Progress since then is reviewed in a *Lancet* editorial (15) which summarizes the multidrug protocols currently recommended for paucibacillary (tuberculoid) and multibacillary (lepromatous) patients. Noting that the WHO made provision for the use of the thioamides (prothionamide and ethionamide) in patients who might find the reddish skin pigmentation of clofazimine unacceptable, the editorial opines that this alternative has seldom been found necessary and points to the gastrointestinal and hepatic toxicity of the thioamides.

Dapsone *(SED-11, 644; SEDA-12, 258; SEDA-13, 263)*

Side effects of dapsone discussed earlier in these volumes include hemolytic anemia and dermatitis. A case of *psychosis* is described (16[c]) in a 12-year-old Indian girl, which appeared to be causally related to dapsone given for leprosy.

Dapsone causes a *peripheral neuropathy*, usually manifest as progressive weakness and wasting of the distal muscles of the extremities. Two patients receiving dapsone for dermatitis herpetiformis developed neurological symptoms (17[c]) but both had normal nerve-conduction in contrast with most reported cases which show delayed conduction. A diagnosis of multiple sclerosis was subsequently made in one patient. The usual message applies; *post hoc, ergo propter hoc*.

REFERENCES

1. Medical Research Council and Chest Diseases Unit (1988) Management and outcome of pulmonary tuberculosis in adults notified in England and Wales in 1983. *Thorax, 43*, 591.
2. Jacobs RF, Abernathy RS (1988) Tuberculosis in children. *Semin. Respir. Med., 9*, 474.
3. Davies PDO, Brown RC, Church HA, Woodhead JS (1987) The effect of antituberculous chemotherapy on vitamin D and calcium metabolism. *Tubercle, 68*, 261.
4. Campbell IA, Ormerod LP (1988) Ethambutol and the eye. *Lancet, 2*, 113.
5. Kahana LM (1988) Ethambutol and the eye. *Lancet, 2*, 627.
6. Li X, Li C (1988) Toxic optic neuritis with ethambutol. *Eye Sci., 4*, 45.
7. Hwang JJ, Liu HW, Wang TH et al (1988) Antinuclear antibodies induced by isoniazid. A prospective study. *Kaohsiung J. Med. Sci., 4*, 345.
8. Chaturvedi SK, Upadhyaya M (1988) Secondary mania in a patient receiving isonicotinic acid hydrazide and pyridoxine. *Can. J. Psychiatry, 33*, 675.
9. White NW (1989) Venous thrombosis and rifampicin. *Lancet, 2*, 434.
10. Umeki S (1988) Rifampicin and pulmonary fibrosis. *Arch. Intern. Med., 148*, 1663 and 1667.
11. Offer O, Nasser VH, Campbell WG, Bourke E(1987) Light chain cast nephropathy and acute renal failure associated with rifampicin therapy. *Am. J. Med., 82*, 1052.
12. Tsuchihashi K, Fukami K, Kishimoto H et al (1988) A case of variant angina exacerbated by administration of rifampicin. *Heart Vessels, 3*, 214.
13. Ediger SK, Isley WL (1988) Rifampicin-induced adrenal insufficiency in the acquired immune deficiency syndrome: difficulties in diagnosis and treatment. *Postgrad. Med. J., 64*, 405.
14. Study Group (1982) Chemotherapy of leprosy for control programmes. *WHO Tech. Rep. Ser.*, 675.
15. Anonymous (1988) Chemotherapy of leprosy. *Lancet, 2*, 487.
16. Bhatia MS, Singhal PK, Dhar NK (1988) Dapsone-induced psychosis. *Indian J. Pediatr., 55*, 153.
17. Fernandez-Obregon AC, Forconi RJ (1988) Neurologic symptoms posing as dapsone-induced polyneuropathy in two patients with dermatitis herpetiformis. *Cutis, 41*, 347.

A.G.C. Bauer

32 Anthelminthic drugs

The treatment of onchocerciasis

Onchocerciasis is one of the major tropical diseases affecting 18 million people in 26 African and 6 Latin American countries. Untreated it may lead to irreversible blindness. The treatment of onchocerciasis has recently been reviewed (1[R]). Treatment has been difficult because of a lack of non-toxic and effective drugs. While diethylcarbamazine is an effective microfilaricidal drug, it does not kill the adult worm and therefore has to be given repeatedly. Furthermore, severe Mazotti-type allergic reactions to antigen from killed microfilaria occur in more than 50% of patients. The new drug ivermectin seems to be as effective as diethylcarbamazine as a microfilaricidal drug and can be given in a single dose, but has much less severe side effects since it kills the microfilaria more slowly while the effects lasts longer. This certainly is an improvement and makes treatment on a larger massive scale possible. However, ivermectin does not kill the adult worm; it can therefore curb the disease but not cure it. In collie dogs, which lack a blood–brain barrier, ivermectin leads to severe hypoventilation due to an inhibitory effect of ivermectin on GABA receptors in the brain. Although in man ivermectin does not cross the blood–brain barrier, its safety in mass treatment has yet to be established.

There still is a sad lack of macrofilaricidal drugs. At this stage only the highly toxic suramin is available to kill the adult worm.

***Diethylcarbamazine** (SED-11, 652; SEDA-12, 262)*

Although diethylcarbamazine (DEC) is an effective microfilaricidal drug in the treatment of onchocerciasis, it may have severe side effects and the effect is only temporary. In a double-blind placebo-controlled chemotherapy trial DEC in a dosage of 30 mg/kg/d over 1 week preceded by 1 week initial treatment with oral doses of DEC or DEC lotion was compared to a single dose of ivermectin (150 μg/kg) and placebo (2[c]). During the initial treatment DEC caused distinctly more frequent and severe reactions than ivermectin. High doses of DEC caused headache, dizziness, nausea and vomiting in about half of the patients while reactions to ivermectin did not differ from those to placebo. DEC markedly increased the number of corneal microfilaria and opacities compared to ivermectin. All changes resolved within 2 months after completion of treatment. In all treatment groups microfilaria counts fell to almost zero after 2 weeks. In the ivermectin group microfilaria counts remained significantly lower than in the DEC patients at 2 and 10 months.

***Ivermectin** (SED-11, 653; SEDA-12, 264; SEDA-13, 266)*

Ivermectin is a semisynthetic macrocyclic lactone active in single dose against many parasites, in particular nematodes and arthropods. It appears to be particularly effective as a microfilaricidal drug in onchocerciasis. Its mode of action is not fully elucidated but seems to involve inhibition of GABA receptors of the parasite, inhibition of muscle contraction and a longer-acting effect on the embryogenesis of microfilaria (3[R]). In a study reported by Albiez (2[c]) from Liberia, ivermectin was found to be as effective as diethylcarbamazine but with no greater side effects while the clinical effect lasted longer. In a further study from Mali, ivermectin was found to be very effective in a group of highly infected onchocerciasis patients (4[c]). The effects of 3 treatment schemes (100, 150, 200 μg in a single dose) were compared during a 12-month follow-up. The results did not differ significantly and varied between 72–79% reduction of parasite counts at 3 days, 91% at 6 months and 87% at 12 months.

Side Effects of Drugs Annual 14
M.N.G. Dukes and L. Beeley, editors

No serious side effects were noted although there were some allergic reactions such as pruritus, edematous swelling of the limbs, rash and arthralgia. However, no symptomatic treatment with cortico-steroids or antihistamines was found to be necessary. In 21 out of 234 patients T-wave inversion in the right precordial leads was found on electrocardiographic examination between days 1 and 4. These findings were not dose-related and did not lead to clinical symptoms. Ivermectin was also found to be very effective in single dose treatment for Wuchereria bancrofti filariasis in 40 Indian patients (5). A complete clearing of blood microfilaria was found within 5–12 days in single dose treatment schemes ranging from 25–200 μg/kg. Microfilaria reappeared at 3 months. Mild side effects occurred in almost all patients and comprised fever in 92%, chills in 64%, headache in 92%, lethargy in 53%, diaphoresis in 54%, myalgia in 79%, lightheadedness in 54%, arthralgia in 33%, anorexia in 54%, abdominal pain in 23%, sore throat in 54%, cough in 74%, chest pain in 28%, nausea in 13% and vomiting in 5%.

Even at their peak intensity however, these effects were found to be generally slight to moderate and were easily managed clinically with simple analgesic medication. There were 2 types of reactions, however, that were of potential greater concern. ***Postural hypotension*** *developed in 3 patients (1 in the 50 μg/kg and 2 in the 200 μg/kg group) with tachycardia and a fall in the standing mean arterial blood pressure after 12–24 hours. Two patients returned to normal after 48 hours, the third after 72 hours. The recumbent blood pressure remained normal and no specific treatment except bedrest was needed. The second, more important side effect, was a transient but significant (> 15%)* ***fall in forced vital capacity*** *or forced 1-second expiratory volume in 11 out of 23 patients evaluated both before and 24–30 hours after administration of ivermectin. This apparent bronchoconstriction disappeared after 48 hours and was not accompanied by radiographic changes. In this group of patients no electrocardiographic changes were found after treatment.*

Oxamniquine *(SED-11, 598, 654; SEDA-12, 261)*

Oxamniquine is a very effective drug in the treatment of *S. mansoni* infections; however, severe *CNS reactions* including epileptic seizures have been described. In a study from Ethiopia (6[C]) in 100 patients oxamniquine was found to be as effective as praziquantel with generally mild and transient side effects, notably dizziness (57%), diarrhea (18%), abdominal discomfort (45%) and itching (15%). In this group of 100 patients one epileptic seizure occurred, further confirming oxamniquine as a drug of second choice after praziquantel in the treatment of *S. mansoni* infections.

Praziquantel *(SED-11, 655; SEDA-12, 262; SEDA-13, 267)*

Praziquantel is generally considered a very effective and safe drug in the treatment of all forms of schistosomiasis and many other trematode infections. It is also effective in neurocysticercosis. In recent years, identification by Ciferri of a delayed cerebrospinal fluid reaction has led to the suggestion being made to treat these patients concurrently with corticosteroids to prevent this complication (SEDA-13, 267). In a comment on this issue, Del Brutto has suggested that in many cases treatment of neurocysticercosis with praziquantel leads to *cerebrospinal reactions* such as headache, nausea and seizures due to the strong inflammatory reaction to the destruction of cysticerci but that these reactions are mostly mild and do not warrant treatment with corticosteroids, the more so since concurrent corticosteroid treatment may reduce the effective plasma levels of praziquantel by up to 50% (7[r]).

The good therapeutic effect of praziquantel in the treatment of *S. mansoni* infections was again confirmed in a study from Ethiopia (2[C]). In a treatment group of 100 patients only mild and transient side effects such as dizziness (58%), abdominal discomfort (50%), itching (30%), diarrhea (6%) and vomiting (20%) were recorded.

Suramin *(SED-11, 658)*

Suramin was originally developed as an antitrypanosomal agent but was found to be effective as a macrofilaricidal drug in filariasis. It is a highly complex chemical which is poorly absorbed from the gut and given by intravenous injection. Suramin is toxic and reactions include stomatitis, buccal ulceration, exfoliative dermatitis, liver function disturbances, proteinuria and renal damage. No recent papers about its use in onchocerciasis have been published. Suramin has recently been found to be an inhibitor of reverse transcriptase of the human immunodeficiency virus and a trial of suramin to treat AIDS patients was started. In 1986 *toxic keratopathy* was described in 5 AIDS patients treated with high-dose suramin (8[c]). A further report of keratopathy caused by suramin treatment concerns a group of 6 patients with adrenal carcinoma treated with suramin because of its toxic effect on the adrenal (9[c]). All 6 patients were treated with high doses of suramin (1400 mg/m^2). In all patients a bilateral vortex keratopathy developed similar to that seen in Fabry's disease and drug-induced lipid storage disease. The mean total dose at the onset of symptoms was 8.3 g.

Triclabendazole

Triclabendazole, a benzimidazole used in veterinary medicine against *Fasciola hepatica*, was studied in 1 patient with a *Fasciola hepatica* infection in Switzerland (10[c]). This patient was at first unsuccessfully treated with albendazole and later with albendazole after initial treatment with praziquantel. Three months later, as egg production was undiminished she was treated with triclabendazole, 625 mg in a single dose. Ten days after treatment fasciola eggs could no longer be found in the stools. During the first 3 days of treatment no side effects were noted. On the 4th day there was a sudden chill and fever to 39°C with upper abdominal colic. The patient was treated with spasmolytic therapy and cotrimazole for 2 days. After 48 hours she was afebrile and after 72 hours all abnormal symptoms had disappeared. Although the symptoms were suggestive of acute cholangitis, no change in alkaline phosphatase or bilirubin levels was found. There was, however, a slight transient leukopenia and a short-lived 3-fold rise of the ALAT. After 1 week these findings had all returned to normal. Five months after treatment there were no signs of recurrence.

REFERENCES

1. Orme M, Awadzi K, Edwards G et al (1988) Drug treatment of onchocerciasis. *Q. J. Med., 251*, 195.
2. Albiez EJ, Newland HS, White AT et al (1988) Chemotherapy of onchocerciasis with high doses of diethylcarbamazine or a single dose of ivermectin: microfilaria levels and side effects. *Trop. Med. Parasitol., 39*, 19.
3. Bennett JL, Williams JF, Dave V (1988) Pharmacology of ivermectin. *Parasitol. Today, 4*, 226.
4. Vingtain P, Pichard E, Ginoux J et al (1988) Ivermectine et onchocercose humaine. *Bull. Soc. Pathol. Exot., 81*, 260.
5. Kumaraswami V, Ottesen EA, Vijayaserakam V et al (1988) Ivermectin for the treatment of *Wuchereria bancrofti* filariasis. Efficacy and adverse reactions. *J. Am. Med. Assoc., 259*, 3150.
6. Del Brutto OH (1988) Delayed CSF reaction to praziquantel. *Lancet, 1*, 341.
7. Taddese K, Zein ZA (1988) Comparison between the efficacy of oxamniquine and praziquantel in the treatment of *S. mansoni* infection on a sugar estate in Ethiopia. *Ann. Trop. Med. Parasitol., 82*, 175.
8. Teich SA, Handwerger S, Mathur-Wagh U et al (1986) Toxic keratopathy associated with suramin therapy. *N. Engl. J. Med., 314*, 1455.
9. Holland EJ, Stein CA, Palestine AG et al (1988) Suramin keratopathy. *Am. J. Ophthalmol., 106*, 216.
10. Markwalder K, Koller M, Goebbel N et al (1988) Infection with *Fasciola hepatica*. Erfolgreiche Therapie mit Triclabendazol. *Schweiz. Med. Wochenschr., 18*, 1048.

M.N.G. Dukes

33 Enzymes and enzyme inhibitors

℞ *Efficacy, risk and chymopapain (SED-11, 660; SEDA-13, 269)*

Twenty-five years have elapsed since Lyman Smith, following experimental work, introduced chemonucleolysis with chymopapain in human subjects in 1964 (1,2[C]), a suitable moment to attempt to assess the efficacy/risk ratio of the procedure as a means of producing lasting benefit in cases of disc herniation.

The notion had in fact originally been advanced in Hirsch in 1959, his hypothesis being that the intradiscal injection of a chondrolytic enzyme would accelerate the degeneration of the disc to the point where it would be stable and asymptomatic (3[c]). Despite various misgivings at what some considered to be an over-simplistic and risky procedure, the initial clinical results proved highly encouraging, and later work convinced even the drug regulatory authorities that the method was defensible. Whether the actual effect indeed corresponded to the hypothesis was not entirely clear. Ultimately it was found that the chymopapain rendered the disc more flexible and decreased its torsional stiffness (4[R]). The height of the disc decreased within a period of weeks or months following the injection, though various studies showed that it might subsequently increase again. The short-term pain relief which was commonly experienced remained unexplained, but it came to be widely believed that the enzyme reduced the water-binding capacity of the proteoglycans, thereby reducing the intradiscal pressure, a view apparently confirmed by animal experiments (5[R]).

Efficacy *The long-term results, against which the acceptability of adverse reactions has to be judged, have remained somewhat controversial, particularly because the studies conducted to assess the clinical improvement have been carried out in different ways; there is also clearly an inconsistency in the selection of subjects, not all of whom have a proven herniated disc. Several studies have claimed a success rate of between 60 and 80%. Certainly at 6 months the results seem better than those attained by the injection of a placebo (6[CR]), insofar as that is relevant. More sceptical workers have however pointed to the fact that the natural history of sciatica and disc herniation has to be taken into account, and it does not appear that any large long-term comparison has yet been completed, but the serious work which has been done does not seem to indicate a great deal of lasting improvement following the treatment (7[C]). Other workers have compared the chemonucleolysis with surgical treatment and generally found that the latter is more effective. This is not the place for a full debate on the subject, but one must conclude that there is no proven spectacular degree of long-term benefit such as would outweigh any serious risk of adverse effects.*

Anaphylactic and allergic reactions *The most prominent risk to have come to the fore with chymopapain, because of its severity rather than its frequency, is that of anaphylaxis, including fatalities and reactions accompanied by permanent neurological sequelae (8[CR]). Figures available at the time when the 11th Edition of Meyler's Side Effects of Drugs was prepared in 1988 suggested an incidence of about 0.7%, and various studies suggest that this level is reached in the United States. European figures seem to be much lower, with a rate of only 0.06% reported by Bouillet in 1984 (9[R]). The incidence of less severe allergic reactions is probably similar to that of anaphylaxis, giving a total for a North American population of about 1.5%. It has been argued*

Side Effects of Drugs Annual 14
M.N.G. Dukes and L. Beeley, editors

that the higher rate of hypersensitivity reactions reported in the U.S.A., unless it is an artefact, could be due to widespread sensitization of the population there by the use of chymopapain in foodstuffs, beverages and even cleaning fluids for contact lenses. However it is also clear that the intradiscal use of chymopapain itself results in the appearance in the circulation of IgE and IgG with reactivity to the enzyme, i.e. sensitization; it is thus sensible to regard this as a one-time treatment which should not be repeated. Beyond that, it is simply necessary to avoid using the treatment in sensitized subjects; sensitivity apparently can and should be tested for in advance (10[C]).

Injury *Injection into a disc can itself prove injurious if it is not performed ideally, and earlier reviews in these volumes have pointed to the occurrence of paraplegia and even conclusions or hemorrhage. Compression of multiple nerve roots may result from extrusion of the disc fragments and necessitate surgical intervention (11[CR]). The effects of injury are aggravated by the enzyme, and particularly if adverse effects appear some weeks later this suggests enzymic injury. Certainly if chymopapain is injected directly into a nerve, severe neural injury is possible; if it is accidentally injected intrathecally, subarachnoid bleeding can occur, as has been shown in animals, and appears to have occurred in a patient described by Anderson in 1988 (12). Wiltse et al even suggested that epidural leakage of the enzyme from the disc is common, perhaps involving a quarter of the treated cases (13[r]), but in the 15 years since they made that suggestion little clear evidence of adverse consequences on this scale has emerged, and animal studies have suggested that the presence of the enzyme is well-tolerated. All in all, there seems to be 1 serious neurological injury per 1800 injections, only some of these being due to the drug rather than the technique (14[R]). Risk factors include '...chymopapain injections at multiple disc levels, the use of general anaesthesia as opposed to local or supplemental local anesthesia, and performing discography at the time of chymopapain injection...' (ibid.). It is not clear whether the neurological complications are more common in sensitized subjects, but the risk of simultaneous discography must be stressed; it could relate to the toxicity of contrast media.*

Conclusion *As is evident from the above, statements both as to the efficacy and the safety of chemonucleolysis remain disputed. Nachemson and Rydevik in Sweden, considering all the evidence available in 1988, concluded that 'at the present time, surgery with removal of the disc hernia through a small laminotomy remains the documented treatment of choice for patients with disc herniation and sciatica in whom conservative treatment has failed' (4[R]). A medico-legal analysis of court cases in the United States relating to the chemonucleolytic technique, its risks, and the reasonableness of a patient's refusing such treatment, has underlined just how much doubt, after a quarter of century of work, remains (15[R]). Chemonucleolysis has been given a great deal of time to prove itself, but even in the United States its use appears to have declined rapidly in recent years because of the known risks and the uncertain results. In experienced hands, use of the method may still be justified, but it is probably not a technique to be pressed upon the patient or taken into use today in centers where other approaches to disc herniation are more familiar.*

REFERENCES

1. Smith L, Garvin PJ, Gesler RM et al (1963) Enzyme dissolution of the nucleus pulposus. *Nature, 198*, 1311.
2. Smith L (1984) Enzyme dissolution of the nucleus pulposus in humans. *J. Am. Med. Assoc., 187*, 137.
3. Hirsch C (1959) Studies on the pathology of low back pain. *J. Bone Jt. Surg. (Br. Vol.) 41*, 237.
4. Nachemson AL, Rydevik R (1988) Chemonucleolysis for sciatica. *Acta Orthop. Scand., 59*, 56.
5. Takahashi K, Inoue S, Takada S et al (1986) Experimental study on chemonucleolysis. With special reference to the change of intradiscal pressure. *Spine, 11*, 617.
6. Dabezies EJ, Langford K, Morris J et al (1987) Safety and efficacy of chymopapain (discase) in the treatment of sciatica due to a herniated nucleus pulposus. *Spine, 13*, 561.
7. Weber H (1983) Lumbar disc herniation. A prospective study of prognostic factors including a controlled trial. Part II. *J. Oslo City Hosp., 28*, 89.
8. Schurch B, Walther C, Chantraine A (1988) Ré-

actions allergiques à la chimionucléolyse; à propos d'un cas de choc anaphylactique sévère suivi de séquelles neurologiques majeures. *Méd. Phys., 31*, 207.
9. Bouillet R (1984) Chemonucleolysis: adverse reactions. Paper presented at the annual meeting of the International Society for the Study of the Lumbar Spine, Montreal, Canada.
10. Grammer LC, Schafer M, Bernstein D et al (1988) Prevention of chymopapain anaphylaxis by screening chemonucleolysis candidates with cutaneous chymopapain testing. A preliminary report. *Clin. Orthop. Rel. Res., 234*, 12.
11. McDermott DJ, Agre K, Brim M et al (1988) Chymodiactin in patients with herniated lumbar intervertebral disc(s). *Spine, 10*, 242.
12. Anderson BA (1988) Acute encephalopathy and third-nerve palsy after chymopapain injection. *Can. Med. Assoc. J., 139*, 422.
13. Wiltse LL, Widell EH, Hansen AY (1975) Chymopapain chemonucleolysis in lumbar disc disease. *J. Am. Med. Assoc., 231*, 474.
14. Agre K (1985) Serious neurological adverse events associated with administration of Chymodiactin. In: Norby EJ (Ed), *Chemonucleolysis*. Slack Inc.
15. Brushwood DB, Kaufman HH, Trumbull WH (1988) New technologies and patient choice. A lesson from the chymopapain experience. *Med. Law, 7*, 211.

S. Dittmann

34 Immunobiological preparations

GENERAL

In 1989, the Immunization Practices Advisory Committee (ACIP) updated the (1983) 'General Recommendations on Immunization' ([1R]). Introducing the recommendations, the Committee stated that the benefits of immunization range from partial to complete protection against the consequences of infectious disease (which range from mild or asymptomatic infection to severe course such as paralysis or death); the risks of immunization range from common, trivial and inconvenient side effects to rare, severe and life-threatening conditions. The recommendations for immunization practices balance the scientific evidence of benefits, costs and risks by providing specific advice on dose, route, injection site, spacing of vaccines and sera, and delineating situations that warrant precautions or contraindicate their use. They are recommendations for use in the United States because epidemiological circumstances and vaccines often differ in other countries. The relative balance of benefit and risks can change as diseases are controlled or eradicated.

Recommendations regarding contraindications for vaccines used in the Expanded Programme on Immunization (EPI) have also been formulated by the European Programme Managers on Immunization, who met in Budapest in April, 1988. The recommendations were drafted for the consideration of national authorities, to be adapted to national circumstances as appropriate. Six categories of disease/health status have to be considered as potential contraindications for a distinct vaccine: acute illness, altered immunity including symptomatic and asymptomatic HIV infection (see SEDA-13, 273), severe adverse events after a previous dose, neurological disorders, pregnancy, and anaphylaxis to egg protein and antibiotics in vaccines ([2R]).

Side Effects of Drugs Annual 14
M.N.G. Dukes and L. Beeley, editors

Immunization of HIV-infected persons *(SEDA-12, 269; SEDA-13, 271)*

Further reports on the efficacy and safety of immunization in HIV-infected persons have been provided.

Side effects following immunization A 13-month-old child who had been immunized with BCG in the neonatal period (mother's HIV-infection unknown at the time of vaccine administration) developed HIV encephalopathy and *Pneumocystis carinii* pneumonia (PCP). Two months later BCG-culture-positive inguinal lymphadenitis occurred. There were no signs of generalization ([3C]). Reports on 5 further lymphadenitis cases in HIV-infected children have been published (SEDA-13, 271).

The first case-reports on disseminated BCG infection were discussed in SEDA-13 (p. 271): a 4-month-old African infant and an infant born in France with suggested generalization. Houde and Dery ([4C]) have described the first case in detail. In addition, Vetter ([5C]) recently reported the development of BCG dissemination in a 31-year-old AIDS patient. *Mycobacterium bovis*, BCG strain, was grown from blood, sputum and urine.

Investigating the effect of hepatitis B immunization (3 doses) on the acceleration of HIV-related disease in 13 HIV-positive (Stages II and III, CDC classification) homosexual men (17 HIV-negative control persons), Gutfreund et al ([6C]) found no detrimental effect on the CD4+ cell count.

A similar study was carried out by Buchbinder et al ([7C]): hepatitis B vaccine administered to homo- and bisexual men in a randomized controlled trial (359 participants) did not cause acceleration of HIV-related disease.

An ongoing retrospective survey (first results published in SEDA-12, 269) was conducted by the New York City Department of Health to evaluate the frequency of serious adverse events following the receipt of live vaccines among children with HIV infection receiving pediatric care in New York City and New Jersey. Outpatient records of 319 children were reviewed; 221 contained immunization histories. Perinatal HIV transmission was suspected for 94% of the 221 cases and infection via transfusion for the remaining 6%; 81% of the 221 cases had received at least 1 dose of live oral poliomyelitis vaccine (OPV) and 32% had received measles, mumps and rubella vaccine (MMR). There were 120 children for whom a temporal relationship between immunization and onset of symptoms of immunodeficiency could be seen: 46 (out of 120) had received at least 1 dose of OPV and 23 had received MMR after onset of symptoms. Follow-up showed no reports of serious adverse events such as typical or atypical measles, paralytic poliomyelitis, or aseptic meningitis in the 4-week period following immunization. In addition, the Departments of Health in New York City and New Jersey State did not find any child with recorded vaccine-associated illness who was noted to have AIDS or HIV-related disease for the period 1979–1986 (8[C]).

In an overview on immunization and HIV infection, Onorato et al (9[R]) analyzed the results of further prospective studies. In New York City and Newark 70 children born to HIV-infected mothers received DTP and IPV without serious adverse effects.

In Haiti 80 children seropositive at birth enrolled in a cohort study received DTP, OPV, and measles vaccine, also without any severe or unusual reactions.

Using a binomial distribution and the observed incidence (0%) of serious adverse events in vaccinees in the available retrospective and prospective studies, Onorato et al (9[R]) estimated the maximum theoretical risk of serious adverse events following immunization. For OPV, based on over 400 HIV-infected immunized children, the risk is 0.8%. For MMR or measles vaccine, based on approximately 300 vaccinated children, the risk is 1.4%.

Immunogenicity In the study mentioned above (7[C]) the authors considered that plasma-derived hepatitis B vaccine is significantly less efficacious in HIV-seropositive than in HIV-negative subjects. The response to Salk booster immunization correlates with the number of circulating T4 cells and to the T4/T8 ratio (10[C]).

On comparing the antibody response to influenze and pneumococcal immunization in homosexuals (20 HIV-negative men, 10 HIV-seropositive men, and 25 men with persistent generalized lymphadenopathy) and heterosexuals (19 vaccinees), no suppressive effect on the number of T-cells or deterioration in the clinical status of HIV-infected vaccinees could be found. The antibody response to pneumococcal polysaccharide vaccine was lowered in vaccinees with lymphadenopathy. There was no difference in influenza antibody response (11[C]).

To evaluate azidothymidine's (AZT) effect on the pneumococcal vaccine-induced antibody response since immunization is suboptimal for untreated AIDS patients, Glaser et al (12[C]) administered the vaccine to 19 patients receiving AZT and to 4 patients not treated with AZT. Vaccinated AIDS/ARC patients receiving AZT developed protective antibody levels, whereas those not receiving AZT did not.

Three HIV-infected Rwandan infants (postnatal infection suggested; clinical status: marasmus, mild malnutrition, 1 infant healthy) developed measles antibody following immunization and none had notable adverse reactions (13[C]).

Onorato et al (9[R]) have summarized the available data on immunogenicity and efficacy of immunization (DTP, MMR, OPV, IPV, pneumococcal vaccine) in HIV-infected children. The data confirm preliminary results (see SEDA-13, 272) showing that antibody responses to immunization are sometimes attenuated or suboptimal in HIV-infected vaccinees when immunodeficiency is present.

Vaccine-preventable disease in HIV-infected children Six children with HIV infection have acquired measles in the United States (5 children already reported in SEDA-13, 273); two died from measles (14[C]). Markowitz et al (15[C]) have published a report on such a fatal case in detail. The authors support the recommendations of the Immunization Practices Advisory

Committee (ACIP) that measles immunization should be considered for children with AIDS and other kinds of HIV infection.

Although the risks of immunization are not known with certainty, the risks of severe complications of vaccine-preventable diseases may exist if children are not immunized. The Centers for Disease Control, Atlanta, evaluated the potential effect of exclusion of HIV-infected children on a hypothetical cohort of 1 million children in a developing country with the use of decision analysis. It was estimated that 3 measles-vaccine-associated deaths in HIV-infected children would be averted by this policy. However, if immunization levels in uninfected children were reduced by 50%, an additional 205 000 measles cases and 5000 measles deaths would occur (16[R]). Therefore, the WHO believes that the benefits of measles immunization outweigh the potential risks (to date, no complications of measles vaccination in HIV-infected children have been reported) and routine measles immunization is recommended for all children (17[R]).

Conclusions and recommendations regarding HIV infection and immunization The Research and Development Group of WHO's Expanded Programme on Immunization (EPI) recently reviewed research conducted on HIV-infected children and immunization (18[R]). The overall impression of the group was that adverse reactions to EPI vaccines in HIV-infected children are generally comparable to those observed in children not infected with HIV. The data reviewed further suggest that immune responses to vaccines are generally adequate, although sometimes suboptimal. The group underlined the current EPI policies for vaccine use in HIV-infected children (cited at length in SEDA-12, 270 and SEDA-13, 273).

Based on the recommendations elaborated by WHO or ACIP, similar recommendations have been published in some countries such as the Federal Republic of Germany (19[R]).

Monitoring of side effects following immunization *(SED-11, 669; SEDA-12, 271; SEDA-13, 273)*

Since March 21, 1988, health care providers in the United States who administer certain vaccines and toxoids [diphtheria and tetanus toxoids and pertussis vaccine (DTP); pertussis vaccine (P); measles, mumps, and rubella single-antigen vaccine and combination vaccines (MMR, MR); diphtheria and tetanus toxoids (DT); tetanus and diphtheria toxoids (Td); tetanus toxoid (T); poliovirus vaccine live, oral (OPV); and inactivated poliovirus vaccine (IPV)] are required by law (20) to report certain events following immunization (Table 1). In the United States, vaccines are either publicly or privately purchased. The method and route for reporting adverse events depend on whether the vaccine administered is publicly or privately purchased. Events occurring after receipt of publicly purchased vaccines are reported through local, county and/or state health departments to the Centers for Disease Control (CDC) which publish their Report of Adverse Events Following Immunization. Events occurring after receipt of a privately purchased vaccine are usually reported directly to the Food and Drug Administration (FDA) which publishes its Adverse Reaction Report (21[R]). Reporting requirements took effect on March 21, 1988. In the future there will be one system for reporting adverse events following immunizations, thus replacing the two separate systems at present (1[R]).

Recently, a report on adverse reactions to vaccines in the national vaccination program in 1987 has been prepared by a special committee of the Health Council of The Netherlands. Reports on adverse reactions to vaccines for the years 1985 and 1986 were published in SEDA-12 (p. 271) and SEDA-13 (p. 278). Details of the tasks of the special committee mentioned above as responsible for elaborating the report, and the use of classification criteria, definitions etc. were also provided in SEDA-12 (p. 271). In 1987, a total of 197 suspected adverse reactions were reported to the National Institute of Public and Environmental Health, Bilthoven, which acts as the focal point for data collection in The Netherlands. This represents a further increase in comparison with 1984 (80 reports), 1985 (124 reports), and 1986 (149 reports). Analyzing the 197 cases of suspected adverse reactions, the committee classified 174 cases as vaccine reactions. Only the 113 major ones are interpreted in Table 2 according to clinical category and vaccine type. The causal relationship between immunization and adverse reaction has been classified as 'convincing' (88%), 'prob-

Table 1. *Reportable events following vaccination*

Vaccine/Toxoid	Event	Interval from vaccination
DTP, P. DTP-polio combined	A. Anaphylaxis or anaphylactic shock	24 hours
	B. Encephalopathy (or encephalitis)	7 days
	C. Shock-collapse or hypotonic-hyporesponsive collapse	7 days
	D. Residual seizure disorder	
	E. Any acute complication or sequela (including death) of above events	No limit
	F. Events in vaccinees described in manufacturer's package insert as contraindications to additional doses of vaccine (such as convulsions)	
Measles, mumps, and rubella; DT, Td, tetanus toxoid	A. Anaphylaxis or anaphylactic shock	24 hours
	B. Encephalopathy (or encephalitis)	15 days for MMR; 7 days for DT, Td and T toxoids
	C. Residual seizure disorder	No limit
	D. Any acute complication or sequela (including death) of above events	No limit
	E. Events in vaccinees described in manufacturer's package insert as contraindications to additional doses of vaccine	
Oral polio vaccine	A. Paralytic poliomyelitis	
	– in a non-immunodeficient recipient	30 days
	– in an immunodeficient recipient	6 months
	– in a vaccine-associated community case	No limit
	B. Any acute complication or sequela (including death) of above events	No limit
	C. Events in vaccinees described in manufacturer's package insert as contraindications to additional doses of vaccine	
Inactivated polio vaccine	A. Anaphylaxis or anaphylactic shock	24 hours
	B. Any acute complication or sequela (including death) of above event	No limit
	C. Events in vaccinees described in manufacturer's package insert as contraindications to additional doses of vaccine	

able' (3%) and 'possible' (9%). As shown in Table 2, 2 major reactions were diagnosed as encephalitis/encephalomyelitis. In 1 case a causal link with the preceding DTP-polio 4 immunization could not be excluded. An abducens paresis with amblyopia occurred in the other case. The committee has classified the causal relationship with the preceding MMR/DTP/polio immunization as 'possible'. In the reporting year in question 1 case met the criteria laid down in the working definition of 'persistent screaming' (inconsolable, loud crying which persists uninterrupted for longer than 3 hours). The committee is doubtful whether persistent screaming is justified as a specific diagnosis. In 1987 there were 5 reports of death temporally related to immunization, but in none of these cases was a causal link likely (22[R]).

Verbrugge (23[R]) has analyzed the 688 reports of side effects registered from 1984 to 1987. About 88% of the reported events were considered as causally related to immunization; nearly 60% were classified as major side effects. Taking into account the number of immunizations carried out, the author assumed a rate of 1 major side effect per 10 000 immunizations. Using the classification according to clinical category (see Table 2), the following major side effects have been registered in The Netherlands

(1984–1987): 120 cases of collapse, 106 cases of convulsions, 7 cases of encephalitis, 79 general major reactions, 52 local major reactions, and 6 cases of 'persistent screaming'. In the first 4 years of operation the national monitoring program collected data on 30 deaths temporally related to immunization. In none of these cases was a causal link with the preceding immunization likely. However, not all the data necessary for final evaluation could be made available to the committee.

National compensation systems for vaccine-induced injury *(SED-11, 670; SEDA-12, 271)*

United States In 1986, Congress enacted the National Childhood Vaccine Injury Act (20) which establishes and administers a program of compensation for children injured by vaccinations. The system is designed to be faultless; manufacturers will no longer be required to prove their lack of negligence. Any part injured by one of the listed vaccines used in childhood immunization programs would be required to make their initial claim through the federal system, and would have to reject the Government compensation settlement before pursuing other options. The Act limits compensation that could be awarded by the court system. While the Act protects the manufacturer from liability, it does not extend the same protection to the physician who has immunized the child; an effort is being made to amend the law in that direction (24[R]). The legislation levies a tax on pediatric vaccines to cover the cost of compensation for vaccine injury. The amount of tax is based on the estimate of the risk of the vaccine. It can be raised or lowered by the Secretary of Health and Human Services in the light of experience (25[R]). To date, no funding has been approved for the compensation program, and it has not yet become operational. Only time will tell if the act will be adequate to stabilize the childhood vaccine industry (26).

BACTERIAL VACCINES *(SEDA-12, 272)*

Bacille Calmette-Guérin (BCG) vaccine *(SED-11, 670; SEDA-12, 272; SEDA-13, 278)*

The results of a world-wide retrospective study of all types of serious BCG complications (1948–1974), organized by the Committee on Prophylaxis of the International Union against Tuberculosis and Lung Disease (IUATLD), were published at length in SED-11 (pp. 670–673). From the study it became obvious that the number of registered cases was an underestimate and that diagnostic criteria were not always documented properly. The IUATLD has therefore carried out a second study (27[R]); it was hoped that a prospective approach would be successful. Six European countries (Denmark, German Democratic Republic, Hungary, Romania, Croatia of the Federal Socialistic Republic of Yugoslavia, some districts of the Federal Republic of Germany) participated in the study. Nearly 5.5 million children and adolescents or young adults were immunized from 1979 to 1981 and followed up till the end of 1983. The classifica-

Table 2. *Classification of major reactions following immunization according to clinical category and vaccine type (The Netherlands, 1987)*

Clinical category	DTP-poliomyelitis				Measles	Measles, mumps, rubella (MMR)	MMR + DT (P)-polio	Total
	1st	2nd	3rd	4th				
Collapse	14	7	6	2	–	–	–	29
Convulsion	2	9	7	8	4	4	–	34
Encephalitis	–	–	–	1	–	–	1	2
General major	9	6	5	7	2	1	–	30
Persistent screaming	1	–	–	–	–	–	–	1
Local major	8	6	3	–	–	–	–	17
Total	34	28	21	18	6	5	1	113

Table 3. *BCG complications—classification system*

1. Abnormal BCG primary complex	1. 1. Ulcer, abscess, Koch phenomenon 1. 2. Regional suppurative lymphadenitis
2. Disseminated BCG-infection: generalized or local lesions; non-fatal cases	2. 1. Otitis 2. 2. Retropharyngeal abscesses 2. 3. Lupus 2. 4. Other cutaneous tuberculous-like lesions 2. 5. Metastatic subcutaneous or intramuscular abscesses 2. 6. Lesions of bones and joints including synovial lesions 2. 7. Renal and urogenital lesions 2. 8. Pulmonary and hilar lesions 2. 9. Mesenteric adenitis 2.10. Multiple adenitis and/or hepatosplenomegaly and other localizations
3. Disseminated BCG infection. Generalized lesions: fatal cases	
4. Post-BCG syndromes or diseases clinically associated with immunization	4. 1. Local chronic cutaneous lesions (keloids, histiocytoma) 4. 2. Acute cutaneous eruptions (erythema nodosum, rashes) 4. 3. Ocular lesions 4. 4. Non-fatal other syndromes 4. 5. Fatal other syndromes

tion system already used in the retrospective study had been applied (Table 3). Interest was focused on disseminated BCG infections and hypersensitivity manifestations clearly related to BCG. Moreover, local complications such as large and persisting ulcer, the Koch phenomenon, local abscess (category 2.1.) and suppurative regional lymphadenitis (category 2.2.) were recorded. There were important discrepancies among participating countries regarding population size, target groups, vaccination schedule and age at the immunization date, and biological qualities of the vaccines (prepared by national manufacturers in Copenhagen, Jena, Behringwerke, Budapest, Bucharest, Belgrade) as regards both strains/substrains and modalities of preparation.

Results of the prospective study *(a) Risk of local complications and suppurative lymphadenitis (Table 4)* The mean risk for about 2 million infants (in 6 countries) is low: 0.387 per 1000 vaccinees or 0.093 per 1000 with positive bacteriological/histological findings, respectively. The marked differences among the countries (very low in the German Democratic Republic and in Romania, 0.01 per 1000; much higher in Croatia, 17.2 per 1000) may be caused by different modalities of case-finding, different diagnostic criteria and, last not least, different vaccines. The mean risk for nearly 3 million vaccinees >1–20 years of age was very low: 0.025 per 1000 and 0.018 for 'positive' cases respectively, there being once again differences among the countries.

(b) Risk of disseminated BCG infection and hypersensitivity manifestations (Table 5) In the countries under study, 21 such complications were notified till the end of 1983. They were recorded in 4 countries, but no complication occurred in Denmark or in the districts under survey in the Federal Republic of Germany. The complications are well-known postvaccinal diseases often described over the years and included in the retrospective IUATLD study. The rarity of serious complications following BCG immunization must therefore once again be underlined.

Summarizing the results of the prospective IUATLD study, the authors concluded that the study has reaped much more information than those of the retrospective study. The estimated risks of serious disseminated BCG infection were higher than calculated previously (except for bone and joint lesions for which the investigations were probably not thorough enough), but very low when comparing benefits and risks of BCG immunization, especially in infants (27[R]). However, with BCG we are dealing with a live vaccine persisting in the body longer than other live vaccine antigens; the duration of persistence is not well known. This may have particular relevance within the context of HIV infection.

Reviewing the factors that may influence the efficacy and safety of BCG vaccine, Milstien and Gibson (28[R]) paid special attention to regional suppurative lymphadenitis and osteitis.

Regional suppurative lymphadenitis The authors remind us once again that the incidence of this complication depends on many factors, including the type and concentration of the vaccine, the age of the vaccinee, and the use of a proper technique in performing the intradermal injection (ranging from 0.1 per 1000 to 10 per 100). There are many reports suggesting that the number of viable units injected had an important effect on the risk of regional complications. A dose–response relationship between the number of culturable particles and the incidence of suppurative lymphadenitis with the Copenhagen-1331 strain has been found in studies in Hungary and the Federal Republic of Germany. Comparing different lots of Pasteur strain vaccine, Guérin (29[C]) found a fairly good correlation between the number of culturable particles and the incidence of fistulated adenitis in newborns ranging from 0–10%. On the other hand, only small differences in the incidence of lymphadenitis were shown between newborns given half doses and those given full doses of BCG vaccine manufactured in Madras, India, using the Copenhagen-1331 strain.

Assuming consistency of immunization technique and manufacturing process, a number of reports show increases in incidence of suppurative lymphadenitis when the BCG strain was changed, e.g. in Saudi Arabia following the introduction of the Tokyo strain (30[C]) or in the Federal Republic of Germany when the Gothenberg strain was replaced by the Copenhagen-1331 strain (see SED-11, 672). A more recent study in Zaire (31[C]) suggested that an outbreak of axillary and epicondylar abscesses was due to the change of BCG vaccine to the Pasteur-1173P2 product.

Comparative studies using different vaccines under similar conditions in the same population gave the following results:
(a) the incidence of enlarged axillary lymph

Table 4. *Abscess, ulcer and regional suppurative lymphadenitis (prospective IUATLD study, 1979–1981)*

Country	Age at the immunization date			
	<1 year		>1 year	
	No. of patients*	Risk per 1000 vaccinees	No. of patients*	Risk per 1000 vaccinees
Denmark	1 (–)	4.0	20 (19)	0.13
German D.R.	5 (3)	0.007	29 (20)	0.05
Romania	12 (9)	0.01	23 (12)	0.01
Hungary (9 counties)	631 (138)	6.2	No enquiry	
F.R. Germany (2 towns)	43 (16)	1.7	in this	
Croatia (1 district)	84 (22)	17.2	age group	
Total	776 (188)	0.387 (0.093)	0.025 (0.018)	

*In parenthesis: cases with bacteriological/histological findings.

Table 5. *Disseminated BCG infection and hypersensitivity manifestations (prospective IUATLD study, 1979–1981)*

Complication category (according to Table 3)	German D.R. <1 year	>1	Romania <1 year	>1	Hungary <1 year	Croatia <1 year
Disseminated non-fatal cases (2):						
Lupus, other cutaneous TB-like lesions (2.3; 2.4)	–	7 (6)*	4(4)	–	–	–
Lesions of the musculoskeletal system (2.5; 2.6)	–	–	–	–	–	1 (1)
Lesions of intrathoracic and intra-abdominal organs, lymph nodes (2.7–2.9.)	1(1)	–	–	–	–	–
Multiple adenitis and/or hepato-splenomegaly and others (2.10)	–	–	–	1(–)	1(1)	–
Disseminated fatal cases (3)	3(3)	–	–	–	1(1)	–
Post-BCG syndromes (4.2–4.4.)	–	1(–)	–	1(–)	–	–
Total Number	4(4)	8(6)	4(4)	2(–)	2(2)	1(1)
Total Risk per million	5.59	13.6	3.46	0.98	4.59	4.29

*In parenthesis: cases with bacteriological/histological findings.

nodes was 5.05% in 1601 newborns receiving Dutch BCG vaccine/Pasteur-1173P2 strain; 0.3% in 1871 newborns immunized with the Copenhagen-1331 vaccine; 3.15% in 1594 newborns immunized with the national product, prepared from the Pasteur-1173P2 strain (study in Cakovec, Yugoslavia (32[C]);
(b) the incidence of non-suppurative lymphadenitis in Togo was 4.3% in newborns receiving the Pasteur-1173P2 vaccine, whereas adenitis was rare in newborns receiving the London F10 strain (33[C]);
(c) in Turkey, the Tokyo strain gave a risk of 0.3 cases of regional suppurative lymphadenitis per 1000 infants compared with 1.3 per 1000 upon use of local vaccine prepared from the Pasteur strain (34[C]);
(d) in Hong Kong, the risk of complications, including abscess and lymphadenitis, was 0.514 per 1000 infants receiving vaccine prepared by using the Pasteur strain and none per 81 304 infants receiving Glaxo strain vaccine.

Considering that some strains (Tokyo strain, Moreau strain in Brazil) are less closely associated with lymphadenitis than others (Pasteur strain, Copenhagen strain), Milstien and Gibson (28[R]) are in agreement with other authors. Recently, Stuckey (35[R]) has found a statisti-
tration of equal doses of Pasteur vaccine (9.9%
of 531 newborns) and Glaxo/Tokyo strain
cally significant difference between the incidence of lymphadenitis following the adminis-
vaccine (0% of 221 newborns), respectively.

In the framework of WHO's Expanded Programme on Immunization the intensitivity of reporting for adverse reactions has been improved. Reports on BCG-associated lymphadenitis in Mozambique (36[C]), Zimbabwe (cited in Ref. 27[R]), Zaire (31[C]), Saint Lucia, Rwanda, Jamaica, Dominican Republic and Kampuchea (28[R]) have been published. The incidence of regional suppurative lymphadenitis ranged from 1.3–7.4%. Changes from the Merieux vaccine (Glaxo strain) to the Pasteur (Paris) vaccine were sometimes related to an increase in the incidence of lymphadenitis. In general, a BCG immunization program will be adversely affected if the reported incidence of postvaccinal regional lymphadenitis rises above approximately 1%.

Osteitis The mean risk of BCG osteitis varies greatly from country to country, with some countries reporting extremely low incidences (e.g. 0.01 per million vaccinees in Japan) compared with a high incidence in others (e.g., more than 300 per million in Finnish newborns). A retrospective study showed that BCG osteitis was present in Sweden from 1949 onwards. The reported incidence was 1 per 40 000 in children born between 1960 and 1969 (37[C]). The increase in incidence of BCG osteitis in Sweden and Finland had coincided with the replacement (1971) of BCG vaccine produced by the Swedish BCG laboratory in favor of a Statens Seruminstitut, Copenhagen, vaccine. Both vaccines were based on the Gothenberg strain. In Sweden, the reported osteitis incidence rose to 1 per 3000 and 1 per 4000 for children vaccinated in the neonatal period during 1972–1975. Compulsory notification of BCG side effects to the Swedish Adverse Drug Reaction Committee was introduced at that time. The increase in incidence of BCG osteitis in Czechoslovakia coincided with the substitution in 1980 of the Prague strain by the Moscow strain. The risk of osteitis rose to 35 per million in the period 1982–1985 (see SED-11, 671). In contrast, no cases were reported in the U.S.S.R., where the same strain was used (28[R]). The IUATLD study mentioned above failed to find any reports in 6 European countries in 1979–1981, while cases are still being reported in Finland (though at a lower rate) where the Glaxo vaccine is now in use. BCG osteitis has never been reported in the United Kingdom with use of the Glaxo vaccine.

In 1988, the (United States) Immunization Practices Advisory Committee (ACIP) updated the 1979 'Recommendations on the use of BCG vaccines in the control of tuberculosis'. With regard to side effects and adverse events, it is said that these occur in 1–10% of vaccinees including usually severe or prolonged ulceration at the vaccination site and lymphadenitis. Risk rates are given for osteitis (1 per million) and for disseminated BCG infection and death (1–10 per 10 million vaccinees), the latter problem being restricted almost exclusively to persons with impaired immunity. The accelerated response to BCG vaccine (in persons with tuberculous infections) is characterized by the appearance of induration >5 mm in diameter within 24–48 hours after immunization, formation of a pustule within 5–7 days, and scab formation and healing in 10–15 days (38[r]).

Miscellaneous Kanwar et al have reported a case of *lupus vulgaris* occurring in a 7-year-old girl 4 years after only a single BCG immunization. The patient was treated with conventional antitubercular therapy with an excellent response (39[C]). Since the initial report of lupus vulgaris following BCG immunization in 1946, fewer than 60 cases have been published, mostly following (multiple) revaccination. The risk of developing lupus vulgaris following primary immunization is extremely low.

Caglayan et al (40[C]) have reported experience in *treatment of regional lymphadenitis* following BCG immunization. Seventy-eight (of the 120) patients were given medical therapy to prevent drainage and suppuration, and 42 patients did not receive such treatment. No statistical difference was found between the groups with different forms of drug therapy (36 patients erythromycin stearate, 21 isoniacid, and 21 isoniacid + rifampin) and the 'no therapy' group. If lymphadenitis developed rapidly (in 2 months), the incidence of spontaneous drainage and suppuration was reported to be significantly higher than in patients with slowly developing processes. Total surgical excision is recommended in these rapidly evolving cases.

Cholera vaccine (including cholera-typhoid vaccine) *(SED-11, 675; SEDA-12, 273; SEDA-13, 279)*

Recently, the (United States) Immunization Practices Advisory Committee (ACIP) has published its 'Recommendations on cholera vaccine' (41[r]). With regard to reactogenicity it is mentioned that immunization often results in 1–2 days of *pain, erythema and induration at the injection site*. Serious reactions following cholera immunization are reported to be extremely rare.

Diphtheria-tetanus-pertussis vaccine *(see under 'Pertussis vaccine')*

Haemophilus influenza vaccine *(SED-11, 675; SEDA-12, 274; SEDA-13, 280)*

Currently, two vaccines against infections caused by *Haemophilus influenzae* are available: *H. influenzae* type b capsular polysaccharide (PRP) vaccine licensed by the U.S. Food and Drug Administration (FDA) in April 1985, and *H. influenzae* type b conjugate vaccine (diphtheria conjugate vaccine) licensed by the FDA on December 22, 1988. Both vaccines are effective and safe, but the conjugate vaccine seems to be more immunogenic (see SED-11, 675; SEDA-12, 274; SEDA-13, 280).

Milstien et al (42[C]) have performed an analysis of side effects occurring after receipt of the vaccine licensed in 1985 during the first year of marketing. From April 1985 to May 1986, the FDA received 152 side effect reports, i.e. 1–7 per 120 000–350 000 doses (1 batch of the vaccine). The vast majority of side effects were benign. Several reports included reactions not previously recognized, e.g. *convulsions* (13 reports), *anaphylactoid reactions* (2 reports), *urticaria* (27 reports), *vomiting*, 1 case of *thrombocytopenic purpura*, and 1 case of *sudden infant death syndrome*. Causality cannot be inferred from any single report.

Comparing the immunogenicity of 4 *H. influenzae* type b capsular polysaccharide vaccines (produced by Merieux, Lederle, Connaught, Praxis) administered in different doses of 25 and 12.7 μg to 24-month-old children, no differences between the 4 vaccines or the two dosage levels have been observed. Käyhty et al (43[C]) registered *soreness* (15% of vaccinees), *redness* (4%), and *systemic reactions* (1–7%) with the same low frequency.

Meningococcal vaccine *(SED-11, 679; SEDA-12, 274; SEDA-13, 281)*

Nine hundred and sixty-seven children (out of 1065 schoolchildren aged 11–18 years vaccinated with bivalent (A and C) meningococcal polysaccharide vaccine) reported reactogenicity data by means of a questionnaire: 544 children (56,3%) reported transient *local soreness*, and 333 (34.4%) *local redness*. Localized symptoms lasting for longer than 72 hours were rare (2–3%). 97 children (10%) were absent from school at some stage in the 2-week period following receipt of the vaccine. The commonest causes of absenteeism were *upper respiratory infections* and *gastrointestinal symptoms* (4.7 and 3.4%, respectively). Practically, all children were vaccinated without any serious problems (44[C]).

Pertussis vaccine (including diphtheria-tetanus-pertussis vaccine (DTP) and DTP-poliomyelitis vaccine)

Whole-cell pertussis vaccine *(SED-11, 680; SEDA-12, 275; SEDA-13, 281)* Further comments on the English High Court Trial regarding permanent brain damage and whole-cell pertussis vaccine (see SEDA-13, 281), have been published (45[C], 46[C]). The 300-page decision of the High Court is divided into 14 chapters; it appears to be an impressive and logical review of the evidence and arguments, supported by full references. Summarizing the results, the High Court found no justification for an association between whole cell pertussis immunization and permanent *brain damage*. The decision endorsed the policy of widespread pertussis immunization in the United Kingdom.

Recommendations from the American Academy of Pediatrics regarding the optimal timing of DTP immunization of pre-term infants were based on limited data. Koblin et al (47[C]) have conducted a further study to determine the immunogenicity and safety of DTP vaccine in pre-term infants. Comparing 110 pre-term and 146 full-term infants receiving DTP at 2, 4, and 6 months after birth, antibody response and incidence of adverse events did not differ significantly in either group. The study supports the current recommendation from the Academy of Pediatrics that the appropriate age for institution of immunization of prematurely born infants is the usual chronological age.

The U.S. Committee on Infectious Diseases has reviewed the data on the relationship between the family history of *convulsions* and immunization with pertussis-containing vaccines. The Committee took into account the risk of seizures (usually febrile seizures) following DTP immunization of approximately 1 per 1750 doses of vaccine. Follow-up of these children had indicated that they rarely, if ever, develop sequelae. Convulsions of this type were differentiated from encephalopathy occurring once per about 140 000 doses of DTP vaccine. Considering in addition that the administration of acetaminophen can reduce febrile reactions, the Committee has supported the recommendation made by the Advisory Committee on Immunization Practices that a family history of convulsions in parents and siblings is not a contraindication to pertussis immunization (48[R]).

The frequency of serious neurological events following the administration of 106 000 doses of DTP vaccine at the Group Health Cooperative of Puget Sound has been determined by Walker et al (49[C]) using a population-based case-control study with ascertainment through pharmacy and hospitalization records. They found no cases of acute unexplained encephalopathies in close temporal relation to immunization. There was the new onset of only 1 serious seizure disorder in the 3 days following receipt of the vaccine, with 1.1 disorder expected on the basis of chance alone.

Barkin et al (50[R]) have underlined the need for developing criteria for the evaluation of children with alleged temporal associations between immunization and sequelae to collect reliable data on severe adverse events to DTP vaccine in the United States. The evaluation should include at least the following elements: a carefully recorded patient's medical history; a detailed history of the vaccine-associated clinical reactions; an exhaustive physical and neurological examination; an electroencephalogram (carried out in the acute phase and repeated serially); CSF analysis; computed tomography; serological investigations to exclude common alternate etiologies; and other tests indicated by the specific clinical features of the case.

Based on the clinical description by Lewis et al (see SEDA-12, 276) of *petechiae* and *urticaria* in a 4-month-old infant following the second DTP immunization presumably caused by circulating immune complexes (51[C]), an interesting discussion on the quantitative aspects of the report has been published. Habig et al (52[C]) expressed some doubts that such large amounts of circulating immune complexes could be due to toxoid antigens. In their reply Lewis et al (53) confirmed the original findings.

Denning et al (54[C]) have provided a case-report on an infant who developed a *maculopapular rash* of the face and trunk 5 days after the 2nd and 3rd DTP immunization, with no pruritus or oral lesions. The mechanism of the rash had not been elucidated; the vaccine's preservative thiomersal was excluded by subcutaneous testing.

Leung and Szabo (55[C]) have provided case-reports on *erythema multiforme* following DTP immunization in 2 children (2 hours and 3 days interval, respectively).

Children with side effects following a previous dose of DTP vaccine have been revaccinated; 69 children received DPT vaccine and 201 children received DT vaccine. Local and/or systemic reactions occurred in 49% of DTP recipients and in 20% of DT recipients, respectively. Neurological symptoms were not reported; in 10 children following DTP immunization restlessness was observed, and in one child a hypotonic-hyporesponsive syndrome (56[C]).

Lewis et al (57[C]) have tried to determine the effect of prophylactic acetaminophen on reactions (fever, local and systemic reactions) following DTP immunization. 282 children received either acetaminophen or placebo in a double-blind, randomized trial before and 3, 7, 12 and 18 hours after receipt of the vaccine. Switching to known acetaminophen was permitted if the patient's temperature was > 38.9°C or for moderate pain. The rates of occurrence of fever and irritability and the degree of pain at the injection site were significantly reduced by acetaminophen administration.

Age-related efficacy has been reported from a study involving 383 infants (2–6 months of age) and 70 children aged 18 months. In the younger age group acetaminophen reduced both local and systemic reactions as well as the incidence of fever > 38.0 °C (from 44 to 27%) following the administration of DTP-poliomyelitis vaccine. Only 0.9% of acetaminophen-treated infants had overall behavioral changes reported as severe by parents compared to 13% of the placebo group. Children vaccinated at 18 months of age had higher rates of systemic reactions and lower rates of local reactions than infants without significant reduction after treatment. The authors recommended acetaminophen at the time of primary DTP or DTP-poliomyelitis immunization (58[C]).

A slightly different note is sounded from Finland. Five-month-old infants immunized with DTP or DTP-poliomyelitis vaccine were randomly allocated to receive either placebo ($n=130$) or 75 mg of acetaminophen ($n=133$) 4 hours after the administration of vaccine. No significant differences were found in the occurrence of fever or other reactions. The authors concluded that acetaminophen given in a single dose is ineffective in reducing the reactogenicity of DTP vaccine (59[C]).

DTP or DTP-poliomyelitis vaccine and sudden infant death syndrome (SIDS) A cluster of 5 cases of SIDS occurred in France among infants who had received DTP-poliomyelitis immunization within the previous 24 hours. The cluster raised questions regarding a possible causal relationship between vaccine administration and death and led to the decision to carry out a case-control study including 228 cases notified as SIDS at the National French Register of Causes of Deaths and controls. A real association between DTP immunization and SIDS could not be detected (60[C]).

Reporting the unexplained sudden deaths of 2 twins, Roberts (61[R]) has estimated the temporal coincidence of immunization and SIDS in the United Kingdom. As in other developed countries, 2–3 SIDS cases per 1000 occur, one-third of them between 3 and 6 months of age. Simply as a result of a temporal coincidence, 9 SIDS cases per year occurring within 24 hours of DTP immunization could be expected, which is much more than the actual reported number. On the other hand, it is known that twins are at a 3-fold greater risk of sudden death.

Walker et al (62[C]) have compared the immunization status of 29 infants who died of SIDS with that of infants matched for age in a group of 26 000 infants born and followed up between 1972 and 1983. The mortality rate was 7.3 times higher for the 3-day period following DTP immunization than for the period beginning 30 days later, and 2.9 times higher for the 29 days following immunization. SIDS in non-immunized infants was 6.5 times more frequent than in immunized infants. For the SIDS cases, the usual social factors in cases of SIDS were found: one-parent family, unemployment, and financial aid.

Summarizing the results of a cohort-study carried out in 4 Tennessee counties during the period 1974–1984, Griffin et al (63[C]) have found no increased SIDS risk following DTP immunization. The study included 129 834 children; 109 deaths classified as SIDS occurred.

Mortimer (64[R]) has evaluated SIDS studies carried out in some countries which have all shown that infants who died had lower immunization coverage than other infants. There are 3 theories explaining the coincidence of SIDS and immunization: immunization might, in rare cases, cause death which would have occurred sooner or later; it might be a pure coincidence; or immunization given later than scheduled might coincide with the period of highest SIDS risk.

Acellular pertussis vaccine *(SED-11, 681; SEDA-12, 276; SEDA-13, 282)* Blennow et al (65[C]) have compared in a double-blind randomized trial (319 6-month-old infants) the rate of adverse reactions and the immunogenicity of acellular pertussis vaccine with a plain whole-cell pertussis vaccine and a placebo. The acellular vaccine produced fewer and milder systemic and local reactions: e.g. *fever* (> 38 °C) occurred in 6–8% of vaccinees receiving acellular vaccine and in 25–37% of vaccinees receiving whole-cell vaccine; *redness* (> 1 cm) occurred in 2–13% and in 24–32%, respectively. An antibody response to pertussis toxin measured in a neutralization test was obtained in 97–100% following the receipt of 2 or 3 doses of acellular vaccine as compared to 59% after 3 doses of whole-cell vaccine.

As already reported in SEDA-13 (p. 283), the circumstances in Sweden, where the immunization program against pertussis has been discontinued since 1979 (because of low protection of the vaccine available there and public concern about rare severe adverse events), offered a unique opportunity to assess clinical efficacy and safety of acellular pertussis vaccines by a randomized controlled trial. Two Japanese acellular vaccines were included in the trial carried out in 1986: one contained formaldehyde-inactivated lymphocytosis-promoting factor (LPF) and filamentous hemagglutinin (FHA), the second contained LPF alone. Recently, the ad hoc group for the study of pertussis vaccines has published a detailed final report (66[C]). Out of 3801 children aged 5–11 months, 1428 received the LPF vaccine, 1419 received the LPF/FHA vaccine, and 954 were randomized to receive placebo. After 7–13 weeks 3724 infants received a second dose. The point estimate of protective efficacy was 54% for the LPF vaccine and 69% for the LPF/FHA vaccine; protection against culture-confirmed whooping cough of over 30 days duration was 80 and 79%, respectively. The rates of systemic reactions within 24 hours of each dose did not differ between the 3 groups with two exceptions (after the first dose fever was more frequent in both vaccine groups than in the placebo group, and persistent crying was somewhat more common in the LPF vaccine group than in either of the other groups). One LPF/FHA vaccine recipient had a febrile convulsion on the 12th day after the second dose. During 14 days of follow-up after each dose a rectal temperature of 40 °C or more was reported in about 2% and

Table 6. *Adverse reactions following the receipt of acellular pertussis vaccines (Japan 1981–1982)*

Dose	No. of vaccinees	Percentage of vaccinees with fever >38°C				Percentage of vaccinees with local reactions				
						Induration at 24 h	Redness			
							1 cm Ø		5 cm Ø	
		6 h	12 h	24 h	Total		24 h	24 h/7th day		24 h/7th day
1st	786	1.3	0.9	0.6	2.0	4.3	9.4	12.0	2.4	1.1
2nd	815	0.8	0.5	0.6	1.5	22.3	43.8	4.8	9.4	0.5
3rd	509	0.2	1.0	0.6	1.0	24.2	40.5	4.5	13.4	0.4
Booster	545	0.7	1.3	0.7	2.4	18.3	36.9	1.7	12.8	0.2
Total	2655	0.8	0.9	0.6	1.7	16.5	31.2	6.2	8.8	0.6

rhinitis was noted in 40–44% of children in all groups. Early local reactions at the injection site were rare and mild after the first dose. Both redness (10–45 mm) and swelling (10–50 mm) occurred significantly more often after the second dose in LPF/FHA recipients than in LPF or placebo recipients (66[C]).

Kimura and Kuno-Sakai (67[R]) have discussed the deaths of 4 children (due to severe bacterial infections) included in the Swedish clinical trial mentioned above. In agreement with the Swedish investigations and experience gained in Japan the authors have suggested that a correlation between acellular pertussis vaccines and deaths from severe bacterial infection is highly unlikely.

Further reports on clinical trials evaluating acellular pertussis vaccines have been provided. Rutter et al (68[C]) have tested a new acellular vaccine in healthy adults. The vaccine contained filamentous hemagglutinin, pertussis toxin and fimbriae bearing agglutinogens 2 and 3. Of 35 vaccinees, none developed a temperature higher than 37 °C or a severe reaction, only 1 had a moderate reaction, and 9 had mild reactions (local discomfort and/or erythema or induration at the injection site). All vaccinees had good serum antibody responses to vaccine antigens.

In the United States, Anderson et al (69[C]) have compared clinical and serological responses following the administration of DTP vaccines containing either a acellular (LPF and FHA) pertussis vaccine (DTP-AC) or a whole-cell pertussis vaccine (DTP-WC). Nineteen infants received DTP-AC vaccine and 20 infants received DTP-WC vaccine. In general, significantly more infants receiving DTP-WC vaccine manifested fever (>37.8 °C), swelling (>20 mm) and reactions that were other than mild. After the first immunization, 4 infants in the DTP-WC group developed severe reactions, 4 manifested unusual crying, and 1 had severe local and systemic reactions. In contrast, only 1 DTP-AC vaccinee had a severe reaction. After the second immunization, adverse reactions other than mild were significantly more common among the infants receiving DTP-WC vaccine. One additional child in this group manifested unusual crying. After the third immunization, there was no significant difference in adverse reactions between the two groups of infants. Summarizing the results, the authors consider the DTP-AC vaccine to be immunogenic and significantly less reactogenic in infants than the currently used DTP-WC vaccine.

Kumura and Kuno-Sakai (70[C]) have summarized the experience gained in Japan since the introduction in 1981 of new DTP vaccines containing acellular pertussis components. The ratios between filamentous hemagglutinin (FHA) and pertussis toxin (PT) and the content of coexisting agglutinogens differed from one manufacturer's vaccine to another. The Takeda vaccine contains FHA and PT in a ratio of 9:1 and a small amount of agglutinogen. Biken vaccine contains FHA and PT in a ratio of 1:1 and no agglutinogen. Kaketsu vaccine contains FHA and PT in a ratio of 8:2. The 3 other manufacturer's vaccines are said to be like Takeda's vaccine. Acellular vaccines

Table 7. *Adverse events to DTP immunization covered through the national compensation system (Japan, 1970–1986)*

Immunization date Type of vaccine Scheduled age	1970–1974 DTP-WC 3–5 months	1975–1980 24 months	1981–1986 DTP-AC
Distributed doses of vaccine (million)	25.1	19.8	30.5
Adverse events with sequelae including deaths (in parenthesis)	57 (37)	8(3)	5 (2)
Rate per million doses (death rate in parenthesis)	2.27 (1.47)	0.40 (0.15)	0.16 (0.07)
Other adverse events without sequelae (encephalopathy, convulsions, severe local reactions etc.)	82	34	20
Rate per million doses	3.27	1.72	0.66

seem to be effective in Japan. In accordance with the increase of coverage (85%), reported cases of pertussis and pertussis deaths have declined. Data on adverse reactions following the receipt of DTP-AC vaccines produced in Japan have been collected (1981–1982) by the study group of immunization (Table 6). The age groups of the vaccinees were as follows: <1 year 321, <2 years 613, <3 years 1383, <5 years 338. In addition to the data mentioned above, Kimura and Kuno-Sakai cited reports on Quincke's edema-like swelling of the whole arm following the third injection (0.17% of vaccinees) and the booster injection (2.61%), respectively. Comparing the results of administration of DTP-AC vaccines in Japan with data obtained in the Swedish trial using monovalent acellular pertussis vaccine, the authors assumed that some of the local reactions may have resulted from tetanus toxoid and diphtheria toxoid.

Table 7 shows a comparison of adverse reactions following the receipt of DTP-WC or DTP-AC vaccine, respectively. Data were collected from 1970 to 1986 in the framework of the National Adverse Reaction Compensation System. Both the rate for adverse events resulting in sequelae or death and the rate for other severe events without sequelae declined after changing the age of immunization (1975); a further decrease followed the replacement of DTP-WC vaccines in 1981. Summarizing their results on the safety and efficacy of Japanese acellular pertussis vaccines, Kimura and Kuno-Sakai consider the vaccines to be safe and effective enough to eradicate pertussis in Japan in the future (70[C]).

Whole-cell pertussis vaccine versus acellular pertussis vaccine Pertussis is a serious respiratory disease in infants preventable through immunization. Whole-cell pertussis vaccine fulfilling WHO requirements has proved to be an effective method of disease control. Whole-cell pertussis vaccine has been associated with febrile and afebrile seizures which are generalized and occur within 72 hours of immunization. Permanent brain sequelae due to immunization are rare; one large study suggested a risk of 1 per 310000 vaccinees. In Japan, acellular pertussis vaccines have been available since 1981 for immunizing children 2 years of age and older. Most of the evidence for their efficacy rests on epidemiological grounds and limited case-control studies. The vaccines (there are currently 6 different manufacturers of acellular vaccines of one type or another) have never been subjected to a rigorous trial. The large Swedish field trial of two acellular pertussis vaccines has not shown levels of efficacy high enough to make these two types or similar types of vaccine a likely candidate for immediate licensing in European or North American countries. In Sweden, an application to register the two-component vaccine, such as was used in the trial, is currently being considered by the health authorities (71[R], 72[R]).

Reports on further developments and clinical trials are provided in the section on acellular pertussis vaccines.

The WHO view A WHO informal consultation on production and control of diphtheria, pertussis, tetanus and combined vaccines was held in Geneva from 30 May to 1 June, 1988. The WHO group noted that whole-cell pertussis vaccines will be used for several years, and certainly at least until acellular vaccines have been proven safe and effective (equally to whole-cell vaccines) and available in sufficient quantity and at affordable prices (73[r]).

Pneumococcal vaccine *(SED-11, 681; SEDA-12, 277, SEDA-13, 283)*

The last (1984) recommendations on pneumococcal polysaccharide vaccine have been updated (1989) by the Immunization Practices Advisory Committee (ACIP) and include new information regarding vaccine efficacy, use in persons with HIV infection and in other groups at increased risk of pneumococcal disease, and guidelines for revaccination. Two 23-valent pneumococcal vaccines are currently available in the United States: Pneumovax 23 produced by Merck Sharp & Dohme, and Pnu-Imune 23 produced by Lederle Laboratories. Each vaccine dose (0.5 ml) contains 25 μg of each polysaccharide antigen. Approximately 50% of persons develop mild side effects following the receipt of the vaccine, such as erythema and pain at the injection site. Fever, myalgia, and severe local reactions have been reported in $<$ 1% of vaccinees. Severe systemic reactions, such as anaphylaxis, have been rarely reported. Patients with AIDS have been shown to have an impaired antibody response to pneumococcal vaccine (see under section on 'Immunization of HIV-infected persons/immunogenicity'). However, asymptomatic HIV-infected men or those with persistent generalized lymphadenopathy responded to the 23-valent vaccine. Side effects in symptomatic and asymptomatic HIV-infected vaccinees were no different from HIV-negative persons (74[r]).

Pseudomonas vaccine

An experimental *Pseudomonas aeruginosa* O-polysaccharide toxin A conjugate vaccine has been tested in humans. The vaccine was well-tolerated and considered as a pseudomonas vaccine (75[c]).

Tetanus vaccine *(SED-11, 685; SEDA-12, 277; SEDA-13, 284)*

Two case-reports of *polyneuropathy* following tetanus immunization have been provided by Grond et al (76[C]). A case of asymmetric polyneuropathy involving the left lower extremity occurred in a 22-year-old man 3 days after the second dose of tetanus toxoid. The patient recovered completely within a few days. The other case showed a generalized chronic relapsing-remitting demyelinating polyneuropathy, hitherto not described in the context of tetanus toxoid side effects. The authors discuss both cases with regard to the relevant literature.

A case of *Guillain-Barré syndrome* following the receipt of purified tetanus toxoid has been described by Newton and Janati (77[C]).

Typhoid vaccine (including typhoid-paratyphoid vaccine) *(SEDA-11, 687; SEDA-12, 277; SEDA-13, 284)*

In addition to reports on the efficacy and safety of live oral typhoid vaccine and Vi capsular polysaccharide vaccine already provided in SEDA-13 (p. 284), the results of two field trials underline the safety of both new vaccines. Three doses of Ty 21a attenuated *Salmonella typhi* oral vaccine in an enteric-coated formulation provided in a randomized placebo-controlled field trial involving 109 000 schoolchildren in Santiago, Chile, the same level of protection as the heat/phenol-inactivated whole cell parenteral vaccine but differed in not causing adverse reactions (78[c]). In a field trial in Nepal, the protective efficacy of Vi capsular polysaccharide vaccine administered to 6907 vaccinees was 72%. Vaccination was associated with minimal local side effects (79[c]).

Erythema multiforme is an acute, self-limited eruption associated with a number of suspected causative factors, including immunization with DTP, measles, mumps and rubella vaccine. Milstien has reported 8 cases connected with the administration of hepatitis B vaccine in the United States (SEDA-12, 279). A case-report on erythema multiforme following typhoid-paratyphoid immunization in a 4-year-old girl has been provided by Bhatia et al (80[C]).

VIRAL VACCINES *(SEDA-12, 278; SEDA-13, 285)*

Hepatitis B vaccine *(SED-11, 676; SEDA-12, 278; SEDA-13, 285)*

In general, no serious side effects have occurred with any of the licensed hepatitis B vaccines. Fears that other viruses existing in the donors, e.g. HIV, might survive the manufacturing inactivation procedures have not been substantiated. Concern has been expressed that residual components from the source material (human plasma components or yeast proteins, respectively) could cause side effects, but no reports have confirmed this theoretical concern. The experience to date with plasma-derived vaccines is now substantial and it seems likely that this is one of the safest vaccines yet developed. Plasma-derived vaccines are now commercially available from many producers, e.g. Pasteur-Merieux (France), Merck (U.S.A.), Red Cross (Netherlands), Green Cross and Kitasato (Japan), Green Cross (South Korea), and several producers in China and in other countries. Yeast-derived recombinant vaccines are now being marketed by Merck and by Smith Kline-RIT; other manufacturers will follow in the very near future (81[R]).

Plasma-derived vaccine The Centers for Disease Control, the Food and Drug Administration, and the manufacturer (MSD) have created a special surveillance system to monitor spontaneous reports of plasma-derived hepatitis B vaccine. In the 3 years between June 1, 1982 and May 31, 1985, approximately 850 000 vaccinees were immunized. During that period, a total of 41 reports were received for one of the following neurological adverse events: *convulsion* (5 cases), *Bell's palsy* (10 cases), *Guillain-Barré syndrome* (9 cases), *lumbar radiculopathy* (5 cases), *brachial plexus neuropathy* (3 cases), *optic neuritis* (5 cases), and *transverse myelitis* (4 cases). Half of these events occurred after the first of 3 required vaccine doses. There were no deaths. Calculations of the relative risks of these illnesses after hepatitis B immunization was highly dependent on the diagnostic classification of the cases, estimates of the size of the immunization population, background incidence of the diseases, and the length and distribution of the hypothetical at-risk interval used in the analysis. In some cases, Guillain-Barré syndrome was reported significantly more often than expected. However, no conclusive epidemiological association could be made between any neurological adverse event and the vaccine (82[C]).

Polakoff and Vandervelde (83[C]) have reported on side effects following immunization of neonates at high (hepatitis B) risk in England and Wales. Follow-up visits were made after 1222 of the 1485 doses of hepatitis B immunoglobulin, 509 of the 783 doses of hepatitis B vaccine (H-B-Vax, MSD), and 251 of the 313 occasions when both passive and active immunization were given. The incidence of any type of manifestation that might be considered to be a reaction (soreness or swelling at the injection site; fever, malaise, or vomiting; rash) was 8% for the immunoglobulin, 11% for the vaccine, and 9% for both at the start of active immunization. No reaction was considered to be severe. Reactions to more than one dose were reported in 17 infants given immunoglobulin and 11 given vaccine.

Recombinant vaccine The efficacy and safety of a recombinant yeast-derived hepatitis B vaccine (Green Cross, Japan) have been evaluated by Ichida et al (84[C]): 209 vaccinees were distributed into 4 groups given 5 μg vaccine subcutaneously (30 vaccinees), 10 μg s.c. (58 vaccinees), 10 μg intramuscularly (66 vaccinees), and 20 μg s.c. (55 vaccinees). Seroconversion (antibody to HBs-antigen) after the third immunization reached 96.6% in the group given 5 μg s.c., and 100% in the other groups. The incidence of minor reactions (transient *pain, fatigue, headache* and *induration at the injection site*) was 9.1% in vaccinees given 5 μg s.c.; 9.4% in those given 10 μg s.c., 14.9% in those given 10 μg i.m. and 14.8% in those given 20 μg s.c. (see Table 8). No major adverse events were observed; no significant increase in yeast antibody titer was detected.

HIV vaccine (AIDS vaccine)

Vaccine development has been a top priority in AIDS research since the human immunodeficiency virus (HIV) was conclusively shown to be the cause of the disease in 1983/1984. Several approaches to HIV vaccines are on the way,

Table 8. *Minor reactions following the receipt of recombinant hepatitis B vaccine*

Dose/Route	Dose 1 (%)	Dose 2 (%)	Dose 3 (%)	Total (%)
5 μg s.c.	10	10.3	6.9	9.1
10 μg s.c.	19	1.7	7.3	9.4
10 μg i.m.	18.2	13.6	12.9	14.9
20 μg s.c.	16.4	9.1	19.2	14.8

but success is far from assured. The unique pathogenicity and variability of HIV have raised new challenges in vaccine design, testing and evaluation.

In 1987, Zagury et al (85[C]) reported on the first clinical trial in humans using vaccinia vaccine expressing glycoprotein gp160.

The process of conducting clinical trials of HIV vaccines poses significant scientific and logistic challenges including strategies for recruitment of volunteers, confidentiality, vaccine-induced seroconversion, other difficult dilemmas and, last not least, very important safety aspects. In order to accelerate the development of a safe and effective HIV vaccine, the Vaccine Research and Development Branch of the (U.S.) AIDS Program has established a multicenter cooperative clinical trials network. The AIDS Vaccine Clinical Trials Network consists of an AIDS Vaccine Selection Committee and the AIDS Vaccine Evaluation Group. The capacity to clinically evaluate multiple HIV vaccine approaches simultaneously has been instituted, and two candidate vaccines are currently being tested utilizing comprehensive protocols. Guidelines and minimal criteria for candidate vaccines entering phase 1 and 2 clinical trials will be discussed (86[R]).

The first HIV vaccine approved for clinical trial status by the U.S. Food and Drug Administration (FDA) was a recombinant gp-160 vaccine produced in a baculovirus-insect cell expression system by MicroGeneSys. Following investigations on simian immunity to the candidate vaccine (87[C]), 12 volunteers have been immunized as part of the multicentered AIDS vaccine evaluation program in a phase 1 randomized, double-blind, placebo-controlled trial. Six volunteers received HIV vaccine, 3 received hepatitis B vaccine, and placebo has been administered to 3 control persons for each participant at 0, 1 and 6 months. The vaccine induced cellular immune recognition, as illustrated by lymphocyte proliferation, prior to detection of antibodies by Western blot (88[C]); the vaccine appeared to have no adverse effect on cell-mediated immunity (89[C]).

Levine et al (90[C]) have administered an irradiated envelope-depleted HIV immunogen to HIV-seropositive viremic persons in an attempt to prolong their asymptomatic state, or to prevent progression to AIDS. During a medium follow-up of 48 weeks no significant toxicity has occurred. A controlled randomized trial is in progress.

A synthetic subunit vaccine based on HGP-30 representing an immunodominant epitope of HIV-p17, produced antibody in different animals which recognized p17, neutralized HIV infection in vitro, and primed the animal to respond to native HIV p17. Based on the study a phase 1 clinical trial will soon be initiated in the United Kingdom (91[C]).

A consultation on criteria for international testing of candidate HIV vaccines was convened by the WHO's Global Programme on AIDS (Geneva, 27 February to 2 March, 1989). After reviewing the current state of HIV vaccine development including ongoing human trials and ethical, legal and social issues that would be involved in international field testing of HIV vaccines, a consensus on the broad scientific and ethical criteria that would justify submitting candidate vaccines to the different levels of testing in man has been reached (92[R]).

Influenza vaccine *(SED-11, 676; SEDA-12, 281; SEDA-13, 286)*

Although already published in 1980, the complete report (93[C]) on a nationwide surveillance system for illness after influenza immunization (United States, 1976–1977) has not yet been mentioned in this series. The findings provided in that report are worth summarizing. Future surveillance programs could benefit greatly from the analysis carried out during the 'swine flu' immunization program. For the over 48 million persons immunized in 1976 with A/New Jersey/76 influenza vaccine, a total of 4733 reports of illness were received including reports of 223 deaths. Since most of the reported deaths occurred within 48 hours of immunization, the rates for the deaths per 100 000 vaccinees (by diagnosis) have been compared with the expected death rate (by the same diagnosis) per 100 000 population for a 2-day period. In general, the crude expected death rate was found to be much higher than the death rate of vaccinees. Other than *Guillain-Barré syndrome* (see SED-11, 677) and rare cases of *anaphylaxis*, no serious illnesses seem to be causally associated with influenza immunization. Widespread underreporting of illness and death in the passive phase of this surveillance system, however, have impared the validity of the study. *Allergic skin diseases* were reported at a rate of 0.3 per 100 000 vaccinees, *severe anaphylaxis* at a rate of 0.024 per 100 000. A cluster of 4 *encephalitis* cases within 1 week of vaccine administration was noted in one state (0.14 per 100 000). Three deaths from cardiovascular disease were noted in chronically ill persons over 70 years of age vaccinated in one clinic. It was not possible to establish a causative link between immunization and death. Persons vaccinated in the clinic died at a rate of 5/100 000/day in contrast to the expected rate of 17/100 000/day for persons 65 years and older in the respective state.

Discussing the role of vaccine in the framework of influenza prevention and control, Ruben (94[C]) stated that *local reactions* (pain, erythema, induration at injection site) occur in 25–60% of vaccinees, depending on age group, type of vaccine used, and route of immunization. *Fever* and *systemic reactions* occur less frequently, in the range of 5–30%. In order to minimize adverse reactions, the author has recommended for children under 13 years split virus vaccine, and generally the intramuscular route of administration.

One hundred and four elderly patients were immunized with 1 or 2 doses of commercially available (1985/86) inactivated influenza vaccine. Split virus vaccine and whole virus vaccine and 1 or 2 doses 1 month apart were given. No difference in local or systemic reactions was noted among the 4 groups. Similar non-significant differences were observed for immunogenicity (95[C]).

A report on a case of *acute disseminated encephalitis* following the receipt of influenza vaccine in a 4-year-old boy has been provided by Nagano et al (96[C]). All symptoms (convulsion, ataxia, facial palsy, cranial computer tomogram showing a low-density area in the right temporal lobe) disappeared within 3 months after onset.

Japanese encephalitis vaccine

In the last half century, Japanese encephalitis has been recognized as an important arboviral disease in man in Japan, China and Korea. Since 1970, Japanese encephalitis has become a new threat to public health in Thailand, India, Nepal, Sri Lanka and Vietnam. In 1954, Japanese encephalitis (JE) vaccine of the mouse brain type for human use was licensed in Japan. However, strong criticism on mouse brain vaccine was raised and has continued for many years. The Nippon Institute of Biological Products and the Biken Foundation therefore implemented more advanced purification procedures, such as alcohol precipitation and ultracentrifugation, to improve production methods. Both procedures have been included in the Japanese minimal requirements since 1965. The number of doses distributed has increased markedly from 1967 and coincidently the morbidity has decreased rapidly. The production of JE vaccine started in Taiwan and Korea in 1968; the transfer of Japanese vaccine manufacturing technology has been considered also in Thailand and India. In 1965, a special survey team was formed by the Japanese Ministry of Health and Welfare to investigate side effects following the administration of JE vaccine. No severe side effect was reported among 21 396 vaccinees including 18 401 adolescents and children under 18 years of age. Some mild reactions (fever, malaise, abdominal symptoms) were noted in 1.2% of the vaccinees. Using a countrywide hospital network, the survey team studied any severe neurological disease occurring within 1 month after receipt of the vaccine. During 1957–1966, 26 cases (9 cases of meningitis, 10 cases of convulsions, 5 cases of polyneuritis, and 2 cases of demyelinization) could be analyzed. No evidence was provided showing an etiological relationship between these clinical syndromes and JE vaccination. The incidence of neurological disease was considered minor compared with the millions of doses distributed annually in Japan (97[C]).

Measles vaccine *(SED-11, 678; SEDA-12, 282; SEDA-13, 287)*

After analyzing data on the increased risk of *convulsions* among children with a prior history of convulsions or those with such a history in siblings or parents, the (U.S.) Immunization Practices Advisory Committee (ACIP) has recommended that children with a history of convulsion should be vaccinated because the benefits of immunization outweigh the risks. Prophylaxis with antipyretics could be given before the expected onset of *fever* (about 5 days after administration of vaccine) and continued for 5–7 days (see SEDA-13, 287). Recently, the Committee on Infectious Diseases of the American Academy of Pediatrics has discussed the same matter (98[R]). Seizures following measles immunization are usually associated with fever and occur 5–11 days after vaccine administration when febrile reactions are most common. The seizures resemble typical febrile seizures which are common at this age and are rarely connected with any sequelae. In one study, the vast majority of children who had seizures after the receipt of measles vaccine had temperature elevations and about half were associated with intercurrent infections. The Committee underlined the ACIP recommendation to vaccinate children with a prior history of seizures. Childred who are receiving anticonvulsant medications should continue to take them after measles immunization. The Committee was reluctant about prevention with antipyretics because after fever onset these are likely to be effective. The Committee mentioned the proposal by British workers to use measles immunoglobulin for these children but did not support such a recommendation because of uncertain efficacy and possible interference with immunogenicity.

In Japan, there are at present 3 further attenuated live measles vaccines licensed for general use. No significant differences have been reported between the 3 vaccines as regards either immunogenicity or adverse reactions. Seroconversion rates are as high as 95% or more. Mild fever for 1–2 days develops in 20–30% and *exanthema* is reported in less than 20% of vaccinees (Table 9). Since 1978, 16 cases of encephalitis/encephalopathy following measles immunization have been reported to the Ministry of Health and Welfare, i.e. one of these severe neurological disorders per approximately 1 million doses of vaccine administered. The rate is lower than the observed incidence of encephalitis due to other causes among age-matched controls. Furthermore, a national study has indicated that the measles immunization program in Japan has resulted in a significant decrease in the incidence of subacute sclerosing panencephalitis (99[R]).

Hassin (100[C]) has analyzed critically a case-report (101[C]) on a 17-month-old boy who developed a right isolated ocular motor nerve palsy 2 weeks after the receipt of measles vaccine. Summarizing the results of careful follow-up examinations at age 3, 5, 6 and 10 years, he concluded that the patient had an ophthalmoplegic migraine with secondary complications of amblyopia and exotropia. In accordance with other authors, Hassin stated that the pupil is usually involved in the oculomotor palsy of oculomotor migraine and suggested that the damage may be the result of compression.

A study of how mothers perceive the reactogenicity of measles immunization was carried out in a rural area of Haryana State, India. Between days 4 and 7, fever was observed in 6%, pain in 4.8%, and in two-thirds of these it was

Table 9. *Adverse reactions following the receipt of Japanese measles vaccine in children observed in the Pediatric Clinic, Nagoya University Hospital, 1980–1986*

Percentage of vaccinees with:	AIK-C vaccine	Biken-CAM vaccine	Schwarz-FFB vaccine
Fever > 37.5 °C	21.4	35.3	24.0
Fever > 39.0 °C	3.4	6.8	5.7
Rash	15.5	10.5	11.2

accompanied by crying and irritability; 7 cases of convulsions (0.46%) were recorded. By giving paracetamol, these symptoms could be treated and the mother's anxiety allayed, with a resulting increase in acceptability (102[C]).

Measles-mumps-rubella (MMR) vaccine *(SED-11, 679; SEDA-12, 283; SEDA-13, 287)*

Since October 1988, MMR vaccine has been implemented in the United Kingdom, replacing the former use of both single antigen measles vaccine and single antigen rubella vaccine. The Communicable Disease Surveillance Centre has followed up over 7000 children aged 1–2 years (some up to 5 years) receiving the immunization in the 3 pilot districts. A comparison has been made with children receiving measles vaccine. Minor symptoms (*fever, rash, malaise*) occurred with a frequency similar to that following the receipt of single antigen measles vaccine, usually after 5–10 days and lasting for 2–3 days. One percent of children developed mild unilateral *parotitis* in the 3rd week after immunization. Occasionally, *febrile convulsions* have been recorded within 3 weeks of immunization. These were similar in clinical course and incidence to those following measles immunization; all the children recovered completely (103[C]).

In Japan, studies on MMR vaccine started as early as 1974. The first clinical trial was performed with MMR vaccines produced by Takeda, Biken and Kitasato. All 3 companies produced the MMR vaccine by using their own single antigen vaccines. Therefore, the 3 measles components, 3 mumps and 3 rubella components were different from each other. In 1980 and 1981, two national field trials coordinated by the MMR vaccine study group have been carried out. Two combined vaccines were chosen for the trial. One combination used in 1980 included AIK-C measles vaccine (Kitasato), Urabe Am9 mumps vaccine (Biken) and To 336 rubella vaccine (Takeda). The other combination used in 1981 included AIK-C (measles), Torii mumps vaccine (Takeda) and To 336 rubella vaccine. The field trials confirmed that the 3 live attenuated vaccines could be mixed safely. The last field trial using the same combination as in 1980 was carried out in 1986. Three manufacturers (Kitasato, Biken, Takeda) produced the same MMR vaccine from the same bulk materials by supplying the bulk materials to each other. AIK-C was supplied by Kitasato, Urabe Am9 by Biken, and To 336 by Takeda. A total of 320 children aged 1–3 years were included. The seroconversion rates were as follows: 98.3% (measles), 99.4% (rubella), and 89.9% (mumps). Fever >37.5 °C was observed in 23% of the vaccinees, >38 °C in 16%, and >39 °C in 3.9%, occurring between 4 and 21 days after immunization and lasting 1–2 days. Rash was seen in 15–19% of the vaccinees (7–9 days after immunization, lasting for 3–4 days); 0.4% of children showed swelling of the parotil gland (104[C]).

Greenberg and Birx (105[C]) have carried out a study to assess the reliability of a negative intradermal skin test using a 1:100 dilution of MMR vaccine in predicting the safety of immunization in egg-allergic children; 17 children aged 15–36 months were evaluated with the skin test; 15 children with positive egg skin test results also had positive intradermal histamine skin test results and negative intradermal saline solution skin test results. In the children evaluated with the skin test, no reaction to a full dose of the vaccine was detected. The results confirm the concept that the MMR vaccine does not contain enough egg protein to cause reactions. The data support a screening protocol using a single intradermal injection of 0.02 ml of a 1:100 dilution of MMR vaccine in physiological saline solution and simultaneous administration of a negative control solution (0.02 ml of physiological saline solution).

A series of 135 children with documented or suspected systemic allergy (atopic eczema, asthma, cow milk's allergy, severe systemic reactions following previous doses of different vaccines) has been prick-tested with undiluted MMR vaccine before immunization: 122 out of 126 prick-test-negative children received the MMR vaccine. No untoward reactions developed, except mild generalized urticaria or fever in 2 vaccinees. The author concluded that allergic diseases should not be considered as contraindications to MMR immunization (106[C]).

Between 1985 and 1986, 1035 children with various underlying diseases received MMR vaccine at the immunization clinic of Osaka University Hospital. A low reactogenicity was recorded and no deterioration of the underlying diseases following immunization (107[C]).

Seventy percent of cases of thrombocytopenic purpura occur following viral diseases. Purpura has been reported also following the receipt of measles vaccine. Azeemuddin (108[C]) has provided 2 case-reports of *thrombocytopenic purpura* occurring 2 weeks and 3 weeks, respectively, after MMR immunization.

Mumps vaccine *(SED-11, 679; SEDA-12, 283; SEDA-13, 287)*

Recently, the (U.S.) Immunization Practices Advisory Committee (ACIP) has updated the 1982 recommendations on mumps prevention (109[r]). The subchapter on adverse effects following mumps immunization includes the following: Mainly episodes of *parotitis* and low-grade *fever* have been reported. Rash, pruritus, purpura and other *allergic reactions* are uncommon, usually mild and of brief duration. The reported incidence of 0.4 encephalitis cases occurring within 30 days after immunization per million doses of mumps-containing vaccine is no greater than the observed background rate of CNS dysfunction in the normal population. Other CNS manifestations have also been infrequently reported. Complete recovery is usual. Although mumps vaccine virus has been shown to infect the placenta and the fetus, there is no evidence that it causes congenital malformations.

An important case-report has been provided by Champagne and Thomas (110[C]). A 14-year-old girl developed mumps *meningitis* 26 days after the receipt of Trivirix vaccine (Schwarz/measles; Urabe/mumps; RA27/3/rubella). Mumps virus was isolated from the cerebrospinal fluid. The patient recovered. There was no known exposure to wild mumps virus. Nevertheless, to establish a causal relationship between immunization and meningitis is difficult. Unfortunately, markers for the differentiation of wild and attenuated mumps virus are not yet available.

Poliomyelitis vaccine *(SED-11, 682; SEDA-12, 283; SEDA-13, 288)*

Oral poliomyelitis vaccine (OPV) Begg et al (111[R]) have collected data on paralytic poliomyelitis in England and Wales, 1970–1984. In 61 of 70 cases occurring in this period, poliovirus was isolated. Using intratypic differentiation, 19 isolates were classified as wild viruses, 5 isolates as intermediate strains, and 10 isolates as unclassifiable. A vaccine-like strain was isolated 27 times: in 10 vaccine recipients, in 9 contacts, and in 2 travellers.

A similar analysis covering the period 1982–1984 has been carried out in Spain by Bernal et al (112[R]). In 43 of the 50 recorded cases poliovirus was isolated and intratypic differentiation using absorbed antisera classified the isolated strains into wild and vaccine-like strains. Wild strains type 1 and type 3 were isolated primarily from gypsies. There was a high incidence of vaccine-associated cases during 1982 and 1983 in the Mediterranean and southern area of Spain. In 1984 both wild and *vaccine-asociated poliomyelitis* dropped dramatically.

Gross et al (113[C]) reported a vaccine-associated contact case of poliomyelitis. A 40-year-old patient with Netherton's syndrome, who was receiving long-term glucocorticoid therapy, developed the illness 51 days after his daughter, aged 2 months, had been given her first dose of OPV. Poliovirus type 3 was isolated from his stools. He had received 2 doses of IPV 27 years previously.

Asindi et al (114[C]) have provided the first fully authenticated case of vaccine-associated poliomyelitis from Scotland. Twenty-five days after the receipt of the first dose of OPV a 6-month-old infant developed paralysis of all limbs, facial muscles and right diaphragm, scoliosis, opsoclonus and ocular flutter. Poliovirus types 1, 2 and 3, isolated from her stool specimens, were all vaccine-like strains. It was unclear whether a selective IgA deficiency contributed to her vulnerability.

Oral poliomyelitis vaccine (OPV) versus inactivated poliomyelitis vaccine (IPV) To compare the results of two poliomyelitis immunization strategies, Hinman et al (115[R]) analyzed an imaginary cohort of 3.5 million children followed up until 30 years of age. With 95% immunization coverage and 98% vaccine efficacy, the model foresees for OPV 10 cases of poliomyelitis, 7.4 of them vaccine-associated, and 1.1% of the population unprotected. For IPV, there would be 74.1 cases due to wild virus and 5.9% of the population unprotected. These data are considered to plead in favor of continuing the present U.S. policy of OPV use as long as the wild virus continues to be imported by travellers into the country.

Salk (116[R]) has analyzed critically Hinman's decision analysis and considerations. Criticism was directed at the values chosen for certain epidemiological parameters, the choice of countries used as reference, and the lack of importance given to social factors. He mentioned that there is no practical proof of conferred immunity in subjects who are in contact with vaccinees. The ethical and economic problems related to vaccine-associated cases seems to him very important. Once again, Salk stressed the need for a change of poliomyelitis immunization strategy.

Rabies vaccine *(SED-11, 683; SEDA-12, 283; SEDA-13, 289)*

Rabies Vaccine Adsorbed (RVA), a new cell culture-derived rabies vaccine for human use was licensed in the United States on March 18, 1988, for both pre- and post-exposure prophylaxis. The vaccine is prepared from the Kissling strain of rabies virus adapted to a diploid cell line of the fetal rhesus lung. The virus is inactivated with β-propiolactone and concentrated by adsorption to aluminium phosphate. Reactions after primary immunization with RVA are similar to those observed with human diploid cell vaccines (HDCV). *Local reactions* (pain, redness, swelling at the injection site) occur in 85–90% of vaccinees, and *mild systemic reactions* (fever, nausea, arthralgia) in 10% after receipt of the vaccine. *Systemic allergic reactions* have been reported in 4 persons after receiving booster doses, at a rate $< 1\%$. The use of pre-exposure prophylaxis with HDCV has been limited because approximately 6% of vaccinees developed a serum-sickness-like allergic reaction following both primary and booster immunizations. There reactions are thought to be due to the presence of a small amount of human serum albumin that has been rendered allergenic by the β-propiolactone used in HDCV (117[R]).

Warrington et al (118[C]) investigated 10 persons with a serum-sickness-like reaction following HDCV booster immunization and made a comparison with 7 controls matched for immunization history and antibody level. Skin biopsy revealed leukocytoclastic vasculitis resulting in urticaria, angioedema and arthralgia; 3 of 7 controls had a hypersensitivity reaction following a booster and very high anti-rabies antibody titers. The authors recommend screening of individuals likely to have reactions.

In France, 7890 individuals received rabies prophylaxis in 1987. The vaccines used were mainly cell culture vaccines (HDCV or bovine embryo kidney cells). When serotherapy was additionally necessary, specific gammaglobulins of human origin were used. Generally, the prophylaxis was well tolerated. In 2.6% of the vaccinees, local reactions (pain, redness at the injection site) were recorded. Systemic reactions (fever, malaise, fatigue) occurred in less than 1% of the vaccinees (119[c]).

There are some new developments aiming to improve 3rd generation rabies vaccines for human use, e.g. purified vero vaccine, purified duck embryo vaccine etc. Comparative trials with HDCV have confirmed similar safety and immunogenicity (120[R]).

Rubella vaccine *(SED-11, 684; SEDA-12, 284; SEDA-13, 289)*

Poyner et al (121[C]) have compared the reactogenicity of two RA 27/3 rubella vaccines, Rudivax (Merieux) and Almevax (Wellcome): 40.8% of 162 schoolgirls aged 11–13 years reported a sore arm, 30.8% some pain in joints or muscles, 14.1% fever, and 3.5% rash. No significant arthralgia occurred. One girl in each group developed rubella-like symptoms. There were no differences in reactogenicity between the vaccines.

Imbs et al (122[c]) made a similar comparison administering Rudivax and Cendevax to 1673 girls aged 10–13 years. *Mild local and systemic reactions* were recorded in 9.1 and 12%, respectively.

Side effects following the receipt of Japanese rubella vaccines (TO 336 and MEQ 11) in 232 women aged 18–30 years were related to the phase of the menstrual cycle: 16% during menstruation, 19% during the estrogen phase, 28.5% during ovulation, and 60% during the progesteron phase. The authors therefore recommend immunization of women at the beginning of the cycle, also avoiding immunization of pregnant individuals (123[C]).

Varicella vaccine *(SED-11, 687; SEDA-12, 285; SEDA-13, 290)*

Live attenuated varicella vaccine (Oka strain) has been tested in 187 healthy adults. The seroconversion rate was 82% after the first dose and 94% after 2 doses. *Mild local reactions* at the injection site were the most commonly reported side effects, occurring in 10% after the first dose and in 9% after the second dose. Vaccine-associated *rashes* developing approximately 1 month after the first dose were reported in 12 vaccinees (6%), *sore throat* in 15 (8%), and *fever* > 37.8 °C in 4 vaccinees (2%). Rash and fever after the second dose of vaccine were reported by less than 1% of individuals (124[c]).

In healthy children aged 12–24 months, the seroconversion rate was 96.6%. A papular rash within 6 weeks of immunization was observed in 19 children. In 15 children the rash was considered vaccine-related. In 4 children a coincident viral illness was diagnosed (125[c]).

Kamiya (126[C]) has collected the experience with Oka-varicella vaccine gained in Japan. Adverse reactions are mainly fever and rash (see Table 10). Reactions are classified according to severity (slight reactions, < 10 vesicles; severe reactions, > 500 vesicles and fever > 40°C; moderate reactions, between slight and severe).

MISCELLANEOUS

Simultaneous administration of vaccines *(SED-11, 687; SEDA-11, 296; SEDA-12, 285)*

Double-blind and placebo-controlled clinical trials to compare the efficacy and safety of single-component vaccines with those of combined vaccines or simultaneous administration of different vaccines have been carried out by several investigators. The results of two further trials have been reported. Deforest et al (127[R]) compared the simultaneous administration of MMR, DTP and OPV (405 children) with the sequential administration of the same vaccines in a control group (410 children). The rates of side effects were low and similar in both groups. Some minor side effects were reported more frequently in the test group, but these differences were judged to be related to study design rather than to differences in reactogenicity of the two vaccine schedules. Seroconversion rates to measles, mumps and rubella exceeded

Table 10. *Immunogenicity and side effects of Oka-varicella vaccine, Japan 1984*

	No. of vaccinees	Seroconversion rate (%)	Side effects	Slight	Moderate	Severe
Acute leukemia	330	92.1				
During remission	251	91.1	46 (18.3%)	36	10	0
'Urgent' immunization	79	95.0	38 (48.1%)	22	15	1
Chronic leukemia	5	100	0			
Malignant lymphoma	20	90.0	8 (40.0%)	2	2	4
Solid tumor	54	90.7	6 (11.1%)	5	1	
Total	409	91.9	98 (24.0%)	65	28	5
Vaccinees with underlying disease	1.602	94.1	40 (2.5%)	40		
Healthy children	2.180	98.7	25 (1.1%)	25		

96% in both groups, and antibody titers to the other antigens were similar in both groups.

Simoes et al (128[R]) have reported that local and systemic reactions were no more frequent in children receiving measles vaccine with either DTP or DTP/polio vaccine than in children receiving DTP or DTP/polio vaccine alone (total 191 children aged 12–18 months).

Malaria vaccine

The first human vaccines against the malaria parasite have been developed. Ballou et al (129[R]) tested a recombinant DNA *Plasmodium falciparum* sporozoite vaccine produced in *Escherichia coli* in 15 volunteers. No serious side effects occurred. The highest antibody titers induced were similar to those resulting from lifelong natural exposure to sporozoite-infected mosquitoes. A synthetic peptide comprising the immunodominant epitope of *P. falciparum* circumsporozoite protein was conjugated to tetanus toxoid, adjuvanted with aluminium hydroxide, and administered intramuscularly in 3 doses at monthly intervals to 35 healthy males. Mild *soreness at the injection site* was the only common symptom. Seroconversion against the peptide occurred in 53% and 71%, depending on the different peptide content of the trial vaccines (130[R]).

Aluminium-adsorbed vaccines

Reporting on *cutaneous reactions* to aluminium in vaccines (pruritus, eczema, hyperpigmentation, hypertrichosis, granuloma formation), Cox and Moss (131[R]) draw attention to the prevention of such events. Patch-testing with metallic aluminium is a simple screen and able to confirm contact hypersensitivity to aluminium. Thereafter, plain vaccines could have been substituted for adsorbed vaccines.

Jet-gun infection-associated infections

Recently published studies (SEDA-12, 286) have documented virus transmission from infected to non-infected animals by means of jet injection. A hepatitis outbreak in California in 1985 was also linked to an injector (SED-11, 687). It was not the type generally used in immunization programs, however. In fact, jet injectors have been used for many years in such programs with no suggestion of their involvement in transmission of infection. Robertson (132[R]) has discussed the California event. He reminds us that the risk is greatest for subcutaneous injections perpendicular to the skin, as the nozzle is likely to be splashed by an accidental reflux of blood. The manufacturers have therefore fitted the injector with a nylon cap which maintains an angle of 45° and a sleeve which protects the nozzle; all this has to be changed each time it is used and sterilized. However, WHO and UNICEF have stated in their 'Guidelines for selecting injection equipment for the Expanded Programme on Immunization' that 'the use of jet injectors should be restricted to circumstances in which reusable or disposable equipment is not feasible because of the large number of persons to be immunized within a short period of time' (133[R]).

Allergen extracts

Ten patients with grass pollen rhinitis were treated with Allpyral extract and 10 with Conjuvac two-grass mixture (both extracts based on pollen from cocksfoot and timothy). Lymphocyte transformation responses to grass antigen have been investigated. Three patients developed side effects (*urticaria* in 2 patients, the other patient stopped treatment when he felt 'more discomfort from the injections than from the season itself'). Cells from the 2 patients with urticaria gave occasional high lymphocyte stimulation indices. The authors considered that the cellular response has predictive value for possible side effects (134[C]).

Biological response modifier

Henrichs and Lubach (135[C]) have provided a case-report on the imitation of tuberculosis cutis colliquativa following receipt of the vaccine 'Utilin S' containing *Mycobacterium phlei*. The preparation is used to activate the immunological system in general. After 20 intramuscular injections the patient developed granulomatous and exudative inflammations at the injection sites. Pus was found to contain acid-fast bacilli, whereas mycobacteria could not be cultured.

In the 1960s, mixed bacterial vaccine (MBV, derived from *Streptococcus pyogenes* and *Serratia marcescens*) was shown to produce partial

Table 11. *Side effects following the receipt of mixed bacterial vaccine (MBV)*

Symptoms	Side effects per MBV administration	%	No. of patients with side effects
Chills	89/130	68	11/13
Increased respiration (> 20)	43/130	33	9/13
Respiratory distress	1/130	<1	1/13
Blood pressure increase	32/130	25	7/13
Blood pressure decrease	7/130	5	1/13
Temperature elevation > 37.8 °C	29/130	23	9/13
Headache	3/130	2	2/13
Wheezing	5/130	4	2/13
Nausea	15/130	11	3/13
Vomiting	4 /130	3	2/13
Cyanosis	4/130	3	2/13

regression in a broad spectrum of advanced human tumors. Clinical trials of the early product caused fever, chills and nausea, which limited the dose and the drug's acceptance. Axelrod et al (136[C]) used a new MBV preparation and treated 13 patients with refractory malignancy (colorectal cancer, pancreatic cancer, chronic lymphatic leukemia, hepatoma, sarcoma, non-small-cell lung cancer). In this pilot study, most of the patients showed objective evidence of immune stimulation with acceptable toxicity. The most common side effect was a shaking chill, lasting several minutes and followed by temperature elevation. A summary of side effects is presented in Table 11. Side effects were mild, with the exception of 1 patient who developed hypertension and respiratory distress; the medication has been interrupted.

Honeybee venom *(SEDA-13, 290)*

Hymenoptera venom has been used since 1975 and has given protection to a large number of allergic subjects. Bousquet et al (137[C]) have provided a report on 5 patients allergic to honeybee venom who experienced *anaphylactic reactions* during maintenance immunotherapy with the relevant venom. One patient had a life-threatening reaction when stung by a honeybee. In most cases these reactions might have been predicted since patients developed large *local reactions* prior to systemic reactions when allergens were injected. Subsequently, using monthly doses of 200–400 μg of honeybee venom, the patients were protected efficiently.

REFERENCES

1. Immunization Practices Advisory Committee (1989) General recommendations on immunization. *Morbid. Mortal. Wkly Rep., 38,* 205.
2. Expanded Programme on Immunization (EPI) (1988) Contraindications for vaccines used in EPI. *WHO Wkly Epidemiol. Rec., 63,* 279.
3. Enenkel S, Kynast I, Cammann U (1989) Lymphadenitis durch *Mycobakterium bovis* 15 Monate nach BCG-Impfung bei einem HIV-infizierten Kind. In: *Programm und Abstracts, 2. Deutscher AIDS-Kongress, Berlin, 1989,* No. 23.
4. Houde C, Dery P (1988) *Mycobacterium bovis* sepsis in an infant with human immunodeficiency virus infection. *Pediatr. Infect. Dis. J., 7,* 810.
5. Vetter N (1989) Personal communication.
6. Gutfreund K, Cheatham-Speth D, Rossol S et al (1989) The effect of vaccination against hepatitis B on the CD4+ cell count in anti-HIV positive man. In: *Abstracts, V International Conference on AIDS, Montreal, 1989,* p. 435.
7. Buchbinder SP, Hessol N, Lifson A et al (1989) The interaction of HIV and hepatitis B vaccination in a cohort of homosexual and bisexual men. In: *Abstracts, V International Conference on AIDS, Montreal, 1989,* p. 259.
8. McLaughlin M, Thomas P, Onorato I et al (1988) Live virus vaccines in human immunodeficiency virus-infected children: a retrospective survey. *Pediatrics, 82,* 229.
9. Onorato IM, Markowitz LE, Oxtoby MJ (1988)

Childhood immunization, vaccine-preventable diseases and infection with human immunodeficiency virus. *Pediatr. Infect. Dis. J.*, *7*, 588.

10. Vardinon N, Handsher R, Zackut V et al (1989) HIV-infected subjects respond to polio vaccination booster according to absolute T4 cell count. In: *Abstracts, V International Conference on AIDS, Montreal, 1989*, p. 435.

11. Kuo-Liang Huang, Ruben FL, Rinaldo CR et al (1987) Antibody responses after influenza and pneumococcal immunization in HIV-infected homosexual men. *J. Am. Med. Assoc.*, *257*, 2047.

12. Glaser JB, Volpe S, Schiffman G (1989) AZT's effect on responses to pneumococcal vaccine. In: *Abstracts, V International Conference on AIDS, Montreal, 1989*, p. 228.

13. Ndikuyeze A, Taylor E, Farzadegan H et al (1987) Measles immunization in children with human immunodeficiency virus infection. *Vaccine*, *5*, 168.

14. Centers for Disease Control (1988) Measles in HIV-infected children. *Morbid. Mortal. Weekly Rep.*, *37*, 183.

15. Markowitz LE, Chandler FM, Roldan EO et al (1988) Fatal measles pneumonia without rash in a child with AIDS. *J. Infect. Dis.*, *158*, 480.

16. Onorato IM, Jones TS, Orenstein WA (1988) Immunizing children infected with HIV. *Lancet*, *1*, 354.

17. Expanded Programme on Immunization (1987) Global advisory group, World Health Organization. *WHO Wkly Epidemiol. Rec.*, *62*, 5.

18. WHO's Research & Development Group of Expanded Programme on Immunization (EPI) (1989) The safety and efficacy of routine childhood immunization of HIV-infected children. *World Immuniz. News*, *5*, 9.

19. Bösel B, Döll M, Ebeling J et al (1988) Zur Schutzimpfung von Kindern mit HIV-Infektion. *AIDS-Forschung*, *3*, 103.

20. The National Childhood Vaccine Injury Act (1986) Section 2125 of the Public Health Service Act as codified at *42 U.S.C. §300aa-25 (Suppl. 1987)*.

21. U.S. Department of Health and Human Services (1988) National Childhood Vaccine Injury Act: requirements for permanent vaccination records and for reporting of selected events after vaccination. *Morbid. Mortal. Wkly Rep.*, *37*, 197.

22. Health Council of The Netherlands (1989) *Adverse Reactions to Vaccines in the National Vaccination Programme in 1987*. Report, Gezondheidsraad, The Hague.

23. Verbrugge HP (1989) Surveillance of adverse reactions to vaccines in the Dutch National Vaccination Programme. Unedited working paper presented at: Workshop on Methodologies on Evaluation of Immunization Programmes, International Children's Center, Paris, 1989.

24. Iglehart JK (1987) Compensating children with vaccine-related injuries. *N. Engl. J. Med.*, *316*, 1283.

25. Marwick C (1988) Pediatric vaccine tax seeks to cover injury: not all manufacturers passing on increase. *J. Am. Med. Assoc.*, *259*, 1292.

26. Marcus LC, Inglehart JK (1988) Liability for vaccine-related injuries (Letters to Editor). *N. Engl. J. Med.*, *318*, 191.

27. Lotte A, Wasz-Hockert O, Poisson N et al (1988) Second IUATLD study on complications induced by intradermal BCG-vaccination. *Bull. Int. Union Tuberc. Lung Dis.*, *63*, 47.

28. Milstien JB, Gibson JJ (1989) Quality control of BCG vaccines by the World Health Organization: a review of factors that may influence vaccine effectiveness and safety. *WHO/EPI/GEN/89.3.*

29. N. Guérin (1989) Personal communication.

30. Abdullah MA (1985) BCG lymphadenitis: a report of eight cases. *Ann. Trop. Paediatr.*, *5*, 77.

31. Colebunders RL (1988) BCG vaccine abscesses are unrelated to HIV infection. *J. Am. Med. Assoc.*, *259*, 352.

32. Bleiker MA (1986) Report of a study into skin sensitivity and into scar diameter after vaccination with BCG in 5000 newborns in Cakovec, Yugoslavia. *Dev. Biol. Stand.*, *58*, 725.

33. Gheorghiu M (1978) Potency and suppurative adenitis in BCG vaccination. *Dev. Biol. Stand.*, *41*, 79.

34. Lotte A (1984) BCG complications. Estimates of the risks among vaccinated subjects and statistical analysis of their main characteristics. *Adv. Tuberc. Res.*, *21*, 107.

35. Stuckey J (1988) *Prevalence of BCG Related Adenitis in Healthy Children, Maputo City, Mozambique*. UNICEF Report, October, 1988.

36. World Health Organization (1988) Lymphadenitis associated with BCG immunization. *Wkly Epidemiol. Rec.*, *63*, 381.

37. Bottiger M (1982) Osteitis and other complications caused by generalized BCGitis. *Acta Paediatr. Scand.*, *71*, 471.

38. Immunization Practices Advisory Committee (1988) Use of BCG vaccines in the control of tuberculosis: a joint statement by the ACIP and the Advisory Committee for Elimination of Tuberculosis. *Morbid. Mortal. Wkly Rep.*, *37*, 663.

39. Kanwar AJ, Kaur S, Bansal R et al (1988) Lupus vulgaris following BCG vaccination. *Int. J. Dermatol.*, *27*, 525.

40. Caglayan S, Yegin O, Kayran N et al (1987) Is medical therapy effective for regional lymphadenitis following BCG vaccination? *Am. J. Dis. Child.*, *141*, 1213.

41. Immunization Practices Advisory Committee (1988) Recommendations on cholera vaccine. *Morbid. Mortal. Wkly Rep.*, *37*, 617.

42. Milstien JB, Gross TP, Kuritsky JN (1987) Ad-

verse reactions reported following receipt of *Haemophilus influenzae* type b vaccine: an analysis after 1 year of marketing. *Pediatrics, 80,* 270.
43. Käyhty H, Peltola H, Eskola J (1988) Immunogenicity and reactogenicity of four *Haemophilus influenzae* type b capsular polysaccharide vaccines in Finnish 24-month-old children. *Pediatr. Infect. Dis. J.,* 7, 574.
44. Roberts JStC, Bryett KA (1988) Incidence of reactions to meningococcal A & C vaccine among U.K. schoolchildren. *Public Health, 102,* 471.
45. Brahams D (1988) Pertussis vaccine: Court finds no justification for association with permanent brain damage: *Lancet, 1,* 837.
46. Dyer C (1989) Whooping cough vaccine on trial again. *Br. Med. J., 295,* 1053.
47. Koblin BA, Townsend TR, Muñoz A et al (1988) Response of preterm infants to diphtheria-tetanus-pertussis vaccine. *Pediatr. Infect. Dis. J., 7,* 704.
48. Committee on Infectious Diseases (1987) Family history of convulsions in candidates for immunization with pertussis-containing vaccines (diphtheria, tetanus, pertussis). *Pediatrics, 80,* 743.
49. Walker AM, Jick H, Perera DR et al (1988) Neurologic events following diphtheria-tetanus-pertussis immunization. *Pediatrics, 81,* 345.
50. Barkin RM, Jabhour JT, Samuelson JS (1987) Immunizations, seizures, and subsequent evaluation (Letter to Editor). *J. Am. Med. Assoc., 258,* 201.
51. Lewis K, Cherry JD, Jordan SC (1986) Circulating immune complexes after DTP immunization. *J. Pediatr., 109,* 1009.
52. Habig WH, Holohan TV, Phillips TM (1986) Circulating immune complexes after DTP immunization. *J. Pediatr., 112,* 162.
53. Lewis K, Cherry JD, Jordan SC (1988) Circulating immune complexes after DTP immunization (Reply). *J. Pediatr., 112,* 163.
54. Denning DW, Peet L, Poole J (1987) Skin rash after triple vaccine. *Arch. Dis. Child., 62,* 510.
55. Leung AKC, Szabo TF (1987) Erythema multiforme following diphtheria-pertussis-tetanus vaccination. *Kobe J. Med. Sci., 33,* 121.
56. Bergmannova V, Stehlikova J, Domorazkova E (1988) Revaccination of children with known side effects following previous doses of DTP vaccine. *Cs. Pediatr. 43,* 522.
57. Lewis K, Cherry JD, Sachs MH et al (1988) The effect of prophylactic acetaminophen administration on reactions to DTP vaccination. *Am. J. Dis. Child., 142,* 62.
58. Ipp MM, Gold R, Greenberg S et al (1987) Acetaminophen prophylaxis of adverse reactions following vaccination of infants with diphtheria-pertussis-tetanus toxoids-polio vaccine. *Pediatr. Infect. Dis. J., 6,* 721.
59. Uhari M, Hietala J, Viljanen MK (1988) Effect of prophylactic acetaminophen administration on reaction to DTP vaccination. *Acta Paediatr. Scand., 77,* 747.
60. Flahault A, Messiah A, Jougla E et al (1988) Sudden infant death syndrome and diphtheria/tetanus toxoid/pertussis/poliomyelitis immunization (Letter to Editor). *Lancet, 1,* 582.
61. Roberts SC (1987) Vaccination and cot deaths in perspective. *Arch. Dis. Childh., 62,* 754.
62. Walker AM, Jick H, Perera DR et al (1987) Diphtheria-tetanus-pertussis immunization and sudden infant death syndrome. *Am. J. Public Health, 77,* 945.
63. Griffin MR, Ray WA, Livengood JR et al (1988) Risk of sudden infant death syndrome after immunization with the diphtheria-tetanus-pertussis vaccine. *N. Engl. J. Med., 319,* 618.
64. Mortimer EA (1987) DTP and SIDS: When data differ. *Am. J. Public Health, 77,* 925.
65. Blennow M, Granström M, Jäätmaa E et al (1988) Primary immunization of infants with an acellular pertussis vaccine in a double-blind randomized clinical trial. *Pediatrics, 82,* 293.
66. Ad Hoc Group for the Study of Pertussis Vaccines (1988) Placebo-controlled trial of two acellular pertussis vaccines in Sweden–protective efficacy and adverse events. *Lancet, 1,* 955.
67. Kimura M, Kuno-Sakai H (1988) Acellular pertussis vaccines and fatal infections. *Lancet, 1,* 881.
68. Rutter DA, Ashworth LA, Day A et al (1988) Trial of a new acellular pertussis vaccine in healthy adult volunteers. *Vaccine, 6,* 29.
69. Anderson EL, Belshe RB, Bertram J (1988) Differences in reactogenicity and antigenicity of acellular and standard pertussis vaccines combined with diphtheria and tetanus in infants. *J. Infect. Dis., 157,* 731.
70. Kimura M, Kuno-Sakai H (1988) Pertussis vaccines in Japan. *Acta Paediatr. Jpn., 30,* 143.
71. Fenichel GM (1988) Pertussis: the disease and the vaccine. *Pediatr. Neurol., 4,* 201.
72. Marwick C (1988) Pertussis vaccines: trials (and tribulations). *J. Am. Med. Assoc., 259,* 2057.
73. WHO (1988) Informal consultation on WHO requirements for diphtheria, pertussis, tetanus and combined vaccines. *Wkly Epidemiol. Rec., 63,* 317.
74. Immunization Practices Advisory Committee (1989) Pneumococcal polysaccharide vaccine. *Morbid. Mortal. Wkly Rep., 38,* 64.
75. Cryz SJ, Furer E, Cross AS et al (1987) Safety and immunogenicity of a *Pseudomonas aeruginosa* O-polysaccharide toxin. A conjugate vaccine in humans. *J. Clin. Invest., 80,* 51.
76. Grond M, Gibbels E, Schädlich HJ et al (1988) Polyneuropathien nach Gabe von Tetanustoxoid. *Nervenartz, 59,* 309.
77. Newton N Jr, Janati A (1987) Guillain-Barré

syndrome after vaccination with purified tetanus toxoid. *South. Med. J.*, *80*, 1053.
78. Levine MM, Ferreccio C, Black RE et al (1987) Large-scale field trial of Ty21a live oral typhoid vaccine in enteric-coated capsule formulation. *Lancet*, *1*, 1049.
79. Acharya IL, Lowe CU, Thapa R et al (1987) Prevention of typhoid fever in Nepal with the Vi capsular polysaccharide of *Salmonella typhi*. A preliminary report. *N. Engl. J. Med.*, *29*, 1101.
80. Bhatia KK, Chaudhary SD, Gupta V et al (1988) Tab vaccine causing erythema multiforme. *Indian J. Dermatol. Venereol. Leprol*, *54*, 40.
81. Beasley RP (1988) Hepatitis B immunization strategies. *WHO/EPI/GEN/88.5.*
82. Shaw FE, Graham DJ, Guess HA et al (1988) Postmarketing surveillance for neurologic adverse events reported after hepatitis B vaccination. Experience of the first three years. *Am. J. Epidemiol.*, *127*, 337.
83. Polakoff S, Vandervelde EM (1988) Immunization of neonates at high risk of hepatitis B in England and Wales: national surveillance. *Br. Med. J.*, *297*, 249.
84. Ichida F, Yoshikawa A, Mizokami M et al (1988) Clinical study of recombinant hepatitis B vaccine. *J. Int. Med. Res.*, *16*, 231.
85. Zagury D, Leonard R, Fouchard M et al (1987) Immunization against AIDS in humans. *Nature*, *326*, 249.
86. Koff WC, Wescott SL, Novak J et al (1989) Clinical evaluation of experimental AIDS vaccines. In: *Abstracts, V International Conference on AIDS, Montreal, 1989*, p. 542.
87. Neumann P, O' Shaughnessy MV (1989) Simian immunity to HIV 1 candidate vaccine. In: *Abstracts, International Conference on AIDS, Montreal, 1989*, p. 541.
88. Keefer MC, Bonnez W, Roberts NJ et al (1989) HIV-1 recombinant gp160 vaccine recipients demonstrate gp160-specific lymphocyte proliferation prior to Western blot reactivity. In: *Abstracts, V International Conference on AIDS, Montreal, 1989*, p. 543.
89. Midthun K, Garrison L, Gershmann K et al (1989) Cellular immunity in HIV-1 rgp160 vaccinees. In: *Abstracts, V International Conference on AIDS, Montreal, 1989*, p. 544.
90. Levine A, Henderson BE, Groshen S et al (1989) Immunization with inactivated envelope-depleted HIV immunogen in HIV-infected men with ARC. In: *Abstracts, V International Conference on AIDS, Montreal, 1989*, p. 219.
91. Goldstein AL, Maylor PH, Kirkley JE (1989) Evaluation of a synthetic HIV-1 p17-based candidate AIDS vaccine. HPG-30. In: *Abstracts, V International Conference on AIDS, Montreal, 1989*, p. 544.
92. WHO'S Global Programme on AIDS (1989) Consultation on criteria for international testing of candidate HIV vaccines. *WHO/GPA/INF/89.8* Geneva.
93. Retailliau HF, Curtis AC, Storr G et al (1980) Illness after influenza vaccination reported through a nationwide surveillance system, 1976–1977. *Am. J. Epidemiol.*, *111*, 270.
94. Ruben FL (1987) Prevention and control of influenza. *Am. J. Med.*, *82*, 31.
95. Gross PA, Weksler ME, Quinnan V et al (1987) Immunization of elderly people with two doses of influenza vaccine. *J. Clin. Microbiol.*, *25*, 1763.
96. Nagano T, Mizuguchi M, Kurihara E et al (1988) A case of acute disseminated encephalomyelitis with convulsion, gait disturbance, facial palsy and with multifocal CT lesions. *No To Hattatsu*, *20*, 325.
97. Oya A (1988) Japanese encephalitis vaccine. *Acta Paediatr. Jpn.*, *30*, 175.
98. Committee on Infectious Diseases (1987) Personal and family history of seizures and measles immunization. *Pediatrics*, *80*, 741.
99. Isomura S (1988) Measles and measles vaccine in Japan. *Acta Paediatr. Jpn.*, *30*, 154.
100. Hassin H (1987) Ophthalmoplegic migraine wrongly attributed to measles immunization. *Am. J. Ophthalmol.*, *2*, 192.
101. Chan CC, Sogg RL, Steinman L (1980) Isolated oculomotor palsy after measles immunization. *Am. J. Ophthalmol.*, *89*, 446.
102. Singhi SC, Kaur A, Khajuria R et al (1987) Side effects of measles vaccine; as perceived by mothers. *Indian Pediatr.* *24*, 215.
103. United Kingdom (1988) Immunization policy–measles/mumps/rubella vaccine (MMR) implementation. *Wkly Epidemiol. Rec.*, *51*, 392.
104. Kuno-Sakai H, Kimura M (1988) Measles-mumps-rubella (MMR) vaccine in Japan. *Acta Paediatr. Jpn.*, *30*, 167.
105. Greenberg MA, Birx DL (1988) Safe administration of mumps-measles-rubella vaccine in egg-allergic children. *J. Pediatr.*, *113*, 504.
106. Juntunen-Backman K, Peltola H, Backman A et al (1987) Safe immunization of allergic children against measles, mumps, and rubella. *Am. J. Dis. Child.*, *141*, 1103.
107. Kanesaki T, Baba K, Tsuda N et al (1986) Protection of mumps in children with various underlying diseases: application of a live attenuated mumps and trivalent measles-rubella-mumps (MMR) vaccines in these children. *Biken J.*, *29*, 63.
108. Azeemuddin S (1987) Thrombocytopenia purpura after combined vaccine against measles, mumps, and rubella. *Clin. Pediatr.*, *26*, 318.
109. Immunization Practices Advisory Committee (1989) Mumps prevention. *Morbid. Mortal. Wkly Rep.*, *38*, 388.

110. Champagne S, Thomas E (1988) A case of mumps meningitis: a complication of vaccination? *Can. Med. Assoc. J., 138,* 135.
111. Begg NT, Chamberlain R, Roebuck M (1987) Paralytic poliomyelitis in England and Wales, 1970–84. *Epidemiol. Infect., 99,* 97.
112. Bernal A, Garcia-Seiz A, Llacer A et al (1986) Poliomyelitis in Spain, 1982–1984: virologic and epidemiologic studies. *Am. J. Epidemiol. 126,* 69.
113. Gross TP, Khurana RK, Higgins et al (1987) Vaccine-associated poliomyelitis in a household contact with Netherton's syndrome receiving long-term steroid therapy. *Am. J. Med., 83,* 797.
114. Asindi AA, Bell EJ, Browning MJ et al (1988) Vaccine-induced polioencephalomyelitis in Scotland. *Scott. Med. J., 33,* 306.
115. Hinman AR, Koplan JP, Orenstein WA et al (1988) Live or inactivated poliomyelitis vaccine: an analysis of benefits and risks. *Am. J. Public Health, 78,* 291.
116. Salk D (1988) Polio immunization policy in the United States: a new challenge for a new generation. *Am. J. Public Health, 78,* 296.
117. Anonymous (1988) Rabies vaccine, adsorbed: a new rabies vaccine for use in humans. *Morbid. Mortal. Wkly Rep., 37,* 217.
118. Warrington RJ, Martens CJ, Rubin M et al (1987) Immunologic studies in subjects with a serum sickness-like illness after immunization with human diploid cell rabies vaccine. *J. Allergy, 79,* 605.
119. Anonymous (1987) Human rabies prophylaxis, 1987. *Wkly Epidemiol. Rec., 13,* 357.
120. WHO (1988) Report of the Second International Symposium on New Developments in Rabies Control, Essen, 5–7 July 1988. *WHO/Rab. Res./89.31,* Geneva.
121. Poyner M, Beaver R, Elton P et al (1986) The reactogenicity of United Kingdom school-girls. *Br. J. Clin. Pract., 40,* 468.
122. Imbs D, Kantoch M, Rudnicka H et al (1987) Comparative studies of immunogenicity and reactogenicity of various rubella vaccines. II. Seroconversion and post-vaccination reactions in girls immunized against rubella with Rudivax and Cendevax vaccines (in Polish). *Przegl. Epidemiol., 41,* 141.
123. Nakazono N, Fujimoto S, Wakisaka A et al (1987) Factors associated with clinical reactions to rubella vaccination in women. *Int. J. Gynaecol. Obstet., 25,* 207.
124. Gershon AA, Steinberg SP, LaRussa P et al (1988) Immunization of healthy adults with live attenuated varicella vaccine. *J. Infect. Dis. 158,* 132.
125. Johnson CE, Shurin PA, Fattlar D et al (1988) Live attenuated varicella vaccine in healthy 12- to 24-month-old children. *Pediatrics, 81,* 512.
126. Kamiya H (1988) Prevention of severe varicella with varicella vaccine. *Asian Med. J., 31,* 380.
127. Deforest A, Long SS, Lischner HW et al (1988) Simultaneous administration of measles-mumps-rubella vaccine with booster doses of diphtheria-tetanus-pertussis and poliovirus vaccines. *Pediatrics, 81,* 237.
128. Simoes EA, Balraj V, Selvakumar R et al (1988) Antibody response of children to measles vaccine mixed with diphtheria-pertussis-tetanus or diphtheria-pertussis-tetanus-poliomyelitis vaccine. *Am. J. Dis. Child., 142,* 309.
129. Ballou WR, Hoffman SL, Sherwood JA et al (1987) Safety and efficacy of a recombinant DNA *Plasmodium falciparum* sporozoite vaccine. *Lancet, 1,* 1277.
130. Herrington DA, Clyde DF, Losonsky G et al (1987) Safety and immunogenicity in man of a synthetic peptide malaria vaccine against *Plasmodium falciparum* sporozoites. *Nature,* 328, 257.
131. Cox NH, Moss C (1988) Cutaneous reactions to aluminium in vaccines: an avoidable problem. *Lancet, 1,* 43.
132. Robertson JS (1987) Jet injector's and infection. *Public Health, 101,* 147.
133. Expanded Programme on Immunization (1986) Immunization policy. *WHO/EPI/GEN/86/7 Rev. 1,* Geneva.
134. Broman P, Möller E (1988) Lymphocyte transformation by grass pollen allergens: a study of atopic patients receiving immunotherapy. *Allergy, 43,* 321.
135. Henrichs J, Lubach D (1988) Imitation einer Tuberculosis cutis colliquativa durch Utilin S. *Aktuel. Dermatol., 14,* 133.
136. Axelrod RS, Havas HF, Murasko DM (1988) Effect of the mixed bacterial vaccine on the immune response of patients with non-small cell lung cancer and refractory malignancies. *Cancer, 61,* 2219.
137. Bousquet J, Menardo JL, Velasquez G et al (1988) Systemic reactions during maintenance immunotherapy with honey bee venom. *Ann. Allergy, 61,* 63.

M.N.G. Dukes

35 Blood and blood products

REACTIONS TO PLASMA PROTEIN FRACTIONS *(SED-11, 699; SEDA-12, 294; SEDA-13, 301)*

Human serum albumin

Rx ***Anaphylaxis to human albumin***

Adverse reactions to human serum albumin are, as pointed out in SED-11, extremely uncommon. When they do occur, however, they tend to be in the form of anaphylactoid reactions (0.011% of cases treated) and about a third of these may be life-threatening (1[R]). The reactions are unpredictable, and it has been known for a patient who has reacted violently to albumin on one occasion to tolerate it well on another after being given diphenhydramine; no evidence for an immunological mechanism was found in that case (2[C]). A newer case in which the mechanism of such a reaction was studied exhaustively has been presented by Stafford and his colleagues (3[CR]):

A woman of 20 in the 26th week of pregnancy and having no prior history of allergic conditions developed severe anti-Kell isoimmunization with an anti-Kell titer of 1:32. Plasmapheresis was performed to reduce the anti-Kill antibody titre. While being transfused with her own erythrocytes mixed with 5% human serum albumin she complained of a sensation of heat and developed generalized pruritus and urticaria. These were relieved with intravenous diphenhydramine. The next day plasmapheresis was repeated after a prophylactic dose of diphenhydramine; this time she developed throat constriction, chest tightness and generalized urticaria which demanded discontinuation of the plasmapheresis and use of additional diphenhydramine. Subsequent intradermal skin testing with 5% human serum albumin produced a wheal and erythema. An enzyme-linked immunoassay was positive for IgE antibody to 5% human serum albumin before and after dialysis for removal of sodium caprylate and despite ultracentrifugation of the albumin to remove any aggregates which might be present. These results were considered to be consistent with an IgE-mediated basis for this patient's reaction to unaltered albumin.

These workers went to great lengths to exclude in their case the various causal factors which have in the past been incriminated in cases of anaphylactoid reactions to albumin. Such reactions have sometimes been shown to be due to albumin aggregates or denatured complexes (which may form during preparation and processing, particularly heat treatment); this patient however reacted to an ultracentrifuged albumin in which aggregates would no longer the present. The possible involvement of the sodium caprylate stabilizer was examined in this patient because of earlier evidence that serum immunoglobulins can react with this stabilizer to form soluble complexes capable of causing agglutination of erythrocytes. A reaction of this type may sometimes be due to contamination of albumin with other proteins, but excess contamination could be ruled out in this case. The albumin used had not been exposed to ethylene oxide (which again can alter albumin to render it antigenic) (4[Cr]). Anaphylactoid reactions can also be related to complement activation caused by circulating immune complexes (CIC). CIC were not measured in the present patient at the time of the event but they were certainly normal 3 weeks later. The possibility of simultaneous complement activation could not be entirely excluded, but it appeared unlikely. All in all, then, with both positive and negative evidence to hand, one must conclude with Stafford and his colleagues that this was a remarkable first instance of IgE-mediated anaphylaxis to unaltered human serum albumin.

Intravenous immune globulin

The incidence of adverse effects to intravenous immune globulins (IVIG) has been discussed by Cunningham-Rundles (5[R]) but also

Side Effects of Drugs Annual 14
M.N.G. Dukes and L. Beeley, editors

by Rousell (6[CR]), the latter both in the light of the literature and by examining reports on suspected adverse reactions submitted to the manufacturer of one product of the current standard (Cutter Biological).

A series of 39 patients with primary immune deficiency were treated at 3 centers; they received a total of 232 infusions of IVIG at a monthly dosage of 400 mg/kg body wt. In this series a non-modified IVIG with a pH of 4.25 produced 2 inflammatory-type reactions in 39 patients (5 reactions in 115 infusions) whereas a modified version which had undergone reduction and alkylation resulting in a pH of 6.8 produced 5 reactions in 39 patients (7 reactions in 117 infusions). These same data have also been published by Pirofsky (7[C]). There were only 6 phlogistic-type reactions spontaneously reported to the manufacturer. All were mild and self-limiting. There was no correlation between the anticomplementary activity of the lot concerned and the reactions observed.

Side effects associated with IVIG may be either *local* or *systemic*. Local reactions are essentially attributable to the technique used and are not specific to IVIG. Of the systemic reactions, those of inflammatory nature are usually mild and influenza-like, and they generally respond to slowing or temporary interruption of the infusion. The more severe reactions are possibly complement-mediated and may be due to spontaneous activation of the complement system by the immune globulin preparation concerned; IgG aggregates may perhaps be involved. The symptomatology can be similar to that of inflammatory reactions though it may be more severe. Finally, there are the rare reactions of anaphylactic type and occasional cases in which the transmission of infection has been suspected, e.g. non-A, non-B hepatitis (8[C]).

Aseptic meningitis occurred in a 2-year-old Japanese girl who was being treated for acute idiopathic thrombocytopenic purpura; since corticosteroids had produced no rise in the platelet count she was given 0.4 g/kg/d of immune globulin prepared with polyethylene glycol for 5 days; the meningitis developed 7 days later and lasted for 1 day. Tests for C-reactive protein were negative. Twenty days later, similar therapy with sulphonated immune globulin and hydrocortisone was administered with precisely the same reaction which however persisted for some days. Corticosteroid treatment alone was well tolerated. The only clue found to the reaction was a rise in eosinophils which accompanied it, suggesting that the patient may have been allergic to some component of the preparation, perhaps human protein (9[Cr]).

Brox et al have described how a young homosexual man with immune thrombocytopenia developed transient *intravascular hemolysis* during IVIG treatment, apparently mediated by anti-A antibody present in the commercial preparation used (10[Cr]). It may be recalled that compensated hemolysis has been described earlier with this treatment (11[C]), but up to this time a clinically significant effect had not been shown.

Barton et al, in a 1987 paper not earlier considered in these volumes, provided serial clinical data on a women who developed *severe renal dysfunction* after the intravenous infusion of IgG for the treatment and prophylaxis of infection; their data provide grounds for a contraindication to such treatment:

A woman of 39 had mixed IgM/IgG cryoglobulinemia, but was later found to have a lymphoma that produced an IgM kappa paraprotein with rheumatoid factor activity. The condition was controlled for some years by immunosuppression, but because of intractable lung infection and hypogammaglobulinemia G she was given an intravenous infusion of gammaglobulin. Within 72 h, renal failure and a sustained decrease in serum concentrations of IgM and IgG began concurrently. Renal biopsy strongly suggested that complexes consisting of IgM kappa rheumatoid factor, IgG and complement initiated the renal damage (12[Cr]).

The report suggests that demonstrable serum rheumatoid factor activity in patients with B-cell neoplasms should be considered a contraindication to the administration of intravenous gammaglobulin.

Kurlander et al however noted generally good tolerance when they treated 17 adults for immune thrombocytopenic purpura with 400 mg/kg IVIG daily for 5 days and a further 10 with 1000 mg/kg daily for only 2 days, in most cases with success. Here again the Cutter preparation Gamimune-N was used. There were no serious side effects in either group, but *thrombophlebitis* was observed in some patients receiving the 5-day regimen when a single intravenous catheter was used for more than 3 days. *Headache* and, less commonly, low-grade *fever* were noted in some patients receiving the 2-day regimen when infusions were given at flow rates in excess of 0.04 ml/kg/min (13[Cr]).

A slightly larger series was treated with IVIG from the Scottish National Blood Transfusion Service; here 37 patients received a total of

1235 immunoglobulin infusions for primary hypogammaglobulinemia. The most satisfactory dose appeared to be 100 mg/kg at the first 2 infusions and 200 mg/kg subsequently, though initially some patients were started at the higher dose. Ten patients experienced adverse reactions during 34 infusions (2.8% of all infusions) but only 5 were moderately severe; all were of similar character (flu-like symptoms, rash, nausea, rigor with wheezing). In this study again, the reactions appeared to be related to the rate of administration, but administration at 5 mg/kg/min (0.1 ml/kg/min) was tolerated well (14[C]).

Good tolerance to IVIG was also found in 16 young patients (aged from 9 months to 22 years) with immune-mediated hematocytopenias (13 with childhood immune thrombocytopenic purpura) who received a total of 210 infusions. Minimal toxicity (transient headaches) was experienced in only 4 infusions, and in 3 of the 4 patients concerned later infusions were free of problems (15).

Granulocyte-macrophage colony stimulating factor *(SEDA-13, 302, 416)*

Recombinant human granulocyte-macrophage colony stimulating factor was primarily reviewed in Chapter 47 of the previous Annual. Work on this cytokinin has continued to be promising.

Gabrilove et al used rHuGM-CSF alongside cytostatics in 27 patients with transition-cell carcinoma of the urothelium, using doses up to 60 g/kg daily at various times in relation to cytostatic treatment. These doses were sufficient to be considered effective. All patients tolerated the first and second courses of rHuGm-CSF well. During the first course, given before chemotherapy, mild to moderate pain localized to the lower back, posterior iliac crests and sternum occurred in two thirds of patients during the infusion and in another tenth of them 4–8 h later. In patients with a history of trigeminy there was a suspicion that the treatment had precipitated an attack. Only a fifth of patients had bone pain during or after a second course of treatment, the symptoms apparently co-inciding with a rebound in the neutrophil count. The leukocyte alkaline phosphatase level increased 1.3–9.8 times in patients during the first and second courses of rhG; during the first course only there was a dose-dependent increase in serum alkaline phosphatase, lactate dehydrogenase and uric acid (16[C]).

Gutterman (17[C]) treated 6 patients with solid tumors, 8 with myelodysplasia and 10 with aplastic anemia. A dose-escalation schedule was planned, with intravenous doses ranging from 15 to 500 g/m^2, but with the dose unchanged during each 14-day cycle of treatment and with treatment-free intervals of a fortnight between cycles. Glycosylated material produced in yeast was used. Doses of this order of magnitude produced a response in the first 2 conditions but not in the third. Constitutional adverse effects were minimal. No episodes of pericarditis, pleuritis or pulmonary edema occurred. Bone pain occurred mostly during or after a bolus infusion or during a continuous infusion when the white blood cell count rose to a very high level.

Although the author concludes that the safety of the preparation appears promising, the latter study above does not exclude the other possible risks discussed earlier in this series, such as the possibility that in cases of myelodysplasia the treatment might give rise to the progression of pre-leukemic conditions (SEDA-13, 302). Of other possible emergent risks, the prospect of *sepsis* has been discussed by various writers (18[r], 19[r]); symptomatic *hypokalemia* has been described by Viens et al in the light of a case involving an elderly woman in whom the acute onset of the complication parallelled the increase in leukocytes (20); and *vasculitis* requiring corticosteroid treatment was precipitated in a male patient, suggesting the need for particular caution in individuals with pre-existing autoimmune disease (21[C]).

Human placenta gamma globulin *(SEDA-12, 300)*

Human gamma globulins derived from placenta (PGG) first appear to have been tried clinically in 1985 by Combe. A study from Beijing reported in 1988 used a Chinese PGG preparation in vitro and demonstrated its ability to inhibit lymphocyte alloreaction. The authors advanced some evidence for the hypothesis that PGG does not act nonspecifically on cellular growth, but selectively affects the process of lymphocyte activation initiated by antigenic stimuli. They stress that PGG must be a heterogenous antibody solution and although it has been shown earlier to be beneficial for graft enhancement and perhaps the remission of severe rheumatoid arthritis it may depress active immunity of patients after frequent use in spite of its simultaneous passive immune augmentation (22[r]).

HEMIN *(SEDA-12, 297)*

Hemin (hematin), used in porphyrias as an exogenous source of heme, is generally well-tolerated in the recommended doses, though *thrombophlebitis, coagulation defects, circulatory collapse* and occasional *renal shutdown* have been reported. A more recent report relates to the infusion of hemin in 9 healthy male volunteers to examine the extent of the thrombophlebitic risk and means of avoiding it. The study suggested that the slower the rate of infusion the lower the risk of thrombophlebitis in the vein used; when a 4 mg/kg dose was given over 20–30 minutes local thrombophlebitis occurred in 3 of 6 volunteers, while lengthening the period of infusion of the same dose to 50–90 minutes produced thrombophlebitis in only 1 of 3 subjects; the numbers are of course too small to provide more than a hypothesis. In the same investigation, degradation materials capable of exerting an anticoagulant effect were found to be present in the product used ('Panhematin') (23[Cr]).

TRANSMISSION OF DISEASE BY BLOOD AND BLOOD PRODUCTS *(SED-11, 702; SEDA-12, 297; SEDA-13, 304)*

In his review already cited above (6[r]) of the clinical safety of *intravenous immune globulin* (IVIG), Rousell has devoted particular attention to the means which can currently be adopted to eliminate the risk of transmitting infection.

Data are presented on 2 series of patients who had been treated with a native (Cutter) IVIG and who were followed-up for periods of up to 18 months. No evidence was found of the transmission of human immune deficiency virus (HIV) in patients, with idiopathic thrombocytopenia, or of the agents of non-A, non-B hepatitis in 41 immune-deficient patients.

For a technical discussion of the treatment of IVIG to eliminate transmission of infection the reader is referred to the original paper. Essentially the Cohn-Oncley cold ethanol fractionation process produces at least a 100 000-fold reduction of HIV when fractionating plasma to fraction II, i.e. the fraction used to manufacture either intramuscular immune serum globulin or (after reduction and alkylation) IVIG. The primary lesson from the material extensively reviewed by Rousell is that a great deal has been and can be done in this respect; those cases in the past where it has been thought that IVIG had been the carrier for infection are, if proven, likely to have been due to the use of less advanced methods of inactivation than those currently available.

It may be noted that in 1988 a national multi-center study was published from the Netherlands in which the effects of donor selection and the use of heat-treated coagulation factor concentrates on seroconversion to HIV was studied in 157 Dutch hemophiliacs. All patients included in the study had been seronegative to HIV in 1983. 13% of them ($n = 20$) seroconverted between 1983 and 1986. Nineteen of the 20 seroconverted following the use during the preceding year of non-heat-treated coagulation factor concentrates. One seroconversion involved a patient using a heat-treated non-donor screened product available from Armour in 1983 (24[C]).

MISCELLANEOUS

Erythropoietin *(SEDA-12, 350; SEDA-13, 303)*

During the early phases of human investigation of recombinant erythropoietin (rHuEPO), which has proved of such value to patients with the anemia of renal failure, the adverse reactions reported were mild. There were occasional references to pruritus, bone pain and mild pyrexia (25[CR]), and much hope that as a physiological substance erythropoietin would be free of adverse effects. That proves to be the case; the problem is primarily to administer it in such a manner that it can act physiologically and so that its effects do not overwhelm the disordered system.

Cardiovascular The most prominent problem appears to be *hypertension* and the sequelae thereof (26[R]). The improvement in the anemia brings with it an increase in blood viscosity (27[Cr]) and it is this which apparently can lead to an increase in blood pressure, an increased need for heparin during dialysis, and an increased risk of blockage of the vessels used for the dialysis shunt. Increase in blood pressure is most likely to occur in patients with pre-existing hypertension, even if this has been well-controlled; normotensive patients are much less likely to be affected.

Nervous system The sudden and extreme rises in blood pressure which occurred in some cases elicited reports of *hypertensive encephalopathy* from 1986 onwards, and occasionally cerebral *ischemia* or the occurrence of other neurological complications has been described.

Zehnder and Blumberg have described 4 of their patients treated with rHu-EPO who developed complications: A woman of 58, dialyzed for 4 years for analgesic nephropathy, was also being treated with atenolol for hypertension with retinopathy and peripheral arterial disease. After 7 months on rHu-EPO she developed disorientation, somnolence and then severe headache followed by unilateral paresis and spasms. There was a diffuse cerebral edema and extreme hypertension. With labetalol and nitroprusside treatment the complication receded and there was full symptomatic recovery, but additional hypertensive maintenance therapy (prazosin) was thereafter needed.

A woman of 64, dialyzed for 10 years for the sequelae of analgesic nephropathy also had hypertension controlled with alpha-methyldopa. After 4 months on rHu-EPO she developed headache and vertigo, then became confused; she was found to be severely hypertensive but responded to nifedipine and clonidine; here too the antihypertensive maintenance treatment thereafter required supplementation with prazosin.

A man of 42, hemodialyzed for the consequences of a late pyelonephritis was poorly controlled for hypertension because of inadequate compliance, and also showed arteriosclerotic changes of the large vessels. After 8.5 months on rHu-EPO he developed a hypertensive crisis similar to that in the second case above and was thereafter maintained on atenolol and minoxidil.

A man of 70 with chronic glomerulonephritis, dialyzed for 10 years, was also receiving nifedipine for hypertension. Two weeks after institution of rHu-EPO treatment he became confused and agitated; the blood pressure was raised but there was no headache. The retina was relatively normal and there were no signs of focal brain disorder. The computer tomogram however showed well-defined ischemic parenchymal damage in the right nucleus caudatus and the right capsula interna. The condition normalized during further dialysis (28[CR]).

All 4 patients thus had a long history of hypertension, and 2 were arteriosclerotic; whilst the first 3 developed a syndrome centered around a sudden extreme hypertension at a time when hemoglobin and risen considerably, the fourth probably had a derangement of cerebral perfusion which occurred before the hemoglobin had greatly changed. The cases are typical of the suddenness with which problems can arise, demanding clear instruction of patients, frequent monitoring and ready availability of emergency treatment.

It is not clear why certain patients develop these problems and others do not, but the above cases suggest some particular risk situations. It is possible that the adaptation of the arterioles of anemic patients to the increase in erythrocyte volume is less adequate in some patients (e.g. those with arteriosclerosis) than others. It has also been suggested that the newly-produced hemoglobin binds to (and blocks the action of) endothelium-derived relaxant factor (EDRF) (29[r]). Vallance et al have challenged this hypothesis, primarily in the light of animal experimental evidence, since hemoglobin-induced inhibition of EDRF has only been demonstrated successfully in vitro (30).

Endocrine, metabolic As the erythrocyte volume increases under the influence of erythropoietin the clearance achieved by the dialyzer may fall, and there can as a consequence be an *increase in creatine, potassium and phosphorus* (31[C]).

Antilymphocyte preparations

Antilymphocyte globulin (ALG) proved in a South African study to produce complete and stable remission in a case of idiopathic pure red cell aplasia in a woman of 25 who was given a single 5-day course of ALG in a dose of 50 mg/kg/d i.v. as the sole treatment. At 2-year follow-up all hematological and marrow measures were normal. The treatment produced only transient *arthralgia* and an asymptomatic *thrombocytopenia* (36×10^9/l) of short duration.

One Rh-positive patient with pure red cell aplasia who was treated with ALG developed a *positive direct anti-globulin test*. The batch of ALG used (Lymphoser, produced by Berna, batch 20586) was found to contain anti-D

(32[Cr]). One earlier case of this type was described in 1983 (33[C]), and there was an incidental suspicion of hemolysis in a series reviewed in SEDA-13.

In a general review of the adverse effects of ALG, Marsh and Gordon-Smith distinguish between early and late sequelae. ALG causes an immediate leukopenia (lymphopenia and neutropenia) and thrombocytopenia (sometimes with significant hemorrhage); though marked neutropenia and thrombocytopenia are less common with more recent preparations it may be wise to give prophylactic platelet infusions. Fever may be due either to an allergic reaction of to infection, and is occasionally accompanied by rigors; anaphylactic reactions can occur at any time. Serum sickness is a late manifestation and may demand more intensive platelet support as well as corticosteroids. Writing in 1988, these authors noted that it was customary to use horse ALG for the first course since this was in greater supply; a second course if needed could consist of rabbit ALG (34[R]).

Antithymocyte globulin (ATG) was used by Palmer et al alongside low doses of cyclosporin in an attempt to improve renal allograft survival in 50 highly sensitized patients (35[C]). ATG was given in a 10-day course with the first dose preoperatively, in a dosage of 2 mg/kg/d. In cases of severe rejection a further course was given. The mean period of follow-up was 23.9 ± 0.35 months and the technique was considered successful. ATG was well tolerated, although a number of patients (unspecified) suffered mild *febrile reactions*. Only one patient, who was receiving a second course of ATG, experienced a severe pyrexia requiring a switch to antilymphocyte globulin.

One continues to be reminded of the risk of infectious complications in patients receiving such treatment:

A Finnish group described a boy of 9 with aplastic anemia for whom no compatible bone marrow donor was available and who therefore received ATG ('ATGAM', Upjohn) in a dose of 20 mg/kg/d for 10 days together with oral prednisolone to abrogate symptoms of serum sickness. Eight days after starting ATG, he developed a severe headache, a clonal left Achilles reflex, and intensified left-sided patellar reflex. Two days later he became highly febrile and a previously taken blood culture proved to be positive for *Listeria monocytogenes*, which could also be cultured from the CSF (36[c]). The authors stress that the risk of listerial infections (e.g. via the food) should be borne in mind by clinicians dealing with immunocompromized patients, especially those on ATG treatment, which impairs cell-mediated immunity.

Interleukin-2 *(SEDA-13, 304)*

This preparation is, because of its indications, primarily dealt with in Chapters 39 and 47, but it is by nature an endogenous glycoprotein lymphokinin. It will suffice to note here the appearance of recent reports of *adrenal hemorrhage and failure* (37[C]), *cardiac toxicity* with pulmonary edema which are both relatively frequent (38[C]–40[C]), *hypothyroidism* (41[C]), (42[c]), and *kidney disorders* (43). Particularly severe risks are becoming manifest where interleukin-2 is used alongside beta-interferon or lymphokine-activated killer cells.

Tin protoporphyrin

Kappas and his colleagues were the first to show that synthetic tin protoporphyrin (Sn-P) was effective in decreasing plasma bilirubin levels in both adult and neonatal animals and humans (44, 45[C]). Their work has been reviewed by Stevenson and Vreman (46), and although the substance is not in fact a blood product it merits brief consideration here.

From this exploratory work it looks as if up to 3 doses of 0.75 mol/kg each are effective in human neonates, moderating the characteristic increase in neonatal plasma bilirubin through inhibition of the enzyme heme oxygenase, and hence reducing the need for phototherapy. The clinical side effects were considered to be negligible, occasional subjects developing transient erythema in instances where the use of Sn-P was followed by phototherapy. This occurred only after 3 doses of Sn-P and in 1 child resolved spontaneously even though phototherapy was continued. Apparently, therefore, the compound is somewhat phototoxic, but as Stevenson and Vreman suggest this problem might be circumvented by moderating the dose or source of irradiation or by using lower doses of less photosensitive, more potent derivatives of Sn-protoporphyrin such as Sn-mesoporphyrin (47).

REFERENCES

1. Ring J, Messmer K (1977) Incidence and severity of anaphylactoid reactions to colloid volume substitutes, *Lancet, 1*, 466.
2. Edelman BB, Straughn MA, Getz P et al (1985) Uneventful plasma exchange with albumin replacement in a patient with a previous reaction to albumin. *Transfusion, 25*, 435.
3. Stafford CT, Lobel SA, Fruge BC et al (1988) Anaphylaxis to human serum albumin. *Ann. Allergy, 61*, 85.
4. Grammer LC, Patterson BF, Roxe D et al (1985) IgG against ethylene oxide-altered human serum albumin in patients with anaphylactic reactions to dialysis. *J. Allergy Clin. Immunol., 76*, 511.
5. Cunningham-Rundles C (1988) Intravenous immunoglobulin treatment in the primary immunodeficiency diseases. *Immunol. Allergy Clin. N. Amer., 8*, 17.
6. Rousell RH (1988) Clinical safety of intravenous immune globulin and freedom from transmission of viral disease. *J. Hosp. Infect., 12, Suppl. D*, 17.
7. Pirofsky B (1987) Clinical use of a new pH 4.25 intravenous immunoglobulin preparation (Gamimune-N). *J. Infect., 15, Suppl. 1*, 29.
8. Williams PE, Yap PL, Gillon J et al (1988) Non-A, non-B hepatitis transmission by intravenous immunoglobulin. *Lancet, 2*, 501.
9. Kato E, Shindo S, Eto Y et al (1988) Administration of immune globulin associated with aseptic meningitis. *J. Am. Med. Asoc., 259*, 3269.
10 Brox AG, Cournoyer D, Sternbach M et al (1987) Hemolytic anemia following intravenous gamma globulin administration. *Am. J. Med., 82*, 633.
11. Salama A, Mueller-Eckhardt C, Kiefel V (1983) Effect of intravenous immunoglobulins in immune thrombocytopenia. *Lancet, 2*, 193.
12. Barton JC, Herrera GA, Galla JH et al (1987) Acute cryoglobulinemic renal failure after intravenous infusion of gamma globulin. *Am. J. Med., 82*, 624.
13. Kurlander R, Coleman RE, Moore J et al (1987) Comparison of the efficacy of a two-day and a five-day schedule for infusing intravenous gamma globulin in the treatment of immune thrombocytopenic purpura in adults. *Am. J. Med., 83, Suppl. 4A*, 17.
14. Leen CLS, Yap PL, Williams PE (1988) Tolerance of Scottish National Blood Transfusion Service Intravenous Immunoglobulin in Patients with Primary Hypogammaglobulinaemia: Report of 1235 Infusions. *Scott. Med. J., 33*, 303.
15. Kurtzberg J, Friedman HS, Chafee S et al (1987) Efficacy of intravenous gamma globulin in autoimmune-mediated pediatric blood dyscrasias. *Am. J. Med., 83*, 4.
16. Gabrilove JL, Jakubowski A, Scher H et al (1988) Effect of granulocyte colony-stimulating factor on neutropenia and associated morbidity due to chemotherapy for transitional-cell carcinoma of the urothelium. *N. Engl. J. Med., 318*, 1414.
17. Gutterman J (1988) Clinical studies of granulocyte-macrophage colony stimulating factor. *Sem. Oncolog., 15*, 52.
18. Antman KH, Elias AM, Cannistra SA et al (1989) Recombinant human GM-CSF in myelosuppression of chemotherapy. *N. Engl. J. Med., 320*, 940.
19. Bar MH, Aronson FR (1989) Recombinant human GM-CSF in myelosuppression of chemotherapy. *N. Engl. J. Med., 320*, 939.
20. Viens P, Thyss A, Garnier G et al (1989) GM-CSF treatment and hypokalemia. *Ann. Intern. Med., 111*, 263.
21. Dreicer R, Schiller JH, Carbone PP et al (1989) Granulocyte macrophage colony-stimulating factor and vasculitis. *Ann. Intern. Med., 111*, 91.
22. Dong Y-H, Lu D-P (1988) Immune blocking activity of human placenta gamma globulin on mixed lymphocyte reaction. *Haematol. Rev., 2*, 171.
23. Simionalto CS, Cabal R, Jones RL et al (1988) Thrombophlebitis and disturbed hemostasis following administration of intravenous hematin in normal volunteers. *Am. J. Med., 85*, 538.
24. Wolfs TFW, Breederveld C, Krone WJA et al (1988) HIV-antibody seroconversions in Dutch haemophiliacs using heat-treated and non heat-treated coagulation factor concentrates. *Thromb. Haemost., 59*, 396.
25. Winearls CHG, Oliver DO, Pippard MJ et al (1986) Effects of human erythropoietin derived from recombinant DNA on the anemia of patients maintained by chronic haemodialysis. *Lancet, 2*, 1175.
26. Frei U, Nonnast-Daniel B, Koch KM (1988) Erythropoietin and hypertension (in German). *Klin. Wochenschr., 66*, 914.
27. Raine AEG (1988) Hypertension, blood viscosity, and cardiovascular morbidity in renal failure. Implications of erythropoietin therapy. *Lancet, 1*, 97.
28. Zehnder C, Blumberg A (1988) Zerebrovaskuläre Ereignisse bei vier mit Erythropoietin behandelten Hämodialysepatienten. *Schweiz Med. Wochenschr., 118*, 1423.
29. Martin W, Moncada S (1988) Erythropoietin, haemoglobin, and hypertensive crises. *Lancet, 1*, 644.
30. Vallance P, Benjamin N, Collier C (1988) Erythropoietin, haemoglobin, and hypertensive crises. *Lancet, 1*, 1107.
31. Zehnder C (1989) Erythropoietin treatment: Influence of hemoglobin concentration on dialyser creatinine clearance in haemodialysed patients. (In press).

32. Sermasi G, Malferrari F, Nucci S et al (1988) Problemi correlati con l'impiego terapeutico della globulina antilinfocitaria. *Trasfus. Sangue, 33*, 159.
33. Shirey RS, Smith B, Denserrbrenner L et al (1983) Red cell sensitization due to anti-D in anti-lymphocyte globulin. *Transfusion, 23*, 396.
34. Marsh JCW, Gordon-Smith EC (1988) The role of antilymphocyte globulin in the treatment of chronic acquired bone marrow failure. *Blood Rev., 2*, 141.
35. Palmer A, Bewick M, Welsh K et al (1988) Low-dose cyclosporine and antithymocyte globulin improve renal allograft survival in highly sensitized patients. *Transplant. Proc., 30*, 198.
36. Saxen H, Heiinheimo M, Rajantie J (1988) Listeriosis associated with antithrombocyte globulin treatment. *Lancet, 2*, 280.
37. VanderMolen LA, Smith JW, Longo DL et al (1989) Adrenal insufficiency and interleukin-2 therapy. *Ann. Intern. Med., 111*, 185.
38. Conant EF, Fox KR, Miller WT (1989) Pulmonary edema as a complication of interleukin-2 therapy. *Am. J. Roentgenol., 152*, 749.
39. Samlowski WE, Ward JH, Craven CM (1989) Severe myocarditis following high-dose interleukin-2 administrations. *Arch. Pathol. Lab. Med., 113*, 838.
40. Pasini FL, Perri T, Van der Plas K et al (1989) Myocardial injury after interleukin-2 therapy. *Lancet, 1*, 674.
41. Van Liessum PA, De Mulder PHM, Mattijssen EJM et al (1989) Hypothyroidism and goitre during interleukin-1 therapy without lak cells, *Lancet, 1*, 224.
42. Hartmann LC, Urba WJ, Steis RG et al (1989) Hypothyroidism after interleukin-2 therapy. *J. Clin. Oncol., 7*, 686.
43. Beldegrun A, Webb DE, Austin HA et al (1989) Renal toxicity of interleukin-2 administration in patients with metastatic cell cancer. *J. Urol., 141*, 499.
44. Drummond GS, Kappas A (1982) Chemoprevention of neonatal jaundice. Potency of tin protoporphyrin in an animal model. *Science, 217*, 1250.
45. Kappas A, Drummond GS, Manola T et al (1988) Sn-protoporphyrin use in the management of hyperbilirubinemia in term newborns with direct Coombs-positive ABO-incompatibility. *Pediatrics, 81*, 485.
46. Stevenson DK, Vreman HJ (1988) Sn-Protoporphyrin: a consideration of the first clinical trial in human neonates. *Pediatrics, 81*, 881.
47. Drummond GS, Galbraith R, Sardana MK et al (1987) Reduction of the C2 and C4 vinyl groups of Sn-protoporphyrin to form Sn-mesoprotoporphyrin markedly enhances the ability of the metalloporphyrin to inhibit in vivo heme catabolism. *Arch. Biochem. Biophys., 255*, 64.

P.I. Folb

36 Intravenous infusions

PLASMA SUBSTITUTES *(SED-11, 725; SEDA-12, 306; SEDA-13, 315)*

Dextrans *(SED-11, 725; SEDA-12, 306; SEDA-13, 315)*

In a recent review of the antithrombotic efficacy of dextran, Ljungstrom (1[R]) points out that the pathophysiological mechanisms of dextran-induced allergic reactions have now been elucidated. Severe anaphylactic reactions only occur in patients with preformed dextran-reactive antibodies. Infusion of dextran causes the formation of large immune complexes that trigger activation of a cascade of enzyme systems, leukocytes and platelets. It may be possible to prevent or minimize these effects by blocking the reactive sites of these antibodies with small dextran fragments (mol. wt. 1 000 daltons, dextran-1); this is hapten inhibition. The value of hapten inhibition with very-low-molecular-weight dextran (dextran–1) has been established. It has led to a marked reduction in the incidence of severe anaphylactic reactions: from 22 per 100 000 units of dextran used between 1983 and 1985, to approximately 1 case in every 40 000 treated patients today.

Haemaccel (Polygeline) *(SED-11, 726)*

A highly unusual Haemaccel *fatality* has been reported by Barratt and Purcell (2[c]).

A 22-year-old male with a previous history of asthma developed refractory bronchospasm following Haemaccel (polygeline, available as a 3.5% colloidal infusion solution, with the following electrolyte content in each liter: sodium 145 mmol, potassium 5.1 mmol, calcium 6.26 mmol, chloride 145 mmol) and bupivacaine epidural anesthesia for reduction of a comminuted spiral fracture of the tibia. Two ml of 0.5% bupivacaine were administered; followed after 4 min by a further 13 ml of 0.5% bupivacaine; 0.5 l of Haemaccel was administered intravenously for a fall in blood pressure that had not responded to intravenous Hartmann's solution. The patient developed pain in the neck, shoulder and abdomen and severe asthma immediately afterwards. There was no urticaria. He became progressively more distressed, cyanosed and unresponsive, despite adequate resuscitative measures, salbutamol given by nebulizer, and aminophylline 250 mg intravenously. There were multiple cardiac arrhythmias, including episodes of ventricular fibrillation, and cardiopulmonary bypass was necessary to achieve adequate oxygenation of the blood and cerebral perfusion. Later the patient developed focal seizures; there was no return of normal neurological function after the operation, and he died 4 days later. The Haemaccel was discarded before it could be analyzed for bacteria or other contaminants.

The allergic reactions that have been described in association with Haemaccel are thought to be caused by direct histamine release as a result of allergenic stimulation of mast cells. This case-report raises the question as to whether Haemaccel is appropriate for bronchoreactive patients, and/or whether such patients should be protected by histamine receptor blockade. The authors reporting the case suggested that inadvertent intravenous injection of bupivacaine may have complicated the resuscitation of this patient.

Hydroxyethyl starch (Hetastarch) *(SED-11, 726; SEDA-13, 316)*

Blood volume was maintained by infusion of 2 liters of hydroxyethyl starch (HES) during, and for the first 28 hours after, a major orthopedic operation in a 13-year-old girl who was a Jehovah's Witness and therefore ineligible for treatment with blood products. This resulted in a generalized hemorrhagic state, a coagulopathy associated with a shortened thrombin, prolonged prothrombin and activated partial

Side Effects of Drugs Annual 14
M.N.G. Dukes and L. Beeley, editors

thromboplastin times, and an acquired Von Willebrand syndrome. The *coagulation disturbance* normalized approximately 72 hours after cessation of the infusion of hydroxyethyl starch (3[c]).

There are several known mechanisms whereby synthetic macromolecular colloids such as hydroxyethyl starch disturb hemostasis. The thrombin time is shortened by a fibrinoplastic effect of the macromolecules in hydroxyethyl starch. This accelerates the conversion of fibrinogen to fibrin, resulting in a less stable thrombus which is more susceptible to lysis. The macromolecules in HES induce an acquired Von Willebrand's syndrome with reduced levels of all three main Factor VIII parameters: Factor VIII:C, vWF and Von Willebrand factor antigen (vWFag). Macromolecules may coat the outer membrane of circulating platelets and cause a qualitative platelet function defect, thus prolonging bleeding time. Minor abnormalities of platelet aggregation have been observed after infusion of low volumes of hydroxyethyl starch, and platelet defects probably contribute to the hemorrhagic state.

In the patient referred to above, platelet function tests were not investigated at the time of the acute illness. The prolonged half-life of HES (25.5 h) delayed correction of the hemostatic defect. Effective clinical hemostasis did not occur until 24 hours after discontinuing the infusion. The patient had received replacement of approximately 60% her total blood volume. This case draws attention to the acute hemorrhagic problems that may develop when blood volume is maintained by infusion of macromolecules as the sole fluid.

Hydroxyethyl starch is produced synthetically by introducing hydroxyethyl groups onto glucose units of starch molecules. This is then subjected to acid hydrolysis, which results in a product with a molecular weight of approximately 450 000 daltons. Metabolism and elimination of the substance is complex, and it is related to the size of the particles. The smaller molecules, with a molecular weight of less than 50 000 daltons, are excreted unchanged by glomerular filtration. Larger molecules are metabolized to smaller molecules, and distributed to various body tissues, where they may undergo hydrolysis in the reticuloendothelial system or enzymatic degradation by amylases. In a patient with normal renal function it is possible that the undamaged kidney presents a selective barrier to all but the smallest of the hetastarch molecules. The breakdown products are then eliminated by urinary excretion.

There has been a recent report of hetastarch causing a *discrepancy between urinary specific gravity and osmolality* (4[c]). Large-molecular-weight molecules present in the hetastarch solution produced a disproportionate rise in urine-specific gravity compared with osmolality. In 2 patients, the combined effects of acute tubular necrosis secondary to hypotension and abnormal glomerular permeability were thought to have allowed large-molecular-weight particles of hetastarch to be excreted in the urine. The hetastarch particles elevated the urine-specific gravity, but had a correspondingly lesser effect on osmolality. It is not thought that hetastarch itself was nephrotoxic. The authors concluded that in the setting of pre-existing renal disease, hetastarch may elevate the urinary-specific gravity without unduly affecting the ability of the kidney to concentrate urine. They recommended that urinary osmolality, rather than specific gravity, should be regarded as the preferred method of evaluating the urine, after the administration of high-molecular-weight colloid solutions.

TOTAL PARENTERAL NUTRITION
(SED-11, 714; SEDA-13, 316)

Micronutrient and enzyme deficiency The time-course for the depletion of red blood cell and plasma glutathione peroxidase activity has been documented in 5 patients receiving home parenteral nutrition (5[c]). There was a decrease in red blood cell glutathione peroxidase, general enzyme activity and protein content in these patients. Plasma and red blood cell selenium content was also decreased, as was cellular metabolism of exogenous peroxide. Once replacement of selenium (as selenious acid) had begun there was a rapid increase (within 6 h) in plasma glutathione peroxidase activity. Platelet and granulocyte glutathione peroxidase activity, which was low prior to treatment with selenium, normalized within a time consistent with the kinetics of platelets and polymorphonuclear production. Red blood cell glutathione peroxidase activity returned to normal within

3–4 months, which is consistent with the time-course for bone marrow red blood cell production. The authors concluded that the repletion of red blood cell glutathione peroxidase in this setting requires the presence of selenium.

Selenium in the form of selenocysteine is part of the active site of glutathione peroxidase, the enzyme which catalyzes glutathione reduction of organic hydroperoxides and hydrogen peroxide, which protects against oxidative damage. The minimum daily selenium requirement for patients receiving parenteral nutrition has not been determined.

Metabolic bone disease In a study of 17 patients who first received total parenteral nutrition (TPN) containing casein hydrolysate with high aluminium and ergocalciferol (25 μg/d) for 6–72 months followed by total parenteral nutrition containing amino acids with reduced aluminium and ergocalciferol (5 μg/d) for 9–58 months, and in a further cross-sectional study of 22 patients receiving casein and ergocalciferol (24 μg/d) compared with 46 patients receiving amino acids and ergocalciferol (5 μg/d) for 6–58 months, the following were found: bone formation was higher and osteoid area, bone-surface stainable aluminium and total bone aluminium were lower with amino acid TPN than with casein TPN; bone formation varied inversely with both plasma aluminium and bone-surface aluminium, suggesting that plasma or bone-surface aluminium, acquired during TPN, reduces bone formation and leads to patchy osteomalacia. Serum levels of immunoreactive parathyroid hormone and 1,25-dihydroxyvitamin D were higher with amino acid TPN (6[c]).

The data in this study demonstrate that the metabolic bone disease associated with long-term TPN improves after a change from casein to amino acids. This is associated with a reduction in the quantities of aluminium, protein and ergocalciferol in the TPN solutions. Bone-formation rate was higher and the osteoid lower in patients who received amino acids compared with casein hydrolysate. Serum levels of 1,25-dihydroxyvitamin D were higher, and the plasma levels of aluminium and urinary excretion of aluminium and calcium were markedly lower, during the administration of amino acids compared with casein hydrolysate.

The changes in the TPN solution made over the time of this study were complex, and the significance of the findings reported here is uncertain. Nevertheless, the inverse relationships between bone-formation rate and both plasma and surface-stainable aluminium support the view that less exposure to aluminium may play a significant role in improving the bone histology in this setting.

Hepatic complications The pathogenesis and management of liver injury caused by both short-term parenteral nutrition and long-term TPN have been reviewed by Baker and Rosenberg (7[R]). Progressive liver injury developing in patients needing prolonged TPN raises serious dilemmas. There is a high prevalence of hepatic complications of TPN in children. Premature or low-weight-for-age infants are at increased risk of *cholestasis*, which is the prominent abnormality both clinically and on biopsy. Infants are at high risk of developing *progressive liver injury* and *liver failure* if TPN is prolonged beyond 5 months. The outcome may be fatal. The pattern and prognosis of liver injury in children is distinct from that seen in adults, despite some overlap.

Increased hepatic lipogenesis and reduced transport function are important in the fatty liver associated with TPN. Providing ample quantities of essential amino acids lessens but does not prevent this. This highlights the importance of total caloric intake. If insufficient amounts of amino acids are taken together with adequate non-protein calories, a situation may develop which is analogous to kwashiorkor. Hepatic lipid accumulates, but lipoprotein synthesis is limited. Carnitine supplementation minimizes fatty infiltration of the liver in patients receiving dextrose-based TPN, which supports the idea that carnitine deficiency plays a role in the development of this complication. However, carnitine can ordinarily be synthesized from the essential amino acids methionine and lysine, which are present in all commercially available TPN formulae. Hepatic tissue requirements may be increased under conditions of stress, contributing to the development of a fatty liver by impairment of transport and oxidation of fatty acids by mitochondria.

Several mechanisms have been proposed to explain the cholestasis that occurs during TPN, but there is little direct evidence to support any of them. Nutrient deficiencies which may be critical for hepatic uptake, biotransformation, and secretion of bile may be involved; taurine, which is important for bile acid conjugation, may cause cholestasis in premature infants when there is a deficiency. Certain amino acids may act as toxins. Decreased hormonal and neural stimulation of hepatic bile secretion may be a factor in patients who are not receiving nutrition enterally. Increased production of lithocholate, which is an hepatotoxic bile acid, by intestinal bacteria, or retention of lithocholate in the liver, might account for the cholestasis.

Elevated levels of lithocholate, portal bacteremia and/or endotoxemia have all been suggested as contributing to *hepatic triaditis* in patients with inflammatory bowel disease receiving TPN. Toxic amino acids or their metabolic products, excessive calorie administration and a disturbed carbohydrate-to-protein ratio may also influence the development of triaditis.

Steatonecrosis is also known to occur when nutritional depletion develops. Inadequate administration of a critical nutrient or combination of nutrients might be involved in the pathogenesis of this lesion.

SODIUM CHLORIDE SOLUTIONS

Central pontine myelinolysis, also known as osmotic demyelination syndrome, has been associated with rapid correction of severe hyponatremia. A case has been presented of a healthy young pregnant woman with hyperemesis gravidarum who developed severe hyponatremia (serum sodium 103 mEq/l). After rapid correction of serum sodium within 12–15 hours using a 0.9% sodium chloride solution, the patient lost consciousness and died of sepsis and respiratory failure. Examination of the brain showed extensive demyelination in pontine and extrapontine areas (18[c]).

This subject has been reviewed in the *Lancet* (9[R]). Pontine and extrapontine myelinolysis are generally considered to be linked with rapid correction of severe hyponatremia. Neurological deterioration is likely to result. It is not clear what rate of sodium repletion is safe. The best data available indicate that correction should not exceed 12 mmol/l/d, although more rapid correction may be safe. The duration of treatment may also be important: 12 mmol/l/d may be excessive if continued for more than 2 or 3 days.

A major difficulty in the setting of severe hyponatremia is accurate control of the serum sodium. The administration of an amount of hypertonic saline calculated to raise the sodium to mildly hyponatremic levels may result in a serum sodium in the normonatremic, or even hypernatremic, range. The serum sodium should not be allowed to rise more than 12 mmol/l over the first 24 hours, and even less over each subsequent 24-hour period. It is clear that an amount of saline calculated to raise the serum sodium by a given amount affects individuals differently. This makes frequent monitoring of serum sodium mandatory.

Cutaneous complications Complications at the needle site have been studied in the short-term and during continuous subcutaneous infusion of aqueous fluid through portable mini-pumps in a number of volunteers. Local complications, such as leakage of fluid, erythema, and bacterial contamination of the hypodermic needle were increasingly frequent with the duration of the indwelling time, but not with total volume (10[R]). These findings may be relevant to the performance of continuous subcutaneous hormone infusion therapy (e.g., insulin pump treatment of Type-1 diabetes mellitus).

Calcinosis cutis A young woman with hypoparathyroidism developed multiple firm white-yellow papules along the path of extravasation of intravenous infusion of calcium chloride. A biopsy specimen obtained 10 days afterwards revealed an urticarial reaction. A subsequent biopsy specimen, obtained 25 days after the extravasation, showed diffuse dermal calcification, confirmed by roentgenographic analysis. Forty days after the extravasation histology was consistent with an elimination reaction. Electron microscopy showed mineral deposits along collagen fibrils without collagenous degeneration. The pathological alteration in this case appeared to be due to factors other than massive collagen degeneration, soft tissue necrosis, and an increase in mast cells. Secondary tissue damage appeared to result from the high local calcium concentration. It follows that parenteral administration of the calcium chloride must be done with caution given the potential hazards (11[c]).

REFERENCES

1. Ljungstrom K-G (1988) The antithrombotic efficacy of dextran. *Acta Chir. Scand., Suppl., 543*, 26.
2. Barratt S, Purcell GJ (1988) Refractory bronchospasm following 'Haemaccel' infusion and bupivacaine epidural anaesthesia. *Anaesth. Intensive Care, 16*, 208.
3. Lockwood DNJ, Bullen C, Machin SJ (1988) A severe coagulopathy following volume replacement with hydroxyethyl starch in a Jehovah's Witness. *Anaesthesia, 43*, 391.
4. Haskell LP, Tannenberg AM (1988) Elevated urinary specific gravity in acute oliguric renal failure due to hetastarch administration. *NY State J. Med., July*, 387.
5. Cohen HJ, Brown MR, Hamilton D et al (1989) Glutathione peroxidase and selenium deficiency in patients receiving home parenteral nutrition: time course for development of deficiency and repletion of enzyme activity in plasma and blood cells. *Am. J. Clin. Nutr., 49*, 132.
6. Vargas JH, Klein GL, Ament ME et al (1988) Metabolic bone disease of total parenteral nutrition: course after changing from casein to amino acids in parenteral solutions with reduced aluminum content. *Am. J. Clin. Nutr., 48*, 1070.
7. Baker AL, Rosenberg IH (1987) Hepatic complications of total parenteral nutrition. *Am. J. Med., 82*, 489.
8. Castillo RA, Ray RA, Yaghmai F (1989) Central pontine myelinolysis and pregnancy. *Obstet. Gynecol., 73*, 459.
9. Laureno R, Karp BI (1988) Pontine and extrapontine myelinolysis following rapid correction of hyponatraemia. *Lancet, 1*, 1439.
10. Emshoff R (1988) Cutaneous complications induced by continuous subcutaneous infusion. Experimental studies with portable mini-pumps. *Infusionstherapie, 15*, 125.
11. Goldminz D, Barnhill R, McGuire J et al (1988) Calcinosis cutis following extravasation of calcium chloride. *Arch. Dermatol., 124*, 922.

J. Vermylen, Ph. Vanhove and M. Verstraete

37 Drugs affecting blood coagulation and hemostasis

COUMARIN CONGENERS *(SED-11, 733; SEDA-12, 311; SEDA-13, 321)*

Bleeding incidence An important consideration before deciding to initiate long-term oral anticoagulation in a given patient is whether the risk of complications may exceed the benefit. Cumulative risks for life-threatening complications and warfarin-related death were calculated to be 1% at 6 months, 5% at 1 year and 7% at 2 and 3 years in a historical cohort study (1[C]).

Bleeding due to overdoses of anticoagulant drugs can affect all organ systems. Spontaneous retroperitoneal hematomas and bleeding in the brain are life-threatening. Any neuropsychiatric abnormality seen during anticoagulant therapy should be regarded as a warning sign and lead to prompt neurological evaluation. The risk of oral anticoagulation in the older patients did not differ substantially from the risk in younger patients in the Sixty Plus Reinfarction Study (2[c]), but others consider that the risks of oral anticoagulants in the elderly usually outweigh the benefits (3[c]). Either way, the starting dose must be lower than that used in younger patients and extra attention must be paid to the possibility of intercurrent illness and the use of the numerous drugs interfering with oral anticoagulants.

Influenza vaccination and coumarin drugs Influenza vaccination has been shown to reduce hepatic elimination of certain drugs and to reduce enzymatic activity of the cytochrome P-450 system (4[r], 5[R]). A case of potentiation of warfarin after influenza vaccination has been reported (6[C]), but other reports have been either less convincing or contradictory (reviewed in Ref. 7[R]).

Side Effects of Drugs Annual 14
M.N.G. Dukes and L. Beeley, editors

Osteoporosis and long-term anticoagulation with coumarin drugs Osteocalcin is a non-collagenous bone matrix protein containing γ-carboxyglutamic acid, the synthesis of which is vitamin-K-dependent. During oral anticoagulation with phenprocoumon, a significantly lower osteocalcin level in serum was found and the proportion of osteocalcin that was non-carboxylated was significantly higher than in normal subjects (8[C]). Since osteocalcin levels reflect bone formation, but not bone resorption, the decreased serum total osteocalcin levels during oral anticoagulation do not necessarily imply that bone loss occurs in these patients. However, decreased bone formation and impaired γ-carboxylation of osteocalcin in patients treated with phenprocoumon may prove clinically important in circumstances such as fracture healing or when there is pre-existing bone disease.

UNFRACTIONATED AND LOW-MOLECULAR-WEIGHT HEPARIN *(SED-11, 749; SEDA-11, 317; SEDA-12, 309; SEDA-13, 322)*

Cutaneous skin necrosis and glomerulonephritis *(SEDA-11, 317, SEDA-12, 309; SEDA-13, 322)* Heparin- or coumarin-induced cutaneous necrosis has been described in the past and while this rare skin reaction to systemic heparin can also be associated with local vasculitis (9[C]), involvement of other organs by vasculitis has not previously been reported. However, glomerulonephritis complicating heparin-induced skin necrosis has now been described (10[C]).

Bleeding risk with fractionated heparin In an overview of clinical trials on the prevention of postoperative deep vein thrombosis, the efficacy of low-molecular-weight heparin fractions was found to be similar to that of unfractionated heparin (11[r]). The bleeding risk with low-molecular-weight heparin is negligible, provided that the antifactor Xa levels do not exceed 0.2 U/ml.

Heparin flush syndrome Heparin is frequently used with saline in the 'flushing' of venous and arterial catheters in order to maintain their patency. A case of serious bleeding necessitating reintervention surgery following repeated flushing with 500–1000 U of heparin has been described (12[C]). This 'heparin flush syndrome' should be considered as a cause of iatrogenic hemorrhage, especially in patients in whom 'no heparin' has been formally ordered.

Heparin-induced thrombocytopenia *(SED-11, 749; SEDA-11, 317; SEDA-12, 309; SEDA-13, 322)* Heparin-induced thrombocytopenia is a well-known complication after administration of unfractionated or low-molecular-weight heparin and pentosan polysulfate. A subgroup of these patients with this complication experience associated thrombotic events. A well-known example is skin necrosis, but numerous other manifestations of heparin-induced thrombosis have been reported: myocardial infarction, venous and arterial graft occlusions, deep venous thrombosis and pulmonary embolism. Heparin-induced thrombocytopenia and ischemic stroke were found in 6 of 2527 patients subjected to carotid endarterectomy (13[C]).

Acute management of unfractionated heparin-associated thrombocytopenia with thrombosis includes surgical thrombectomy, thrombolytic therapy, dextran, ancrod, low-molecular-weight heparin or aspirin (14[r]–16[r]); more recently plasmapheresis has been proposed (17[r]). It should be recognized that heparin-coated catheters can sustain the thrombocytopenia in patients with heparin-associated antiplatelet antibodies (18[C]). Heparin-coated catheters serve as a source of heparin and must be removed from such patients.

Low-molecular-weight heparin associated with dihydroergotamine *(SED-11, 733; SEDA-11, 749; SEDA-12, 309; SEDA-13, 323)* This combination is in clinical use in several countries. The risk of arterial spasm to the dihydroergotamine component was investigated in a prospective trial involving 33 421 surgical or gynecological patients receiving this drug combination (Embolex) as a routine antithrombotic agent. The number of patients experiencing thrombotic events was remarkably low, with 17 myocardial infarctions (7 fatal), 63 instances of pulmonary embolism (12 fatal) and one reversible vasospastic reaction reported (19[R]).

DESMOPRESSIN *(SED-11, 779)*

Desmopressin (dDAVP), a synthetic analog of the neurohypophyseal nonapeptide, arginine–vasopressin, has enhanced antidiuretic potency, markedly diminished pressor activity, and a prolonged half-life and duration of action compared to the natural hormone. This compound has become the most effective agent available for the treatment of diabetes insipidus. More recently, it has also been used to increase plasma levels of endogenous coagulation factors and to reduce bleeding episodes in patients with coagulation disorders such as hemophilia and von Willebrand's disease (20–24). Following the report of a fatal postoperative myocardial infarction during infusion of dDAVP and Factor VIII concentrate in an elderly patient with hemophilia (25[C], 26[C]), other reports indicated a risk of thrombosis when desmopressin is given to patients with coronary atherosclerosis (27[C], 28[C]). It is likely that the thrombotic effect is related to the release of stored endothelial factors and of abnormally large multimers of von Willebrand factor. The latter can aggregate platelets during conditions of artificially raised fluid shear stress that resemble those found in partially obstructed atherosclerotic arteries (29[r], 30[r]).

PLATELET SUPPRESSANTS *(SED-11, 760; SEDA-13, 324)*

Anagrelide

Anagrelide is a member of the imidazoquinazolin series of compounds with a powerful antiaggregating effect on platelets. During studies in humans, anagrelide in small doses has been found to produce thrombocytopenia. This drawback became an advantage in patients with thrombocytosis, a clinical condition in which an agent lacking mutagenicity and leukemogenic potential has long been needed (31).

THROMBOLYTIC DRUGS *(SED-11, 753; SEDA-12, 312; SEDA-13, 323)*

Streptokinase *(SED-11, 753; SEDA-12, 312; SEDA-13, 323)*

Since streptokinase is a natural product of the streptococcus and thus a foreign protein in humans, most of the population have anti-streptokinase antibodies. Sufficient quantities of streptokinase must be infused to overcome the neutralizing effects of these antibodies, and in most patients a dose of 1.5 million units administered intravenously over 60–90 min is adequate. Anaphylactic reactions (urticaria, bronchospasm, angioedema) as a result of preexisting antibodies to streptokinase appear to be rare, occurring in less than 1% of the patients in the GISSI-I (32[c]) and ISIS-2 (33[c]) trials to 1.6% reported by Taylor et al (34[c]). However, streptokinase, used alone or in combination with human plasminogen (anistreplase, APSAC, BRL-26 921, Eminase), is immunogenic and repeat administration should not be considered in patients who have received a prior dose of streptokinase or APSAC between 5 days and 6–12 months previously. Serious *allergic reactions* resembling serum sickness can occur and cases of plasmocytosis and renal failure after early readministration of streptokinase have been described (35[R], 36[r], 37[C]).

The incidence of transient *hypotensive reactions* to the infusion of streptokinase is higher, at 5–7%, but these are not necessarily antibody-related, and may be due to either histamine release or kinin production. They occur shortly after the initiation of infusion, may be accompanied by flushing and anxiety, and are reversible with fluid administration and temporary discontinuation of the infusion (38[R]). The more rapidly streptokinase is infused, the more likely a hypotensive reaction will occur (38[R]). The incidence of such reactions does not seem to be affected by premedication with steroids. Rapid injection of anistreplase (APSAC) can also cause transient hypotension, which is much less common if the injection is given over 4–5 minutes (39[c]). Alteplase (recombinant tissue-type plasminogen activator) does not appear to be associated with a risk of either anaphylactic or hypotensive reactions.

The most common manifestation of the non-anaphylactic reactions to streptokinase or anistreplase are transient *skin rashes* which are seen in about 5% of patients receiving streptokinase, but rarely, if ever, with alteplase. A more serious type of reaction is antibody-mediated *platelet aggregation* (40), which has been suggested as a cause of streptokinase-enhanced thrombosis in patients with specific types of antistreptokinase antibodies.

Vasculitic reactions probably result from the formation of antigen–antibody complexes either in plasma or, more commonly, in perivascular tissues. The mechanism is therefore analogous to that of serum sickness. Onset is usually delayed 6–21 days after initiation of treatment. Clinical manifestations include purpuric rash, joint and abdominal pains, and in some cases, microscopic hematuria. These features resemble the clinical syndrome of Henoch-Schönlein purpura. Vasculitic reactions have been described, rarely, after streptokinase or anistreplase (41[C]–43[C]) but not after urokinase or alteplase. The reactions have usually been mild and self-limiting, and symptomatic treatment may be all that is necessary. In severe episodes steroid therapy or plasmapheresis might be useful. A few cases go on to develop serious renal complications, as discussed below.

Acute renal failure has very rarely been described as a complication of streptokinase therapy and glomerular damage by immune complexes has been suggested as the etiology. A case of irreversible renal failure due to crescentic *glomerulonephritis* following streptokinase thrombolysis for myocardial infarction has been reported (41[C]). *Hemolysis* after intravenous streptokinase or anistreplase is rare (44[c], 45[C]).

ANTIDOTES TO THROMBOLYTIC TREATMENT *(SED-11, 758)*

Tranexamic acid *(SED-11, 759)*

There is a theoretical risk of an increased thrombotic tendency during treatment with fibrinolysis inhibitors. A few patients have developed intracranial (46[C], 47[C]) or mesenteric (48[C]) *thrombosis*, or evidence of thrombosis in other vascular areas during treatment with tranexamic acid (49[r]). Recently, tranexamic acid was suspected of causing thrombosis in a patient with acute myelogenous leukemia who underwent autologous bone marrow transplantation (50[C]). She received two 3-day courses of aminocaproic acid (500 mg i.v. b.i.d.) for cyclophosphamide-induced hemorrhagic cystitis, but did not tolerate the medications. Ten days later, tranexamic acid was administered (750 mg i.v. b.i.d.) for persistent hemorrhage. On the 5th day of therapy, the patient reported blurred vision which was due to a retinal artery occlusion.

Overall, the association between tranexamic acid and thrombosis may be fortuitous and the risk of this potential hazard very small. Indeed, the adverse reaction follow-up data of the Swedish National Board of Health and Welfare did not find an increase of thromboembolic complications in women with menorrhagia treated with tranexamic acid. During a 9-year period, corresponding to 238 000 women-years, 11 thromboembolic complications were reported. This corresponds to an annual incidence of 0.005%, which is not higher than the spontaneous incidence of thrombosis in fertile women.

REFERENCES

1. Petty GW, Lennihan L, Mohr JP et al (1988) Complications of long-term anticoagulation. *Ann. Neurol., 23,* 570.
2. Sixty Plus Reinfarction Study Research Group (1982) Risks of long-term oral anticoagulant therapy in elderly patients after myocardial infarction. *Lancet, 1,* 64.
3. Scott PJW (1988) Anticoagulant drugs in the elderly: the risks usually outweigh the benefits. *Br. Med. J., 297,* 1261.
4. Levine M, Jones M, Gribble M (1988) Increased serum phenytoin concentration following influenza vaccination. *Clin. Pharmacol., 3,* 505.
5. Meredith CG, Christian CD, Johnson RF et al (1985) Effects of influenza virus vaccine on hepatic drug metabolism. *Clin. Pharmacol. Ther., 37,* 396.
6. Kramer P, Tsuru M, Cook CE et al (1984) Effect of influenza on warfarin anticoagulation. *Clin. Pharmacol. Ther., 35,* 16.
7. Bussey HI, Saklad JJ (1988) Effect of influenza vaccine on chronic warfarin therapy. *Drug Intell. Clin. Pharm., 22,* 198.
8. Pietschmann P, Woloszczuk W, Panzer S et al (1988) Decreased serum osteocalcin levels in phenprocoumon-treated patients. *J. Clin. Endocrinol. Metab., 66,* 1071.
9. Stavorovsky M, Lichenstein D, Nissim F (1979) Skin petechiae and ecchymoses (vasculitis) due to anticoagulant therapy. *Dermatologia, 158,* 451.
10. Jones BF, Epstein MT (1987) Cutaneous heparin necrosis associated with glomerulonephritis. *Aust. J. Dermatol., 28,* 117.
11. Levine MN, Hirsh J (1988) An overview of clinical trials of low molecular weight heparin fractions. *Acta Chir. Scand., Suppl. 543,* 73.
12. Passannante A, Macik BG (1988) Case report: the heparin flush syndrome—a cause of iatrogenic hemorrhage. *Am. J. Med. Sci., 296,* 71.
13. Atkinson JLD, Sundt Jr TM, Kazmier FJ et al (1988) Heparin-induced thrombocytopenia and thrombosis in ischemic stroke. *Mayo Clin. Proc., 63,* 353.
14. Leroy J, Gruel Y, Delahousse B et al (1988) Les thrombocytopénies à l'héparine. *Rev. Pract., 15,* 937.
15. Vitoux J-F, Aïach M (1988) Les héparines en pratique quotidienne: indications, complications, surveillance. *Rev. Prat., 38,* 927.
16. Chong BH (1988) Heparin-induced thrombocytopenia. *Blood Rev., 2,* 108.
17. Nand S, Robinson JA (1988) Plasmapheresis in the management of heparin-associated thrombocytopenia with thrombosis. *Am. J. Hematol., 28,* 204.
18. Laster J, Silver D (1988) Heparin-coated catheters and heparin-induced thrombocytopenia. *J. Vasc. Surg., 27,* 667.
19. Wolf H, Welzel D, Kaiser H et al (1988) Bewertung der perioperativen Thromboembolie-Prophylaxe mit niedermolekularem Heparin und Dihydroergotamin: eine Untersuchung zur Frage der Inzidenz tödlicher Lungenembolien sowie unerwünschter Begleiterscheinungen, insbesondere des Vasospasmus- und Herzinfarktrisikos. *Arzneim.-Forsch./Drug Res., 38,* 1516.
20. Mannucci PM, Remuzzi G, Pusineri F et al (1983) Deamino-8-D-arginine–vasopressin shortens the bleeding time in uremia. *N. Engl. J. Med., 308,* 8.
21. Mannucci PM, Vicente V, Vianello L et al (1986) Controlled trial of desmopressin (DDAVP) in liver cirrhosis and other conditions associated with a prolonged bleeding time. *Blood, 67,* 1148.
22. Salzman EW, Weinstein MJ, Weintraub RM et al (1986) Treatment with desmopressin acetate to reduce blood loss after cardiac surgery. *N. Engl. J. Med., 314,* 1402.

23. Schulman S, Johnsson H, Egberg N, Blombäck M (1987) DDAVP-induced correction of prolonged bleeding time in patients with congenital platelet function defects. *Thromb. Res., 45,* 165.
24. Mannucci PM (1988) Desmopressin: a nontransfusional form of treatment for congenital and acquired bleeding disorders. *Blood, 72,* 1449.
25. Salzman EW, Weinstein M, Weintraub R et al (1988) Myocardial infarction in a patient with hemophilia treated with DDAVP. *N. Engl. J. Med., 318,* 121.
26. Bond L, Bevan D (1988) Myocardial infarction in a patient with hemophilia treated with DDAVP. *N. Engl. Med., 318,* 121.
27. O'Brien JR, Green PJ, Salmon G et al (1989) Desmopressin and myocardial infarction. *Lancet, 1,* 664.
28. Van Dantzig JM, Duren DR, Ten Cate JW (1989) Desmopressin and myocardial infarction. *Lancet, 1,* 664.
29. Moake JL, Turner NA, Stathopoulos NA et al (1986) Involvement of large plasma von Willebrand factor (vWF) multimers and unusually large vWF forms derived from endothelial cells in shear-stress induced platelet aggregation. *J. Clin. Invest., 78,* 1456.
30. Editioral (1989) Desmopressin and arterial thrombosis. *Lancet, 1,* 938.
31. Silverstein MN, Petitt RM, Solberg Jr LA et al (1988) Anagrelide: a new drug for treating thrombocytosis. *N. Engl. J. Med., 318,* 1292.
32. Gruppo Italiano per lo Studio della Streptochinasi nell'Infarto Miocardico (GISSI) (1986) Effectiveness of intravenous thrombolytic treatment in acute myocardial infarction. *Lancet, 1,* 397.
33. ISIS-2 (Second International Study of Infarct Survival) Collaborative Group (1988) Randomised trial of intravenous streptokinase, oral aspirin, both, or neither among 17 187 cases of suspected acute myocardial infarction: ISIS-2. *Lancet, 2,* 349.
34. Taylor GJ, Mikell FL, Moses HW et al (1984) Intravenous versus intracoronary streptokinase therapy for acute myocardial infarction in community hospitals. *Am. J. Cardiol., 54,* 256.
35. McGrath K, Patterson R (1985) Immunology of streptokinase in human subjects. *Clin. Exp. Immunol., 62,* 421.
36. Dyckewicz MS, McGrath KG, Davison R et al (1986) Identification of patients at risk for anaphylaxis due to streptokinase. *Arch. Intern. Med., 148,* 305.
37. Chan NS, White H, Maslowski A, Cleland J (1988) Plasmacytosis and renal failure after readministration of streptokinase for threatened myocardial infarction. *Br. Med. J., 297,* 717.
38. Lew AS, Laramee P, Cercek B et al (1985) The hypotensive effect of intravenous streptokinase in patients with acute myocardial infarction. *Circulation, 72,* 1321.
39. Been M, De Bono DP, Muir AL et al (1986) Clinical effects and kinetic properties of intravenous APSAC—anisoylated plasminogen streptokinase activator complex (BRL26 921)—in acute myocardial infarction. *Int. J. Cardiol., 11,* 53.
40. Vaughan DE, Krishenbaum JM, Loscalzo J (1988) Streptokinase induced, antibody mediated platelet aggregation: a potential cause of clot propagation in vivo. *J. Am. Coll. Cardiol., 11,* 1343.
41. Murray N, Lyons J, Chappell M (1986) Crescentic glomerulonephritis: a possible complication of streptokinase treatment for myocardial infarction. *Br. Heart J., 56,* 483.
42. Ong ACM, Handler CE, Walker JM (1988) Hypersensitivity vasculitis complicating intravenous streptokinase therapy in acute myocardial infarction. *Int. J. Cardiol., 21,* 71.
43. Sorber WA, Herfst V (1988) Lymphocytic angiitis following streptokinase therapy. *Cutis, 42,* 57.
44. Mathiesen O, Grunnet N (1989) Haemolysis after intravenous streptokinase. *Lancet, 1,* 1016.
45. Vanier MT, Rousson RM, Mandon G et al (1989) Haemolysis after intravenous streptokinase. *Lancet, 1,* 1016.
46. Davies D, Howell DA (1977) Tranexamic acid and arterial thrombosis. *Lancet, 1,* 49.
47. Agnelli G, Gresele P, Decunto M et al (1982) Tranexamic acid, intrauterine contraceptive devices, and fatal cerebral arterial thrombosis. *Br. J. Obstet. Gynaecol., 89,* 681.
48. Razis PA, Coulson IH, Gould TR, Findley IL (1986) Acquired C_1-esterase inhibitor deficiency. *Anaesthesia, 41,* 838.
49. Verstraete M (1985) Clinical application of inhibitors of fibrinolysis. *Drugs, 29,* 236.
50. Parsons MR, Merritt DR, Ramsay RC (1988) Retinal artery occlusion associated with tranexamic acid therapy. *Am. J. Ophthalmol., 105,* 688.

M.N.G. Dukes

38 Gastrointestinal drugs

ANTACIDS *(SED-11, 781; SEDA-12, 316; SEDA-13, 328)*

Aluminium hydroxide *(SEDA-13, 328)*

Risk situations An infant boy of 17 days with recurrent apnea was thought to be suffering from gastrointestinal reflux. Treatment included the use of aluminium hydroxide in the form of 'Infant Gaviscon' 53 mg daily. After a week of treatment the plasma aluminium was found to be 3 times higher than normal; the antacid was withdrawn and the level normalized within 2 weeks. As the authors point out, this product is not recommended for young infants, but it does appear to be commonly used in this age group. Because aluminium is apparently absorbed much more readily in such infants, it seems wise to avoid using it in *premature babies or during early infancy* (1[c]). In this respect one should realize that there are reports of seizures and death in young infants attributed to aluminium intake in the form of parenteral feeding (2[cr]), a topic primarily dealt with in Chapter 23 of this series of volumes.

Interactions The 'Metals' section of these Annuals has likewise dealt in recent years with some risks of aluminium in renal patients. In this connection a recent report suggests that there may be a particular risk in combining aluminium hydroxide with *citrate*:

A woman of 50 with a long history of severe hypertension and renal failure was admitted with cerebral hemorrhage. She received sodium nitroprusside to lower the blood pressure as well as other antihypertensive agents and ranitidine. Aluminium hydroxide 30 ml suspension was administered 4-hourly for 3 weeks and later in somewhat reduced frequency. Citric acid 334 mg/15 ml and sodium citrate 500 mg/5 ml were given in the form of Shohl's solution from days 16–28 for metabolic acidosis and then replaced by sodium bicarbonate 4.8 g/d. On days 21 and 36, serum aluminium levels were found to the 3124 and 479 g/l, respectively. In view of the fact that the other treatment had not varied, it seems likely that it was the concomitant use of citrate which had produced the excessively high aluminium levels on the first occasion (3[C]).

Sodium bicarbonate *(SEDA-13, 328)*

Nervous system Reif et al have described an unusual case of *absence seizures* in a young girl treated with sodium bicarbonate:

The patient, a 2 year-old girl, was initially admitted with metabolic acidosis, hypercarbonemia and hyperchloremia and a general failure to thrive. It was considered that she had a renal tubular acidosis and she was treated with 4 mmol/kg sodium bicarbonate daily p.o. After a month of treatment she experienced 4 absence seizures, with diffuse, slow brain activity on the EEG; serum pH was normal. The bicarbonate dose was halved and seizures did not recur during the next 6 months of follow-up (4[c]).

ANTIEMETICS *(SED-11, 782; SEDA-12, 316; SEDA-13, 328)*

Domperidone *(SED-11, 783; SEDA-12, 316)*

The same cautions relating to *'neuroleptic'-type effects* as have been discussed for metoclopramide apply to domperidone; though it has been thought that the reported frequency is lower (5[R], 6[r]), this may reflect no more than the fact that domperidone has been much less widely used. In 1988 Meyboom and Huijbers noted that of 55 reports on possible suspected reactions to domperidone reported up to that date to the Netherlands National Centre for Adverse Reaction Monitoring 9 concerned extrapyramidal reactions. The time-frame and absence of other causal factors pointed very

(Biomedical Division)
Side Effects of Drugs Annual 14
M.N.G. Dukes and L. Beeley, editors

strongly to a relationship with the drug. Seven of these cases were children less than 3 years of age and 5 were younger than 1 year. The neurological picture is alarming, with athetotic movements, hypertonia and a varying level of consciousness, perhaps reflecting the drug's passage through the blood–brain barrier. The symptoms can develop even with normal doses, and there is too little publicly available information on the absorption of the drug in its various forms (7[CR]).

Metoclopramide *(SED-11, 783; SEDA-12, 316; SEDA-13, 329)*

Nervous system Continuing failure by some practitioners to realize that metoclopramide is related to the benzamide family of neuroleptics (8[R]) results in an unnecessarily high incidence of *parkinsonian complications*, many instances of which have been reported earlier in these volumes. A particularly clear case of an acute dystonic reaction with asterixis and myoclonus has been described recently (9[C]). Some indication of the incidence of the problem of extrapyramidal adverse effects has been obtained by the Newcastle-on-Tyne group who obtained information from a large group of general practitioners:

Data were provided on 2557 patients taking metoclopramide and 2811 taking prochlorperazine. Metoclopramide was generally used for gastrointestinal symptoms, and of the 71 adverse effects recorded 25 were extrapyramidal complications. Dystonia and dyskinesia were present in 12 cases and were significantly more frequent in patients below the age of 30. Typically parkinsonian reactions were seen in 5 cases and did not appear to be age-related. The incidence of extrapyramidal reactions was similar when using prochlorperazine (16, including 8 of parkinsonism) (10[Cr]).

In a much smaller series of 12 patients reported from Italy who were receiving metoclopramide over a variable period to reduce the gastric effects of cytostatic drugs, 4 experienced *akathisia* after 3 doses given around the time of cytostatic therapy; akathisia was absent in a comparison group given a corticosteroid instead (11[C]).

The risk is naturally higher in the presence of predisposing factors. Eisele, for example, demonstrated a case with both *multiple myoclonus and generalized seizures* in a patient with renal failure; although patients on dialysis may exhibit several neurological syndromes, the course of events in his case seems to show that metoclopramide had lowered the threshold for both seizures and myoclonus and that it must be used judiciously in renal failure (12[Cr]).

Another typically neuroleptic effect which metoclopramide like other dopamine blockers can induce is the *neuroleptic malignant syndrome*; in a case from Missouri this condition appeared 4 days after starting treatment of a 55-year-old man with 10 mg 3 times daily. The symptoms were typical and worsened rapidly over 24–28 hours to the point where he required dantrolene and bromocriptine to relieve what had become a life-threatening condition (13[C]).

HISTAMINE H_2-ANTAGONISTS *(SED-11, 783; SEDA-12, 317; SEDA-13, 330)*

The relative safety of the various H_2-blockers will no doubt be debated for as long as they are used. Currently the only two which have been employed on a sufficiently wide scale and for a long enough time to make valid comparisons possible are still cimetidine and ranitidine. A lengthy review by Freston (14[R]), which looks carefully at some of the subtleties, concludes that there is a not a great deal of difference between the adverse reaction or interaction profiles of any of these substances and that age does not greatly influence the incidence of adverse effects. Surprisingly, his figures for the incidence of *CNS reactions* (somnolence, lethargy, confusion, agitation, visual hallucinations, headache, slurred speech) are higher for ranitidine (1.8%) than for cimetidine (0.4–0.7%) which is the reverse of what was originally claimed by the initiators of ranitidine. However, the figures remain very low and highly dependent upon the doses employed; one has the impression that claims as to the greater safety of ranitidine actually led to its being preferred in situations of risk and hence to an increase in the adverse reaction figures, a phenomenon not unknown in the adverse reaction world. As Freston points out, some of the CNS effects reported are typical of the 'intensive care unit syndrome' and not necessary drug-associated at all.

Cimetidine *(SED-11, 783; SEDA-12, 317; SEDA-13, 331)*

Cardiovascular It is indeed clear that, while *bradycardia* has repeatedly been reported with cimetidine and *hypotension* has followed intravenous use, a wider variety of cardiac effects can occur, particularly with parenteral use and in high-risk patients.

Drea et al described a case associated with the intravenous use of cimetidine in a hypertensive woman of 75 having a history of angina pectoris and who had just undergone a coronary bypass operation; after the 5th infusion of cimetidine 300 mg given over 30 min she experienced *junctional rhythm, bradycardia and hypotension.* The reaction, which demanded calcium chloride treatment, was reproduced on rechallenge. There was no evidence of allergy and the patient had previously tolerated oral cimetidine well (15[Cr]).

The cardiac history in this case clearly created a high-risk situation for cardiovascular complications. The authors themselves speculate on the possible role of phenol (used as a preservative) in producing the cardiac reaction since it does have some cardiotoxic potential, but the doses used only amounted to 10 mg per 300 mg infusion of cimetidine.

Some idea of the *incidence* of cardiovascular effects with cimetidine and ranitidine was provided by the FDA's Division of Epidemiology in 1988, which up to that time had received 39 spontaneous domestic reports of bradycardia associated with the use of these drugs, 24 being associated with cimetidine and 15 with ranitidine (16[CR]); 11 of the reports described positive dechallenge, and in 2 there was a positive rechallenge. A further 32 reports had been received from foreign sources. Atrioventricular block was recorded alongside the bradycardia in 6 cases in the total series available to the FDA, but its presence or absence was not specified in the remainder. While, as the FDA points out, the American figures represent an incidence of only 1.6 reports per 10 million prescriptions for cimetidine and 3.6 for ranitidine, one has to bear in mind the gross under-reporting of adverse effects to national agencies; the reporting rate in the United States has sometimes been estimated at 1:1000 or less, rising to 1:10 in the case of very severe incidents, and one certainly must apply a very large multiple to the figures if one is to approach reality.

Nervous system See general section above.

Hematological Some cases in which patients developed hematological reactions to both cimetidine and ranitidine are considered under 'ranitidine' below.

Respiratory A case of *interstitial lung disease* which may have been due to cimetidine has been reported by Höltman et al:

A man of 55 with a long asthmatic history was treated with cimetidine gel (200 mg daily) for progressive gastroesophageal reflux. Within 3 months he noted worsening dyspnea due to diffuse interstitial pulmonary changes which did not respond to corticosteroids. A further 3 months later he was hospitalized for his condition and ceased to take cimetidine. He was treated with cyclophosphamide and high doses of prednisolone. Because of worsening reflux esophagitis and a peptic ulcer cimetidine was recommenced in high dosage (1500 mg/d) and sucralfate added. There was a rapid further aggravation in his lung symptoms. Cyclophosphamide was withdrawn and the prednisolone dose raised. The cimetidine dose was halved after 3 weeks and the drug then withdrawn, after which his lung condition progressively improved and he could in due course be discharged on a lower prednisolone dose (17[C]).

The time-course and the apparently positive rechallenge are striking, but, as the authors point out, cyclophosphamide can play a role in interstitial lung disease as can chronic aspiration of esophageal material in reflux states.

Gastrointestinal The question as to whether cimetidine can induce *pancreatitis* has not answered consistently. SEDA-13 provided a convincing case (p. 332) and another suggestive one was published by Nott and De Sousa in 1989; the elderly woman involved was taking 400 mg cimetidine twice daily and the acute pancreatitis with raised serum amylase, urea and creatinine levels worsened in spite of supportive treatment until cimetidine was withdrawn. There was no rechallenge (18[C]).

Metabolic, endocrine Some degree of breast enlargement without a change in prolactin levels is a relatively common problem with cimetidine; *galactorrhea with prolactin increase* is highly unusual though recognized:

In a case reported by Ehrinpreis et al, a woman taking cimetidine 300 mg 4 times daily was hospitalized because of bilateral milky discharge from the breast which had been present for a month. There was elevated serum prolactin. The cimetidine was replaced by ranitidine 150 mg twice daily; the breast discharge ceased and serum prolactin was normal within 2 months (19[C]).

One should note that this patient was also receiving spironolactone which also has some stimulant effect on the breast and could have potentiated that of cimetidine.

Interaction For a possible interaction with spironolactone see 'Metabolic, endocrine' above.

Famotidine *(SED-11, 785; SEDA-12, 317; SEDA-13, 333)*

The more one learns about famotidine the more closely it seems to resemble the earlier H_2-blockers. One recent report points to its having induced *mental confusion* in 2 elderly patients with the reduced renal and hepatic function typical of the age group; each of these subsequently tolerated other H_2-blockers, but the latter were given orally and in relatively low doses whereas famotidine had been given intravenously in an acute situation (20[C]). There are also well-documented reports of thrombocytopenia (21[C]) and of throbbing *headache*, the latter being observed in the same patient with ranitidine but not cimetidine (22[C]); neither case was rechallenged, but the time-frame was strongly suggestive of a drug effect.

The question of whether there is less propensity to interactions with famotidine than with earlier H_2-blockers also requires a clearer answer; the lack of effect on cytochrome P-450 continues to suggest that this might prove to be an advantage.

Nizatidine *(SEDA-13, 333)*

The relatively limited experience with nizatidine means that there are still doubts as to any particular safety characteristics which it may have. The overview literature notes that a slight *increase in the platelet count*, which remains stable for as much as a year, has been described (23[r]).

Ranitidine *(SED-11, 785; SEDA-12, 317; SEDA-13, 334)*

Cardiovascular The question of cardiovascular effects and their incidence with the principal H_2-blockers has been considered above when discussing cimetidine. Cases relating to ranitidine continue to appear, with a clear tendency to occurrence where there are predisposing factors. When a man of 47 described by Hart was given a series of intravenous ranitidine doses (50 mg t.i.d.) for a perforated duodenal ulcer, the 5th dose was followed by *cardiac arrest* requiring resuscitation; before recovery he experienced a hypoxic seizure (24[c]). Both *shock* and *bradycardia* have been reported before in similar situations and careful cardiac monitoring is demanded when ranitidine is given intravenously in acute conditions.

Occasional patients without any apparent predisposing factor will however also suffer cardiac complications on ranitidine, apparently because they are sensitive to the cholinergic-like effects of the drug; one must recall the case of well-proven *first-degree atrioventricular block* described in the previous Annual which was entirely specific to this particular compound (25[C]).

Nervous system Ranitidine is capable of producing *behavioral disturbances* and, although they are very uncommon in patients in general good health, they can easily occur where there are serious predisposing risk factors:

A woman of 60 with a history of alcoholism, various forms of seizures and ultimately right hemiparesis involving both epileptic and atrophic brain changes was admitted for treatment with clonazepam and carbamazepine. Shortly after they had been discontinued, hematemesis occurred and a duodenal ulcer was found, for which ranitidine 300 mg daily was prescribed. Two days later she became manic with euphoria, logorrhea and flight of ideas, and the symptoms persisted until a few hours after ranitidine was withdrawn. On rechallenge the manic state recurred (26[C]).

A case of throbbing *headache* is discussed in connection with famotidine above.

Hematological The conclusion of earlier volumes in this series was that the occasional instances of *blood dyscrasias* described over the years with ranitidine or other H_2-blockers related to patients in a very poor state of health, generally with other direct risk factors, and that cause and effect had not been demonstrated.

That interpretation also holds for a recent case of bone marrow aplasia in a woman of 83, in whom the blood condition was somewhat deranged even before ranitidine treatment began, though it became much worse during the 9 days of therapy, at which time she also developed myalgia and polyarthralgia (which might indeed have been drug-associated in view of experience with cimetidine). By the time the patient developed clear pancytopenia she had also received cefaprim and thiamphenicol (27[C]).

Ranitidine may well have triggered thrombocytopenia and agranulocytosis in a case reported by Bader et al (28[C]), the prior condition in that particular man having been impaired by heavy alcohol abuse with chronic liver disease, duodenal ulcer and diabetes; in this case too the blood picture was somewhat deranged before ranitidine was given, but there was indeed a marked and sudden fall in leukocyte and platelet counts during the brief period of ranitidine treatment. There is also a case reported by List et al in which a man recently operated for a brain tumor and receiving phenytoin developed granulocytopenia within 3 weeks of being given ranitidine for his gastritis; the blood disorder recurred within a month of his being prescribed cimetidine and receded when the latter drug was withdrawn (29[C]).

In passing, one may note that there has been a further case of *thrombocytopenia* where a patient similarly seemed to be hypersensitive to both ranitidine and cimetidine (30[C]), while Pixley et al have sought to detect mechanisms which could explain the occasional occurrence of *anemia* during ranitidine treatment (31[r]).

Metabolic, endocrine Another of the sporadic cases of gynecomastia attributed to ranitidine comes from Spain; the breast enlargement, which like that reported by Tosi in 1982 was painful, was not in this case accompanied by raised prolactin levels, and it receded fully within 2 months of stopping the drug (32[cr]).

Risk of infection The arrival of alternative treatments to the H_2-blockers has stimulated a critical approach by those examining the newer agents to points on which they may score against the established products. In a study of perenzepine for the prevention of stress ulcer bleeding in patients in intensive care it was set against ranitidine 200 mg i.v. in reasonably equivalent doses. In the subgroup of 61 patients requiring ventilation there was a higher incidence of pneumonia (28.6%) with ranitidine than with pirenzepine (9.1%), the difference being significant at the 5% level. The difference is attributed by the authors to the increased gastric colonization with Gram-negative organisms during ranitidine treatment, particularly in the light of earlier published findings on this score with cimetidine (33[CR]).

Miscellaneous It is difficult to interpret a case of *chest pain* reported by Shimp et al in 1989:

The 45-year-old woman concerned had chronic duodenal ulcer disease unresponsive to cimetidine and an antacid (which were however given for only 5 days) and was therefore treated with ranitidine 150 mg twice daily. Within an hour of the first dose she experienced a dull, pounding chest pain to the left of the sternum which resolved after an hour. She thereafter took a half dose without complications, but when taking the 150 mg dose again, the pain recurred. She was subsequently maintained on cimetidine and sucralfate (34).

It is possible that one is dealing with one of the very occasional instances of referred pain from the primary lesion when treated, or even with an acute cardiac effect (see 'Cardiovascular' above).

Interactions Bearing in mind that ranitidine probably does not share most of the interactions of cimetidine, it is important to identify any specific interactions which it can have. Bramhall and Levine have provided evidence that ranitidine did in a case which they observed raise blood levels of *phenytoin* by reducing its metabolic clearance. If that is true, it could also reduce clearance of other drugs eliminated by hepatic cytochrome P-450 (35[C]). A similar effect of ranitidine on the clearance of *theophylline* has been claimed by some but denied by others (36[C], 37[r]–39[r]), suggesting that the effect is not consistent.

OTHER ANTISECRETORY DRUGS

Omeprazole *(SED-11, 786; SEDA-12, 317)*

For a new type of antisecretory drug which has been promoted actively for the last 2 years as a rival to the H_2-blockers, and which has acquired a corresponding share of the market, there is a surprising dearth of adverse reaction reports. The debate has centered more upon the drug's very high price than on its safety, which may indeed indicate that it is well tolerated in the conditions of use, overuse and careless use which are inevitably associated with the treatment of peptic disorders. An acrimonious debate beteen manufacturers on relative safety seems to have centered more on the supposed risks of the H_2-blockers than on those of omeprazole; the occurrence of carcinoid tumors in rats has generally been dismissed as irrelevant to man (40[R]). However, doubts persist as to the long-term safety of such thorough inhibition of gastric section in long-term use; clinical trials with omeprazole and drugs of comparable potency have been short, licenses have been issued mainly for short-term use, and even though in practice such drugs will often be used long-term, a decade could pass before any late risks emerge. A thoughtful review by Wormsley in 1988 (41[R]) takes as its starting point the fact that all the powerful gastric secretion inhibitors currently known produce cancer of the stomach in experimental animals. This applies to the potent H_2-blocker, loxtidine, as well as to the proton pump blocker, omeprazole. Both stimulate generalized proliferation of gastric mucosal cells in animal studies, with subsequent development of benign and malignant neoplasms. In the rat, the onset of the mitogenic response to this type of drug is virtually immediate. If this sort of epigenetic carcinogen exerts promoting effects in man, then irrespective of the duration of exposure, sufficiently mutated cells may be triggered into malignant proliferative activity. In Wormsley's view the possible long-term risks of this process outweigh the benefits of drugs such as omeprazole, since the small proportion of patients who do not respond to the established H_2-blockers of the ranitidine generation can and should be treated surgically rather than being transferred to more powerful drugs.

Experience with the short-term use of omeprazole is still reassuring. A review in the *Drugs and Therapeutics Bulletin* which appeared as this volume went to press remarked that the drug was well-tolerated, side effects merely comprising occasional nausea, headache, diarrhea, constipation and rash. As was pointed out, omeprazole inhibits the cytochrome P-450 enzyme system in the liver, so reducing the clearance of diazepam, phenytoin and warfarin, but this effect is minor at clinically relevant doses (42[R]).

MUCOSAL PROTECTIVE AGENTS *(SED-11, 786)*

Bismuth subcitrate

Bearing in mind much older instances of bismuth encephalopathy, the medical community has been agreeably surprised by the lack of such problems with the newer bismuth preparation, De-Nol (colloidal bismuth subcitrate), during its decade of use (43[R]). One may however note the theoretical warning by Locke et al, in the light of their biochemical studies, that even when bismuth is used in such low doses accumulation in the body does occur, and that if used sufficiently long, even this form of bismuth treatment could result in adverse effects (44[r]).

OTHER ULCER-HEALING AGENTS

Sucralfate *(SED-11, 786; SEDA-12, 318; SEDA-13, 335)*

As a basic aluminium salt of sucrose octasulfate, sucralfate is not pharmacologically very active, its most relevant property being its ability to bind to inflamed surfaces. Some practical problems result from its physical rather than its chemical nature. They generally comprise no more than a little gastric discomfort, nausea or meteorism (45[C]), but they can be more subtle:

Anderson described in 1989 the case of a man with Guillain-Barré syndrome who required enteral feeding through a nasogastric tube, through which he also received sucralfate (1 g every 6 h) and various drugs. After 2 weeks of protein supplementation in this way it proved impossible to remove the tube and it was found to be embedded in a large *gastric bezoar* which had to be broken down using a 'Water Pik' pressure spray, followed by gastric lavage. The bezoar was composed of 29% protein but also of sucralfate (46[C]).

Not dissimilar is a report on a woman of 48 who received sucralfate 1 g 4 times daily by mouth, but was given various other medications intravenously because she was suffering from dysphagia. After 3 days on sucralfate she was unable to swallow at all, and the esophagus proved to be obstructed by a foreign body composed largely of sucralfate, requiring dissolution by a water jet (47[C]).

As a review points out (48[R]), the way in which sucralfate acts can result in a decrease in plasma phosphate (though osteomalacia as a result of long-term use is only a theoretical possibility so far) and in a decrease in absorption of some drugs including phenytoin, warfarin and cimetidine (though subject to a reservation advanced in SEDA-13, this has not usually been shown to be significant).

Risk situations Because of its aluminium content, sucralfate can result in *absorption of aluminium ions* and while this is not usually a problem it may become so in the presence of severely *impaired renal function*. In one recent case a girl of 13, with terminal renal disease and an existing history of aluminium intoxication from aluminium carbonate used in connection with dialysis, was given sucralfate 3 g daily in divided doses for her gastritis; aluminium levels again rose sharply, resulting in bone pain, seizures and muscular weakness; the symptoms and blood levels reacted rapidly to withdrawal of sucralfate (49[C]).

Interactions See above under the general introduction to this section.

LAXATIVES *(SED-11, 788; SEDA-12, 318; SEDA-13, 336)*

Laxative abuse was reviewed in SEDA-13. One may note here a case of a type which is easily missed for a long time when the doctor is confronted with vague symptoms:

A girl 4 months of age was admitted because of poor feeding, lethargy, weight loss and passage of 6–10 loose stools daily. No abnormalities were found and she was discharged after 6 days. At the age of 7 months she was readmitted because of continued failure to gain weight, repeated minor infections and continuing diarrhea; the mother was admitted with her. After a weekend at home she was readmitted in a severely dehydrated state and required resuscitation followed by intravenous feeding. Only when the stool electrolytes were examined was it clear that some noxious influence was present and at this point the mother admitted to administering the child Epsom salts so that symptoms were maximalized and 'the doctors would take her more seriously' (50[Cr]).

ANTI-INFLAMMATORY AGENTS *(SED-11, 789; SEDA-12, 319; SEDA-13, 337)*

5-Aminosalicylic acid (mesalazine, fisalamine) *(SED-11, 790; SEDA-12, 319; SEDA-13, 337)*

Since mesalazine is the active principle of sulfasalazine, it is increasingly replacing it, and one might expect a reduced incidence of those adverse effects ascribable to the sulfa moiety. On the other hand, some newer preparations of mesalazine allow for greater absorption in the upper gastrointestinal tract with higher blood levels, and this could result in changes in the pattern of adverse reactions originally described. Certainly such symptoms as *diarrhea, pyrexia, exanthema, arthralgia and pruritus* now seem more prominent than was originally hoped (51[Cr]).

Cardiovascular In a case reported by Agnholt et al a young man with Crohn's disease developed *chest pains with ECG changes* when he was treated with sulfasalazine and mesalazine, but not when he subsequently received sulfasalazine alone. The adverse effect reappeared on rechallenge with the two drugs given together, suggesting that mesalazine can in some patients affect the myocardium (52[c]).

Nervous system A little evidence from the past suggests that the nervous system can occasionally react to this type of product, and a striking case now relates mesalazine to a *neuropathy*:

A woman of 38 received 400 mg mesalazine 3 times daily for what was first thought to be ulcerative colitis but later diagnosed as non-specific colitis. During the first month of treatment she complained of numbness in the feet at night. For this reason she was (curiously) transferred to sulfasalazine, but this produced gastrointestinal problems and mesalazine was reinstated. After 16 months of treatment the patient presented with impaired memory and concentration, numbness in the feet and fatigue of the leg muscles. Neurological examination showed the presence of a mixed sensorimotor neuropathy, primarily but not exclusively involving the legs. The condition (and the findings in nerve conduction studies) resolved within 2 months of withdrawing mesalazine (53[c]).

Gastrointestinal *Pancreatitis* has several times been ascribed to sulfasalazine, and it is not surprising to see two recent reports firmly associating mesalazine with the same complication, perhaps reflecting the arrival of preparations with greater bioavailability. In both recent reports there was a positive rechallenge and the condition was manifest both clinically and biochemically (54[C], 55[C]).

Second-generation effects There is now firm evidence that mesalazine, which is excreted in the breast milk, can affect the infant. In a case described in the *Lancet* early in 1989, a young woman had been treated during pregnancy with rectal mesalazine for relapsing ulcerative proctitis, and treatment was resumed during breast-feeding. Twelve hours after the first maternal dose the breast-fed child developed diarrhea, which vanished when the drug was discontinued. On 4 subsequent occasions resumption of treatment was attempted and each time the infant's diarrhea recurred (56[c]).

Olsalazine *(SED-11, 790)*

As pointed out earlier in this series, olsalazine (disodium azodisalicylate) represents a further attempt to retain the usefulness of sulfasalazine while dissociating the adverse effects of the sulfapyridine moiety. It consists of two molecules of 5-aminosalicylic acid linked by a diazo bond; the bond is broken by colonic bacteria, liberating 5-aminosalicylic acid, i.e. mesalazine. One would expect the adverse effects to correspond closely to those of mesalazine and, although experience is still limited, this seems to be the case. *Diarrhea* has been described and from Rotterdam there is a well-documented instance of *pancreatitis* with positive dechallenge and rechallenge (57[C]).

Salazosulfapyridine (sulfasalazine) *(SED-11, 789; SEDA-12, 319; SEDA-13, 337)*

An impressive historical overview of work on sulfasalazine makes the point that the drug does not exist in a pure state in currently used tablets, capsules and suppositories. The purity has been of the order of 85%; the identity of the remaining 15% is not clear, but experience gained in the field indicates that the impurities are harmless, most adverse effects being attributable to the sulfapyridine component of the molecule. However, since the U.S. Food and Drug Administration was concerned about the high percentage of impurities, a product of 95–97% purity has now been prepared (58[R]). It will be interesting to see whether this changes its safety record as the purer product comes into general use.

Nervous system An unusual mental reaction, perhaps due to some unusual sensitivity to sulfasalazine, was considered in SEDA-13. One can add to that a case of *severe depressive illness* which seems to have been triggered on 3 occasions by the drug in a girl of 17 with Crohn's disease. The girl was already suffering from a masked depression of cyclic character, but the time schedule with repeated positive rechallenge and dechallenge clearly shows that a mental disorder to which the patient was prone was released by taking this drug (59[C]).

Respiratory One more case of '*sulfasalazine lung*' was reported from Germany, involving a woman of 36 with early rheumatoid arthritis but a much earlier history of pulmonary tuberculosis. It is an example of very early development of the complication:

During the first 4 weeks of treatment on doses rising from 1500 to 2000 mg sulfasalazine daily, she developed severe dyspnea, mild fever, dry cough with chest pain, marked hypoxemia and severely abnormal restrictive lung functions. The first symptoms had appeared only 14 days after the start of treatment. Chest X-ray demonstrated diffuse alveolar-interstitial infiltrates. After discontinuing the drug and employing short-term treatment with corticosteroids, the blood gases and chest X-ray normalized over the next 4 weeks, but the abnormal lung functions persisted at the time of discharge. The total dose ingested by the time of admission and discontinuation of sulfasalazine was 48 g (60[Cr]).

Skin and appendages Rashes and more serious skin reactions, even extending to *toxic epidermal necrolysis* or similar states (61[CR], 62[CR]), are a recognized complication of the sulfa moiety in this substance. *Lupus erythematosus* has been well documented in a Spanish case (63[Cr]). Some statistics on dermatological complications were provided when Hoffmann et al reported on 260 patients with rheumatoid arthritis or psoriatic arthritis treated with sulfasalazine. Skin effects occurred in 7 of them, comprising variously a *macular, papular, vesicular of hemorrhagic-bullous rash, a systemic eczematous contact-type dermatitis or a photoallergic dermatitis.* In all cases the skin reaction caused termination of treatment (64[R]). Naturally one must bear in mind the particular spectrum of patients involved; the psoriatic element may have rendered some of them more susceptible to skin complications.

Antibiotic resistance Lane et al provided in 1988 a reminder, not only of the earlier evidence that sulfasalazine could induce resistance to sulfonamides, but also some new evidence suggesting that it could raise antibiotic resistance (65[cr]). When they examined the resistance pattern of *E. coli* taken from rectal mucosal swabs of 43 patients treated with sulfasalazine they found a very broad increase in antibiotic resistance as compared with patients having similar conditions but not taking the drug; there was a marked improvement in the picture (except for the sulfonamides) where the drug had been withdrawn for more than 6 months. In the ulcerative colitis series the changes were noted with respect to sulfonamides (76% resistance vs. 21% in controls), tetracycline (48% vs. 14%), kanamycin and neomycin (19% vs. 0%) and chloramphenicol (15% vs 0%). If these findings are confirmed, they could provide an additional reason to move to the 5-aminosalicylate.

OTHER DRUGS

Activated charcoal *(SED-11, 790; SEDA-12, 319; SEDA-13, 339)*

The description of another *fatality* due to pulmonary aspiration of activated charcoal (with a brief reference to another instance of aspiration) (66[C]) raises the question as to why these things occur and how they can be avoided. To quote the authors:

'Repeated oral administration of activated charcoal is considered to be a simple, safe and effective means of increasing the elimination of many drugs taken in overdose. The charcoal is, however, unpalatable and must be given by nasogastric tube in unconscious patients. Vomiting can occur, and although pulmonary aspiration of charcoal is rare, it can cause obstruction, shunting of blood, and hypoxemia, which may be exacerbated by aspiration of gastric acid. Medicoal [the charcoal preparation used in this case – *Ed.*] contains povidone as a non-absorbable suspending agent. This can cause chronic inflammatory reactions and has been implicated in pneumonitis after inhalation of hairsprays. In our patient aspiration of activated charcoal resulted in progressive and ultimately fatal respiratory failure. The pronounced reaction in the pulmonary alveoli and associated lymph nodes presumably accentuated pre-existing damage and precipitated respiratory failure. The airway should be protected when activated charcoal is given, particularly when the preparation contains povidone.'

ACKNOWLEDGEMENTS

The author would like to acknowledge the support which he received in the preparation of this Chapter from a specialized section of the Working Group on Human Toxicological Assessment at the University of Copenhagen.

REFERENCES

1. Puntis JWL, Ballantine NE, Durbin GM (1989) Raised plasma aluminium in an infant on antacid. *Lancet, 2*, 923.
2. Bishop NJ, Robinson MJ, Lendon M et al (1989) Increased concentration of aluminium in the brain of a parenterally fed preterm infant. *Arch. Dis. Child., 64*, 1316.
3. Kirchbaum BB, Schoolwerth AC (1989) Hyperalbuminaemia associated with aluminium hydroxide. *Hum. Toxicol., 8*, 45.
4. Reif S, Holzmann M, Barak S et al (1989) Absence seizures associated with bicarbonate therapy and normal serum pH. *J. Am. Med. Assoc., 262*, 1328.
5. Champion MC (1988) Domperidone. *Gen. Pharmacol., 18*, 499.
6. Anonymous (1988) Domperidone. *Drugs Ther. Bull.*, 59.
7. Meyboom RHB, Huijbers WAR (1988) Acute extrapyramidale bewegingsstoornissen bij jonge

kinderen en bij volwassenen tijdens het gebruik van domperidon. *Ned. Tijdschr. Geneeskd., 132*, 1981.
8. Cabrera Bonet R, Cabrera Forneiro J (1988) Efectos indeseables de las benzamidas. *Pharmaklinik, 2(4)*, 23.
9. Roquer J, Herraiz J (1989) Acute dystonic reaction with asterixis and myoclonus following metoclopramide therapy. *Neurosurg. Psychiatry, 52*, 248.
10. Bateman DN, Darling WM, Boys R et al (1989) Extrapyramidal reactions to metoclopramide and prochlorperazine. *Q. J. Med., 71*, 307.
11. Roila F, Basurto C, Minotti V et al (1988) Methylprednisolone versus metoclopramide for prevention of nausea and vomiting in breast cancer patients treated with intravenous cyclophosphamide methotrexate 5-fluorouracil: a double-blind randomized study. *Oncology, 45*, 346.
12. Eisele G (1988) Neurologic complications of metoclopramide therapy. *NY State J. Med., 88*, 332.
13. Patterson JF (1988) Neuroleptic malignant syndrome associated with metoclopramide. *South. Med. J., 81*, 674.
14. Freston JW (1989) Perspectives on safety issues and drug interactions with H_2-receptor antagonists. *J. Drug. Dev., 2, Suppl 3*, 61.
15. Drea EJ, Mutnick AH, Lam W (1990) Cimetidine-associated adverse reaction. *DICP Ann. Pharmacother., 24*, 581.
16. Tanner LA, Arrowsmith JB (1988) Bradycardia and H_2-antagonists. *Ann. Intern. Med. 109*, 434.
17. Höltmann BJ, Schött D, Ulmer WT (1989) Diffuse interstitial pulmonary disease after usage of cimetidine in a patient with severe reflux disease of the oesophagus (in German). *Med. Klin., 84*, 405.
18. Nott PT, De Sousa BA (1989) Suspected cimetidine-induced acute pancreatitis. *Br. J. Clin. Pract., 43*, 264.
19. Ehrinpreis MN, Fhar R, Narula A (1989) Cimetidine induced galactorrhoea. *Am. J. Gastroenterol., 84*, 563.
20. Henann NE, Carpenter DU, Janda SM (1988) Famotidine-associated mental confusion in elderly patients. *Drug. Intell. Clin. Pharm., 22*, 976.
21. Comer JB, Evans JA, Kerns A (1989) Possible famotidine-induced thrombocytopenia. *DICP Ann. Pharmacother., 23*, 507.
22. Hirsch E (1989) Famotidine and ranitidine but not cimetidine cause severe, disabling headache. *Am. J. Gastroenterol., 84*, 202.
23. Anonymous (1988) Nizatidine – an H_2-antagonist. *Hosp. Pharm., 23*, 413 and 430.
24. Hart AM (1989) Cardiac arrest associated with ranitidine. *Br. Med. J., 299*, 519.
25. Allegri G, Pellegrini K, Dobrilla G (1988) First-degree atrioventricular block in a young duodenal ulcer patient treated with a standard oral dose of ranitidine. *Agents Actions, 24*, 237.
26. Delerve O, Muller JP, Destee A (1988) Mania-like episodes associated with ranitidine. *Am. J. Psychiatry, 145*, 271.
27. Dubois A, Nakache N, Zerbib A et al (1988) Aplasie médullaire et ranitidine. *Ann. Gastroentérol. Hépatol., 24*, 261.
28. Bader A, Carrigan T, Gopalswamy N et al (1989) Reversible hematologic suppression during ranitidine treatment. *DICP Ann. Pharmacother., 23*, 508.
29. List AF, Beaird DH, Kummet T (1988) Ranitidine-induced granulocytopenia: recurrence with cimetidine administration. *Ann. Intern. Med., 108*, 566.
30. Gafter U, Zevin D, Komlos L et al (1989) Thrombocytopenia associated with hypersensitivity to ranitidine; possible cross-reactivity with cimetidine. *Am. J. Gastroenterol., 84*, 560.
31. Pixley JS, MacKintosh FR, Sahr EA et al (1989) Mechanism of ranitidine associated anemia. *Am. J. Med. Sci., 297*, 369.
32. Lópes Herce A, Lópes-Herce JA, López-Herce J (1988) Ginecomastia secundaria a tratiamento con ranitidina. *Gastroenterol. Hepatol., 11*, 315.
33. Tryba M, Zevounou F, Wruck G (1988) Stressblutingen und postoperative Pneumonien bei Intensivpatienten unter Ranitidin oder Pirenzepin. *Dtsch. Med. Wochenschr., 113*, 930.
34. Shimp LA, Smith MA, Wahr DW (1989) Ranitidine-induced chest pain. *DICP Ann. Pharmacother., 23*, 224.
35. Bramhall D, Levine M (1988) Possible interaction of ranitidine with phenytoin. *Drug Intell. Clin. Pharm., 22*, 979.
36. Muir JG, Powell JR, Bauman JH (1989) Induction of theophylline toxicity and inhibition of clearance rates by ranitidine. *Am. J. Med., 86*, 513.
37. Roy AK (1989) Induction of theophylline toxicity and inhibition of clearance rates by ranitidine. *Am. J. Med., 86*, 513.
38. Kelly HW (1989) Lack of evidence for reduction of theophylline clearance by ranitidine. *Am. J. Med., 86*, 629.
39. Roy AK (1989) Lack of evidence for reduction of theophylline clearance by ranitidine. *Am. J. Med., 86*, 630.
40. Delvaux M (1987) Les médicaments inhibiteurs de la sécrétion gastrique: mode d'action et pharmacologie. *Méd. Chir. Dig., 16*, 547.
41. Wormsley KG (1988) Is chronic long-term inhibition of gastric secretion really dangerous? *Scand. J. Gastroenterol., 23, Suppl. 146*, 166.
42. Anonymous (1990) Omeprazole: blocks gastric acid secretion completely. *Drugs Ther., Bull., 28*, 49.
43. Börsch G (1988) Alte and neue Magentherapie mit Wismutsalzen. *Med. Klin., 83*, 605.
44. Locke M, Nichol H, Ketola-Pirie C (1988) Binding of bismuth to cell components: clue to mode of action and side effects. *Can. Med. Assoc. J., 138*, 1099.
45. Cabriéres F (1988) Étude clinique, endosco-

pique et histologique de l'activité du sucralfate sur des patients atteints de gastrites sympatomatiques. *Méd. Chir. Dig., 17*, 55.
46. Anderson W, Weatherstone G, Veal C (1989) Esophageal medication bezoar in a patient receiving enteral feedings and sucralfate. *Am. J. Gastroenterol., 84*, 205.
47. Hart RS, Levin B, Gholson CF (1989) Esophageal obstruction caused by sucralfate impaction. *Gastrointest. Endosc., 35*, 474.
48. Bartle B, Cornish P (1988) Sucralfate update. *On Contin. Pract., 15*, 2.
49. Robertson JA, Saluksy IB, Goodman WG, et al (1989) Sucralfate, intestinal aluminium absorption, and aluminium toxicity in a patient on dialysis. *Ann. Intern. Med., 111*, 179.
50. Fenton AC, Wailoo MP, Tanner MS (1988) Severe failure to thrive and diarrhoea caused by laxative abuse. *Arch. Dis. Child., 63*, 978.
51. Fardy JM, Lloyd DA, Reynolds RPE (1988) Adverse effects with oral 5-aminosalicylic acid. *J. Clin. Gastroenterol., 10*, 635.
52. Agnholt J, Sörensen HT, Rasmussen SN et al (1989) Cardiac hypersensitivity to 5-aminosalisylic acid. *Lancet, 1*, 1135.
53. Woodward DK (1989) Peripheral neuropathy with mesalazine. *Br. Med. J. 299*, 1224.
54. Sachedina B, Saibil F, Cohen LB et al (1989) Acute pancreatitis due to 5-aminosalicylate. *Ann. Intern. Med., 110*, 490.
55. Deprez P, Descamps Ch, Fiasse R et al (1989) Pancreatitis induced by 5-aminosalicylic acid. *Lancet, 2*, 445.
56. Nelis GF (1989) Diarrhoea due to 5-aminosalicyclic acid in breast milk. *Lancet, 1*, 383.
57. Poldermans D, Van Blankenstein M (1988) Pancreatitis induced by disodium azodisalicylate. *Am. J. Gastroenterol., 83*, 578.
58. Svartz N (1988) Sulfasalazine. II. Some notes on the discovery and development of salazopyrin *Am. J. Gastroenterol., 83*, 497.
59. Scherer J (1988) Durch Salazosulfapyridin ausgelöste Depression bei Zyklothymie und M. Crohn. *Nervenarzt, 59*, 371.
60. Klein HO, Rupp M, Thiele-Fishbach A (1988) Arzneimittelinduzierte Alveolitis durch Salazosulfapyridin. *Dtsch. Med. Wochenschr., 113*, 1239.
61. Guerra R, Trevisanuto E, Corradin MT (1988) Un caso di sindrome di Lyell: contributo alle casistica. *Chron. Dermatol., 19*, 31.
62. Krakamp B, Beinhoff U, Knöpfle G et al (1988) Flächenhafte Nekrosen der Haut nach Sulfasalazin-Therapie bei Colitis ulcerosa. *Med. Klin., 83*, 611.
63. Capdevila JA, Ocana I, Ribera E et al (1988) Lupus eritematoso inducio por sulfasalazine. *Ann. Med. Interne, 5*, 363.
64. Hofmann C, Voigtländer Ch (1988) Unerwünschte Sulphasalazinwirkungen an der Haut unter besondere Berücksichtigung photoallergischer Reaktionen. *Aktuel Rheumatol., 13*, 121.
65. Lane MR, Allan RN, Pease PE (1988) Antibiotic resistance in *Escherichia coli* from patients on sulphasalazine. *Lancet, 1*, 1403.
66. Menzies DG, Busuttil A, Prescott LF (1988) Fatal pulmonary aspiration of oral activated charcoal. *Br. Med. J., 297*, 459.

J. Descotes and J.-C. Evreux

39 Immunomodulating agents

The field of pharmacological immunomodulation is progressing slowly. Recent studies have mainly focussed on the therapeutic application of cytokines, e.g. interleukin-2 (1[R]).

INDIVIDUAL COMPOUNDS OF NATURAL ORIGIN *(SED-11, 795; SEDA-12, 323; SEDA-13, 341)*

Bacillus Calmette-Guérin (BCG) *(SED-11, 795; SEDA-12, 323)*

Favorable results have been demonstrated with intravesical BCG in patients with superficial bladder tumors. However, toxicity may occur particularly in the *bladder*. El-Housseiny et al (2[C]) reported for example, on 12 out of 17 patients who developed cystitis symptoms after receiving intravesical BCG 120 mg (Montreal Armand Frappier strain). Similarly, when 95 patients were given 6 weekly intravesical injections of 120 mg Pasteur strain BCG, Kavoussi et al (3[C]) noted that *dysuria* was the most frequent complaint (91% of patients), followed by *hematuria* (47%). *Fever and chills* were seen in 39% of cases. *Granulomas, hemorrhagic cystitis, leukopenia* and *elevated liver function*, were noted in 1–4% of patients.

Corynebacterium parvum *(SED-11, 795)*

Casali et al (4[C]) have shown that intracavitary injection of *Corynebacterium parvum* may more effectively control neoplastic pleural effusion. Interestingly, side effects, namely *fever*, *pain* and *coughing*, were also promising to be milder.

Side Effects of Drugs Annual 14
M.N.G. Dukes and L. Beeley, editors

Interleukin-2 *(SED-11, 795; SEDA-12, 323)*

Interleukin-2 (IL-2), a glycoprotein normally produced by T-lymphocytes, serves as the second signal in antigen-induced T-lymphocyte proliferation. It also stimulates tumor cell lysis by certain lymphocytes, a phenomenon called lymphocyte-activated killing (LAK). Objective responses to the administration of recombinant IL-2 alone or in conjunction with LAK cells have recently been documented in patients with a variety of cancers and numerous clinical trials of IL-2 are under way. Unfortunately, IL-2 proved to be markedly toxic (5[R]).

As with most cytokine preparations, IL-2 infusions were associated with ***fever, chills, malaise, nausea, vomiting and diarrhea*** *in the majority of patients (6[C]–9[C]).*

However, cardiovascular toxicity is the main dose-limiting toxicity (10[R], 11[R]). Lee et al (12[C]) reported the cardiorespiratory effects of rIL-2 alone or in association with LAK cells in 317 patients: the majority of patients (65%) had ***hypotension*** *and* ***tachycardia*** *requiring vasopressors and intravenous fluids to maintain systolic blood pressure to a sufficient level. Severe* ***peripheral edema*** *was seen in 1.8% of patients while* ***ascites and/or pleural effusions*** *developed in approximately 3%.*

Weight gain *of 10% or more was observed in 32% of patients during the period of IL-2 administration. Vasopressors were also useful to avoid pulmonary edema due to increased capillary permeability, but severe* ***respiratory distress*** *was noted in 9.2% of patients and 6.4% required intubation.* ***Arrhythmias****, mostly supraventricular in nature, were present in 9.7% of patients.* ***Coronary ischemic changes*** *or* ***anginal pain*** *were noted in 2.6%. However,* ***myocardial infarction*** *may occur (13[c], 14[c]). A mild reversible* ***depression of cardiac function*** *similar to that seen in septic shock, with a significant decrease in the left ventricular end-diastolic volume index and ejection fraction, was associated with IL-2* *treatment (15[C]). Interestingly, release of tumor necrosis factor by either IL-2 or bacterial endotoxins has been thought to account for the similar cardiac complications of IL-2 administration and septic shock (11[R], 15[C]). However, it remains to be conclusively established whether direct cardiotoxicity or increased vascular permeability (or both) account for the cardiopulmonary side effects of IL-2 (16[R]).*

***Azotemia** and **creatinine elevation** were also common findings in IL-2 treated patients. Among their 317 patients, Margolin et al (9[C]) found creatinine levels between 5 and 10 times the upper limit of normal in 37% of cases and more than 10 times in 6%. **Anuria** was observed in 38% of patients but renal function rapidly returned to normal after cessation of IL-2 administration. Renal toxicity with oliguria, fluid retention, azotemia, low urinary excretion of sodium, phosphorus, calcium and magnesium (17[C]), is indeed often a dose-limiting effect. Direct tubular toxicity and fluid retention due to increased vascular permeability probably account for this severe side effect of IL-2 (18[c]).*

Hypothyroidism is another recently reported complication of IL-2 therapy (19[C]–22[C]). The mechanism is unknown but direct cellular lysis of the thyroid gland by LAK cells or alterations in MHC Class II antigen expression on thyroid cells might be involved.

***Erythematous rash with pruritus** was noted in most patients (9[C]). **Erythema nodosum** was reported in a 26-year-old woman 2 weeks after a second course of IL-2 plus LAK cells (23[c]). A case of fatal **pemphigus** despite concurrent high-dose corticosteroid therapy was reported in a 48-year-old lymphoma patient treated with IL-2 and β-interferon (24[C]). Exacerbation of pre-existing psoriasis is another possible complication of IL-2 therapy as shown by a recent report on 3 such patients (25[C]).*

***Muscle pain, joint aching, swollen and stiff joints** were also noted in 8 patients out of 13 given IL-2 infusion for 5 continuous days (26[C]). Finally, intrahepatic **cholestasis** has been described (27[C]).*

OK-432 (picibanil) *(SED-11, 795; SEDA-12, 323)*

While comparing intradermal versus intramuscular injections of OK-432, a hemolytic streptococcus preparation, Hanaue et al (28[C]) noted a 4.8% incidence of *fever* and a 52.4% incidence of *abscess* at the injection site among 42 gastric cancer patients given intradermal injections, and a 90% incidence of fever but no abscess among 40 patients given intramuscular injections.

Fever, chest pain, pleural effusion and thickening were observed in nearly all 155 patients with spontaneous pneumothorax treated with intrapleural administrations of OK-432 (29[c]).

Thymic hormones *(SED-11, 796; SEDA-12, 324)*

Thymosin fraction 5 *(SED-11, 796; SEDA-12, 324)* Gossain et al (34[c]) have shown that thymosin fraction 5 administration did not change glucose tolerance in 8 patients. However, an increased baseline plasma level of cortisol and ACTH was noted in 6 patients, suggesting a possible influence of thymosin on the hypothalamic pituitary/adrenal axis.

Tumor necrosis factor (TNF) *(SEDA-13, 343)*

A large body of experimental evidence suggests that TNF has marked cytolytic or cytostatic effects on tumor cells. A Phase I trial of intravenous recombinant TNF in 19 cancer patients (35[C]) showed marked toxicities: *fever* and *chills* occurred in nearly all patients. *Nausea* and *vomiting* were noted in 40% of patients receiving doses above 100 $\mu g/m^2$ and were severe in half. *Hypotension* was noted in 5 patients whilst one patient developed *myocardial infarction* followed by *acute cortical blindness*. Slight *elevation of serum transaminase and bilirubin levels* were noted in 6 patients. There was an absolute *granulocyte reduction* and a dose-related *platelet reduction*. Interestingly, antibodies to rTNF as determined by radioimmunoassay were not observed.

These results were confirmed in another Phase I trial of recombinant TNF (36[C]): severe hypotension, *fluid retention, watery diarrhea* and central nervous system toxicity (*confusion and dysphasia*) were dose-limiting. Nearly all patients experienced fever and chills. Nausea and vomiting were noted in half of the 15 patients. Platelet reduction was present in 3.

INDIVIDUAL SYNTHETIC COMPOUNDS

Ciamexon

No side effects were noted during a pilot study of 7 patients with Type I diabetes given 300 mg ciamexon daily for up to 9 months (37[c]).

Dithiocarb (sodium diethyldithiocarbamate) *(SED-11, 796)*

Dithiocarb was shown to slow progression to acquired immunodeficiency syndrome (38[C]) in a study of 83 patients given 10 mg dithiocarb/kg orally once a week. An *unpleasant taste* was the most frequent complaint (32%), followed by *abdominal discomfort* (26%), *nausea* (15%), *sensation of malaise* (8%), *anorexia* (7%), *excitement* (5%), *somnolence* (4%) and *vomiting* (2%).

Levamisole *(SED-11, 797; SEDA-12, 324; SEDA-13, 344)*

Administration of 2.5 mg/kg/d levamisole on days 1 and 2 of each week for 18 consecutive months was not associated with longer survival in patients with colorectal cancer (39[c]), but there was only minimal toxicity.

Poly I:C *(SED-11, 797; SEDA-12, 325)*

Fever and *chills* are commonly observed in patients treated with interferon inducers, e.g. poly I:C. Fever has been considered as a major limiting side-effect in patients treated with poly I:C. Interestingly, Bever et al (40[c]) did not find any correlation between interferon levels and temperature rise in 18 patients with progressive multiple sclerosis.

REFERENCES

1. Goey SH, Wagstaff J, Pinedo HM (1988) Biological approaches to the treatment of cancer. *Neth. J. Med., 33*, 41.
2. El-Housseiny II, Ghoneim MA, Nigam V et al (1988) Prophylactic maltose tetrapalmitate and Bacillus Calmette-Guérin immunotherapy of recurrent superficial bladder tumors: preliminary report. *J. Urol., 140*, 498.
3. Kavoussi LR, Torrence RJ, Gillen DP et al (1988) Results of 6 weekly intravesical Bacillus Calmette-Guérin instillations on the treatment of superficial bladder tumors. *J. Urol., 139*, 935.
4. Casali A, Gionfra T, Rinaldi M et al (1988) Treatment of malignant pleural effusions with intracavitary *Corynebacterium parvum. Cancer, 62*, 806.
5. Fent K, Zbinden G (1987) Toxicity of interferon and interleukin. *Trends Pharmacol. Sci., 8*, 100.
6. Javadpour N, Lalehzarian M (1988) A phase I–II study of high-dose recombinant human interleukin-2 in disseminated renal-cell carcinoma. *Semin. Surg. Oncol., 4*, 207.
7. West WH, Tauer KW, Yannelli JR et al (1987) Constant-infusion recombinant interleukin-2 in adoptive immunotherapy of advanced cancer. *J. Engl. J. Med., 316*, 898.
8. Rosenberg SA, Lotze MT, Muul LM et al (1987) A progress report on the treatment of 157 patients with advanced cancer using lymphokine-activated killer cells and interleukin-2 or high-dose interleukin-2 alone. *N. Engl. J. Med., 316*, 889.
9. Margolin KA, Rayner AA, Hawkins MJ et al (1989) Interleukin-2 and lymphokine-activated killer cell therapy of solid tumors: analysis of toxicity and management guidelines. *J. Clin. Oncol., 7*, 486.
10. Glauser FL, DeBlois G, Bechard D et al (1988) Cardiopulmonary toxicity of adoptive immunotherapy. *Am. J. Med. Sci., 296*, 406.
11. Isner JM, Dietz WA (1988) Cardiovascular consequences of recombinant DNA technology: interleukin-2. *Ann. Intern. Med., 109*, 933.
12. Lee RE, Lotze MT, Skibber JM et al (1989) Cardiorespiratory effects of immunotherapy with interleukin-2. *J. Clin. Oncol., 7*, 7.
13. Osanto S, Cluitmans FHM, Franks CR et al (1988) Myocardial injury after interleukin-2 therapy. *Lancet, 2*, 48.
14. Pasini FL, DePerri T, Van der Plas K, Palmer P, Franks CR (1989) Myocardial injury after interleukin-2 therapy. *Lancet, 2*, 674.
15. Ognibenee FP, Rosenberg SA, Lotze M et al (1988) Interleukin-2 administration causes reversible hemodynamic changes and left ventricular dysfunction similar to those seen in septic shock. *Chest, 94*, 750.
16. Conant EF, Fox KR, Miller WT (1989) Pulmonary edema as a complication of interleukin-2 therapy. *Am. J. Roentgenol., 152*, 749.
17. Webb DE, Austin HA, Billdegrun A et al (1988) Metabolic and renal effects of interleukin-2 immunotherapy for metastatic cancer. *Clin. Nephrol., 30*, 141.

18. Cochat P, Brunet J, Philip T et al (1988) Étude de la néphrotoxicité du traitement par l'interleukine-2 chez l'enfant. *Thérapie, 43*, 129.
19. Atkins MB, Mier JW, Parkinson DR et al (1988) Hypothyroidism after treatment with interleukin-2 and lymphokine-activated killer cells. *N. Engl. J. Med., 318*, 1559.
20. Van Liessum PA, De Mulder PHM, Mattijssen EJM, Corstens FHM, Wagener DJ (1989) Hypothyroidism and goitre during interleukin-2 therapy without LAK cells. *Lancet, 1*, 224.
21. Beuzeboc P, Escourolle H, Dorval T et al (1989) Hypothyroïdie après traitement par l'interleukine-2. *Presse Méd., 18*, 727.
22. Hartmann LC, Urba WJ, Steis RG et al (1989) Hypothyroidism after interleukin-2 therapy. *J. Clin. Oncol., 7*, 686.
23. Weinstein A, Bujak D, Mittelman A, Davidan M (1987) Erythema nodosum in a patient with renal cell carcinoma treated with interleukin-2 and lymphokine-activated killer cells. *J. Am. Med. Assoc., 258*, 3120.
24. Ramseur WL, Richards F, Duggan DB (1989) A case of fatal pemphigus vulgaris in association with beta interferon and interleukin-2 therapy. *Cancer, 63*, 2005.
25. Lee RE, Gaspari AA, Lotze MT et al (1988) Interleukin-2 and psoriasis. *Arch. Dermatol., 124*, 1811.
26. Wallace DJ, Margolin K, Waller P (1988) Fibromyalgia and interleukin-2 therapy for malignancy. *Ann. Intern. Med., 108*, 909.
27. Hoffman M, Mittelman A, Dworkin B et al (1989) Severe intrahepatic cholestasis in patients treated with recombinant interleukin-2 and lymphokine-activated killer cells. *J. Cancer Res. Clin. Oncol., 115*, 175.
28. Hanaue H, Kim DY, Machimura T et al (1987) Hemolytic streptococcus preparation OK-432; beneficial adjuvant therapy in recurrent gastric carcinoma. *Tokai J. Exp. Clin. Med., 12*, 209.
29. Ishihara K, Hasegawa T, Okazaki M et al (1988) OK 432 Chemical pleurodesis as a standard therapy of spontaneous pneumothorax. *Jpn. J. Thorac. Dis., 26*, 10.
30. Hertler AA, Spitler LE, Frankel AE (1987) Humoral immune response to a ricin A chain immunotoxin in patients with metastatic melanoma. *Cancer Drug Deliver, 4*, 245.
31. Von Wussow P, Spitler L, Block B, Deicher H (1988) Immunotherapy in patients with advanced malignant melanoma using a monoclonal antimelanoma antibody ricin A immunotoxin. *Eur. J. Cancer Clin. Oncol., 24*, S-69.
32. Gepner P (1988) Immunotolérance du RU 41740. *Presse Méd., 17*, 1421.
33. Grazia Bernengo M, Doveil GC, Meregalli M et al (1988) Immunomodulation and Sézary syndrome: experience with thymopentin (TP-5). *Br. J. Dermatol., 119*, 207.
34. Gossain VV, Dimitrov N, Ashby D et al (1988) Effect of thymosin (fraction 5) on the plasma levels of glucose and glucoregulatory hormones in humans. *J. Med. (N.Y.), 19*, 335.
35. Feinberg B, Kurzrock R, Talpaz M et al (1988) A phase I trial of intravenously administered recombinant tumor necrosis factor-alpha in cancer patients. *J. Clin. Oncol., 6*, 1328.
36. Steinmetz T, Schaadt M, Gähl R et al (1988) Phase I study of 24-hour continuous intravenous infusion of recombinant human tumor necrosis factor. *J. Biol. Response Modif., 7*, 417.
37. Hogan M, Beyer J, Stuermer W et al (1988) Influence of ciamexon on blood glucose and insulin requirement in newly manifested type I diabetes. *Arzneim.-Forsch., 38*, 1185.
38. Lang JM, Touraine JL, Trep C et al (1988) Randomised, double-blind, placebo-controlled trial of dithiocarb sodium ('Imuthiol') in human immunodeficiency virus infection. *Lancet, 2*, 702.
39. Chlebowski RT, Nystrom S, Reynolds R et al (1988) Long-term survival following levamisole or placebo adjuvant treatment of colorectal cancer: a Western cancer study group trial. *Oncology, 45*, 141.
40. Bever CT, McFarland HF, McFarlin DE, Levy HB (1988) The kinetics of interferon induction by poly ICLC in humans. *J. Interferon Res., 8*, 419.

H.D. Reuter

40 Vitamins

GENERAL TOPICS

Vitamin supplementation in children *(1[r])* It is generally accepted that the diets of most children contain enough vitamins to prevent deficiency diseases. Full-term babies who are either breast-fed or bottle-fed are not likely to develop vitamin deficiencies. Very premature infants do, however, need supplementary vitamins because they do not have the stores normally laid down during the last trimester of pregnancy; they particularly need vitamin D and folic acid during the first 6 months of life. Vitamin supplementation is also needed in babies of lactating mothers with low vitamin intake, who as well as providing insufficient vitamins in their breast milk are likely to have transferred inadequate amounts of vitamins across the placenta during late pregnancy. Babies of vegetarian mothers may, for example, develop megaloblastic anemia and rickets from deficiency of vitamin B_{12} and D. The heat-labile vitamin C may be destroyed in formula feeds and during the preparation of food. There is thus good reason for all babies and toddlers to receive supplements of vitamins A, C and D as multivitamin drops.

A more controversial question is whether subclinical vitamin deficiencies can have various non-specific effects. The provision of 'freedom of choice' for youngsters in meals they buy and the growth of the 'junk food' industry have led to concern that school-age children may not be getting enough vitamins. A double-blind placebo-controlled trial showed that non-verbal intelligence was improved by supplements of vitamins and minerals. This finding would have wide implications if correct, but it has been criticized on methodological and statistical grounds. Unfortunately, the study included both vitamins and minerals in the supplement, so the effect of either alone is unknown.

There are considerable attractions for both parents and health professionals in ascribing often intractable and worrying problems to causes that might be amenable to simple dietary solutions and that carry no pejorative implications. It should however be kept in mind that treatment with high doses of vitamins, particularly with the fat-soluble vitamins A and D, may have side effects. Though water-soluble vitamins are safer, they can also have undesired effects. Thus, huge of doses of ascorbic acid may cause hematuria and a massive intake of pyridoxine has been associated with peripheral neuropathy.

Vulval pruritus caused by oral vitamin preparations Vulval pruritus can be caused by a wide variety of conditions and provocative factors. Among others it can be induced by oral vitamin preparations (2[c]).

VITAMIN A (RETINOL) *(SED-11, 799; SEDA-12, 327; SEDA-13, 346)*

Even moderate amounts of vitamin A, when ingested over a prolonged period of time, can cause significant hepatocellular injury. This is emphasized by a report of vitamin A *hepatotoxicity* in several members of a family. Three out of 5 family members experienced symptoms and biochemical evidence of hepatitis that could not be explained on the basis of infectious, metabolic or immunological disorders of the liver. A history of prolonged ingestion of 20 000–45 000 IU per dag for 7–10 years was obtained in each of the 3 family members (father, 62 years old; mother, 63 years old; son 33 years old) and was absent in the remaining 2 unaffected individuals. Vitamin A toxicity in one family member was confirmed by liver biopsy (3[C]).

An update of vitamin A toxicology is summarized by Biesalski and Seelert (4[R]). Accord-

Side Effects of Drugs Annual 14
M.N.G. Dukes and L. Beeley, editors

ing to the review by Bauernfeind (5[C]), symptoms of toxicity develop more quickly when very high daily doses are ingested. With daily intake of 1 000 000 IU toxicity develops within days or weeks. Intake of 400 000–700 000 IU per day produces symptoms of hypervitaminosis after 1–36 months and daily doses of 150 000–200 000 IU produce toxicity only after 6–85 months.

The frequency and severity of toxicity in general depend on the vitamin status of the individual. Thus, in persons with low hepatic vitamin stores, high daily doses are tolerated much better than in persons with normal stores.

Because the development of toxic symptoms depends on various factors such as liver stores, age, protein intake and underlying diseases, an absolute real therapeutic range cannot be defined. Goodman et al (6[C]) found that daily intake of 200 000 IU vitamin A per m^2 body surface corresponding to about 330 000 IU per patient for up to 4 months did not result in important side effects. Precautions have however to be taken in pregnant women and in women capable of childbearing.

In animals both deficiency and massive overdose with vitamin A can be teratogenic. In humans only a few cases of teratogenicity associated with vitamin A (in the form of retinol or retinylester) have been observed. Rosa and colleagues from the Food and Drug Administration (FDA) have reported 18 cases of malformations correlated with high doses of vitamin A taken long before and during pregnancy (7[C]). They conclude that: ‘though the data so far do not provide human dose/risk estimates, findings in laboratory studies and human experience with other vitamin A analogues provide reason for cautioning against long term intake of 25 000 units per day or more in women who may become pregnant.’ On the basis of laboratory studies, of experiences with retinoids in man and of the few cases of fetal lesions during 1987 recommendations have been issued by several institutions concerning dosage of vitamin A in pregnant women. The FDA, the Teratology Society and the American College of Obstetricians and Gynecologists recommend that pregnant women and women who may become pregnant limit their daily vitamin A intake for food supplementation to a maximum of 8000 IU. 10 000 IU of vitamin A per day is the recommendation issued by the Council of Responsible Nutrition and the International Vitamin A Consultative Group (IVACG). The limits of 8000 and 10 000 IU per day for pregnant women cannot be substantiated scientifically. They result from the high safety consciousness of all responsible institutions.

The hepatic complications of long-term ingestion of vitamin A include hepatomegaly, abnormal biochemical tests, portal hypertension, and even cirrhosis. The role of perisinusoidal cells in the genesis of fibrosis linked to vitamin A ingestion was first suggested when electron microscopy showed collagen deposits in close contact with perisinusoidal cells in Disse’s space in chronic hypervitaminosis A with portal hypertension and ascites. Since then, in several cases of hypervitaminosis A, investigators have stressed that an excessive amount of vitamin A in perisinusoidal cells may stimulate fibrinogenesis but have not given further evidence. There is much evidence showing that perisinusoidal cells (Ito’s cells) store vitamin A and are involved in fibrinogenesis. The presence of vimentin attests to their mesenchymal origin and the presence of desmin is in favor of their myoid differentiation. Moreover, perisinusoidal cells acquire certain characteristics of fibroblasts or myofibroblasts, as shown by electron microscopy, in diseases with progressive liver fibrosis (e.g. alcoholic cirrhosis), in diseases with liver cell necrosis (e.g. after CCl_4 administration) and in miscellaneous conditions (including chronic venous congestion). A report of the chance discovery of hepatic fibrosis in a patient with asymptomatic hypervitaminosis A (8[c]) is the first in which the liver ultrastructure has been investigated before clinical or liver function abnormalities have occurred.

A liver biopsy specimen was obtained from a 50-year-old patient who had taken approximately 40 000 IU per day of vitamin A for 4 years (4 times the maximum required). Liver architecture was normal with slightly dilated perisinusoids in zone 2 and numerous and enlarged perisinusoidal cells. On Sirius red staining, there was mild fibrosis of the central veins, portal tracts, and terminal portal venules and perisinusoidal fibrosis in zone 1 of the acinus. Liver vitamin A level was increased. On electron microscopy, perisinusoidal cells filled with numerous lipid droplets had slightly dilated rough endoplasmatic reticulum, numerous minute filament condensations below the plasma membrane, and stellate-shaped processes giving them the appearance of fibroblast-myofibroblast-like cells. Numerous collagen bundles, fibrils, amorphous material, and fragments of basement-membrane-like material were identified in Disse's space. Immuno-cytochemistry showed increased amounts of collagen types I, III, IV, laminin, and fibronectin. This observation suggests that vitamin A *per se*, and not the cellular damage often seen in hypervitaminosis A, is responsible for fibrosis.

β-Carotene

A transitory dose-dependent *carotenodermia* was seen in the course of treatment of erythropoietic protoporphyria with β-carotene (100 mg/d by mouth for 20 days) in an 18-year-old male patient (9[c]).

VITAMIN B *(SED-11, 801; SEDA-12, 328; SEDA-13, 347)*

Nicotinic acid (*SED-11, 802)*

A case of self-administered intra-arterial injection of nicotinic acid in a patient with dystrophia myotonica is reported (10[c]). A 27-year-old former male nurse presented 3 hours after accidentally injecting a suspension of several tablets of nicotinic acid (niacin) in tap water into his right ulnar artery. The injection resulted in a continuous blockade of the brachial plexus via the axillary route with severe *peripheral ischemia.* Severe peripheral ischemia also has been reported following intra-arterial injection of many drugs. The vascular damage is probably the result of a combination of vasospasm, endothelial damage and occlusion of the vessel by embolization or thrombus. Further, the injected drug may crystallize at body pH and a direct toxic effect may result in a vasculitis with further reduction in blood flow.

Niacin *maculopathy* is reported in 4 patients who had been taking daily doses of 3.0–4.5 g niacin as a serum-cholesterol-lowering drug (11[C]). Three of the patients with niacin-induced visual symptoms (blurring of central vision, seeing haloes round lights) had cystoid maculopathy without leakage on fluorescein angiography, the 4th patient exhibited no fundus abnormality. In all patients the visual symptoms disappeared upon cessation of niacin therapy. An additional 15 asymptomatic patients who were receiving daily doses of 1.0–1.6 g niacin for the treatment of hypercholesterolemia were evaluated for evidence of subclinical macular disease. None of these patients had cystic or other significant macular changes. Over the last 9 years in the Lipid Disorders Clinic at the Oregon Health Sciences University approximately 300 patients have been treated with niacin for hyperlipidemia. In only 2 cases was definite cystoid maculopathy observed. Thus the incidence of documented niacin maculopathy in these patients is estimated at 0.67%. Reports in the literature of loss of vision due to high-dose niacin are likewise rare.

Folic acid *(SED-11, 803; SEDA-13, 348)*

The existence of a relationship between some anticonvulsant compounds and folic acid is now common knowledge. Phenytoin, primidone and phenobarbital affect folate absorption at the level of the intestinal mucosa, and low levels of folate have been observed in serum, red cells and cerebrospinal fluid of patients on long-term anticonvulsant therapy. It has been suggested that the antiepileptic action of some drugs may be partly mediated by their antifolate action. Though the vast majority of patients with epilepsy are not adversely affected by folic acid supplementation, the apparent deleterious effect of folic acid on individual epileptic patients should not be ignored. Sensitivity to the epileptogenic effect of folic acid may be quite rare, but when present it represents a major therapeutic problem. In a study reported here, 19 epileptic patients (16 on chronic antiepileptic treatment and 3 untreated at the time of observation) and 10 age-matched healthy volunteers were slowly infused with 50 ml saline containing 10 mEq of 5-methyltetrahydrofolate with continuous EEG monitoring to detect a possible increase in epileptic activity. Folate infusion had no clinical effect in healthy volunteers and 16 epileptic patients. Two of 19 patients (with partial seizures secondarily generalized and on carbamazepine and phenobarbital therapy) exhibited a slight increase in spike focal activity in comparison with the baseline recordings. Another patient with secondary generalized seizures and on treatment with carbamazepine and phenobarbital, 4 min after the beginning of folate intravenous administration showed a marked slowing of the basal EEG activity and the presence of multiple spike and wave generalized discharges, accompanied by diffuse myoclonic jerks and a reduced level of consciousness. This situation was followed by serveral (4–6 per day) elementary partial and partial complex seizures, which lasted for the next 9 days despite intensive treatment with intravenous diazepam. The data confirm the presence of an *epileptogenic* effect of folic acid. This effect, occurring in a small percentage of patients, may produce early changes on the EEG which can prevent such patients being exposed to the dangerous side effects of folate therapy (10[C]).

VITAMIN C (ASCORBIC ACID) *(SED-11, 803; SEDA-13, 348)*

A premature infant, born after 27 weeks gestation, developed anemia and jaundice 2 days after receiving a multivitamin preparation. 20% of the red blood cells contained Heinz bodies. Numerous 'bite cells' and other abnormally shaped erythrocytes were noted in a blood film. When the medication was stopped, the hemolysis ceased and Heinz body numbers decreased to 2%. On rechallenge with the multivitamin preparation (Poly-Vi-Sol) Heinz bodies reappeared in the red blood cells. This observation, together with the fact that ascorbic acid can act as an oxidant, suggested to the authors that vitamin C might have been responsible for the *erythrocyte damage*. A study was therefore undertaken to investigate the effect of ascorbic acid on erythrocytes obtained from premature infants, full-term infants and adults. In vitro incubation of erythrocytes of premature infants with 0.1 mg/ml sodium ascorbate for 3 hours significantly raised the percentage of Heinz-body-containing cells from 17.6 ± 5.7 to 27.2 ± 8.2 (mean $\pm$ SD). Erythrocytes of term infants and those of adults developed Heinz bodies after exposure to higher sodium ascorbate concentrations (1.0 mg/ml). Erythrocytes of adult and newborn guinea-pigs were similarly affected by sodium ascorbate. Daily intraperitoneal injections of 500 mg of sodium ascorbate, given for 7 days to 4 adult guinea pigs, caused significant Heinz-body formation. These studies indicate that the erythrocytes of premature infants are uniquely sensitive to the development of Heinz bodies after exposure to sodium ascorbate. The levels required to produce Heinz bodies in vitro are in the range of those found in vivo after routine administration of vitamin C to premature infants. The significance of these observations for the development of hyperbilirubinemia in premature infants and the safety of vitamin C remains to be determined (13[C]).

VITAMIN D (CALCIFEROL) AND ANALOGS *(SED-11, 805; SEDA-12, 334)*

Hypervitaminosis D with *hypercalcemia* and *acute renal failure* developed in 4 female patients with osteoporosis or osteomalacia. All patients were given pharmacological doses for 6 weeks to 5 years. 25-Hydroxyvitamin D levels were elevated in 3 patients (mean 247 ng/ml; range 142–322). Levels were not determined in the 4th patient who became normocalcemic when vitamin D was discontinued (14[C,R]).

The hypothesis that reversal of the negative calcium balance associated with senile, postmenopausal and glucocorticoid-induced osteoporosis with vitamin D metabolites could lead to skeletal stabilization or healing has been extensively tested. The use of pharmacological doses of vitamin D has become common clinical therapy, despite lack of clearcut efficacy and safety. Hypervitaminosis D reported in patients with osteoporosis suggests that pharmacological doses of vitamin D should be avoided in patients suffering from any form of osteoporosis. Published data on the use of vitamin D for prophylaxis or treatment of osteoporosis fail to document benefits superior to those of calcium alone or calcium with estrogens and fluoride. Data on the use of 25-hydroxyvitamin D show no greater benefit than for vitamin D. The use of 1,25-dihydroxyvitamin D plus calcium may be superior to the use of calcium alone in some forms of osteoporosis (14[R]).

VITAMIN E (α-TOCOPHEROL) *(SED-11, 723; SEDA-12, 330; SEDA-13, 349)*

Postrhinoplasty *epistaxis* occurred in 2 patients who had been ingesting megadoses of vitamin E (>400 mg/d). The rate of vitamin E consumption in a population of 100 uncomplicated nasal operations during the same period was 16%. Seven patients ingested daily doses of 100 g, 9 patients 400 mg (15[c,r]).

Although vitamin E does not have significant effects on the coagulation factors of healthy humans and animals (16[R]) vitamin E therapy in vitamin-K-deficient subjects and subjects on anticoagulant therapy has a marked effect on hemostasis by decreasing active plasma *prothrombin* levels (17[C]). A statistically significant increase in retinal hemorrhage with parenteral vitamin E was found in premature infants (18[C]). Investigations on the potential role of vitamin E as an inhibitor of platelet aggregation in healthy volunteers given vitamin E in dosages of 400–1200 mg/d showed a small but sigificant reduction in collagen-induced platelet aggregation. Even more striking was the reduction of platelet adhesion to collagen (19[C]). These results were recently confirmed using a dynamic flow chamber (20[C]). An almost complete lack of platelet adhesion was observed at the 400 mg/d dose. This effect was amplified with vitamin E ingestion up to 1200 mg/d. Vitamin E exerts its antiaggregating effect without inhibiting the enzymes of the arachidonic acid cascade in the platelets (21[C]).

A further side effect of vitamin E supplements in premature infants is *necrotizing enterocolitis*. Determination of the α-tocopherol concentrations in 52 preterm infants receiving $<$ 25 mg/kg/d α-tocopherol acetate supplements in intravenous hyperalimentation solutions, lipid and oral α-tocopherol showed concentrations of $>$ 3.5 mg/100 ml at least once in 25% of the infants. Another 25% of the infants had concentrations $<$ 0.5 mg/100 ml through the first postnatal week. The highly variable serum tocopherol concentrations correlated with total serum lipid content but not with plasma α-tocopherol hydrolysis activity (22[C]). A correlation was found between concentrations of α-tocopherol exceeding 3.5 mg/100 ml and necrotizing enterocolitis.

VITAMIN K *(SED-11, 809; SEDA-13, 349)*

Vitamin K (phytomenadione) *(SED-11, 758, 809; SEDA-12, 330; SEDA-13, 349)*

Localized *pseudoscleroderma (Texier's syndrome)* occurring around the sites of intramuscular injection of phytomenadione in a female with drug-induced liver disease is reported (23[c]). The patient had been treated with 10 mg phytomenadione daily intramuscularly into the thighs for 13 days. This is the first report on Texier's syndrome to appear in the Britisch literature.

REFERENCES

1. Taitz LS (1988) Which children need vitamins? *Br. Med. J., 296,* 1753.
2. Commens C (1988) Vulval pruritus caused by mouth vitamin preparation. *Med. J. Aust., 148,* 658.
3. Minuk GY, Kelly JK, Hwang W-S (1988) Vitamin A hepatotoxicity in multiple family members. *Hepatology, 8,* 272.
4. Biesalski HK, Seelert K (1988) Vitamin A: Neue Erkenntnisse, Nutzen und Risiko. *Dtsch. Apoth.-Z., 128,* 1662.
5. Bauernfeind JC (1980) *The Safe Use of Vitamin A.* The Nutrition Foundation, Washington DC.
6. Goodman GE, Alberts DS, Ernest DL (1983) Phase I trial of retinol in cancer patients. *J. Clin. Oncol., 1,* 394.
7. Rosa FW, Wilk AL, Kelsey FO (1986) Teratogen update: vitamin A congeners. *Teratology, 33,* 355.
8. Bioulac-Sage P, Quinton A, Saric J et al (1988) Chance discovery of hepatic fibrosis in patient with asymptomatic hypervitaminosis A. *Arch. Pathol. Lab. Med., 112,* 505.
9. Pravettoni C, Pinelli S, Veraldi S, Bertani E (1988) Trattamento della protoporfiria eritropeoietica con beta-carotene. *Chronic Derm., 19,* 45.
10. Dyson A, Henderson AM (1987) Continuous axillary brachial plexus blockade following intra-arterial injection of nicotinic acid. *Anaesth. Intensive Care, 15,* 462.
11. Millay RH, Klein ML, Illingworth DR (1988) Niacin maculopathy. *Ophthalmology 95,* 930.
12. Bramanti P, Ricci RM, Bagala S et al (1987) Does folic acid exert a provocative action on the EEG of epileptic patients? A preliminary report. *Acta Neurol., 42,* 250.
13. Ballin A, Brown EJ, Koren G, Zipursky A (1988) Vitamin C-induced erythrocyte damage in premature infants. *J. Pediatr., 113,* 114.
14. Schwartzman MS, Franck WA (1987) Vitamin D toxicity complicating the treatment of senile, postmenopausal, and glucocorticoid-induced osteoporosis: four case reports and a critical commentary

on the use of vitamin D in these disorders. *Am. J. Med., 82,* 224.
15. Churukian MM, Zemplenyi J, Steiner M et al (1988) Postrhinoplasty epistaxis. *Arch. Otolaryngol. Head Neck Surg., 114,* 748.
16. Hale WE, Perkins LL, May FE et al (1986) Vitamin E effect on symptoms and laboratory values in the elderly. *J. Am. Diet Assoc., 114,* 625.
17. Helson L (1984) The effect of intravenous vitamin E and nenadiol sodium diphosphate on vitamin K-dependent clotting factors. *Thrombos. Res., 35,* 11.
18. Rosenbaum AL, Phelps DL, Isenberg SJ et al (1985) Retinal hemorrhage in retinopathy of prematurity associated with tocopherol treatment. *Ophthalmology, 92,* 1012.
19. Steiner M (1983) Effect of alpha tocopherol administration on platelet function in man. *Thromb. Haemost, 49,* 73.
20. Jandok J, Steiner M (1986) An effective inhibitor of platelet adhesion. *Blood, 68,* 1153.
21. Srivastave KC (1986) Vitamin E exerts antiaggregatory effects without inhibiting the enzymes of the arachidonic acid cascade in platelets. *Prostglandins Leukotrienes Med., 21,* 177.
22. Friedman CA, Wender DF, Temple DM et al (1988) Serum alpha-tocopherol concentrations in preterm infants receiving less than 25 mg/kg/day alpha-tocopherol acetate supplements. *Dev. Pharmacol. Ther., 11,* 273.
23. Brunskill NJ, Beth-Jones J, Graham-Brown RAC (1988) Pseudosclerodermatous reaction to phytomenadione injection (Texier's syndrome). *Clin. Exp. Dermatol., 13,* 276.

S. Erill

41 Corticotrophins and corticosteroids

CORTICOSTEROIDS *(SED-11, 815; SEDA-12, 332; SEDA-13, 352)*

Case-reports of adverse effects of corticosteroids continue to appear regularly. Along with these, more sophisticated articles dealing with dose–effect relationships, identification of early markers of severe effects or elucidation of biochemical mechanisms certainly contribute to our understanding of the incidence and nature of adverse effects of corticosteroids, and may hopefully lead to the safer use of these very valuable drugs.

MISCELLANEOUS REPORTS

Psychiatric syndromes *(SED-11, 817; SEDA-12, 334; SEDA-13, 352)* Episodes of *acute psychosis* during treatment with high doses of corticosteroids (1[c]) are not necessarily surprising, but it is perhaps worth insisting upon the notion that these episodes may occur a few days after termination of treatment (2[c]). On the other hand, recognition of this side effect may be more difficult if the condition being treated can itself lead to the development of psychosis, as in the case of systemic lupus erythematosus (3[c], 4[c]).

Mood elevation is a recognized effect of corticosteroids and therefore one should not be surprised to read, in a recent report from Canada (5[Cr]), that a patient who experienced moderate euphoria and decreased fatigue while taking prednisone for an acute asthmatic episode subsequently managed to obtain prescriptions for this drug from different physicians during the ensuing year. Periods of temporary abstinence resulted in dysphoric symptoms (depressed mood, irritability and fatigue) and these would prompt him to escalate his steroid intake when the drug became available. Interestingly, this patient presented with a psychotic behavior when 3 years later he was given high doses of prednisone for the treatment of temporal arteritis.

Development of *mania* in patients treated with high doses of steroids is well documented, but this complication seldom occurs after treatment is discontinued. A recent communication (6[C]) adds one more case to the very short list of reports of mania associated with *steroid withdrawal.* Nevertheless, new steroid-induced psychiatric disorders continue to be reported, and an article from Hungary (7[C]) presents the case of a 32-year-old patient in whom *panic attacks* developed during maintenance corticosteroid therapy.

Endocrine, metabolic *(SED-11, 817; SEDA-12, 334; SEDA-13, 353)*

Corticosteroids and growth

The growth-inhibiting effects of corticosteroids in children have long been recognized, but there is still much to be learned about this phenomenon. For instance, it is generally acknowledged that use of single doses of prednisone on alternate mornings minimizes growth retardation, but there are cases in which children treated with this regimen are definitely short or show delay in their sexual maturation. A very interesting paper in the Archives of Disease in Childhood (8[C]) deals with the endocrine function of children with steroid-sensitive nephrotic syndrome, and shows that long-term steroid treatment given throughout adolescence has an adverse effect on the rate of growth in boys, despite

(Biomedical Division)
Side Effects of Drugs Annual 14
M.N.G. Dukes and L. Beeley, editors

the use of a low-dose alternate regimen for the major part of the treatment course (effects in girls were not significant, perhaps because the number was smaller and the duration of treatment shorter). Mean age at diagnosis in the boys studied was 3 years, and the beginning of a fall in growth velocity occurred at the age of 10 years, with a sudden sharp decline in all the boys at the age of 13 years. This, together with a high incidence of delayed appearance of secondary sex characteristics, strongly suggests an independent effect of steroids on the onset and progression of puberty and the pubertal growth spurt. In fact, the authors were able to show, by means of overnight profile analysis, that steroid treatment considerably affects physiological secretion of growth hormone and gonadotrophins with reduction in pulse amplitude, but not in pulse number, in both cases. As the authors rightly point out, despite the evidence in the literature that final height is usually acceptable, there is a definite clinical problem with associated emotional difficulties, and their findings clearly suggest that some sort of therapeutic intervention could be envisaged.

It is of interest to note that by means of a knemometer, a device designed to measure changes in tibial length with great accuracy, authors from England have recorded a variation in lower leg growth with alternate-day prednisolone treatment in a 11.6-year-old boy with Crohn's disease (9[C]). It is claimed that the precision of measurement is 0.2 mm and that the magnitude of the observed changes in lower leg length were well within the capabilities of the device. Were these observations confirmed, this could represent the first direct observation of the growth-sparing effect of alternate-day steroid treatment.

As recently pointed out in an editorial (10[R]), our understanding of the pathogenesis of growth inhibition by corticosteroids is limited. In this context, an article in The Journal of Pediatrics (11[CR]), exploring the relationship of Type I procollagen to corticosteroid therapy in children with inflammatory bowel disease, provides very valuable data. In this study, growth velocity and serum concentrations of the C-terminal propeptide of Type I procollagen were evaluated for 2–6 months in a group of 60 children with ulcerative colitis or Crohn's disease. For each of the two categories of disease severity considered (mild and moderate/severe), procollagen concentrations and growth velocity were lower in patients receiving daily corticosteroid therapy than in patients treated with alternate-day steroids or not receiving any corticosteroid. In this study, there were no differences between the alternate-day and the non-steroid groups. On the other hand, the authors were able to study 7 asthmatic children, currently receiving only theophylline therapy, 24–48 hours after the initiation of intravenous methylprednisolone therapy to control an acute attack. In these children, the administration of the steroid was associated with a dramatic decrease in procollagen concentrations. In view of the results of this study, and of previous data from the same group showing that serum procollagen is a biochemical marker of growth in children with inflammatory bowel diseases, it seems logical to conclude that longitudinal measurement of procollagen concentrations may provide rapid assessment of the effects of different corticosteroids regimens on growth.

Addisonian crises are usually very easy to recognize in patients with a known diagnosis of hypoadrenalism, but, as illustrated by a recent report of 2 cases (12[C]), the diagnosis may be notoriously problematic in patients taking high doses of glucocorticoids. Both patients presented on more than one occasion in an acutely ill state with what were recognized subsequently as episodes of addisonian crisis, despite taking relatively high doses (30–40 mg daily) of prednisone for an underlying inflammatory disease (recurrent pleuropericarditis and sarcoidosis, respectively) rarely associated with primary hypoadrenalism. One cannot refrain from borrowing the words of an editorial in the same issue of the journal reporting these cases (13) and refer to the emerging nature of the corticosteroids as 'great camoufleurs, great deceivers'.

Patients treated with corticosteroids are at increased risk for *atherosclerotic vascular disease* and a recent study (14[C]) of plasma lipids and apolipoprotein levels in steroid-treated patients with systemic lupus erythematosus (SLE) casts some light on the factors leading to this increased risk. In this study of 38 women with SLE (28 treated with steroids and 10 not receiving these drugs), compared with 15 normal women, there were significant differences between the corticosteroid-treated group and the other two groups with regard to plasma concentrations of triglycerides, total cholesterol and apolipoprotein B levels. It has been reported (15) that the production rates of VLDL triglycerides and apolipoprotein B are enhanced in animals treated with prednisone. Since the level of apolipoprotein B may be an independent risk factor for the development of atherosclerosis, the association of increased levels of apolipoprotein B and dyslipoproteinemia may explain the increased risk of atherosclerosis in patients (particularly women) treated with corticosteroids.

Lipomatosis *(SEDA-11, 338)* Spinal cord compression secondary to epidural lipomatosis is a rare complication of corticosteroid treatment, but isolated reports continue to appear (16[C]). In these cases, laminectomy is regularly called for to achieve decompression, but a report from Japan (17[C]) describes the second patient in the literature in which reduction of steroid dosage alone sufficed to achieve recovery of neurological function.

The spinal canal is not the only site of steroid-induced fat deposition. Apart from the well-known features of Cushing's disease, fat deposition in the central body axis is a recognized effect of corticosteroids, and a recent report (18[C]) of cough and shortness of breath in a 73-year-old man treated with dexamethasone, as adjuvant therapy for an astrocytoma, shows that fat envelopment of the mediastinal structures is indeed a possible complication of steroid therapy.

Myopathy and effects on myasthenia gravis *(SED-11, 822; SEDA-12, 333)* Cases of acute myopathy in patients with severe asthma treated with high doses of corticosteroids continue to be reported (19[C], 20[C]) and some suspicion has arisen that the conditions of mechanical ventilation might increase in some unknown way the potential of corticosteroids to cause myopathy. Interestingly, an antagonistic interaction between corticosteroids and anticholinesterase agents has been described in experimental studies in animals, and this has led to the investigation of the potential need to discontinue anticholinesterase drugs when starting high-dose corticosteroid therapy in patients with myasthenia gravis. In this study (21[C]), the improvement in neuromuscular function after single doses of prednisone + pyridostigmine was more marked than after pyridostigmine alone, while prednisone alone had no effect. Thus, there does not seem to be any evidence for an adverse interaction between corticosteroids and anticholinesterase drugs in patients with myasthenia gravis.

Osteonecrosis and osteoporosis *(SED-11, 821; SEDA-12, 332; SEDA-13, 354)* Not surprisingly, the effects of steroids on bone continue to attract wide attention, and reviews of the problems created (22[R]) as well as descriptions of cases (23[C]) continue to appear in the literature. Curiously enough, even in this somewhat crowded field there is room for novelty, and an article from Japan (24[C]) describes, apparently for the first time, 2 cases of steroid-induced *necrosis of the patella*, precisely in patients who had previously experienced necrosis of the femoral head.

As mentioned in SEDA-12 (p. 332), controversy continues regarding the dose and duration of treatment necessary to induce *osteoporosis*. In this context, it is worth noting a recent study (25[c]), in healthy young men, that clearly shows that administration of daily 60 mg doses of prednisone rapidly results in a fall in serum osteocalcin, a bone matrix protein that appears to correlate with bone formation rate. In this study, an attempt was made to obtain dose–response relationships. Twenty healthy subjects were divided into 4 groups and received either 5, 10, 15 or 20 mg of prednisone at 8 a.m. on 2 consecutive days. No effects on serum osteocalcin were seen 48 hours after the last dose in subjects receiving the 5 mg dose, while there were significant and roughly dose-related falls in the other groups. Osteocalcin is synthesized by osteoblasts and, therefore, it is obvious that effects of corticosteroids on bone cells can be demonstrated long before clinical evidence of osteoporosis becomes apparent.

Acute effects of steroids on calcium and bone metabolism have also been assessed in a group of 10 patients with rheumatoid arthritis treated with pulses of 1 g methylprednisolone on 3 alternate days (26[C]). This study, from a group that had previously reported only minor and transient changes in bone metabolism in patients receiving methylprednisolone pulse therapy (see SEDA-12, 333), further illustrates the complexity of the effects of corticosteroids on bone in patients with diseases that themselves affect bone metabolism, and shows that decreases in serum calcium and subsequent increases in serum parathyroid hormone concentration are evident 24 hours after methylprednisolone pulses.

Mention was made in SEDA-12 (p. 332) that total body calcium may be reduced in patients treated with *inhaled* steroids. A new study (27^C), focusing on calcium and phosphate metabolism in healthy subjects receiving two different formulations of budenoside, fails to detect clear detrimental effects on this metabolism, even at high dosage. However, and in contrast with previous findings, both doses of budenoside (0.6 and 2.4 mg/d, inhaled via a cone spacer) did induce a state of functional hypogonadism, as evidenced by a reduction in the output of endogenous cortisol. Therefore, high-dose budenoside treatment cannot be assumed to be free of the risk of bone complications, since direct effects on bone cell function are possible.

The extent of the benefit afforded by *calcium and vitamin D supplements* in the prevention of steroid-induced osteoporosis is a matter of continuing controversy. The last link in the chain of partially contradictory findings is a study (28^C) which evaluated the effects of oral calcium or calcium + vitamin D in preventing bone loss in patients treated with more than 10 mg prednisone per day.

Fourteen patients were treated daily with 500 mg calcium and 16 patients with daily 500 mg calcium plus 0.1 mg dihydrotachysterol on alternate days. Twenty-one patients completed 2 years of the study and when changes in bone mineral mass, measured by dual photon absorptiometry, were analyzed it was found that both regimens were equally effective. There was a non-significant small increase in bone mineral mass in the lumbar spine in both groups, and a marginal decrease in the bone mineral content of both femoral necks in the calcium group, with a marginal increase in the calcium plus vitamin D group. There was no control group, but these data compare favorably with the expected decrease in bone mineral content during 2 years of treatment with corticosteroids.

Since the dose of vitamin D used in this study is considered quite adequate, the argument in favor of adding vitamin D to a calcium supplementation regimen seems to weaken.

Avascular necrosis of bone is a serious complication of corticosteroid therapy and there is some evidence suggesting that bolus steroids pose less risk than regular oral administration (see SEDA-12, 332). However, steroid pulse therapy cannot be proclaimed safe with regard to the risk of osteonecrosis. In a study (29^{Cr}) aimed at establishing the dose-range for effectiveness of methylprednisolone pulses in patients with rheumatoid arthritis it was found that avascular necrosis developed in 3 patients.

In 1 patient, bilateral humeral avascular necrosis became symptomatic 11 months after receiving a 40 mg and a 1 g methylprednisolone pulse 6 weeks apart. In this case, previous intra-articular injections may have played a role, but in the other 2 cases, necrosis of the femoral head ensued 8 months after a single 40 mg pulse and 6 months after a single infusion of 1 g. The protocol excluded patients who had received oral steroids during the preceding 6 months and the authors only mention that there were no obvious contributory factors in these 2 cases.

Since avascular necrosis of the bone can occur many months after treatment with steroids, it would be of interest to know the medication history of these 2 patients, but, at any event, there are grounds for worrying about the possible development of osteonecrosis in patients treated with pulse steroids.

Blood cells and lymphoid tissue *(SED-11, 819)* A new case (30^C) of *very high white blood cell counts and neutrophilia* in a pre-term infant whose mother had received 2 doses of betamethasone prenatally, to enhance fetal lung maturation, adds one more report to the very short list of leukemoid reactions associated with antenatal steroid treatment. Another unusual reaction is described in a report of a case of *acute tumor lysis syndrome* after steroid therapy for anaphylaxis (31^C). This patient, who suffered a leukemic relapse of a mediastinal lymphoblastic lymphoma, had an anaphylactic reaction after a platelet transfuction and was treated with adrenaline, diphenhydramine and intravenous methylprednisolone. This resulted in rapid tumor lysis with hyperuricemia, hyperphosphatemia, hypocalcemia and a rise in creatinine, requiring treatment with allopurinol and high-volume alkaline diuresis to achieve normal renal function.

Infections and infestations *(SED-11, 822; SEDA-12, 335)* Unusual forms of infections and infestations continue to be described in association with steroid therapy. Thus, another case of *cutaneous alternariasis* (32[C]) in a 78-year-old patient with temporal arteritis treated with prednisone, a case of *Q-fever-endocarditis* exacerbated by cardiac surgery and corticosteroid therapy (33[C]) and the description of 2 cases of *brain abscess* as a complication of esophageal dilatation and corticosteroid treatment of alkali-induced strictures (34[C]) can be found in the recent literature. However, as discussed in SED-11 (p. 822), the role of corticosteroids in infections arising in patients treated with these drugs can often be qualified, since the underlying disease may itself impair the immune response. *Amebic disease* may be precipitated by corticosteroids prescribed for tuberculous pleural effusions, as in 2 cases from Nepal (35[C]), and *trichophytic granuloma* may be associated with steroid treatment of bullous pemphigoid (36[C]), but one may always wonder what is the relative role of the well-known immunosuppressive effects of corticosteroids (37[R]), of the underlying disease, or even of other factors. Nevertheless, very rare infections are described in patients on steroids. A recent case-report from Sweden (38[Cr]) refers to a 51-year-old female farmer with sarcoidosis who suffered fever episodes, recurrent hemoptyses, general malaise and loss of weight after 28 months of continuous treatment with prednisolone in low doses. A chest roentgenogram showed a left upper lobe infiltrate (which later cavitated) and rib destruction. Diagnosis could only be made 22 months later, when blood and sputum cultures and cultures from the destroyed rib showed growth of *Rhodococcus equi*, a common soil organism which can cause infections in foals and other animals. Only a few cases of this type of infection, which can be treated successfully with erythromycin and rifampicin, have been described. In every case, immunosuppression attributable to the underlying disease or to its treatment seems to have played a role.

Pancreatitis Among the rare complications of steroid therapy, pancreatitis remains controversial, in spite of the numerous case-reports in the literature. A recent case-report, (39[CR]) of a 50-year-old male with Stage IIIB Hodgkin's disease, who developed clinically evident pancreatitis on 3 occasions after treatment with dexamethasone for symptoms of spinal cord compression, may finally settle the issue. On each occasion, epigastric abdominal pain, with elevations of serum amylase and lipase values, developed shortly after administration of dexamethasone (2 days after starting high doses of the steroid and 5 days after a more modest dose). These episodes rapidly resolved upon discontinuation of steroid therapy. There is some anecdotal evidence that corticoids may be beneficial in some patients with acute pancreatitis. Whatever the weight of this evidence, it now seems clear that corticosteroids may be an etiological factor in this disorder.

Kaposi's sarcoma This is widely known as a complication of AIDS, but the association should not obscure the link between these lesions and immunosuppressive therapy. A recent report from Philadelphia (40[Cr]) describes an elderly man with Wegener's granulomatosis treated with cyclophosphamide and corticosteroids who developed rapidly progressing cutaneous Kaposi's sarcoma 10 weeks after the start of immunosuppressive therapy with cyclophosphamide and corticosteroids. Interestingly, marked improvement of all skin lesions was noted 1 week after discontinuation of prednisone therapy, and nearly complete resolution was noted several weeks later, despite uninterrupted treatment with cyclophosphamide. Less documented, but also worth mentioning, is the case (41[Cr]) of a 57-year-old man in whom Kaposi's sarcoma occurred in conjunction with rheumatoid arthritis and polymyositis treated with corticosteroids.

Kaposi's sarcoma occurs in over 20% of patients with AIDS, and although the exact mechanism of development of this complication is not known, evidence is mounting that steroid treatment may play some role. A recent study (42[Cr]) of 7 patients who experienced an accelerated growth of Kaposi's sarcoma lesions during corticosteroid therapy clearly suggests that steroids may alter the biological behavior of this disease. In this series, rapid progression of lesions within 2 weeks of continuous steroid use or after 30 days of intermittent steroid therapy was detected in all patients. This progression manifested as enlargement of pre-existing lesions, as well as development of new ones. In one patient, who first developed Kaposi's sarcoma during treatment for non-Hodgkin's lymphoma with corticosteroids and cytotoxic chemotherapy, all lesions resolved spontaneously within 8 weeks of discontinuation of this treatment. Hydrocortisone accelerates the growth of cell lines derived from AIDS-Kaposi's sarcoma cultured in vitro (43) and this may partially explain the above-reported findings. With so many intriguing aspects in the events surrounding AIDS, even this bit of information is quite welcome.

Panniculitis The appearance of erythematous, firm, warm, subcutaneous nodules within 2 weeks of discontinuation of large doses of steroids is recognized as post-steroid panniculitis. This is an infrequently reported complication of steroid therapy and a new case (44[C]) confirms that restitution without scarring is the rule, and that reinstitution of corticosteroids is not necessary for improvement of this condition.

SPECIAL FORMS OF ADMINISTRATION *(SED-11, 824; SEDA-12, 336; SEDA-13, 355)*

Pulse therapy *(SED-11, 825; SEDA-12, 336)*

Bradycardia can develop in patients receiving methylprednisolone pulse therapy for rheumatoid arthritis (see SEDA-12, 336) and a recent report from Canada (45[C]) indicates that this complication can also be observed in babies with bronchopulmonary dysplasia treated with intravenous or even oral dexamethasone. In the 4 cases described, heart rate returned to baseline about 24 hours after dexamethasone was discontinued. Although a role for hypertension in the development of bradycardia cannot be ruled out in these patients (all 4 infants showed an increase in blood pressure) the observation of neurological effects after dexamethasone in some of these children raises the possibility of CNS involvement in the genesis of this complication.

Intravenous corticosteroids *(SEDA-12, 336; SEDA-13, 355)*

There is hardly anything new in the cadence of reports (46[C], 47) of *anaphylactic reactions* after intravenous injection of corticosteroids, but the case of a patient who suffered from an exanthema with pustules after intravenous administration of prednisolone sodium succinate, and who developed contact dermatitis 4 years later after application of an ointment with prednisolone, is worth mentioning. Acute anaphylaxis and contact dermatitis are quite different manifestations of hypersensitivity, but this case somehow strengthens the notion (see SEDA-11, p. 336) that many allergic-like reactions to systemic corticosteroids do qualify as true hypersensitivity reactions.

Inhaled and intranasally applied corticosteroids *(SED-11, 824; SEDA-12, 336; SEDA-13, 355) (see also discussion of osteoporosis above)*

'Not serious if care is taken' is the subtitle of a recent editorial (49[R]) in the *British Medical Journal* on the adverse effects of inhaled steroids, and although a new report (50[C]) tends to confirm that some degree of adrenal suppression can occur in adults receiving moderate doses of beclomethasone dipropionate, there is not, in fact, much new or alarming to contrast to the benefits of inhaled corticosteroids compared with long-term daily doses.

Reports from Italy about *hypercorticism syndromes* associated with nasal sprays continue to appear with regularity (51[c]), and it is again from Italy (52[C]) that we hear of development of cushingoid features resulting from *occupational exposure* to corticosteroids in the pharmaceutical industry.

Locally applied corticosteroids *(SEDA-12, 337)*

Subcutaneous atrophy following local corticosteroid injection is well known, but there are some peculiar forms worth mentioning. A recent report (53[CR]) describes 2 cases of *perilesional linear atrophy and hypopigmentation* in 2 black children, developing after intralesional injection of corticosteroids for treatment of cheloids. In both cases the hypopigmentation resolved in about 3 months. Whatever the exact pathogenesis (lymphogenous spread of the corticosteroid is suspected), perilesional linear atrophy or hypopigmentation (or both) seems a distinct complication of locally injected steroids.

CORTICOTROPHINS *(SED-11, 813; SEDA-13, 356)*

There is no doubt that corticotrophins share all the adverse effects of corticosteroids, including reduction of the body's defenses against infection and infestation (54[C]), while they may have unwanted effects of their own. As an example, one could mention the recent report (55[C]) of 2 cases of myoclonic encephalopathy in which ACTH induced a dramatic behavioral response that disappeared almost directly after changing the medication to prednisone. In these 2 patients (15 and 20 months old) behavior deteriorated to a state of *extreme dullness and depression* after starting treatment with ACTH (40 i.v. daily) and this abnormal behavior persisted during 3–4 weeks of therapy, even though clinical signs of myoclonic encephalopathy improved markedly. However, a striking behavioral improvement was noted 2 days after replacing ACTH by prednisone. As the authors point out, ACTH itself hardly passes the blood–brain barrier, but ACTH fragments do, and this may have desirable as well as undesirable consequences.

REFERENCES

1. Carden PA, Mitchell SL (1988) Acute psychosis plus neuroleptic malignant syndrome as complications of therapy in an adolescent with acute lymphoblastic leukaemia. *Aust. J. Hosp. Pharm., 18,* 205.
2. Vitas J, Jakovljevic M, Vitas M, Car N (1988) Akutna paranoidna psihoza kao posljedica ustezanja deksametazone. *Lijec. Vjesn., 110,* 94.
3. Hirohata S, Iwamoto S, Miyamoto T et al (1988) A patient with systemic lupus erythematosus presenting both central nervous system lupus and steroid induced psychosis. *J. Rheumatol., 15,* 706.
4. Hasegawa T, Miyakoshi T, Takahashi T et al (1987) SLE psychosis and steroid psychosis. *Tohoku Igaru Zasshi, 100,* 1.
5. Parker WA (1988) Corticosteroid-induced addiction and psychosis. *Can. J. Hosp. Pharm., 41,* 153.
6. Venkatarangam SHM, Kutcher SP, Notkin RM (1988) Secondary mania with steroid withdrawal. *Can. J. Psychiatry, 33,* 631.
7. Perényhi A, Frecska E, Badgy G, Barcs G (1988) Panic attacks as a consequence of chronic corticosteroid therapy? *Eur. J. Psychiatry, 2,* 69.
8. Rees L, Greene SA, Adlard P et al (1988) Growth and endocrine function in steroid sensitive nephrotic syndrome. *Arch. Dis. Child., 63,* 484.
9. Wales JKH, Milner RDG (1988) Variation in lower leg growth with alternate day steroid treatment. *Arch. Dis. Child., 63,* 981.
10. Hyams JS, Carey DE (1988) Corticosteroids and growth. *J. Pediatr., 113,* 249.
11. Hyams JS, Moore RE, Leichtner AM (1988) Relationship of type I procollagen to corticosteroid therapy in children with inflammatory bowel disease. *J. Pediatr., 112,* 893.
12. Jacobs TP, Whitlock RT, Edsall J, Holub DA (1988) Addisonian crisis while taking high-dose corticosteroids. An unusual presentation of primary adrenal failure in two patients with underlying inflammatory diseases. *J. Am. Med. Assoc., 260,* 2082.
13. Christy NP (1988) Corticosteroid therapy and unintentional camouflage. *J. Am. Med. Assoc., 260,* 2107.
14. Ettinger WH, Hazzard WR (1988) Elevated apolipoprotein-B levels in corticosteroid-treated patients with systemic lupus erythematosus. *J. Clin. Endocrinol. Metab., 67,* 425.
15. Ettinger WH (1987) Model of VLDL apoB metabolism in the corticosteroid treated rabbit. *Arteriosclerosis, 7,* 540A.
16. Buthiau D, Piette JC, Ducerveau MN et al (1988) Steroid-induced spinal epidural lipomatosis: CT survey. *J. Comput. Assist. Tomogr., 12,* 501.
17. Maehara T, Tanohata K, Noda M, Nakayama D (1988) Medically treated steroid-induced epidural lipomatosis. *Neuroradiology, 30,* 281.
18. Reed DH, Morgan S (1988). The changing mediastinum. *Br. J. Radiol., 61,* 695.
19. Sury MRJ, Russell GN, Heaf DP (1988) Hydrocortisone myopathy. *Lancet, 2,* 515.
20. Picado C, Montserrat J, Agustí-Vidal A (1988) Muscle atrophy in severe exacerbation of asthma requiringmechanicalventilation. *Respiration,53,*201.
21. Miller RG, Milner-Brown HS (1987) Is there an adverse interaction betwen corticosteroids and anticholinesterase drugs in patients with myasthenia gravis? *Ann. NY Acad. Sci. 505,* 847.
22. Hardouin P, Delcambre B (1988) L'ostéoporose cortisonique. *Lille Méd., 28,* 152.
23. Preston-Thomas A, Home G (1988) Avascular necrosis of the femoral head in neurosurgical patients: a report of two cases. *NZ Med. J., 101,* 567.
24. Yamaguchi H, Masuda T, Saski T, Majima T (1988) Steroid-induced osteonecrosis of the patella. *Clin. Orthopaed. Rel. Res., 229,* 201.
25. Godschalk MF, Downs RW (1988) Effect of short-term glucocorticoids on serum osteocalcin in healthy young men. *J. Bone Miner. Res., 3,* 113.
26. Bijlsma JWJ, Duursma SA, Bosch R et al (1988) Acute changes in calcium and bone metabo-

lism during methylprednisolone pulse therapy in rheumatoid arthritis. *Br. J. Rheumatol., 27,* 215.
27. Toogood JN, Crilly RG, Jones G et al (1988) Effect of high dose budenoside on calcium and phosphate metabolism and the risk of osteoporosis. *Am. Rev. Respir. Dis., 138,* 57.
28. Bijlsma JWJ, Raymakers JA, Mosch C et al (1988) Effect of oral calcium and vitamin D on glucocorticoid-induced osteopenia. *Clin. Exp. Rheumatol., 6,* 113.
29. Shipley ME, Bacon PA, Berry H et al (1988) Pulsed methylprednisolone in active early rheumatoid disease: a dose-ranging study. *Br. J. Rheumatol., 27,* 211.
30. Lorca P, Mena P (1988) Reacción leucemoide neonatal asociada a administración prenatal de corticoides. *Rev. Chil. Pediatr., 59,* 279.
31. Smith T (1988) Tumor lysis syndrome after steroid therapy for anaphylaxis. *South. Med. J., 81,* 415.
32. Rainfaing E, Billerey C, Barale T et al (1988) Alternariose cutanée. Aspets anatomopathologiques: à propos d'un cas et revue de la litérature. *Sem. Hôp., 64,* 3117.
33. Lev B, Shachar A, Segev S et al (1988) Quiescent Q fever endocarditis exacerbated by cardiac surgery and corticosteroid therapy. *Arch. Intern. Med., 147,* 1531.
34. Bautista-Casanovas A, Nieto B, Villanueva A et al (1988) Brain abscess: a complication of esophageal dilatations. *Pediatr. Surg. Int., 3,* 354.
35. Ratcliffe GE (1988) Amoebic disease precipitated by corticosteroids prescribed for tuberculous pleural effusions. *Tubercle, 69,* 219.
36. Ueda-Furukawa M, Kitano Y, Hashimoto K (1988) Trichophytic granuloma associated with bullous pemphigoid. *J. Dermatol., 15,* 339.
37. Mukwaya G (1988) Immunosuppressive effects and infections associated with corticosteroid therapy. *Pediatr. Infect. Dis. J., 7,* 499.
38. Hillerdal G, Riesenfeldt-Orn I, Pedersen A, Ivanicova E (1988) Infection with *Rhodococcus equi* in a patient with sarcoidosis treated with corticosteroids. *Scand. J. Infect. Dis., 20,* 673.
39. Levine RA, McGuire RF (1988) Corticosteroid-induced pancreatitis: a case report demonstrating recurrence with rechallenge. *Am. J. Gastroentol., 83,* 1161.
40. Erban SB, Sokas RK (1988) Kaposi's sarcoma in an elderly man with Wegener's granulomatosis treated with cyclophosphamide and corticosteroids. *Arch. Intern. Med., 148,* 1201.
41. Weiner SR, Noritake DT, Paulus HE (1988) Kaposi's sarcoma in a patient with rheumatoid arthritis and polymyositis treated with corticosteroids. *West. J. Med., 148,* 702.
42. Gill PS, Loureiro C, Bernstein-Singer M et al (1989) Clinical effect of glucocorticoids on Kaposi sarcoma related to the acquired immunodeficiency syndrome (AIDS). *Ann. Intern. Med., 110,* 937.
43. Nakamura S, Salahuddin SZ, Biberfeld P et al (1988) Kaposi's sarcoma cells: long-term culture with growth factor from retrovirus-infected $CD4^+$ T cells. *Science, 242,* 426.
44. Silverman RA, Newman AJ, LeVine MJ, Kaplan B (1988) Poststeroid panniculitis: a case report. *Pediatr. Dermatol., 5,* 92.
45. Ohlsson A, Heyman E (1988) Dexamethasone-induced bradycardia. *Lancet, 2,* 1074.
46. Al Mahdy H, Hall M (1988) Anaphylaxis and hydrocortisone. *Ann. Intern. Med., 108,* 487.
47. Lindmaier A, Lindemayr H (1988) Allergien gegen Korticoide. 2. Fallberichte von Soforttypreaktionen. *Aktuel. Dermatol., 14,* 161.
48. Voss M (1988) Eine Prednisolon-Allergie mit pustulösen Exanthem. *Dermatol. Monats. schr., 174,* 221.
49. Stead RJ, Cooke NJ (1988) Adverse effects of inhaled corticosteroids. Not serious if care is taken. *Br. Med. J., 298,* 403.
50. Sánchez Varilla JM, Díaz Gálvez M, Villa Arellano F et al (1988) Función suprarrenal en asmáticos tratados con sodis altas de dipropionato de beclometasona. *Arch. Bronconeumol., 24,* 60.
51. Gugliemi R, Sebastiani N, Marino L et al (1987) Iperaldosteronismo secondario da uso di spray nasale. Descrizione di un caso. *G. Med. Mil., 137,* 112.
52. Moroni P, Pierini F, Cazzaniga R et al (1988) Osservazioni su una casistica di lavoratori professionalmente esposti a corticosteroidi. *Med. Lav., 79,* 142.
53. Friedman SJ, Butler DF, Pittelkow MR (1988) Perilesional linear atrophy and hypopigmentation after intralesional corticosteroid therapy. *J. Am. Acad. Dermatol., 19,* 537.
54. Debussche X, Toublanc M, Camillieri JP, Assan R (1988) Overwhelming strongyloidiasis in a diabetic patient following ACTH treatment and keto-acidosis. *Diabetes Metabol., 14,* 294.
55. Rutgers AWF, Links TP, Coultre R, Begeer JH (1988) Behavioural disturbances after effective ACTH-treatment of the dancing-eyes syndrome. *Dev. Med. Child Neurol., 30,* 407.

K.-W. von Eickstedt

42 Sex hormones and related compounds including hormonal contraceptives

HORMONAL CONTRACEPTIVES *(SED-11, 828; SEDA-13, 370)*

Steroid metabolism in correlation with side effects Individual variations in the metabolism of the hormonal components of oral contraceptives (OCs) can affect the chances of side effects. This may be correlated to the plasma levels of the estrogen component. Induction of hypercoagulability by estrogen is thought to be the mechanism responsible for the thrombogenic activity of OCs (SED-11, 830). While the progestogen component of OCs does not seem to affect the incidence of venous thromboembolism, data have been assembled that demonstrate a correlation between the amount of estrogens contained in OCs and the risk of this disorder (1^R, 2^R). Estrogens have until recently been thought to be responsible for the increased blood pressure associated with OCs. Recent evidence implicates progestogens as well (2^R).

Pharmacokinetic studies on two OCs of the new generation investigated the extend to which the elimination of the ethinylestradiol (EE) component could be inhibited by the progestogen component (3^C-6^C). In these 12-months studies on healthy volunteers the serum concentrations of the progestogens desogestrel (DG) and gestodene (GSD) were measured as well as the concentrations of sex-hormone-binding globulin (SHBG) and corticosteroid-binding globulin (CBG). There were large interindividual variations in the concentrations, but during treatment with EE/GSD the EE levels were higher and the EE peaks occurred 30 min later than during treatment with EE/DG. The serum levels of CBG, which is known to be influenced only by the estrogenic component of the OC, increased significantly more during treatment with EE/GSD than with EE/DG. Moreover, the increase in serum cortisol was higher. There was no difference between the effects of EE/GSD and EE/DG on the SHBG levels which rose by 250–300%. Since the hepatic production of SHBG is stimulated by EE and reduced by progestogens with a partial androgenic effect the SHBG levels were compensated to a certain degree by high serum concentrations of GSD which rose more than the DG levels.

The studies cited above showed a progressive rise in EE levels during each OC cycle. This was interpreted as a reduction in oxidative metabolism by EE itself and possibly by the respective progestogen. The oxidation of EE by human liver cytochrome P-450 has recently been studied (7^c). This study demonstrated that the P-450 heme disappears and that P-450 is a major target for inactivation by EE which is called 'suicide inhibition'. This enzyme inhibition also concerns the retardation of the clearance of prednisolone and many other drugs and can be relevant for women who develop hypertension during OC intake: elevated EE (and also caffeine) serum levels have been described in women who developed hypertension during OC use (8^C). The wide interindividual variations in EE serum levels which have been found in studies with GSD and GD were suggested to be mainly due to a genetic disposition as it was supposed by Stadel (9^C). The identification of slow and fast metabolizers of sex steroids such as EE in women taking OCs may help to reduce untoward side effects of the hormonal contraceptives.

Side Effects of Drugs Annual 14
M.N.G. Dukes and L. Beeley, editors

Hemostatic and cardiovascular effects *(SED-11, 830; SEDA-12, 340; SEDA-13, 370)* The new progestogen gestodene has been studied as a component of a low-dose OC containing 78 μg of the progestogen and 32 μg EE and was compared with an OC containing 92 μg levonorgestrel and 32 μg EE.

Twenty-six healthy women aged 16–30 years were randomly allocated to receive during 6 treatment cycles one of the two OCs. Both groups showed increases in biological activities of procoagulant factors fibrinogen, X and XII and decreased activity of the naturally occurring coagulation inhibitor, antithrombin III.

The findings in this study indicate that both low-dose OCs induced increases in procoagulant factor activities which were not balanced by increased biological levels of the two most important physiological coagulation inhibitors antithrombin III and protein C. Neither OCs differed generally with respect to this kind of side effect (10[c]).

In a randomized study 50 healthy young women were included to determine the hemorheological effects of 2 different OCs.

The women took no medication for 3 cycles. Subsequently they were randomized into Group A which took an OC containing 35 μg EE and 2.0 mg cyproterone acetate and Group B which took an OC containing 30 μg EE and 150 μg levonorgestrel, each for 6 cycles. Finally 3 cycles without medication followed. Blood viscosity was quantified by ex vivo measurements of hematocrit, blood and plasma viscosity, red cell filterability, fibrinogen and colloid oncotic pressure. In Group A fibrinogen rose at the end of the medication phase. In Group B fibrinogen, blood and plasma viscosity increased on medication. The former 2 variables remained elevated even after discontinuation of the oral contraceptive.

These data combined with those from the literature suggest that low-dose OCs do not lead to any biologically meaningful changes in blood rheology whereas higher doses induce limitations of blood fluidity which could be involved in the increase in cardiovascular risk due to these medications (11[C]).

In a retrospective cross-sectional study selected hemostasitic parameters were assayed in 131 women taking different kinds of OCs and in 36 control women. Protein C and plasminogen levels were significantly higher and the fibrinonectin levels were lower in the OC users. The other main coagulation factors remained unchanged (12[c]). The conclusion of this report that OC use does not cause thromboembolic diseases cannot be correlated to distinct OCs.

In 2 prospective controlled studies with 2 low-dosed OCs an activation of coagulation was observed in the group of pill users. The one study group consisted of 16 healthy women, 7 of whom were smokers. They took an OC with 50 μg EE and 50–125 μg desogestrel in a 2-phase preparation. The other study group consisted of 24 healthy women, 12 of whom were smokers. They took a 3-phase preparation with 30–40 μg EE and 50–125 μg levonorgestrel. Factors such as antithrombin III, protein C, antiplasmin, fibrinogen, fibrinopeptid A, thrombocytes and ELT were investigated. Activation of coagulation showed no differences between smoking and non-smoking OC users (13[C]).

Several case-reports have recently been published:

The first case concerned a 21-year-old woman using a triphasic OC with 35 μg EE and 0.5–1.0 mg norethindrone. She had a deep venous thrombosis in the right leg with no flow in the deep venous system. The second concerned a 30-year-old woman using the same OC formulation. She showed a portal venous thrombosis with extension to the splenic and superior mesenteric veins (14[C]). A 3rd case was a 26-year-old woman using 35 μg EE and 0.5–1.0 mg norethindrone for $2^1/_2$ years. She had smoked more than 25 cigarettes daily for about 10 years. A thrombus was found in the superior mesenteric artery which was eliminated by operation. The inferior mesenteric artery was also occluded at its origin. This thrombus was also eliminated. A bowel ischemia persisted and the patient died a few days later (15[c]). A 4th case concerned a 16-year-old girl who developed pulmonary emboli and subsequently died. She received an OC with 30 μg EE and 150 μg desogestrel for 2 months (16[C]). A 5th case was of cerebral deep venous thrombosis in a 21-year-old woman. She took an OC containing 35 μg EE and 0.5–1.0 mg norethindrone. She recovered completely during 1 week of clinical treatment (17[c]).

In an integral report 22 cases of cerebral infarction involving arteries or veins (2 cases of thrombophlebitis) are described with respect to OC use; 7 of these cases were probably and 15 cases possibly correlated with the use of OCs. 17 patients were under 30. In 55% of cases the cerebral infarction occurred within the first 2 years of treatment. All contraceptives involved contained low dosages of ethinyl estradiol. Attention is drawn to the role of immune factors, with circulating immune complexes and/or specific anti-hormone antibodies found in significant concentrations in 15 of 20 patients evaluated (18[C]).

The use of OCs is an established risk factor for cardiovascular events, which again was evaluated in a hospital-based case-control study of myocardial infarction in young women.

A total of 58 women with infarction, aged 30–50 years, were compared with 174 aged-matched controls. Smoking of 15 or more cigarettes per day, diabetes, hypertension, angina pectoris and hypercholesterolemia all significantly raised the risk of myocardial infarction. Relative risk among past users of oral contraceptives (crude RR = 2.48, 95% CI = 0.98–6.23) remained elevated after stratification for the other 5 significant risk factors.

Although small, this study is consistent with already published work on the subject (19[C]).

The risk factors which influence coronary artery disease in women are less well characterized than those associated with ischemic heart disease in men. Former studies have tended to confirm smoking, hypertension, clotting variables and serum lipid concentrations as major risk factors in both men and women (SEDA-10, 359); (20[R]). The Royal College of General Practitioners' oral contraceptive study, although primarily designed to investigate the effects on health of OCs, provided a valuable opportunity to examine other influences on myocardial infarction in women. A nested case-control study was therefore carried out on the cohort data of the cited study to determine solely in women the pattern of risk factors for acute myocardial infarction. Smoking (adjusted relative risk 1.7 for light smokers and 4.3 for heavy smokers), hypertension (2.4), toxemia of pregnancy (2.8), and diabetes mellitus (6.9) were associated with a significantly increased risk of myocardial infarction. No significant trend of risk was seen in relation to social class. Current use of the pill increased the risk only among women who also smoked (relative risk 20.8 for heavy smokers). Previous use of the pill did not affect the risk of myocardial infarction. If heavy smokers also had a history of toxemia of pregnancy, their risk of myocardial infarction was further increased (relative risk 41.0). Other variables associated solely with women, such as parity, hysterectomy and hormone replacement therapy, had little effect on the risk of having a myocardial infarction. Overall, smoking was the most important independent risk factor and had a strong influence on the risks associated with other factors (20[C]).

Effects on lipids *(SED-11, 833; SEDA-13, 370)* Estrogens and progestins for contraception or hormonal replacement therapy are widely used. These steroids have substantial effects on lipids and lipoproteins that appear to be primarily related to the chemical structure of the compound, dosage, and a patients hormonal status (21[r]). Natural fluctuations in concentrations of physiological sex hormones in the course of a woman's life affect lipoprotein levels; such effects may be compared with those induced by exogenous hormone therapy. During the progesterone-dominated luteal phase of the menstrual cycle, high-density lipoprotein (HDL) concentrations do not fall, but low-density lipoprotein (LDL) concentrations usually decline. During pregnancy both estrogen and progesterone levels are extremely high; LDL concentration gradually increases to a maximum value at term of 50% above the non-pregnant level. Total HDL and HDL-2 concentrations also increase, reaching a maximal 30% increase at 20 weeks of gestation. These physiological fluctuations have not been associated with increased arteriosclerosis. Oral contraceptives that combine C21 progestins and certain C19 progestin derivatives with estrogen have little or no effect on HDL-2; however, those with a marked progestogenic or androgenic effect are more likely to lower HDL and HDL-2. Increases in LDL concentration during oral contraceptive use are not consistently proportional to the estrogen/progestin ratio and may reflect progestin androgenicity or a progestin–estrogen interaction. In postmenopausal women estrogen alone benefits lipoproteins, whereas cyclical administration of progestin with estrogen appears to lower HDL-2–cholesterol in proportion to the progestin dose. These exogenous-hormone-induced changes are associated with the expected changes in arteriosclerosis risk when they have been looked for. In summary, estrogen–progestin regimens that do not affect LDL– and HDL-2–cholesterol concentrations are most desirable in terms of long-term cardiovascular risk (22[R]).

In a 12-month controlled prospective clinical trial the effects of 2 triphasic OCs on lipid/lipoprotein metabolism were compared in 8 volunteers ranging in age from 21 to 35 years.

One triphasic OC contained 35 μg EE and 0.5–1.0 mg norethindrone, the other 30–40 μg EE and 50–125 μg levonorgestrel. The data of the trial indicated that use of both estrogen–progestin preparations were accompanied by increases in cholesterol, low-density lipoprotein and high-density lipoprotein, cholesterol, apolipoproteins A and B, and triglycerides. A decline in high-density lipoprotein cholesterol and greater decreases in high-density lipoprotein-2, cholesterol levels were also observed; the latter were below the lower limits of the laboratory reference range. All other changes remained within clinically acceptable limits.

There were no statistically significant differences between the test preparations, suggesting that the impact on lipid metabolism of the triphasic preparations is similar and, given the dynamic balance between the various fractions, is unlikely to impart an adverse cardiovascular risk (23[C]). The authors conclude: Since the individual metabolic response to an oral contraceptive varies and the long-term effect of oral contraceptives regarding atherogenesis are still to be defined, high-risk women taking OCs (including the low-dose, triphasic oral contraceptives) should be monitored with annual lipid and lipoprotein profiles.

In a cross-sectional study at the John Radcliffe Hospital in Oxford the glucose metabolism and lipoprotein levels of 198 women taking 10 different combined and progestogen-only oral OCs were compared.

The women were aged 16–40 and had been taking OCs for at least 6 months. Glucose metabolism, as assessed by fasting glucose and HbAlc, was not significantly different from controls using alternative contraceptive methods. Plasma cholesterol concentration was higher in women using ethinylestradiol (EE) 35 + norethisterone (NE) 1000, but not when the estrogen content was higher (EE-50 + NE-1000). Low-density lipoprotein (LDL) cholesterol concentration was raised in women using EE-35 + NE-500 and EE-30 levonorgestrel (LN) 250; high-density lipoprotein (HDL) cholesterol and log HDL/LDL were also lower in the latter group. Plasma triglycerides were highest in those using EE-35 + NE-1000, EE-30 + ED-2000 and triphasic gestodene.

Women on progestogen-only preparations (LN-30 + NE-350), EE-30 + LN-150 and the triphasic preparations (EE-30/40 + LN-50/75/125) had lipid levels which did not differ significantly from non-users. All OC users had significantly lower cholesterol, LDL-cholesterol and trigylceride levels than the pregnant women (24[C]).

The women in this study were not randomized to the pill groups and the results could therefore suffer from unknown bias. The numbers in each group are relatively small, and minor differences could be missed, or their significance overestimated in the analysis (24[C]).

In a relatively short clinical study the difference in the effects of 2 OCs containing desogestrel (DG) + EE or levonorgestrel (LNG) + EE on lipoprotein metabolism in smoking and non-smoking women was investigated.

The authors measured the changes in plasma lipoprotein levels in a group of healthy young women stratified for smoking and non-smoking, before and after 3 cycles on either an OC containing 150 μg DG + 30 μg EE (n = 12 and 17, respectively) or one containing 150 μg LNG and 30 μg EE (n = 20 and 21, respectively). The baseline characteristics did not differ significantly from each other in the 4 groups.

The expected lower plasma level of HDL in smoking women compared with non-smoking controls was not observed in this study. Except for triglyceride, the serum levels of (lipoprotein-) lipids and apolipoproteins (i.e. cholesterol, HDL–cholesterol, LDL–cholesterol, apolipoprotein A-1, A2 and B) were not dependent on smoking (25[c]).

A recently published paper presented the results of a randomized clinical trial of healthy young women utilizing 3 different types of OCs as changes in mean lipid, lipoprotein and apolipoprotein B and A-1 levels during a 9-month period:

Sixty-seven women used an OC with 50 μg EE + 1.0 mg norethindrone (NE), 61 women an OC with 35 μg EE + 1.0 mg NE and 64 women an OC with 35 μg EE + 0.5 mg NE. Fasting lipids and lipoproteins were measured at baseline, 3, 6 and 9 months. All groups showed an increase in plasma total cholesterol, triglycerides, LDL/apolipoprotein B and apolipoprotein A-1. The group taking the preparation with 0.5 mg NE was the only one to show an elevation of HDL–cholesterol; the other two groups showed declines in the mean levels of this lipoprotein over the study period. The mean changes in lipid/lipoprotein levels associated with oral contraceptive use appeared to be at least partially related to the doses of the contraceptive steroids (26[C]).

The authors of the above study conclude that examinations of the mean changes suggest an early 'impact' on certain lipid/lipoproteins followed by a leveling off for some groups. For example, the 35 μg EE + 1 mg NE mean results for total cholesterol and apolipoprotein A-1 showed this phenomenon. Further, when we examined some of the individual records, this type of pattern was shown for many individuals among all 3 oral contraceptive groups. Although most OC users may not face an increased risk in the future, there may be subgroups of users whose risk could be different. For example, the relationship between lipid/lipoprotein levels and risk of coronary heart disease is curvilinear, suggesting that individuals at the extremes may face increased risk. Thus, analysis directed towards such subgroups may be important. Further, since the initial 'first pass' to the liver by contraceptive steroids may influence subsequent changes in systems highly dependent on this organ (e.g. lipids/lipoproteins, antithrombin III), analysis of certain measurements of contraceptive steroid metabolism in relationship to changes in these systems may also be of importance in defining potential risk (26[C], 27[r]).

Effects on carbohydrate metabolism *(SED-11, 833; SEDA-12, 341)* A wide variability in blood glucose and insulin responses during the oral glucose tolerance test (OGTT) has been reported in women using the low-dose combination type of OC for short- and long-term contraception (28[c], 29[R]). Some of the problems mentioned in the beginning that led to conflicting results have been eliminated in a clinical study by administering only one type of low-dose combinated of OC in a homogeneous population and followed-up for 1 year.

Carbohydrate metabolism was evaluated in 20 healthy women volunteers using a low-dose combined OC containing 30 μg EE and 500 μg *dl*-norgestrel by measurent of serum glucose and insulin levels during 3-hour OGTT before and after 3, 6 and 12 months of medication. There were no significant differences in body weight or blood pressure pre- or post-treatment. Fasting serum glucose levels were slightly reduced, although not significantly, during all periods of treatment. However, serum glucose levels were increased at 1, 2 and 3 hours in association with high insulin responses during OGTT in all periods of OC therapy, indicating mild to moderate insulin resistance.

These data suggest that the low-dose combined OC used in the study exerts changes in carbohydrate metabolism in women during 1 year of OC use (30[C]). Several mechanisms have been postulated to explain impaired glucose tolerance in OC users. Alterations in liver morphology and function have been demonstrated in oral contraceptive users, as this could affect carbohydrate metabolism through gluconeogenesis and glycogenolysis. OCs have been reported to increase insulin-antagonistic hormones such as growth hormone, cortisol and glucagon, although the role played by some of these hormones on carbohydrate metabolism in OC users is still controversial (30[C]).

A clinical comment to the effects of OCs on carbohydrate metabolism concludes that changes in carbohydrate metabolism in women taking OCs are essentially related to the dose and type of progestin used; low-dose OCs mainly with estrogen are those which induce the least adverse effects from this point of view. It is unlikely that their administration induces or aggravates in an irreversible manner poor glucose tolerance or diabetes. Subjects presenting with this clinical picture are more likely to suffer from vascular disease; in these patients, oral contraception should be limited to avoid increasing the risk of vascular disease (31[r]).

Liver *(SED-11, 854; SEDA-13, 362)* The effects of OCs on the liver concern not only benign liver tumors and hepatocellular carcinomas but also peliosis hepatis, sinusoid dilatations and, not least, icterus and gall stones. Two cases of *icterus* with *cholestasis* have been reported which occurred in women taking OCs with levonorgestrel and EE. The women recovered after about 1 month (32[c]). Peliosis hepatis, a condition characterized by the presence of blood-filled lacunar spaces in the liver, has been described primarily in patients on androgenic steroid medication and patients with tuberculosis. It has never been reported as a complication of the use of oral contraceptives, except in association with and localized in contraceptive-induced hepatic tumors. A recently published case-report concerned a 43-year-old women with generalized *peliosis hepatis* that developed during long-term use of oral contraceptives. Extensive examination did not reveal a hepatic tumor. Liver cirrhosis and portal hypertension developed, although the oral contraceptives had been withdrawn. The patient finally underwent successful orthotopic liver transplantation (33[c]).

In a cross-sectional study in Copenhagen the prevalence of *gall stone disease* in a random sample of a Danish population was ascertained by ultrasonography. Estimates were made of possible associations between the gall stones and menarche, menopause, pregnancies and exogenous female sex hormones. The random sample comprised 2301 women of Danish origin aged 30, 40, 50 and 60 years, of whom 1765 (77%) attended the investigation. Gall stone disease was significantly associated with young age at menarche, abortions, and multiple childbirth. Use of oral contraceptives was significantly associated with gall stone disease in univariate analysis, but not in multivariate analysis. Breastfeeding, age at menopause and menopausal hormone therapy were not associated with gall stones. These determining variables seemed sufficient to explain the higher prevalence of gall stone disease in women than in men (34[C], 35[r]).

Sinusoid dilatations in the liver were reported in a 23-year-old woman who developed an acute painful syndrome of the right hypochondrium with hepatic cytolysis. She had been taking an OC (Minidril) for 7 years. The liver biopsy showed a periportal and mediolobular dilatation of the sinusoids. After cessation of OC intake she recovered in less than 1 day with normalization of the plasma enzyme levels (36[c]).

A causal association between OC use and benign *liver tumors* is well documented. Recent evidence suggests that a similar relationship may exist between OCs and *hepatocellular carcinoma* (37[r]). A statistical analysis of the association between long-term OC use and hepatocellular carcinoma has been performed in Italy. There were 4 women who had used OCs compared with 11 controls. The relative risk was 1.8 for up to 5 years' use and 8.3 for over 5 years. The trend in risk was statistically significant (38[r]). Different types of liver tumors have been reported recently such as a giant liver *adenoma* which developed after 13 years of uninterrupted OC use in a 37-year-old woman. The advantage of this type of tumor is not as much its known low prevalence but its clinical diagnosis. The diameter of this tumor was 14 cm. It was diagnosed sonographically (39[c]). A ruptured tumor which measured about 15 $\times$ 10 cm was removed in a 36-year-old woman who took OCs with 50 μg EE + 0.5 mg norgestrel for 6 years (40[c]). In a summarising report 10 liver tumors were described as diagnosed and treated in the hospital center in Angers (France). Among these 10 liver tumors in patients on OCs 8 were removed (wedge or segmental resection, lobectomy). Pathological examination showed focal nodular hyperplasia (FNH) in 6 cases, hepatocellular adenoma (HCA) in 1 case, and HCA with FNH in 1 case. The authors give the therapeutic recommendation: Removal is preferable in tumors that fail to shrink following prolonged discontinuation of oral contraceptives, especially in adenomas which carry a high potential for bleeding, in large symptomatic tumors, and in peripheral or pedunculated tumors that can be readily and safely removed. Uncertainty as to the benign or malignant nature of the tumor and planned pregnancy are two additional indications for surgical removal (41[C]). In a report from Pittsburgh (Pennsylvania) 10 patients with *hepatic epitheloid hemangioendothelioma* are described, 6 of whom were women. There was an association of OC use with this tumor in 4 of the 6 female patients in this series and in 37% of such reported cases (42[C]). A case of *intrahepatic biliary cystadenoma* in a young woman who had no prior history of liver disease and who had taken OCs for 1 year has been reported from Japan. A 27-year-old woman was admitted to hospital with a firm epigastric mass. At laparotomy, a large cystic mass was resected from the left hepatic lobe, and diagnosed as biliary cystadenoma. In the tumor tissue, the estrogen receptor content was 14.0 fmol/mg cytosol protein, which was much higher than the 3.0 fmol/mg cytosol protein in the surrounding liver tissue. This is the first case of biliary cystadenoma in which the estrogen receptor content was increased (43[c]). Three cases of *hepatic cellular adenomas* (HCA) were reported from New Haven (Michigan). In 2 of the cases the liver tissue was tested for estrogen receptors; both were found to be negative. With respect to the results of their clinical investigations the authors state that although the technique as well as the observed progression of these lesions or development of new lesions after the discontinuance of steroids may account for this negative finding, it suggests that induction of this process may be caused by means other than direct cellular stimulation by the exogenous hormones. Finally, these 3 cases call attention to a potential subgroup of patients having OC-associated HCA who may have progression of their liver tumors when no longer receiving steroids and who require an aggressive treatment program and non-invasive follow-up examinations (44[C]).

Tumors of sex-organs *(SED-11, 855; SEDA-12, 339; SEDA-13, 358)* *Breast cancer* The relationship between OC use and breast cancer is still under discussion, since there is concern about the possible association between OC use and breast cancer risk in selected populations or subgroups of women (SEDA-12, 339, SEDA-13, 362). The results of different studies which have in the meantime been published are still contradictory and therefore the statement of the U.K. Committee on Safety of Medicines may be helpful for prescribing doctors: 'the newly reported findings do not indicate the need to change at this time the current advice regarding the use of the presently available contraceptive agents... The committee remains of the view that women receiving oral contraceptives should be prescribed a product with the lowest suitable content of both estrogen and progestogen.' In addition, 10 members of the International Committee for Research in Reproduction noted in a letter to the journal in which the British study appeared that 'an uncritical response to the present data may lead to unjustified anxiety and an unnecessary change of contraceptive practice...' Nevertheless, similar careful analysis are still needed to resolve any relationship between breast cancer and pill use (45[r]).

An analysis of the occurrence of breast cancer in women taking OCs has been based upon data available from the Royal College of General Practitioners' OC study (46[C]). This analysis shows a significant relative risk of 3.33 in women aged 30–34 at diagnosis who have ever used OCs and a relative risk of 5.88 in those who were primiparous at the time of diagnosis. In women below the age of 35 years the relative risk of 2.38 was not significant. There was no increased risk in women over the age of 35 years. A significant trend relating to duration of use was demonstrable in women who were primiparous in the analysis of both current and ever-users. An analysis by time since stopping OC use revealed a significant trend in all ever-users, but the trends were much steeper in primiparous women or those aged 30–34 years at diagnosis. There was no evidence that the increased rates in OC users were related to the estrogen or progestogen dose. The 5-year survival rate in users diagnosed under the age of 35 years was significantly poorer than in comparable non-users.

It is possible that the increased rates in younger OC users might be due to an accelerated presentation of breast cancer in those women who would otherwise have been diagnosed at a later stage. The non-significant excess risk in non-users under 35 years of age was approximately 1 in 7000 users per year (46[C]). The authors conclude: The unresolved discrepancies between the results of the published studies make it impossible at the present time to decide whether or not OC use is associated with an increased risk of breast cancer.

Another analysis performed in Oxford was based on the data gained in 17 large family planning clinics in England and Scotland. During the interval 1968–1974, 17 032 women aged 25–39 years were recruited, more than half of whom were using OCs. These women have been followed up over the years and breast cancer has been diagnosed in 189 of them. The available data were analysed in two ways. First were the standardized breast cancer incidence rates calculated in non-users and users of OCs according to total duration of use, interval since first use, interval since last use, duration of use before first-term pregnancy and duration of use before age 25. Second was a case-control conducted within cohort analyses to examine the possible effects of different types of pill and to search for evidence of a latent effect of OC use before first-term pregnancy on breast cancer risk. There was no evidence found of any adverse effect of OC use on the risk of breast cancer in this study. There was, however, little exposure to the pill before first-term pregnancy among the participants and virtually no such exposure at a very young age (i.e. below 20 years). Accordingly, the results of this study strengthen the evidence that OC use by mature women does not increase breast cancer risk, but add little to the uncertainty about the effects of early use (47[C]).

In the U.K. National Case-Control Study (published in 1989) which investigated the relation between OC use and breast cancer risk, 755 cases each with a matched control were interviewed in their homes by trained interviewers. General practitioner notes and family planning clinic records were abstracted and combined with the interview data. There was a highly significant trend in risk of breast cancer with a total duration of OC use with a relative risk of 1.43 (95% confidence interval 1.15–2.62) for 97 or more months of use. The relative risks were similar for use before and after first full-term pregnancy. There is some evidence that OCs containing less than 50 μg estrogen have a lower risk associated with their use than higher estrogen dose OCs and that there may be some protective effect of use of progestagen-only pills (48[C]).

In 1987 the final results of an epidemiological study were published based on 351 case-control pairs aged under 45 years with and without OC use (49[C]). Shortly after this publication a histopathological review of as many as possible of these neoplasms was performed.

> A detailed review was made of the histopathology of 227 tumors taken from 261 women under 45 years of age with breast cancer. The tumors were classified as follows: whether OCs had been used at any time, and whether OCs had been used before the first term of pregnancy. All analyses were adjusted for the effects of age. Overall, 201 (88.5%) of tumors were infiltrating ductal in type, 19 (8.4%) were infiltrating lobular, and 7 (3.1%) were in situ ductal. Of the infiltrating ductal tumors, 28 (14%) were Grade I, 88 (44%) Grade II, and 84 (42%) Grade III. Various other tumor characteristics were also examined (percent of carcinoma in situ, lymphatic permeation, necrosis, lymphoplasmocytic reaction and tumor edge).

None of the histopathological features assessed showed any significant association with OC use. Some characteristics of the areas of breast tissue adjacent to the tumors were also studied. The degree of cyst formation was considerably less pronounced in those using OCs before first-term pregnancy than in those not doing so (50[C]).

A population-based case-control study in Sweden and Norway showed an increased risk of breast cancer with increasing duration of OC use with the exception of that for women with more than 15 years since the first use. The study consisted of 317 Swedish and 105 Norwegian cases diagnosed 1984–1985 with 317 Swedish and 210 Norwegian controls (51[C]). The authors state that the results suggest that long-term use of OCs may increase the risk of breast cancer in young women.

A hospital-based case-control study in Northern Italy evaluated the risk of breast cancer in relation to OC use including 1517 cases below the age of 60 and 1351 controls. In this study the breast cancer risk was significantly elevated among short-term OC users and the point estimate was 0.9 among users for 5 years or more. The elevated risk among short-term users, if not due to residual confounding or selection mechanisms, is probably explainable in terms of recall bias (i.e. more careful report of short or very short use by cases) (52[C]). The authors state that a major limitation of their study lies in the low prevalence of OC use in Italy with a consequently reduced statistical power.

A population-based case-control study called the ‘Cancer and Steroid Hormone Study’ was conducted in 8 geographic areas of the United States.

> The cases consisted of 2945 women who were premenopausal and 20–54 years of age when breast cancer was diagnosed between December 1, 1980, and December 31, 1982; controls consisted of 2646 women with no history of breast cancer who were also premenopausal and 20–54 years of age when selected during the same period. Among nulliparous women who experienced menarche before age 13, the relative risk of developing breast cancer in the age interval 20–44 years was estimated to be 1.0 for never-users of OCs, 1.3 for >0–3 years of use, 1.3 for 4–7 years, 2.7 for 8–11 years and 11.8 for 12 years or longer.

These findings suggest that prolonged OC use may accelerate the onset of breast cancer in a small group of susceptible women while having no appreciable impact on overall risk (53[C]). The authors state that their findings should be regarded as tentative but they suggest that high-risk women (those who experience menarche before 13 years of age and remain nulliparous) are at increased risk of developing premenopausal breast cancer before the age of 45 if they use OCs for 8 years or longer. And they further comment: 'Nonetheless, in the analysis of high-risk women 45–54 years of age, we found no increased risk of premenopausal breast cancer among long-term OC users; the risk is non-significantly decreased, although based upon small numbers of long-term users.' This suggests that their findings for the high-risk group before age 45 are either due to a tendency among physicians to diagnose breast cancer earlier among OC users than among non-users, or to a promotional effect of OC use which advances the clinical onset of breast cancer by a few years but does not appreciably alter subsequent risk. Finally, in view of their findings for high-risk women being restricted to those under 45 years of age, they suggest a need for cautious interpretation when studies of OCs and breast cancer are limited to disease in young women and the results then projected to older ages (53[CR]).

A population-based case-control study of OC use and breast cancer was carried out among young women (<43 years of age) in Seattle (Washington). The study was based on 127 women with breast cancer and on matched controls. Use of OCs before first pregnancy did not materially differ between cases or controls. The rate ratio estimate of breast cancer incidence in women who had used OCs before first pregnancy compared to those who had not was 0.9. There were no meaningful patterns of association between breast cancer and duration of use or formulation of OC used before first pregnancy (54[C]). The study yielded results for other breast cancer risk factors which are consistent with those often found by others. Women with breast cancer were more likely to be nulliparous, to have a later age of first pregnancy, an earlier age of menarche, a family history of breast cancer and a history of breast lumps than were controls.

In Adelaide (South Australia) a population-based case-control study was conducted which involved 395 cases of OC users and 386 controls. These women were aged 20–69 years. The results of this study suggest that, in women in Australia who are aged less than 70 years, the use of OC agents is not associated with an alteration in the over-all risk of breast cancer. Ever use of OC agents was associated with an adjusted relative risk of 1.06; there was no evidence of a dose–response relationship between the total duration of use of OC agents and the risk of breast cancer; the risk of breast cancer did not increase with an increasing interval since first use of OC agents; and no clear evidence was found of a reduction in risk with an increasing interval since last use of OC agents (55[C]).

The International Committee for Research in Reproduction stated in a letter to the Editor: After 30 years of human use of OCs we still do not know for certain if they have an adverse effect on breast cancer.

(1) The overwhelming proportion of the current rise in cases of breast cancer is among women who are too old to have taken OCs when they were younger.
(2) Population-based data on the incidence of breast cancer in the United States confirm the protective effect (demonstrated in case-control studies) of OCs on ovarian and endometrial cancers in women now less than 45–50 years of age, but leave open the possibility of a small rise in breast cancer in a subset of women less than 45 years of age.
(3) Calculations suggest that even if an adverse effect among younger users of OC were proved, it would still only account for a few percent of all breast cancers occurring in Western countries (56[r]).

Cervical cancer The incidence of cervical cancer in women who had used OCs and in never-users was evaluated from long-term data of the Royal College of General Practitioners' Oral Contraception Study with the following results: Of 47 000 women followed since 1968, those who had used OCs (ever-users) had a significantly higher incidence rate of cervical cancer than never-users. After standardization of rates by age, parity, smoking, social class, number of previously normal cervical smears, and history of sexually transmitted disease, the excess was 41 per 100 000 woman-years for carcinoma-in-situ and 8 per 100 000 woman-years for invasive cervical cancer. Incidence increased with increasing duration of use: the standardized incidence rate for cervical cancer in women who had taken the pill for more than 10 years was 4 times that in never-users. Ever-users had a lower incidence of other uterine cancers; a lower incidence of ovarian cancer was also found, but was not statistically significant. The findings from this cohort study of 47 000 women confirm other published data that women who have used OCs have a higher incidence of cervical cancer and a lower incidence of endometrial and ovarian cancer than women who have never used OCs (57[C]).

Endometrial cancer OC use and the risk of endometrial cancer was investigated in a multinational trial. The WHO Special Programme of Research, Development and Research Training in Human Reproduction published a report on the relationship of combined OCs to risk of endometrial cancer from a multinational hospital-based case-control study of various steroid contraceptives and 5 different cancers. Based on data on 130 cases and 835 matched controls from 9 participating centers in 7 developing countries and 2 participating centers in 2 developed countries, the relative risk of endometrial carcinoma in women who ever took combined OCs was estimated to be 0.55. This value is similar to estimates from prior investigations in the United States and Italy, and the protective effect observed in this study was at least as great in the developing countries with low incidence rates as in the developed countries with higher rates. The reduction in risk was observed for adenocarcinomas with and without squamous elements (59[C]). The results of this study are consistent with previous reports in showing about a 50% lower incidence of endometrial cancer in women who had ever used combined OCs compared with those who had not. Moreover, the protective effect of OCs against endometrial cancers was as strong, if not stronger, in women from developing countries.

Ovarian cancer The relationship between use of combined OCs and risk of epithelial ovarian cancer was investigated in a hospital-based case-control study conducted from 1979–1986 in 7 countries by the WHO:

A total of 386 women with histologically confirmed epithelial ovarian cancer were compared to 2397 hospital controls matched for age, study center, hospital and year of interview. The relative risk in women who had ever used combined OCs, controlling for the confounding effect of the number of pregnancies, was 0.75. The relative risk decreased with increasing duration of OC use and with increasing time since cessation of use. Except for mucinous tumors, OC use was associated with lower risk of all histological subtypes of epithelial ovarian cancer. While a reduced risk associated with OC use was present in parous women (relative risk = 0.85), it was most pronounced in nulliparous women (relative risk = 0.16). The magnitude of the negative association between OCs and ovarian cancer in 5 developing countries (relative risk = 0.77) was similar to that reported in developed countries.

These results indicate that combined OCs are associated with reduced risk for epithelial ovarian cancer. Risk in ever-users is about 75% of that in non-users, and women who use OCs for 5 or more years experience about a 50% reduction in risk (59[C]).

Second-generation effects *(SED-11, 840)* In a review of the available literature published in Yugoslavia the causal relation between birth defects and contraception of different kinds was discussed. The conclusion of this publication is: It appeared that the use of contraception before intended pregnancy does not have any teratogenic effect on the fetus. The use of contraception (mainly oral contraception) during pregnancy is suspected to be teratogenic to some small degree (60[R]).

A case-control study investigated the correlation of OC use and smoking with the incidence of malformations. Intrauterine exposure of the embryo to the sex steroids of OCs involved pregnant women who had taken the pill during early pregnancy; 2834 pregnant women had taken OCs during pregnancy or became pregnant within 6 menstrual cycles after discontinuation of the OC; 3032 pregnant women without OCs served as controls. The authors of the study conclude that smoking in relation to malformations represents a higher risk than the intake of OCs (61[C]).

Implanted hormonal contraceptives *(SED-11, 845; SEDA-12, 342)*

Norplant is a system of subdermal implants that release a steady dose of levonorgestrel for long-term, reversible contraception. Norplant consists of 6 Silastic capsules, each of which measures 36 mm in length by 2.4 mm in diameter and contains 36 mg of levonorgestrel crystals. The capsules release about 30 μg of levonorgestrel per day and provide effective contraception for approximately 5 years. A newer system, Norplant-2, consists of only 2 capsules, each of which measures 44 mm in length and contains 35 mg of levonorgestrel.

Norplant-2 is effective for approximately 3 years. The primary mechanism of action of Norplant is suppression of ovulation. Studies have shown a pregnancy rate of 0.6/100 woman-years after 1 year and a cumulative rate of 1.5/100 woman-years at 5 years. Principal side effects are *irregular menstrual bleeding* and *headaches*. No changes in carbohydrate metabolism, blood coagulation or liver function have been reported. Lipid levels decreased by 5–15%. About 5–20% of patients have experienced headaches, which are considered a method-related side effect with Norplant use. Other side effects considered method-related include *acne* and *breast discharge*, both of which have an incidence of 5–20%. Acne often subsides as irregular bleeding patterns return to normal. 5% of Norplant users have experienced slight *weight gain*. *Amenorrhea* has been reported in as many as 25% of patients. Transient *ovarian cysts* have been noted in as many as 10% of users. Other side effects include leukorrhea, dizziness, nervousness, hirsutism, mastalgia, pruritus, nausea, and hair loss, although their relationship to Norplant is not proven (62[R]).

A longitudinal study on different long-term effects of Norplant subdermal implants has been performed in 100 women in Singapore.

Menstrual irregularities were the main complaint associated with the use of this implant during the first year (63[C]). During the first year the implant acceptors also had an enhanced potential for *hypercoagulation* with a significant shortening of their prothrombin time and activated partial thromboplastin time. They had moreover an *increased predisposition to thrombosis* as evidenced by significant increases in platelet count and aggregability (64[C]). At the end of 2 years of use, results from this ongoing study indicate that these acceptors continue to have an increased predisposition to thrombosis as evidenced by significant increases in platelet count and aggregability. The shortened but stable prothrombin time and activated partial thromboplastin time and increase in certain coagulation factors indicate that Norplant acceptors still have a possible potential for hypercoagulation at the end of 2 years of use (65[C], 66[C]). With respect to liver function, the results at the end of 2 years indicated the presence of possible *hepatocellular dysfunction*. Despite a 4.5% decrease in serum bilirubin during the second year, the mean serum bilirubin still remained significantly raised ($P < 0.001$). Furthermore, there was a significant fall in total proteins and globulin during the period under review ($P < 0.001$). However, mean levels of all 3 parameters remained within the normal clinical range. Total triglycerides and total cholesterol remained significantly decreased at the end of 2 years ($P < 0.001$). The LDL–cholesterol, which was significantly decreased at the end of 1 year, increased by 2.2% during the second year. However, this rise in LDL–cholesterol was not significant and was still below the pre-insertion level. The HDL–cholesterol levels returned to the pre-insertion levels after a significant increase in the first year. The HDL–cholesterol/total cholesterol + HDL–cholesterol ratio returned to its pre-insertion value at the end of 2 years whereas the LDL–cholesterol/HDL–cholesterol ratio was still significantly lower than the pre-insertion ratio (67[C], 68[C]).

In Rio de Janeiro 175 Norplant users were interviewed at home, and their answers compared with those of two control groups (levenorgestrel pill-users and non-hormonal method users). The results show increased relative risks in Norplant users in *menstrual disorders, hypertension*, severe *weight disturbances* and *hypertrichosis*, all of which had statistical significance. Other non-statistically significant findings were angina pectoris, hypertensive encephalopathy, acne and duodenites. Some severe symptoms such as headaches and behavioral disturbances were mentioned and these disappeared after the capsules had been withdrawn (69[C]).

In a preliminary clinical study, Capronor, a single-capsule, biodegradable, subdermal contraceptive that releases levonorgestrel over a 12–18-month period, has been evaluated in 48 healthy women, aged 18–40 years; 16 participants received a 2.5 cm capsule (12 mg of levonorgestrel), and 32 received a 4.0 cm capsule (21.6 mg of levonorgestrel). Serum levonorgestrel levels were significantly lower in the 2.5 cm group. Ovulation occurred in all cycles in the 2.5 cm group and in 26.3% of cycles in the 4.0 cm group. Levonorgestrel levels with the shorter capsule were too low for reliable contraception in all users, and 4 cm may be a minimal functional length. Bleeding patterns were regular in most women who ovulated and irregular in most remaining subjects. It is assumed that changes in cervical mucus and the endometrium contributed to effective contraception despite the frequency of ovulation. Four patients among the early participants in the trial experienced *local swelling or itching* of the skin at the capsule insertion site. The symptoms were relieved by topical corticosteroids and resolved spontaneously in all subjects (70[C]).

Intercervical hormonal contraceptives

The clinical performance during the first 2 years of the use of a progestogen-releasing intracervical device (ICD) was studied in 198 women in Helsinki. The ICD released 20 μg levonorgestrel per day. A total of 7 pregnancies occurred during the study period, all of them during the first year; 6 pregnancies occurred after unnoticed expulsion of the device. One pregnancy occurred in an epileptic woman using carbamazepine, with the ICD remaining in situ. The ICD was removed because of *infection* in 3 cases. They all took place during the first year of LNG-ICD use. In one case, *Neisseria gonorrhea* was found, and in another *Chlamydia trachomatis*. In the 3rd case the result of culture was negative. Two subjects were lost to follow-up. During the study period of 2 years, the mean body weight increased. Statistically significant *decreases in both the mean diastolic and systolic blood pressures* were observed after 1 and 2 years of ICD use compared to the pre-insertion values (71[C]).

Intrauterine devices *(SED-11, 846)*

Steroid-releasing intrauterine devices (IUDs) have been reviewed by Odlind (72[R]). One of the main disadvantages of conventional IUDs is the increased menstrual blood loss associated with their use. Progesterone-releasing IUDs have a life-span of about 1 year and are therefore impractical and moreover have been associated with an increased risk of ectopic pregnancy. Devices releasing different doses of levonorgestrel have been tried both by the WHO and the Population Council. In a randomized multicenter study in Sweden, Finland, Norway, Denmark and Hungary 1821 women were fitted with the 20 μg levonorgestrel IUD and 937 with a copper-bearing IUD, the Nova-T. The women have now been followed for 3 years. The cumulative net pregnancy rates at 12 months were 0.1% and 0.8%, respectively. The main mechanism of action of the 20 μg levonorgestrel IUD is due to its pronounced effects on the endometrium, whereas the ovarian hormone pattern is usually unaffected. As a result of the direct action of levonorgestrel, the endometrium is suppressed with atrophic glands and predecidual stromal changes. Effects on the cervical mucus are also likely to contribute to the contraceptive performance. The reported side effects are usually due to the low dose of levonorgestrel. The side effect pattern, however, clearly reflects that the levonorgestrel IUD is a hormonal method. The gross termination rate at 12 months for *acne, weight gain, headache, mood changes* and *breast tension* was 2.7% among levonorgestrel IUD users compared with 0.1% among users of Nova-T.

In a Birth Control Clinic in Rome 600 IUD users were examined; 339 of them had completed the scheduled usage period successfully. In 21.8% this contraceptive technique was a failure. The most common reason for IUD removal was *bleeding*. There were 18 pregnancies, 3 of them ectopic in the group as well as 4 cases of PID. The failure rate was higher among nulliparous women. Progesterone IUDs were effective and well tolerated, though it must be borne in mind that these were mostly used by multiparous women over 30 (73[C]).

At the Margaret Pyke Centre in London 50 women have been fitted with an IUD releasing 20 μg of levonorgestrel daily. In this group 6 women have developed functional *ovarian cysts*, giving an incidence of 12%, associated with this method of contraception. The cysts varied in size between 3 and 7 cm diameter and were all confirmed with ultrasound examination. Laparoscopy was undertaken in 2 cases. In one woman the ovarian cyst remained unchanged in size and the dyspareunia persisted. When reviewed 4 weeks post-aspiration she was no longer troubled by painful intercourse. In the 2nd case abdominal pain had persisted for a few weeks, although the cyst had been reabsorbed at operation. Symptoms improved after laparoscopy, so the precise cause of the pain remains uncertain. The ovarian cysts in the 4 remaining women were asymptomatic and all resolved spontaneously within 6 weeks. In one of these women a second asymptomatic cyst developed on the opposite ovary 4 months later. This also resolved spontaneously. Five of the 6 women are continuing with their devices. One device was removed for personal reasons unrelated to the ovarian cyst.

Other progestogen-only methods of contraception are associated with functional ovarian cysts. One study demonstrated an incidence of 57% in progestogen-only OC users and 10% of women using Norplant are said to develop transient ovarian cysts. It appears that progestogen-only methods that disturb, rather than inhibit, ovulation are associated with an increased incidence of functional ovarian cysts. It would also suggest that the levonorgestrel IUD, although principally active at the uterine level, also has an effect on ovarian function (74[c]).

Two case-reports of *abdominopelvic actinomycosis* associated with an IUD have been published. They were successfully treated with antibiotics (75[c]).

ESTROGENS *(SED-11, 860; SEDA-12, 344; SEDA-13, 363)*

Diethylstilbestrol (DES) *(SED-11, 854; SED-11, 352; SED-12, 346)*

The fact that DES taken in pregnancy has fatal second-generation effects is continuing to have consequences: 30% of DES in utero exposed girls present a cervical vaginal adenosis (76[r]). In France 150 000–200 000 pregnancies are involved. The young women who have been exposed to DES in utero are now aged 13–35 (77[r]). The doctors will be confronted with their problems until 2010. In The Netherlands 180 000–380 000 pregnant women had been treated with DES up to 1976 (78[r]). In France a case-control study was performed in which 110 pregnancies with DES treatment were identified after the distribution of questionnaires to 500 gynecologists. The outcome of these 110 pregnancies were 57 patients exposed in utero to DES. Of particular note is the high level of extrauterine pregnancies in these women (15%). Also a high level of 1st and 2nd trimester *miscarriages* was noticed (42%). Only 41% of these women exposed to DES delivered a live baby (79[C]). New cases of *clear-cell adenocarcinoma* of the vagina of DES-exposed second-generation women are still being diagnosed accidentally in different countries (79[R]–81[R]). The Connecticut State Tumor Registry listed an incidence of 10 clear-cell adenocarcinomas in their region. Ten new cases were detected by an incidence study. The authors conclude that the finding of stable (or rising) incidence rates for clear-cell adenocarcinomas occurring nearly 30 years after the market decrease in DES sales emphasizes the need for continued clinical and epidemiological studies of the etiology and clinical course of this carcinoma (82[C]).

In a clinical study on 200 women with a history of DES exposure in utero 5 volunteered to undergo magnetic resonance (MR) imaging of the pelvis. Hysterosalpingography showed *uterine and cervical abnormalities* in all 5 patients. Abnormalities included hypoplasia of the uterine cavity, a T-shaped uterine cavity, constrictions of the uterine cavity, irregular margins of the uterine cavity, bilateral hydrosalpinges and a diverticulum of a fallopian tube. MR images showed abnormalities in all 5 patients. These included hypoplasia of the uterine cavity, uterine corpus, and cervix; a T-shaped uterine cavity; constrictions of the uterine cavity; and bilateral hydrosalpinges (83[c]).

Soon after recognition of the increased risk of vaginal clear-cell adenocarcinoma in women with in utero exposure to DES, the National Cancer Institute funded a large multicenter epidemiological cohort study, the DESAD Project. The purpose of this national project was to describe the prevalence of DES-associated genital tract changes among women exposed in utero and to compare these findings with an unexposed control group. In addition, the study sought to determine the incidence of cancer and other diseases in the exposed and unexposed cohorts. Because of the possibility that prenatal exposure to DES might adversely affect the adult immune system, the participants in the DESAD Project were surveyed to determine the prevalence of autoimmune diseases. The result was that women with vaginal epithelial changes had nearly 50% more autoimmune diseases than exposed women without vaginal changes (84[C]).

A single case of a young azoospermic patient is described whose spermatogenesis reflected an abnormality of meiosis. A diagnosis of asynapsis of chromosomes during early spermatogenesis was made by cytogenetic examination of a testicular biopsy. Standard histological examination gave no indication of this abnormality. An incidental history of intrauterine DES exposure of the patient was elicited. Attention is called to the dearth of cytogenetic studies of spermatogenesis in DES-treated male progeny and the usefulness in general of meiotic cytogenetic studies for obtaining accurate diagnoses in human infertility (85[c]).

Estrogen replacement therapy *(SED-11, 860; SEDA-13, 363)*

In a clinical study of 250 healthy women there was a decrease observed in estrone to 35 pg/ml and of estradiol to 10 pg/ml serum between the 49th and 54th year of age. Thereafter no further decline occurred because the androgen precursors of the estrogens were secreted by the adrenal cortex until an advanced age. In a period of 30 years there was a decrease in androgen levels of only 25%. In 200 patients with severe obesity no differences were found in peripheral steroid concentrations, but the SHBG concentrations were significantly lowered; the amount of free active estradiol and the effect on the target organ is therefore higher in these patients. The consequence of these results is that substitution of estrogens is indicated. The authors state that estriol has no effects on the endometrium but also no sufficient effects on the climacteric syndrome (86[C]).

Concerning the endometrium, a new publication shows that the present opinion should probably be revised. Contrary to some other authors, the data showed that local therapy with conjugated estrogens did not affect the development of endometrial hyperplasia and that estriol promoted endometrial proliferation in postmenopausal women. In this study the endometrial proliferation may be due to the fact that estriol was administered twice daily (87[C]).

To determine whether there is an association between the use of hormonal replacement therapy (HRT) and the risk of *stroke* and *myocardial infarction* (MI) a case-control study of women with stroke or MI was undertaken.

The cases were notified from 83 general practices to the coordinating center at Northwick Park Hospital, where the diagnoses were independently confirmed. The cases comprised 603 white women aged 45–69 matched to 2 controls for age. A research nurse completed a questionnaire for each case and both controls, which included information obtained from the medical notes on the prescriptions of HRT. An independent quality control check on the selection of controls and on the abstraction of information from the medical notes was made. More than one HRT prescription had been given to 109 cases (18%) and 174 controls (14%), showing a weak association between the risk of stroke and MI and the past use of HRT (relative risk 1.36). There was a stronger association with preparations containing progestogen alone. On average, HRT had been used 9 years before recruitment to the study and for 15 months.

However, the observed gradients of risk according to the duration of HRT use and time since HRT use do not support a causal interpretation. The conclusion is: There is no evidence that the use of HRT as recently prescribed in the United Kingdom constitutes a major cardiovascular risk or benefit (88[C]). The authors state: 'It should be noted that the women who had used HRT in the present study had used it, on average, only for 15 months some 9 years before. More evidence is certainly required on the use of HRT containing progestogen, since the frequency and duration of use of such preparations may well increase over the next few years, particularly as a treatment for postmenopausal osteoporosis.'

In a retrospective cohort study the authors re-evaluated 10 366 consecutive breast biopsy specimens of benign lesions performed between 1950 and 1968.

Follow-up information was obtained on 3303 women with a median duration of follow-up of 17 years. This sample comprised 84% of the patients originally selected for follow-up. The relative risk of developing breast cancer was 0.98 for women who took exogenous estrogens as compared to 1.8 for women who did not. Exogenous estrogens lowered the observed breast cancer risk in women with atypical hyperplasia (relative risk = 3.0 vs. 4.5), proliferative disease without atypia (relative risk = 0.92 vs. 1.9), and in women without proliferative disease (relative risk = 0.69 vs. 0.91). Women who took estrogens before 1956 were at 2.3 times the risk of other estrogen users, presumably due to a dose effect. There was no significant association between breast cancer risk and birth control pills, cigarette smoking, or alcohol consumption.

Exogenous estrogens are not associated with increased breast cancer risk in women with benign breast disease. A previous history of benign breast disease does not contraindicate replacement estrogen therapy (89[C]).

A prospective clinical study was performed in Montreal to investigate the clinical responses and *lipoprotein lipid changes* in perimenopausal women who received different doses of conjugated estrogens and medroxyprogesteroneacetate for 1 year.

A total of 95 healthy women who had been amenorrheic for at least 6 months were randomly assigned to 1 of 4 cyclic, sequential hormone regimens for 1 year. Groups A and C received 0.625 or 1.25 mg conjugated equine estrogen, respectively, from days 1–25 and 5 mg medroxyprogesterone acetate from days 15–25. Groups B and D were given 0.625 or 1.25 mg conjugated equine estrogen, respectively, from days 1–25 and placebo from days 15–25. Plasma estrone levels were physiological after the lower dose of conjugated equine estrogen and supraphysiological after ingestion of the higher dose. All 4 treatment regimes successfully controlled hot flushes, but patients who received 1.25 mg conjugated equine estrogen with or without medroxyprogesterone acetate had a higher energy level and a more enhanced sense of well-being. The 4 treatments all had favorable effects on lipid metabolism, albeit in a dose-related manner: After 1 year of treatment, high-density lipoprotein levels increased 4.3, 13.7, 13.4 and 19% in groups A, B, C and D, respectively, compared with pre-treatment values. The high-density lipoprotein/low-density lipoprotein ratios, an antiatherogenic index, increased by 7.3, 13.6, 24 and 43% in Groups A, B, C and D, respectively.

The authors state: It is important to note that the lower dose of conjugated equine estrogen (0.625 mg) provides physiological replacement, whereas the higher estrogen dose induces supraphysiological plasma E1 levels.

The authors conclude: 'Finally, it should be noted that the impact of oral estrogens on lipoprotein lipids may be only one of the mechanisms that explains its protective effect against heart disease. The possibility that estrogen use is protective through mechanisms additional to any effects on high-density lipoprotein in humans awaits confirmation by future studies' (90[C]).

In a 1-year clinical trial in Göteborg 60 postmenopausal women with climacteric complaints were randomly allocated to 4 treatment groups.

Without interruption, each patient was given 1 tablet daily containing 2 mg 17β-estradiol along with either norethisterone acetate 1 and 0.5 mg or megestrol acetate 5 and 2.5 mg. Blood samples were obtained before treatment and then after 1, 4 and 12 months of treatment. Serum was analyzed for cholesterol and triglycerides in serum and for cholesterol in the ultracentrifugally separated lipoproteins. Significant reductions in serum cholesterol were found in all treatment groups except for that given 2.5 mg megestrol acetate. After 1 and 4 months of treatment, low-density lipoprotein cholesterol was 7–22%, whereas high-density lipoprotein cholesterol was reduced by 2–16% in the 4 groups.

No significant differences could be demonstrated among the groups in low-density lipoprotein cholesterol or high-density lipoprotein cholesterol during treatment, as assessed by analysis of variance. Thus, cholesterol metabolism was equally affected by both progestin types (91[C]). In this study, progestins derived from the 2 groups were compared in 4 different doses during a 1-year trial. Both norethisterone acetate and megestrol acetate induced a decrease in serum cholesterol and high-density lipoprotein and low-density lipoprotein cholesterol. However, the lipoprotein lipid levels varied greatly with time in most subgroups. These variances may be explained in part by the relatively low number of patients in each treatment group.

In a case-control study in California all prescriptions concerning estrogen replacement therapy which were made between 1968 and 1973 at the San Francisco Medical Center of the Kaiser Foundation Health Plan were recorded in a computer file.

Review of this file yielded 1110 women who had received at least 2 prescriptions for an oral estrogen preparation and were aged at least 53 years in 1968; 181 estrogen users and 220 controls who had undergone spontaneous menopause and who were subsequently at risk for development of endometrial abnormalities remained in the study. The aim of this study was to evaluate the *gynecological risks* of unopposed, long-term estrogen use in postmenopausal women. The medical record review showed that unopposed estrogen users (mean dose, 0.9 mg of conjugated estrogens) had a significantly higher ($P < 0.001$) incidence of abnormal vaginal bleeding, curettage, hysterectomy, and endometrial cancer. The ratios of occurrence of these events among users compared with non-users were 7.8, 4.9, 6.6 and 7.7. The prevalence of hysterectomy reached 28.2% of users compared with 5.3% of non-users, and endometrial carcinoma developed in 9.9% of users compared with 1.4% of non-users (92[C]).

A case of *postmenopausal endometriosis* associated with estrogen/progestogen replacement therapy was reported in a 62-year-old woman. She had taken conjugated estrogens (0.625 mg) and medroxyprogesterone acetate (10 mg) for 7 years (93[c]). Comparable cases in the literature are discussed.

Estrogen treatment of prostatic cancer *(SED-11, 862; SEDA-13, 363)*

In a Finnish multicenter study 151 patients with locally advanced prostatic cancer (T3-4 MO), representing 38% of the 404 cancer patients, were randomly assigned to 1 of 3 treatment arms: orchidectomy, estrogens or radiotherapy.

The estrogen therapy consisted of polyestradiolphosphate 160 mg i.m. as an initial dose, followed by 80 mg monthly. In addition, ethinylestradiol 1 mg p.o. was given for 2 weeks, followed by 150 μg daily. During the 4-year follow-up period there were no significant differences in the progression rates (appearance of metastases in bone scan) between the therapy groups. The frequency of thromboembolic and other cardiovascular complications was highest in the estrogen group (13/15 patients). In the radiotherapy group, 19 of 45 patients had bowel or bladder complications. On the other hand, orchidectomy resulted in few, if any, complications (94[C]).

The authors conclude that the high risk of complications associated with estrogens and radiotherapy has to be taken into consideration in the selection of treatment.

In a clinical study, 20 patients with prostatic cancer were randomized to therapy with either 160 mg polyestradiolphosphate i.m. per month plus 1 mg ethinylestradiol per day during the first 2 weeks (10 patients) or orchidectomy (10 p.).

Activators and inhibitors of coagulation were studied before treatment, and 1.5 months and 6 months after the start of treatment. The patients in the estrogen group had already increased their Factor VII level after 1.5 months and this increased level persisted after 6 months. Factor X tended to increase after 1.5 months and this increase reached significance after 6 months. In the orchidectomy groups there was a significant increase in Factor X at 6 months and, in addition, antithrombin III was increased at this time. Furthermore, there was a parallelism between the increase in Factor VII and ECG evidence of increased coronary insufficiency. A significant increase in thromboxane as evidenced by the major urinary metabolite 2,3-dinorthromboxane B_2 in the estrogen group as compared to the orchidectomy group was found (95[C]).

The authors summarize: Patients with prostatic cancer during long-term estrogen treatment were found to have increased levels of Factor VII. Factor VIII:C and fibrinogen. In addition, these patients showed increased formation of thromboxane. The changes imply a *hypercoagulable state* and *platelet activation.* No such signs were found after orchidectomy. The findings in the estrogen group might explain the continuously increased risk of cardiovascular complications during long-term estrogen therapy.

PROGESTOGENS *(SED-11, 865; SEDA-12, 343; SEDA-13, 365)*

Medroxyprogesterone acetate *(SED-11, 865; SEDA-12, 343; SEDA-13, 365)*

In a clinical study 3 groups of patients with pelvic endometriosis were treated with medroxyprogesterone acetate (MPA) 50 mg/d (n = 10), lynestrenol (LYN) 10 mg/d (n = 25) and danazol (DAN) 600 mg/d (n = 25), respectively.

Total cholesterol, triglycerides, α-lipoprotein, pre-β-lipoprotein, β-lipoprotein cholesterol, high-density (HDL) and low-density (LDL) lipoprotein and apolipoprotein A_1 and B concentrations were determined before treatment and after 3 and 6 months of therapy. Whereas lipid, lipoprotein and apolipoprotein levels did not change in the MPA group, the patients on LYN and in particular those on DNA showed marked *changes in lipoprotein* patterns. α-Lipoprotein, HDL and apolipoprotein A_1 levels fell, whereas β-lipoprotein, LDL and apolipoprotein concentrations rose, these changes being statistically significant. No alterations were seen in the serum levels of cholesterol, triglycerides or pre-β-lipoprotein cholesterol.

The authors concluded that progestogen-induced alterations in lipoprotein patterns should be avoided as far as long-term treatment is concerned and where additional risk factors are present (96[C]).

The therapeutic efficacy of medroxyprogesterone acetate in hypernephroma was evaluated in a clinical study.

Patients with disseminated and progressive renal carcinoma were treated with high-dose medroxyprogesterone acetate (MPA) using the following regimen: loading dose 1000 mg i.m. for 10 days; maintenance 200 mg t.i.d., p.o. The patients had not been pretreated with hormones and/or cytostatics; 20 patients were evaluable. No objective remission was achieved. 11 patients showed stable disease lasting 3–12 months (median, 7 months). These patients were primarily characterized by a longer disease-free interval (median, 9 months) than patients with progressive disease (median, 2 months). Median survival was 22 months for patients with stable disease and 7 months for patients with progression. Toxicity of MPA treatment was low. However, in 3 patients the blood pressure increased for more than 30 mmHg, 2 cases of deep vein thromboses were registered, 3 cases of dyspnea after physical strain and 3 cases of leg edema. Pulmonary embolism possibly related to high-dose MPA occurred in 1 patient (97[c]).

The authors state that based on their results treatment with high-dose MPA in patients with metastatic renal cell carcinoma cannot be recommended.

On the basis of known dose-regimens for MPA in cancer treatment a study was designed to assess the efficacy and toxicity of high-dose oral MPA in women with clinical parameters suggesting potentially hormonally sensitive metastatic breast cancer.

The first 28 patients received 800 mg/d; 11 of them had received no previous hormone (NPH) therapy. The response rate (complete plus partial) was 63% for those receiving NPH and 12% for those receiving previous hormone (PH) therapy. Toxicity was significant at these doses, especially for women treated for more than 5 weeks. Toxic effects included *excessive weight gain, cushingoid facies, worsening of diabetes mellitus*, and other stigmata suggestive of hypercorticism. 19 other patients were treated at 400 mg/d with a 60% response rate for 10 NPH patients and 44% for patients with PH treatment. Toxicity was less severe in these patients. Moderately high (400 mg/d) and higher dose (800 mg/d) oral MPA are capable of inducing reasonable response rates in patients with NPH treatment.

The toxicity of these regimens was significant; profound weight gain was dose-limiting in some patients (98[C]).

Megestrol acetate *(SED-11, 866; SEDA-12, 344; SEDA-13, 367)*

The efficacy of combined treatment with megestrol acetate and diethylstilbestrol (DES) was studied in 62 men with previously untreated metastatic carcinoma of the prostate. The patients received oral megestrol acetate (80 mg twice daily) and a minidose estrogen (DES 0.1 mg or ethinyl estradiol 0.05 mg once daily) as a means of achieving total androgen ablation (testicular and adrenal). A high incidence of *feminizing side effects* (70–74%), a higher-than-expected rate of *cardiovascular complications* (18%), an unexpected need for cortisone replacement (13%), and failure of patients with Stage D_2 disease to obtain results better than those of standard therapy during the first year of observation suggest that this regimen offers no advantage over other more conventional therapy (99[C]).

In a Phase I–II clinical study with high doses of 480 up to 1600 mg megestrol acetate per day in 47 postmenopausal patients with advanced pretreated breast cancer the following side effects were noted during the treatment period of median 6 (range 2–12) months: *weight gain* (38 pts.), *edema* (16 pts.), *dyspnea* (10 pts.), *hypertension* (8 pts.), *constipation* (8 pts.), *hyperglycemia* (6 pts.), *urinary frequency* (5 pts.), *diarrhea* (3 pts.), *G.I. upset* (3 pts.), *congestive heart failure* (2 pts.), *phlebitis* (2 pts., 1 deep vein thrombosis, 1 superficial phlebitis) and *chest pressure* (2 pts.). A complete response was seen in 6 of the 47 patients, a partial resonse in 6, stable disease in 19 and progressive disease in 16 patients (100[C]).

A randomized clinical trial with megestrol acetate versus observation was performed in 67 patients with high-risk respected Stage I and II (nodal) malignant melanoma. The dosage was 80 mg megestrol acetate orally 4 times daily for 2 years versus 2 years observation. The most troublesome side effect from megestrol acetate was *weight gain*. The median gain in weight by 6 months was 8.2 kg for patients receiving megestrol acetate and 2.6 kg for patients on the observation arm, a significant difference in weight gain. *Impotence* and *decreased libido* affected 3 men. An additional man became *hypertensive*, and treatment was abandoned. A statistical significance in survival advantage for megestrol acetate was observed that approached 7.6 versus 2.6 years (101[C]).

PROGESTERONE ANTAGONISTS *(SEDA-13, 369)*

Mifepristone *(SEDA-13, 369)*

Heavy bleeding as a relevant side effect of this progesterone antagonist has been reported (SEDA-13, 369). This anti-fertility agent is used for the termination of early pregnancy by a single dose of 600 mg p.o. In a clinical study on 150 healthy women applying for legal abortion this dose was used.

The mean length of amenorrhea was 38 days; 131 of the 150 women had a complete abortion. The remaining 19 women included 2 curettages for heavy bleeding, 2 missed abortion, 1 extrauterine pregnancy and 14 developing pregnancies; 3 women of the 150 reported bleeding over 2 weeks (19–30 days) after abortion; 16 women had a hemoglobin level of less than 11 g/100 ml, justifying iron therapy. Other side effects were *uterine contractions* and *pelvic pain* (in 4 women), transient *asthenia* (3 pts.) and *nausea* (2 pts.).

The authors recommend mifepristone as an ambulatory treatment under medical supervision (102[C]).

ANDROGENS *(SED-11, 866; SEDA-12, 348; SEDA-13, 371)*

The approved indications for androgen therapy concern their substitution in hypogonadism during which side effects should be avoidable. Treatment with testosterone enanthate (TE) of male hypogonadism is also generally approved. A case of severe *priapism* has been recently reported concerning a 20-year-old otherwise healthy man with idiopathic hypogonadotrophic hypogonadism (serum testosterone level 0.90 nmol/l, LH and FSH both 1 IU/1).

The patient was treated with TE 250 mg i.m. every 2 weeks. Following the first 2 injections the patient experienced an increase in frequency and duration of erections, 3 days after the 3rd injection the patient had painful erections and 4 days after was admitted to hospital, where severe priapism with strong congestion of the corpora cavernosa and flaccid corpus spongiosum was diagnosed. Conservative treatment failed and operations followed.

The authors observe that among drugs suspected of causing priapism testosterone has not been noted in the literature (103[cr]).

Anabolic androgens are generally restricted in their indications (SEDA-13, 371) and are used only for life-saving treatment such as in aplastic anemia. A further 8 cases of aplastic anemia have been reported.

Pancytopenia with low reticulocyte count was found in all patients. All patients were treated with oral oxymethalone 2 mg/kg body wt./d and oral prednisolone 10 mg/d. In cases where a response occurred, the oxymetholone remained at a level at which the hematological response could be maintained. Prednisolone was reduced to alternate-day therapy and finally stopped. The post-therapy follow-up ranged from 6 to 32 months. Six of the 8 patients responded to therapy; 2 patients did not respond and died of septicemia. One of the patients who had achieved hematological improvement with androgens developed HBsAg-negative *cholestatic hepatitis* requiring stoppage of androgens and a relapse occurred. Renewed hematological recovery was seen after re-administration of androgen therapy (104[c]). The treatment duration of these 6 patients was too short for to calculate the risk of toxic effects on the liver or the induction of liver tumors.

A comparable case of aplastic anemia has been reported in an 8-year-old child who was treated with oxymetholone 0.3 mg/kg body wt. daily for 5 years. After this period of treatment a tumor in the left lobe of the liver was diagnosed histopathologically as *hepatic adenoma*. The tumor was operated and the androgen treatment terminated. For this reason androgen treatment had no further consequences (105[c]).

Discussion of anabolic steroid abuse in body-builders or so-called power lifters continues to appear in the literature. Anabolic steroids are associated with a long list of potentially toxic effects. The effects already mentioned on the liver include benign and malignant *tumors, toxic hepatitis*, and *peliosis hepatis*, the latter bring a rare disturbance in the liver in which multiple blood lakes develop that can rupture spontaneously and cause severe hemorrhage. A recently recognized side effect is a *decrease in serum high-density lipoprotein levels*, which produces an atherogenic lipid profile with consequent possible increased risk of coronary artery disease. Effects on the male reproductive system include oligospermia, azoospermia, decreased testicular size, and reduction of serum testosterone levels, all resulting from suppression of gonadotrophic hormone production. Although serum lipid levels and *testicular changes* are reversible there is still some concern about their long-term effects. *Psychological changes* attributed to steroids include mood swings, aggressive behavior, and changes in libido. Of particular concern to pediatricians is the *premature closure of the epiphyses* in prepubertal and early pubertal youth. *Virilization* in women is a common side effect (106[R]).

A case of a world-class powerlifter using anabolic steroids is reported who presented with acute *myocardial infarction*, marked *hypercholesterolemia* and an *abnormal LDL/HDL ratio*. The clinical circumstances suggest a causal relationship to anabolic steroid use (107[c]).

Other cases of side effects concerning anabolic steroid abuse are *gynecomastia* (108[C]), *cardiomyopathy, cerebrovascular accident* (109[c]), *hypercholesterolemia* (110[c]) and *suicide* (111[c]).

REFERENCES

1. Melis GB, Fruzzetti F, Ricci C et al (1988) Oral contraceptives and venous thromboembolic disease: the effect of the oestrogen dose. *Maturitas, Suppl. I,* 131.
2. Woods JW (1988) Oral contraceptives and hypertension. *Hypertension 11, Suppl. II,* 11.
3. Kuhl H, Jung-Hoffmann C, Heidt F (1988) Serum levels of 3-keto-desogestrel and SHBG during 12 cycles of treatment with 30 μg ethinylestradiol and 150 μg desogestrel. *Contraception, 38,* 381.
4. Kuhl H, Jung-Hoffmann C, Heidt F (1988) Alterations in the serum levels of gestodene and SHBG during 12 cycles of treatment with 30 μg ethinylestradiol and 75 μg gestodene. *Contraception, 38,* 477.
5. Kuhl H, Jung-Hoffmann C, Heidt F (1988) Serum levels of 3-keto-desogestrel and SHBG during 12 cycles of treatment with 30 μg ethinylestradiol and 150 μg desogestrel. *Contraception, 38,* 381.
6. Jung-Hoffmann C, Kuhl H (1989) Interaction with the pharmacokinetics of ethinylestradiol and progestogens contained in oral contraceptives. *Contraception, 40,* 299.
7. Guengerich FP (1988) Oxidation of 17-ethinylestradiol by human liver cytochrome P-450. *Mol. Pharmacol., 33,* 500.
8. Kaul L, Curry CL, Ahluwalia BS (1981) Blood levels of ethinylestradiol, daffeine, aldosterone and desoxycorticosterone in hypertensive oral contraceptive users. *Contraception, 23,* 643.
9. Stadel BC, Sternthal PM, Schlesselman JJ et al (1980) Variation of ethinylestradiol blood levels among healthy women using oral contraceptives. *Fertil. Steril., 33,* 257.
10. Cohen C, Mackie IJ, Walshe K et al (1988) A comparison of the effects of two triphasic oral contraceptives on haemostasis. *Br. J. Haematol., 69,* 259.
11. Ernst, E., Schmölzl CH, Matrai A, Schramm W (1989) Hemorheological effects of oral contraceptives. *Contraception, 40,* 571.
12. Farag A, Bottoms SF, Mammen EF et al (1988) Haemostasis and oral contraceptives. *Folia Haematol., 115,* 340.
13. Von Hugo R, Briel RC, Schindler AE (1989) Wirkung oraler Kontrazeptiva auf die Blutgerinnung bei rauchenden und nichtrauchenden Probandinnen. *Aktuel. Endokrinol. Stoffwechsel, 10,* 6.
14. Miwa LJ, Edmunds AL, Shaefer MS, Raynor SC (1989) Idiopathic thromboembolism associated with triphasic oral contraceptives. *DICP Ann. Pharmacother., 23,* 773.
15. Lamy L, Roy PH, Morissette JJ, Cantin R (1988) Intimal hyperplasia and thrombosis of the visceral arteries in a young woman: possible relation with oral contraceptives and smoking. *Surgery, 103,* 706.
16. Scolding NJ, Gibby OM (1988) Fatal pulmonary embolus in a patient treated with Marvelon. *J. R. Coll. Gen. Pract., 38,* 568.
17. Granato DB, Archer CR, Awwad EE (1989) Magnetic resonance imaging of cerebral venous thrombosis secondary to 'low-dose' birth control pills. *Clin. Imag., 13,* 220.
18. Chopard JL, Moulin T, Bourrin JC et al (1988) Contraception orale et accident vasculaire cérébral ischémique. *Sem. Hôp. Paris, 64,* 2075.
19. Ananijevic-Pandey J, Vlajinac H (1989) Myocardial infarction in young women with reference to oral contraceptive use. *Int. J. Epidemiol., 18,* 585.
20. Croft P, Hannaford PC (1989) Risk factors for acute myocardial infarction in women: evidence from the Royal College of General Practitioners' oral contraception study. *Br. Med. J., 298,* 165.
21. Burkman RT (1988) Lipid and lipoprotein changes in relation to oral contraception and hormonal replacement therapy. *Fertil. Steril., 49, Suppl.,* 39.

22. Knopp RH (1988) Cardiovascular effects of endogenous and exogenous sex hormones over a woman's lifetime. *Am. J. Obstet. Gynecol., 158,* 1630.
23. Notelovitz M, Feldman EB, Gillespy M, Gudat J (1989) Lipid and lipoprotein changes in women taking low-dose, triphasic oral contraceptives: a controlled, comparative, 12-month clinical trial. *Am. J. Obstet. Gynecol., 160,* 1269.
24. Ball MJ, Ashwell E, Jackson MC et al (1989) Which Pill? The effect of various modern preparations on lipoproteins and glucose metabolism. *Br. J. Fam. Plan., 14,* 110.
25. Leuven JAG, Drijkoningen GJA, Alers J et al (1988) The effect of low dose oral contraceptives on lipoprotein lipid and apolipoprotein levels in smoking and non-smoking women. *J. Drug Ther. Res., 13,* 355.
26. Burkman RT, Zacur HA, Kimball AW et al (1989) Oral contraceptives and lipids and lipoproteins. I. Variations in mean levels by oral contraceptive type. *Contraception, 40,* 553.
27. Burkman RT (1989) Oral contraceptives, lipid and lipoprotein changes, and risk of coronary heart disease. *Semin. Reprod. Endocrinol., 7,* 224.
28. Wingerd J, Tuffy TJ (1977) Oral contraceptive use and other factors in the standard glucose tolerance test. *Acta Obstet. Gynaecol. Scand. Suppl. 105,* 25.
29. Kasdorf G, Kalkhoff RK (1988) Prospective studies of insulin sensitivity in normal women receiving oral contraceptive agents. *J. Clin. Endocrinol. Metab., 66,* 846.
30. Ramamoorthy R, Saraswathi TP, Kanaka TS (1989) Carbohydrate metabolic studies during twelve months of treatment with a low-dose combination oral contraceptive. *Contraception, 40,* 563.
31. Gaspard U (1988) Contraception orale, métabolisme glucidique et critères de surveillance. *Contracept. Fertil. Sex., 16,* 113.
32. Ancey P, Saint-Cyr M, Paliard P (1989) Ictère sous contraceptif oral, cholestase gravidique et élévation des transaminases. *Presse Méd., 18,* 1480.
33. Van Erpecum KJ, Janssens AR, Kreuning J et al (1988) Generalized peliosis hepatis and cirrhosis after long-term use of oral contraceptives. *Am. J. Gastroenterol. 83,* 572.
34. Jorgensen T (1988) Gall stones in a Danish population: fertility period, pregnancies, and exogenous female sex hormones. *Gut, 29,* 433.
35. Jorgensen T (1988) Oral contraceptives and gallstones. *Lancet, 2,* 335.
36. Heresbach D, Deugnier Y, Brissot P, Bourel M (1988) Dilatations sinusoidales et prise de contraceptifs oraux. *Ann. Gastroentérol., 24,* 189.
37. Ross RK, Bernstein L, Garabrant D, Henderson B (1988) Avoidable nondietary risk factors for cancer. *Am. Fam. Physician, 38,* 153.
38. La Vecchia C, Negri E, Parazzini F (1989) Oral contraceptives and primary liver cancer. *Br. J. Cancer, 59,* 460.
39. Dreyfus M, Jaeck D, Dreyfus J (1989) Adénomes du foie et contraception orale. *Rev. Fr. Gynécol. Obstét., 84,* 761.
40. Ferrara BE, Rutland ED (1988) Liver tumor in long-term user of oral contraceptives. *Postgrad. Med., 84,* 107.
41. Lorimier G, Delaby J, Rive C et al (1988) Tumeurs du foie et contraceptifs oraux: problèmes diagnostiques, indications thérapetiques. *Sem. Hôp. Paris, 64,* 2216.
42. Kelleher MB, Iwatsuki S, Sheahan DG (1989) Epithelioid hemangioendothelioma of liver. *Am. J. Surg. Pathol. 13,* 999.
43. Suyama Y, Horie Y, Suou T et al (1988) Oral contraceptives and intrahepatic biliary cystadenoma having an increased level of estrogen receptor. *Hepato-gastroenterology, 35,* 171.
44. Marks WH, Thompson N, Appleman H (1988) Failure of hepatic adenomas (HCA) to regress after discontinuance of oral contraceptives. *Ann. Surg., 208,* 190.
45. Anonymous (1987) British study suggests long-term pill use before first term pregnancy raises risk of breast cancer. *Int. Fam. Plan. Perspect., 13,* 146.
46. Kay CR, Hannaford PC (1988) Breast cancer and the pill – a further report from the Royal College of General Practitioners' oral contraception study. *Br. J. Cancer, 58,* 675.
47. Vessey MP, McPherson K, Villard-Mackintosh L, Yeates D (1989) Oral contraceptives and breast cancer: latest findings in a large cohort. *Br. J. Cancer, 59,* 613.
48. Chilvers C, McPherson K, Peto J et al (1989) Oral contraceptive use and breast cancer risk in young women. *Lancet, 1,* 973.
49. McPherson K, Vessey MP, Neil A et al (1987) Early oral contraceptive use and breast cancer: results of another case-control study. *Br. J. Cancer, 56,* 653.
50. Miller N, McPherson K, Jones L, Vessey M (1989) Histopathology of breast cancer in young women in relation to use of oral contraceptives. *J. Clin. Pathol., 42,* 387.
51. Lund E, Meirik O, Adami HD et al (1989) Oral contraceptive use and premenopausal breast cancer in Sweden and Norway: possible effects of different pattern of use. *Int. J. Epidemiol., 18,* 527.
52. La Vecchia C, Parazzini F, Negri E et al (1989) Breast cancer and combined oral contraceptives: an Italian case-control study. *Eur. J. Cancer Clin. Oncol., 25,* 1613.
53. Stadel BV, Lai S, Schlesselman JJ, Murray P (1988) Oral contraceptives and premenopausal breast cancer in nulliparous women. *Contraception, 38,* 287.
54. Jick SS, Walker AM, Stergachis A, Jick H

(1989) Oral contraceptives and breast cancer. *Br. J. Cancer 59,* 618.
55. Rohan TE, McMichael J (1988) Oral contraceptive agents and breast cancer: a population-based case-control study. *Med. J. Aust., 149,* 520.
56. Beaulieu EE, Benagiano G, Brosens I et al (1989) Oral contraceptives and breast cancer (Letter to Editor). *J. Am. Med. Assoc., 262,* 206.
57. Beral V, Hannaford R, Kay C (1988) Oral contraceptive use and malignancies of the genital tract. *Lancet, 2,* 1331.
58. Armstrong BK, Ray RM, Thomas DB (1988) Endometrial cancer and combined oral contraceptives. *Int. J. Epidemiol., 17,* 263.
59. The WHO Collaborative Study of Neoplasia and Steroid Contraceptives (1988) Epithelial ovarian cancer and combined oral contraceptives. *Int. J. Epidemiol., 18,* 538.
60. Ananijevic-Pandej J, Jarebinski M, Vlajinac i Zagorka Radojkovic H (1988) Congenital malformations and contraception. *Jugosl. Pedijatr., 31,* 115.
61. Nikschick S, Göretzlehner G, Boldt O et al (1989) Fehlbildungshäufigkeit nach Anwendung hormonaler Kontrazeptiva. *Zentral bl. Gynäkol., 111,* 1152.
62. Shoupe D, Mishell DR (1989) Norplant: subdermal implant system for long-term contraception. *Am. J. Obstet. Gynecol., 160,* 1266.
63. Singh K, Viegas OAC, Liew D et al (1988) Norplant-2 rods: one year experience in Singapore. *Contraception, 38,* 429.
64. Singh, K, Viegas OAC, Koh S et al (1988) The effects of norplant-2 rods on clinical chemistry in Singaporean acceptors after 1 year of use: haemostatic changes. *Contraception, 38,* 441.
65. Singh K, Viegas OAC, Koh S et al (1989) Two-year follow-up of changes in clinical chemistry in Singaporean Norplant acceptors: haemostatic changes, *Contraception, 39,* 137.
66. Singh K, Viegas OAC, Koh S et al (1989) Two-year follow-up of changes in clinical chemistry in Singaporean Norplant-2 rod acceptors: haemostatic changes. *Contraception, 39,* 155.
67. Singh K, Viegas OAC, Liew D et al (1989) Two-year follow-up of changes in clinical chemistry in Singaporean Norplant acceptors: metabolic changes. *Contraception, 39,* 129.
68. Singh K, Viegas OAC, Liew D et al (1989) Two-year follow-up of changes in clinical chemistry in Singaporean Norplant-2 rod acceptors: metabolic changes. *Contraception, 39,* 147.
69. Koifman S, Primo Paes SJ, Oliveira DP et al (1987) Avaliacão do anticoncepcional Norplant no Municipio do Rio de Janeiro. *Rev. Saude Publica, 21,* 513.
70. Darney PD, Monroe SC, Klaisle CM, Alvarado A (1989) Clinical evaluation of the Capronor contraceptive implant: preliminary report. *Am. J. Obstet. Gynecol., 160,* 1292.
71. Ratsula K (1989) Clinical performance of a levonorgestrel-releasing intracervical contraceptive device during the first two years of use. *Contraception, 39,* 187.
72. Odlind V (1987) Review: New methods for fertility regulation in women. *Clin. Reprod. Fertil., 3,* 221.
73. Calzolari E, Girolametti C, Parisi C et al (1988) Esperienze di contraccezione intrauterina. *Minerva Ginecol., 40,* 317.
74. Robinson GE, Bounds W, Kubba AA et al (1989) Functional ovarian cysts associated with the levonorgestrel releasing intrauterine device. *J. Fam. Plan., 14,* 131.
75. Mäenpää J, Taina E, Grönroos M et al (1988) Abdominopelvic actinomycosis associated with intrauterine devices. Two case reports. *Arch. Gynecol. Obstet., 243,* 237.
76. Sopena-Bonnet B (1989) L'adénose cervico-vaginale: l'une des conséquences possibles de l'exposition in utero au DES. *Contracept. Fertil. Sex., 17,* 461.
77. Kahn-Nathan J (1989) Les effets de l'exposition in utero au DES chez les filles. *Contracept. Fertil. Sexual., 17,* 243.
78. Van Erp EJM, Zalmstra HAM, Hanselaar AGJM, Van Hall EV (1989) La politique de diéthylstilboestrol (DES) aus Pays-Bas. *Contracept. Fertil. Sex., 17,* 517.
79. Pons JC, Goujard J, Derbanne C, Tourmaire M (1988) Devenir des grossesses des patientes exposées in utero au diéthylstilboestrol. *J. Gynecol. Obstet. Biol. Reprod., 17,* 307.
80. Focchi J, Ribalta JCL, Sakano CRB et al (1988) Adenose de vagina. Consideracões sobre 10 casos. *J. Bras. Ginecol., 98,* 635.
81. Flamant F, Goujard J, Castaigne D et al (1989) Risque d'adénocarcinome à cellules claires du vagin chez l'adolescente et la femme jeune. *Contracept. Fertil. Sex., 17,* 239.
82. Horwitz RI, Viscoli CM, Merino M et al (1988) Clear cell adenocarcinoma of the vagina and cervix: incidence, undetected disease, and diethylstilbestrol. *J. Clin. Epidemiol., 41,* 593.
83. Van Gils APG, Tjon RTO, Tham A et al (1989) Abnormalities of the uterus and cervix after diethylstilbestrol exposure: correlation of findings on MR and hysterosalpingography. *Am. J. Roentgenol., 153,* 1235.
84. Noller KL, Blair PB, O'Brien PC et al (1988) Increased occurrence of autoimmune disease among women exposed in utero to diethylstilbestrol. *Fertil. Steril., 49,* 1080.
85. Hembree WC, Nagler HM, Fang JS et al (1988) Infertility in a patient with abnormal spermatogenesis and in utero DES exposure. *Int. J. Fertil., 33,* 173.

86. Von Holst T, Klinga K, Runnebaum B (1989) Endokrinologie des Klimakteriums. *Arch. Gynaekol. Obstet.*, *245*, 952.
87. Montoneri C, Zarbo G, Garofalo A, Giardinella S (1987) Effects of estriol administration on human postmenopausal endometrium. *Clin. Exp. Obstet. Gynecol.*, *14*, 178.
88. Thompson SG, Meade TW, Greenberg G (1989) The use of hormonal replacement therapy and the risk of stroke and myocardial infarction in women. *J. Epidemiol. Commun. Health*, *43*, 173.
89. Dupont WD, Page DL, Rogers LW, Parl FF (1989) Influence of exogenous estrogens, proliferative breast disease, and other variables on breast cancer risk. *Cancer*, *63*, 948.
90. Sherwin BB, Gelfand MM (1989) A prospective one-year study of estrogen and progestin in postmenopausal women: effects on clinical symptoms and lipoprotein lipids. *Obstet. Gynecol.*, *73*, 759.
91. Sporrong T, Hellgren M, Samsioe G, Mattsson LA (1989) Metabolic effects of continuous estradiol–progestin therapy in postmenopausal women. *Obstet. Gynecol.*, *73*, 754.
92. Ettinger B, Golditch IM, Friedman G (1988) Gynecologic consequences of long-term, unopposed estrogen replacement therapy. *Maturitas*, *10*, 271.
93. Goodman JM, Kredentser D, Deligdisch L (1989) Postmenopausal endometriosis associated with hormone replacement therapy. *J. Reprod. Med.*, *34*, 231.
94. Aro J, Haapiainen R, Kajanti M et al (1988) Comparison of endocrine and radiation therapy in locally advanced prostatic cancer. *Eur. Urol.*, *15*, 182.
95. Henriksson P, Blombäck M, Bratt G et al (1989) Effects of oestrogen therapy and orchidectomy on coagulation and prostanoid synthesis in patients with prostatic cancer. *Med. Oncol. Tumor Pharmacother.*, *6*, 219.
96. Teichmann AT, Cremer P, Wieland H et al (1988) Lipid metabolic changes during hormonal treatment of endometriosis. *Maturitas*, *10*, 27.
97. Doberauer C, Becher R, Kurschel E et al (1988) Hochdosierte Behandlung mit Medroxyprogesteronazetat beim metastasierenden Hypernephrom. *Tumor Diagn. Ther.*, *9*, 210.
98. Davila E, Vogel CL, East D et al (1988) Clinical trial of high-dose oral medroxyprogesterone acetate in the treatment of metastatic breast cancer. *Cancer*, *61*, 2161.
99. Johnson DE, Babaian RJ, Swanson DA et al (1988) Medical castration using megestrol acetate and minidose estrogen. *Urology*, *31*, 371.
100. Tchekmedyian NS, Tait N, Abrams J, Aisner J (1988) High-dose megestrol acetate in the treatment of advanced breast cancer. *Semin. Oncol.*, *15*, 44.
101. Creagan ET, Ingle JN, Schutt AJ, Schaid DJ (1989) A prospective, randomized controlled trial of megestrol acetate among high-risk patients with resected malignant melanoma. *Am. J. Clin. Oncol.*, *12*, 152.
102. Maria B, Stampf F, Foepp A, Ulmann A (1988) Termination of early pregnancy by a single dose of mifepristone (RU 486), a progesterone antagonist. *Eur. J. Obstet. Gynecol. Reprod. Biol.*, *28*, 249.
103. Zelissen PMJ, Stricker BHCh (1988) Severe priapism as a complication of testosterone substitution therapy. *Am. J. Med.*, *85*, 273.
104. Pandita R, Quadri MI (1988) Constitutional aplastic anemia. *Ind. Pediatr.*, *25*, 469.
105. Sanchez JMC, Becerra EP, Martin AA et al (1988) Adenoma hepático después del tratamiento con oximetolona. *Rev. Esp. Pediatr.*, *44*, 195.
106. Dyment PG, Goldberg B (1989) Anabolic steroids and the adolescent athlete. *Pediatrics*, *83*, 127.
107. McNutt RA, Ferenchick GS, Kirlin PC, Hamlin NJ (1988) Acute myocardial infarction in a 22-year-old world class weight lifter using anabolic steroids. *Am. J. Cardiol.*, *62*, 164.
108. Aiache AE (1989) Surgical treatment of gynecomastia in the body builder. *Plast. Reconstr. Surg.*, *83*, 61.
109. Mochizuki RM, Richter KJ (1988) Cardiomyopathy and cerebrovascular accident associated with anabolic-androgenic steroid use. *Physician Sportsmed.*, *16*, 109.
110. Cohen JC, Noakes TD, Benade AJS (1988) Hypercholesterolemia in male power lifters using anabolic androgenic steroids. *Physician Sportsmed.*, *16*, 51.
111. Brower KJ, Blow FC, Eliopulos GA, Beresford TP (1989) Anabolic androgenic steroids and suicide. *Am. J. Psychiatry*, *146*, 1075.

R. Bouillon

43 Thyroid hormones, iodine and antithyroid drugs

THYROID HORMONES *(SED-11, 876; SEDA-12, 353; SEDA-13, 375)*

The exact amount of thyroxine needed for optimal substitution of hypothyroid patients has received widespread attention during recent years and the mean dose in use has been reduced (SED-11, 876; SEDA-12, 353; SEDA-13, 375). The importance of this in improving tolerance is evident. Since measurements of TSH, T4 and T3 in serum are used for monitoring the optimal dose, it is necessary to define the timing of the blood sampling in relation to the time of intake of thyroxine. In a careful study by Browning et al of 12 patients with primary hypothyroidism, only total and free T4 increased between 2 and 8 hours after thyroxine intake whereas T3 and TSH remained unchanged. Moreover, the increase in total and free T4, although statistically significant, was small and the overall T4 concentration during the observation period was more stable than the spontaneous fluctuations in serum T3 and TSH (1[C]). The authors, therefore, recommend T4 measurements as the primary method for monitoring thyroxine substitution (1[C]).

Thyroid hormones have a profound effect on bone metabolism, increasing both bone resorption and formation (2[R]). Since prolonged hyperthyroidism may be associated with high-turnover *osteoporosis*, and because methods to improve quantitation of bone mass have improved, the effects of substitution therapy with thyroid hormones on bone have been re-evaluated (SEDA-13, 375). The bone mineral density measured in 31 postmenopausal women treated with thyroxine for at least 5 years was normal in the lumbar spine but markedly decreased in the femoral neck (−13% vs. age-matched controls) (3[C]). Since the serum T4 concentration was significantly higher and TSH concentration significantly lower in the T4-substituted women than in the controls, chronic oversubstitution with thyroid hormones might be a causal factor for osteoporosis although chronic calcitonin deficiency, commonly found in patients with hypothyroidism, might also be a contributing element (4[c]). Since similar results were already reported last year (SEDA-13, 375) it seems wise to follow the advice given by Cooper (5[R]) to choose carefully the dosage of T4, avoiding TSH suppression except for the follow-up of thyroid malignancy. Moreover, the concept of prolonged use of thyroxine for benign, thyroid nodulus may need re-evaluation, especially since its effectiveness for such disorders is questionable (SEDA-13, 375). Some workers, however, found a slight increase in the bone mineral content of the spine and forearm of hypothyroid patients on long-term thyroxine substitution despite the fact that their TSH concentrations were also suppressed (6[c], 7[c]). It might well be that the primary thyroid disease, especially long-standing Graves' disease, may be a confounding factor in the later evaluation of bone mineral content during thyroxine substitution. Until late effects on bone are better known, it seems prudent to use thyroxine in a dose which keeps T4 detectable within the normal range (5[R]).

Early treatment of subclinical hypothyroidism (no clinical signs of hypothyroidism but increased serum TSH concentrations) was evaluated in a double-blind cross-over study. Serum TSH normalized during the T4 substitution period and increased again during the placebo period. Ventricular injection function and serum collagen metabolism increased during thyroxine treatment and 1 in 4 women reported an improved physical condition and better performance during psychometric testing (8[c]).

(Biomedical Division)
Side Effects of Drugs Annual 14
M.N.G. Dukes and L. Beeley, editors

A case of *Graves' disease* developing during treatment with thyroxine for documented autoimmune hypothyroidism has been reported (9[c]). Thyroid-stimulation blocking antibodies disappeared whereas thyroid-stimulating antibodies were detected during the hyperthyroid phase. In view of the rarity of such an observation it seems unlikely that this complication is due to thyroid substitution therapy itself; it probably represents the reverse sequence of what is more commonly found: Graves' disease later replaced by autoimmune hypothyroidism.

Several *cardiac side effects* of thyroid hormone therapy are well documented (SED-11, 877; SEDA-11, 356; SEDA-13, 375). A complete atrioventricular block developed in a 60-year-old hypothyroid woman during treatment with T4 200 μg/d. The conduction disturbances disappeared after stopping the drug and did not resume after restarting it later in the more physiologic dosage of 100 μg/d (10[c]).

Thyroid overdosage *Syncope* attacks and diffuse *vasospasm* of the right coronary artery were observed in a 44-year-old woman shortly after introduction of thyroid hormone therapy for hypothyroidism (11[c]) but the causal effect is disputable. Severe *myocardial ischemia* (documented by echocardiography and scintigraphy) and *shock* were reported in a 68-year-old woman treated with thyroxine 0.3 mg/d. She was clinically and biochemically hyperthyroid. After subsequent reduction of the thyroid dosage cardiac echography, scintigraphy and catheterization revealed normal coronary arteries and ventricular function (12[c]). Myocardial ischemia and infarction have indeed been reported previously during hyperthyroidism or thyroxine overdosage but usually not in patients without pre-existing cardiac diseases (SED-11, 877).

Overdosage An extensive review of the literature on the effects of excess thyroid hormone ingestion has drawn a distinction between inadvertent excessive use of thyroid hormones (by eating ground beef contaminated with thyroid hormones), the incorrect use of these drugs for the treatment of obesity, excessive thyroid substitution therapy and factitious use of thyroid hormones for psychiatric reasons (13[R]). Mild hyperthyroidism is likely to result from such practices but serious short-term side effects are rare. Accidental or suicidal injection of large amounts of thyroid hormones is more exceptional and the literature data are well presented in several tables. Clinical symptoms do not necessarily correlate well with plasma T4 levels and the clinical symptoms observed, if present at all, range from anxiety, confusion coma to tachycardia, atrial fibrillation and angina. No lethal cases of accidental thyroid hormone overdosage were found during the reviewer's survey but one would point out that at least 3 such cases have been reported previously (SEDA-8, 371). Treatment of thyroid overdosage is not well-standardized and may include gastric lavage, sedatives, beta-blockers, hydrocortisone or specific antiarrhythmic drugs. Plasmapheresis and exchange transfusion have successfully been used to treat life-threatening cases. More recent studies have found beneficial effects of iodine-containing organic radiographic agents (ipodate) since they are potent inhibitors of the peripheral conversion of T4 to T3 but rebound effects are not impossible (13[c]).

Second-generation effects During recent decades it has been widely believed that thyroid hormones do not cross the human placenta. More recent data in rat and man however cast doubt on this assumption and confirm that small amounts of thyroxine can cross the placenta and result in detectable, although below normal, levels of T4 in the fetus and rat (14[C], 15[c]). These data will probably not change earlier recommendations for the treatment of Graves' disease during pregnancy (SEDA-11, 357; SED-11, 880). Since hypothyroidism in the mother may result in low T4 levels in the fetus before its own thyroid autonomy is well established and might therefore be associated with disturbances in fetal neural development, these new data are of utmost importance; they underline the need for optimal thyroid substitution in hypothyroid pregnant woman (16[c]).

ANTITHYROID DRUGS *(SED-11, 879; SEDA-12, 354; SEDA-13, 376)*

The use of antithyroid drugs for the treatment of Graves' disease is currently competing with the increased use of ^{131}I (see below). If, however, relapses after a course of antithyroid drugs could be better predicted their use would be greatly extended. Patients with persistent TSH receptor antibodies, an abnoral TSH response to TRH and large goiters at the end of antithyroid therapy are the most likely to relapse but the high sensitivity of this combination of tests is offset by its low specificity so that it is clinically not very useful (17[C], 18[C]). Fairly similar conclusions were reached by others (19[C]) but patients with small goiters and less severe disease (T3 concentrations below 54 mol/l) can usually be expected to have a long-term remission. In neither study did HLA typing prove to be a useful predictor.

Such data may help to guide treatment at an earlier stage so as to avoid consecutive exposure to the side effects of both antithyroid drugs and ^{131}I in young patients with Graves' disease. When only propranolol was used for treatment of Graves' disease, 8 out of 26 patients showed a spontaneous remission lasting for 30–48 months (20[C]). Such spontaneous recovery was not predictable by biochemical tests but disappearance of TSH receptor antibodies and mild disease tended to predict a better outcome. This 25% spontaneous remission rate is quite similar to previous experience (SEDA-2, 337; SEDA-5, 381) and should be compared to an overall relapse-free cure rate of about 50% for antithyroid drugs.

Using a higher than conventional dose of carbimazole (100 mg/d instead of 45 mg/d) it has proved possible to correct the biochemical symptoms of hyperthyroidism significantly more rapidly (4 weeks) than with the conventional dose (6 weeks) without significant side effects (21[C]). It is, however, unlikely that this favorable view of side effects will be confirmed when a large number of patients are studied and such high-dose therapy will best be reserved for patients with very severe forms of the disease.

Allergic reactions to antithyroid drugs are well-known. Moreover, drug-induced *lupus syndrome* can be observed during treatment with antithyroid drugs (22[R]). Some common features include fever, arthralgia, myalgia, pleurisy and pericarditis without involvement of central nervous system or kidneys and usually also without the typical rash or mucosal ulcers. Such occasional cases have been regularly reported in most previous editions of SEDA (SEDA-4, 295; SEDA-7, 398; SEDA-8, 896; SEDA-11, 357; SEDA-13, 376). Cats treated with propylthiouracil can similarly develop anti-DNA antibodies and a clinical picture resembling lupus (23[c]). Such an animal model is important for studying the mechanism of this exceptional but severe drug-induced complication.

Allergic acute hepatitis developed in a 50-year-old patient within 5 hours after accidental re-exposure to methimazole. The jaundice was severe (bilirubin 44 mg/dl) but disappeared uneventfully after about 3 weeks. Lymphocyte transformation tests demonstrated the allergic origin of this disease (24[C]). Although the patient had used methimazole some years earlier without noticeable side effects, allergic reactions to other drugs and to food had occurred previously (24[C]).

Skin and mucosal allergy to methimazole is not exceptional (SED-11, 880; SEDA-9, 345) and was observed together with *agranulocytosis* in a 34-year-old hyperthyroid female (25[c]). Marked improvement was observed after about 2 weeks. As usual the reaction was observed within the first three months after the start of the therapy.

Antithyroid drugs and pregnancy An exceptional case of diabetes and Graves' disease complicating pregnancy in a 27-year old-woman was reported. Since she was known to be allergic to both methimazole and propylthiouracil and because a rash recurred after sequential trial of methimazole and propylthiouracil it was necessary to employ surgery, following pre-treatment with propranolol (26[c]).

Last year's special review on the supposed teratogenic effects on methimazole cast doubt on its causal relationship with fetal scalp defects (SEDA-13, 377) but a new case of *aplasia cutis* and elevated α-fetoprotein levels has since been reported in a child exposed to methimazole during early pregnancy (27[C]). This brings the total number of reported cases of aplasia cutis during methimazole treatment to 13 according to the authors, while our own count rises now to 16. This, nevertheless, does not prove a causal relationship since most prospective or retrospective studies failed to find a significant association (SEDA-13, 377).

IODINE AND THE IODIDES *(SED-11, 881; SEDA-12, 355; SEDA-13, 378)*

Iodine-deficiency disorders (IDD) are a

worldwide problem affecting more than 200 million people in at least 40 countries. In 1986 the WHO General Assembly passed a resolution for the prevention and control of IDD seeking to have these disorders controlled before the end of this millenium (28[R]). Iodine can either be given as potassium iodide or iodate added to salt but this is not always feasible in remote and poor areas of the world. Intramuscular and oral iodized unsaturated fatty acids have, therefore, been introduced and both methods have been found to be effective and remarkably safe. Indeed, long-term evaluation of intramuscular lipiodol administration in the highlands of Papua New Guinea prevented the nervous type of cretinism at least when given prior to conception. Moreover, the survival and the motor and intellectual development of children of treated mothers were significantly better than in the untreated controls after 15 years of follow-up (29[CR]). Oral lipiodol may have similarly beneficial effects and avoids the costs of injections and the associated risks of communicable diseases such as viral hepatitis or AIDS (30[R]). Iodine-induced hyperthyroidism is exceptionally low in such populations, especially when the large dose of iodine ($\pm$500 mg I) is considered (28[R]).

The use of iodide-containing antiseptic drugs for mouth rinsing results in a significant iodide absorption but was not associated with significant thyroid dysfunction (31[C]). Previous observations have, however, indicated that such therapy can occasionally result in iodine-induced hyperthyroidism (SED-11, 882).

Local treatment with potassium iodide can also (although only exceptionally) cause serious *allergic* reactions. Systemic *vasculitis* with impaired kidney function and papillitis of the eyes were observed in a patient treated with KI (3×300 mg/d) for an erythematous dermatosis known as Sweet's syndrome (32[C]). The complications reacted well to subsequent corticoid therapy.

Since amiodarone contains a high amount of iodine and is increasingly used as an antiarrhythmic drug, its thyroid side effects continue to be reported (33[R]–35[R]) (SEDA-13, 4; SEDA-11, 360). Aside from its effect as supplier of excess iodine resulting in increased thyroid gland iodine content (36[c]) it also influences peripheral thyroid hormone metabolism (37[c]) and action (38[c]). It might, therefore, be possible to develop amiodarone analogs with specific thyroid hormone antagonistic effects (38[c]).

Radioactive iodine (^{131}I) *(SED-11, 883; SEDA-12, 356; SEDA-13, 378)*

Radioactive iodine is increasingly chosen as a first option for the treatment of hyperthyroidism due to Graves' disease and even when due to single or multiple thyroid nodules. This therapy is indeed simpler, more effective and less costly than the medical or surgical alternatives (39[CR]). The trend to lower or eliminate the minimum age limit for ^{131}I is therefore increasing though it is not accepted worldwide. For children and young adults ^{131}I is not generally advised in Germany (40[R]) or Belgium (41[R]) whereas its use in children is advocated in the U.S.A. as the first therapeutic option (42[R]).

Such changing attitudes along with better iodide intake in most civilized countries have reduced the frequency of thyroid surgery; an indirect consequence of this shift away from operative treatment could be a loss of experience in many centers; as a result, thyroid surgery for hyperthyroidism might again become associated with increased risks (42[R], 43[R]).

The minimal age limits for safe administration of ^{131}I, however, should not be discussed from such theoretical standpoints but must be assessed on the basis of very long-term evaluation of children exposed to radioiodine or other radioactive products. No really long-term (>30 years) data have been published, despite the fact that a lag period as long as this has been observed between low level thyroid irradiation and thyroid cancer (SED-11, 883). Second generation effects, however, seem to be minimal. Among the 217 offspring of 208 patients treated with ^{131}I for childhood hyperthyroidism, four congenital malformations were observed (clubfoot in 2; tracheoesophageal fistula and patent ductus arteriosus in 1). Disorders diagnosed later in these offspring include diabetes mellitus (2), hypothyroidism (2) and asthma (2), cystic fibrosis (1), leukemia (1), nephrotic syndrome (1), petit mal epilepsy (1) and congenital deafness (1). No increased chromosomal instability was observed in the karyotype of 114 examined progeny of patients treated with ^{131}I (42[C]). The authors reporting these findings, however, recommend for children high dose ^{131}I therapy (3.7–7.4 MBq/g of thyroid tissue) followed by life-long thyroid substitution therapy so as to destroy most of the thyroid tissue and avoid slowly evolving and unrecognized hypothyroidism; this approach should avoid late carcinogenic effects (42[C]).

The need for such a cautious approach to the use of this radio-isotope in children is underlined by what we do know as to the late effects of irradiation at this age. Low dose irradiation (1–2 Gy) in childhood has for example been shown to result in brain tumors, developing up to 30 years after the initial irradiation (44[C]). Benign and malignant thyroid nodules are known to be inducible by low-dose thyroid irradiation (SED-11, 883) and it now seems that after removal such thyroid nodules may recur in the remaining apparently normal thyroid tissue (45[C]). Of these nodules 19% were malignant. Treatment with thyroid hormones reduced the incidence of benign nodules but not that of thyroid cancer. Such data are extremely relevant for the discussion of long-term safety of higher doses of ^{131}I.

The long-term incidence of *hypothyroidism* after ^{131}I is dependent on the dose used but probably also population-dependent. When a high dosage was used (10–15 mCi) hypothyroidism developed in 68% at 12 months follow-up (46[C]), whereas a 10-fold lower incidence (6.6%) was found at 1-year follow-up with a subsequent annual incidence of 3% in France after a mean dose of $\pm$10 mCi (39[C]). This latter incidence is remarkably similar to that noted in previous surveys in other countries (SED-11, 883). Still lower long-term incidence of hypothyroidism after ^{131}I was reported in the Philippines (47[C]). Thyroid irradiation with ^{131}I also results in irradiation of surrounding tissues.

Parathyroid lesions (both hypo- and hyperfunction) have been reported previously (SED-11, 884) while in a retrospective study of 1550 patients with hyperparathyroidism, 0.7% of the patients reported previous neck irradiation. This incidence is probably higher than the prevalence of primary hyperparathyroidism in the general population, which is estimated at not more than 0.4% (48[C]). The C-cells of the thyroid may also be destroyed, resulting in (near)-total calcitonin deficiency (4[c]). Whether this contributes to long-term osteoporosis is disputed (see section on thyroxine substitution). The secretion and enzyme production of the parotid glands may also be affected by ^{131}I therapy since the parotid gland is known transiently to accumulate this ion (49[c]). This side effect was however only significant when very high doses (>470 mCi) were given for thyroid carcinoma (49[c]).

Iodine is also concentrated in (human) milk, and *breast-feeding* is therefore contra-indicated after therapeutic ^{131}I therapy. From a careful study in lactating woman receiving ^{131}I therapy the authors concluded that even the diagnostic use of ^{131}I in 100 mCi (3.7 MBq) is inadvisable if breast-feeding is to be continued (50[C]).

REFERENCES

1. Browning MCK, Bennet WM, Kirkaldy AJ, Jung RT (1988) Intraindividual variation of thyroxine, triiodothyronine and thyrotropin in treated hypothyroid patients: implications for monitoring replacement therapy. *Clin. Chem., 34*, 696.
2. Auwerx J, Bouillon R (1986) Mineral and bone metabolism in thyroid disease: a review. *Q. J. Med., 232*, 737.
3. Paul TJ, Kerrigan J, Kelly AM et al (1988) Long-term L-thyroxine therapy is associated with decreased hip bone density in premenopausal women. *J. Am. Med. Assoc., 259*, 3157.
4. Body JJ, Demeester-Mirkine N, Corvilain J (1988) Calcitonin deficiency after radioactive iodine treatment. *Ann. Intern. Med., 109*, 590.
5. Cooper DS (1988) Thyroid hormone and the skeleton: a bone of contention. *J. Am. Med. Assoc., 259*, 3175.
6. Hurley DL, Tiegs RD, Wahner HW et al (1987) Axial and appendicular bone mineral density in patients with long-term deficiency or excess of calcitonin. *N. Engl. J. Med., 317*, 537.
7. Heath H (1988) Decreased bone density and thyroxine. *J. Am. Med. Assoc., 260*, 2219.
8. Nyström E, Caidahl K, Fager G et al (1988) A double-blind cross-over 12-month study of L-thyroxine treatment of women with 'subclinical' hypothyroidism. *Clin. Endocrinol., 29*, 63.
9. Takeda K, Takamatsu J, Kasagi K et al (1988) Development of hyperthyroidism following primary hypothyroidism: a case report with changes in thyroid-related antibodies. *Clin. Endocrinol., 28*, 341.
10. Daoud ZF, Al-Kaseeh Z, Al-Khateeb H (1988) Possible atrioventricular conduction defect in L-thyroxine-treated patients. *Curr. Ther. Res., 43*, 1190.
11. Ohyagi Y, Kira J, Kobayashi T (1988) A case of syncope attack due to vagal reflex of rest angina. *Clin. Neurol., 28*, 883.

12. Bergeron GA, Goldsmith R, Schiller NB (1988) Myocardial infarction, severe reversible ischemia and shock following excess thyroid administration in a woman with normal coronary arteries. *Arch. Intern. Med., 148*, 1450.
13. Cohen JH, Ingbar SH, Braverman LE (1989) Thyrotoxicosis due to ingestion of excess thyroid hormone. *Endocrine Rev., 10*, 113.
14. Vulsma T, Gons MH, De Vijlder JJM (1989) Maternal-fetal transfer of thyroxine in congenital hypothyroidism due to a total organification defect or thyroid agenesis. *N. Engl. J. Med., 321*, 13.
15. Morreale de Escobar GM, Obregon MJ, Ruiz de Ona C, Escobar del Rey F (1989) Comparison of maternal to fetal transfer of 3,5,3′-triiodothyronine versus thyroxine in rats, as assessed from 3,5,3′-triiodothyronine levels in fetal tissues. *Acta Endocrinol., 120*, 20.
16. Mano MT, Potter BJ, Belling GB et al (1989) The effect of thyroxine, 3,5-dimethyl-3′-isopropyl-L-thyronine and iodized oil on fetal brain development in the iodine-deficient sheep. *Acta Endocrinol., 121*, 7.
17. Schleusener H, Schwander J, Holl G et al (1987) Do HLA-DR-typing and measurement of TSH-receptor antibodies help in the prediction of the clinical course of Graves' thyrotoxicosis after antithyroid drug treatment? *Acta Endocrinol., (Suppl.) 281*, 318.
18. Schleusener H, Schwander J, Fischer C et al (1989) Prospective multicentre study on the prediction of relapse after antithyroid drug treatment in patients with Graves' disease. *Acta Endocrinol., 120*, 689.
19. Young ET, Steel NR, Taylor JJ et al (1988) Prediction of remission after antithyroid drug treatment in Graves' disease. *Q. J. Med., 250*, 175.
20. Codaccioni JL, Orgiazzi J, Blanc P et al (1988) Lasting remissions in patients treated for Graves' hyperthyroidism with propranolol alone: a pattern of spontaneous evolution of the disease: *J. Clin. Endocrinol. Metab., 67*, 656.
21. O'Malley BP, Rosenthal FD, Northover BJ et al (1988) Higher than conventional doses of carbimazole in the treatment of thyrotoxicosis. *Clin. Endocrinol. 29*, 281.
22. Hess E (1988) Drug-related lupus. *N. Engl. J. Med., 318*, 1460.
23. Aucoin DP, Rubin RL, Peterson ME et al (1988) Dose-dependent induction of anti-native DNA antibodies in cats by propylthiouracil. *Arthritis Rheum., 31*, 688.
24. Federmann G, Becker EW, Tautorat H et al (1988) Nachweis der allergischen Genese einer akuten Hepatitis durch den Lymphozytentransformationstest. *Dtsch. Med. Wochenschr., 113*, 1676.
25. Hou GL, Tsai CC (1988) Oral manifestations of agranulocytosis associated with methimazole therapy. *J. Periodontol., 59*, 244.
26. Bruner JP, Landon MB, Gabbe SG (1988) Diabetes mellitus and Graves' disease in pregnancy complicated by maternal allergies to antithyroid medication. *Obstet. Gynecol., 72*, 443.
27. Farine D, Maidman J, Rubin S, Chao S (1988) Elevated alphafetoprotein in pregnancy complicated by aplasia cutis after exposure to methimazole. *Obstet. Gynecol., 71*, 996.
28. Hetzel BS (1988) *The Prevention and Control of Iodine Deficiency Disorders.* Nutrition policy discussion paper no. 3, United Nations ACC/SCN, Rome.
29. Pharoah POD, Connolly KJ (1987) A controlled trial of iodinated oil for the prevention of endemic cretinism: a long-term follow-up. *Int. J. Epidemiol., 16*, 68.
30. Eltom M, Karlsson FA, Kamal AM et al (1984) The effectiveness of oral iodized oil in the treatment and prophylaxis of endemic goiter. In: *Endemic Goiter in the Sudan.* Uppsala.
31. Ader AW, Paul TL, Reinhardt W et al (1988) Effect of mouth rinsing with two polyvinylpyrrolidone–iodine mixtures on iodine absorption and thyroid function. *J. Clin. Endocrinol. Metab., 66*, 632.
32. Eeckhout E, Willemsen M, Deconinck A, Somers G (1987) Granulomatous vasculitis as a complication of potassium iodide treatment for Sweet's syndrome. *Acta Derm. Venereol., 67*, 362.
33. Leger A (1987) L'iode, la thyroide et le radiologiste. *J. Radiol. 68*, 745.
34. Volpe R, Loffredo R, Rinaldi S et al (1987) Funzionalità tiroidea ed amiodarone. *Q. Med. Chir., 3*, 321.
35. De Rosa G, Corsello SM, Testa A, Cecchini L (1987) Amiodarone e funzione tiroidea. *Clin. Ther., 123*, 205.
36. Fragu P, Schlumberger M, Davy JM et al (1988) Effects of amiodarone therapy on thyroid iodine content as measured by X-ray fluorescence. *J. Clin. Endocrinol. Metab., 66*, 762.
37. Safran M, Fang SL, Bambini G et al (1986) Effects of amiodarone and desethylamiodarone on pituitary deiodinase activity and thyrotropin secretion in the rat. *Am. J. Med. Sci., 292*, 136.
38. Norman MF, Lavin TN (1989) Antagonism of thyroid hormone action by amiodarone in rat pituitary tumor cells. *J. Clin. Invest., 83*, 306.
39. Gibold C, Delisle MJ, Maes B et al (1988) Traitement des hyperthyroidies par l'iode radioactif: évolution des méthodes et difficultés de la surveillance. *Presse Méd., 17*, 1397.
40. Becker W, Börner W, Reiners C, Roedler HD (1988) Die Radiojodtheapie der Immunhyperthyreose in Abhängigkeit vom Lebensalter. *Dtsch. Med. Wochenschr., 113*, 954.
41. Jonckheer MH, Glinoer D (1988) Rapport betreffende een enquête, uitgevoerd in België over de modaliteiten van de behandeling van hyperthyreoidie met radiojood. *Nucl. Geneeskd. Bull., 10*, 34.

42. Levy WJ, Schumacher OP, Gupta M (1988) Treatment of childhood Graves' disease. *Cleveland Clin. J. Med.*, *55*, 373.
43. Hennemann G, Krenning EP (1989) Minder schildklieroperaties in Nederland. *Ned. Tijdschr. Geneeskd.*, *133*, 1299.
44. Ron E, Modan B, Boice JD et al (1988) Tumors of the brain and nervous system after radiotherapy in childhood. *N. Engl. J. Med.*, *319*, 1033.
45. Fogelfeld L, Wiviott MBT, Shore-Freedman E et al (1989) Recurrence of thyroid nodules after surgical removal in patients irradiated in childhood for benign conditions. *N. Engl. J. Med.*, *320*, 835.
46. Johansen K, Khan M, Woodhouse NJY (1988) High-dose iodine-131-treatment of hyperthyroidism: experience at King Faisal Specialist Hospital and Research Centre. *Ann. Saudi Med.*, *8*, 466.
47. Bandong-Reyes E, De la Cruz C, Gonzales VL (1988) Transient hypothyroidism in iodine-131 treated thyrotoxicosis: a review of cases from 1970–1984 and JRRMMC. *Phil. J. Intern. Med.*, *26*, 97.
48. Christmas TJ, Chapple CR, Noble JG et al (1988) Hyperparathyroidism after neck irradiation. *Br. J. Surg.*, *75*, 873.
49. Deeg M, Maier H, Bihl H, Adler D (1988) Klinisches Bild und mögliche Ursachen der Funktionsstörungen der Glandula parotis bei der Radiojodtherapie des differenzierten Schilddrüsenkarzinoms. *Laryng. Rhinol. Otol.*, *67*, 362.
50. Dydek GJ, Blue PW (1988) Human breast milk excretion of iodine-131 following diagnostic and therapeutic administration to a lactating patient with Graves' disease. *J. Nucl. Med.*, *29*, 407.

H.M.J. Krans

44 Insulin, glucagon and hypoglycemic drugs

INSULIN *(SED-11, 889; SEDA-12, 358; SEDA-13, 381)*

A recent review of insulin replacement (1[R]) includes the complications and side effects of the various forms of insulin therapy.

Hypoglycemia A study of factors contributing to hypoglycemia in children (up to 19 years old) revealed that 6.8% of 150 children had severe hypoglycemic attacks (2[r]), defined as episodes requiring outside assistance and loss of consciousness. No relation to HbA_1 concentration or age was found. A relation existed to previous attacks, indicating that some patients are more at risk. 64% of the attacks were related to deviations from routine treatment such as missing or delaying meals, failure to take extra food for extra work or maintenance of the same insulin dosage when low blood glucose is measured. Relatively few episodes were seen in the first 5 years of diabetes except for the first year in which the incidence was high. In the first year the necessity for the child and the family to accommodate to insulin treatment may play a role. In longer-standing diabetes changes in the contraregulatory hormones may be of importance.

The frequency of nocturnal hypoglycemia (blood glucose < 3 mmol/l) was determined by hourly blood glucose estimations in patients on intensive therapy (3[r]). Patients with continuous subcutaneous insulin infusion (CSII) showed more frequent hypoglycemia. The periods were of longer duration than those in patients on multiple injections. The periods were mostly seen at the late night hours. Low HbA_{1c} and low blood glucose in the evening and the morning were indicative of hypoglycemia. No Somogyi effect could be demonstrated. Only 1 of 3 patients with hypoglycemic values showed subjective symptoms. This report may be a reflection of the fact that the mean blood glucose is in general lower in patients on CSII than in those on treatment with multiple injections.

To study the role of low blood glucose values in the early night for fasting hyperglycemia, extra insulin was given from 22.00–02.00 hours in a series of CSII patients (4). This extra amount of insulin was in certain patients compensated by extra intravenous glucose (resulting in a blood glucose of 5.5 mmol/l at 3 h) and in the others it was not (blood glucose 2.4 ± 0.2 mmol/l at 03.00 h). All patients were asymptomatic. The fasting and postprandial blood glucose levels in the insulin-only group were significantly higher than in those in the group with normal glucose levels at night. This supports the belief that in elevated morning blood glucose a Somogyi effect has to be taken into account.

The chance of subclinical hypoglycemia in older NIDDM (Type II) patients after the institution of treatment with insulin may also depend on the type of insulin used. Hypoglycemia is especially likely to be induced by long-acting preparations. In 12 patients treated with Humulin-zinc (comparable in duration of action to Lente preparations, in structure to Ultralente preparations) 46 episodes were seen in 6 months as compared to 4 episodes in 10 patients treated with a beef zinc suspension insulin (Neulente). The insulin was given as a single injection in the morning (5[C]).

The symptoms of overinsulinization without overt hypoglycemia are often similar to those of hyperglycemia, namely excessive thirst, nycturia, polyuria, hunger, dizziness, fatigue and headaches (6[r]).

Increased sensitivity to insulin was reported in a patient in whom human insulin was substi-

Side Effects of Drugs Annual 14
M.N.G. Dukes and L. Beeley, editors

tuted for beef insulin (7[C]). Hypoglycemia developed. As in other reports the patient was poorly controlled on animal insulin.

Laron et al (8[c]) note that treatment of 30 newly-diagnosed diabetics with either human or porcine insulin resulted in a similar incidence of hypoglycemic episodes.

Factitious hypoglycemia (9[C]) was reported in a nurse and in a non-diabetic in a family with frequent diabetes. Low (endogeneous) C-peptide during hypoglycemia, the absence of hypoglycemia during fasting and (sometimes) the presence of insulin antibodies are factors that must raise suspicion.

Insulin allergy Two cases of insulin allergy were reported by Plantin et al (10[C]). One was a pregnant patient treated with bovine NPH insulin who developed an urticarial reaction and the other a 52-year-old patient, with known atopic constitution and a history of intermittent treatments with porcine insulin, who developed urticarial lesions when she was regularly treated with porcine insulin. Replacement with human insulin produced no improvement.

In another patient with a history of allergic reactions to purified porcine insulin, generalized urticaria (11[C]) with Quincke's edema, tachycardia and strong dyspnea developed on the third injection of human semisynthetic insulin after the patient had been transferred to that product. She had been treated during earlier periods with bovine insulin. The skin tests were positive to all types of insulin.

Eight patients who had been treated intermittently (12[c]) with animal insulins and who developed generalized allergic reactions (urticaria and non-thrombocytopenic purpura) and local reactions and/or lipohypertrophy were followed for 3 years after the start of treatment with human insulin. Systemic allergy disappeared, local allergy was reduced or disappeared, insulin-specific IgE decreased significantly and insulin-specific IgG decreased. The intradermal skin tests were positive in all persons except one.

In a patient (13[C]) with both an immediate (pruritic wheal and flare) reaction subsiding in 2 hours and a delayed reaction consisting of a pruritic indurated and painful lesion with maximal intensity after 24 hours and subsiding in the next few days normal desensitization had no success. Insulin + diphenhydramine reduced the immediate reaction. Insulin + hydrocortisone reduced the delayed reaction. A combination of insulin + hydrocortisone + diphenhydramine was successful but could not be given permanently when the patient was at home, since hydrocortisone is unstable and the instability increases when diphenhydramine is present. Addition of 1 mg of dexamethasone to 1 unit of insulin resulted in reduction of those side effects which were most bothersome for the patient. To suppress the immediate effects systemic antihistamines were necessary. The patient had a satisfactory HbA_{1c}, demonstrating that the combination of dexamethasone + insulin was effective in lowering blood glucose.

Specific allergic reactions (14[C]) to protamine were seen in 3 patients, a brother and sister both with diabetes and a non-diabetic man from a separate family. The latter developed anaphylactic shock when protamine was used to neutralize heparin. Skin tests were only positive with high concentrations of protamine.

Other side effects *Amyloid-fibril protein* (15[C]) was found in a young man of Afro-Caribbean ancestry at two sites where purified porcine insulin (Actrapid) had been injected. When an abcess occurring at the injection site after more than a year of injections into the abdominal wall was incised, an amount of firm tissue could be excised. Moreover a lump was excised from a hypertrophic nodule on the leg at a previous injection site. The amyloid-fibril protein extracted from both lumps contained intact insulin molecules (amino acid composition and sequence). This appears to be the first report of a foreign protein detected in amyloid protein. The rectum biopsy showed no amyloid. More hypertrophic reactions on insulin may contain insulin amyloid.

Lipoatrophy has become a rare complication since highly purified and synthetic insulins were introduced. Lipoatrophy observed during the use of purified bovine insulin (16[C]) became worse with biphasic purified porcine insulin, but was reversed when biphasic recombinant insulin was used.

Flocculation in insulin vials (see SEDA-12, 360; SEDA-13, 383) was reported by the manufacturer of Humulin-N to have occurred only once in 30 000 vials (17). The phenomenon was further investigated by asking 444 patients if they had ever encountered insulin bottles resembling a bottle with flocculated insulin which was shown to them. Questionnaires were mailed to 1400 patients: 38 patients reported flocculation of Humulin-N insulin. Some had noted a concomitant decrease in the efficacy of their insulin requiring an increased insulin dose or resulting in ketosis. When compared to a group of patients with no complaints it appeared that the risk of flocculation increased when insulin was carried in a briefcase or purse; it was also more likely when low doses of insulin were used and when intermediate and short-acting insulins were mixed. The formulation of Humulin-N has since been changed. It is too early to conclude that this has stopped flocculation. Patients and doctors have to be aware of the risk of flocculation; they should continue to inspect the vials and to replace any vial containing insoluble precipitate.

In a study on the effect of storage temperature on insulin (18) it was concluded that refrigerated storage negatively influenced the pharmacokinetics and pharmacodynamics of Lente/regular mixtures but not of NPH/regular mixtures. It is unclear if the zinc present in Lente insulins affects insulin differentially after refrigeration. Other publications confirmed that the zinc content of insulin renders the effects of mixtures less predictable than it is when mixtures of NPH and short-acting insulins are used (19, 20, 21).

CSII and intensive therapy

In a study on staphylococcal infections at the infusion site in CSII (22[r]), no correlation was found with the carriage rate of *Staphylococcus aureus*, the indwelling needle or the amount of injected insulin. There was, however, a relation with the preservatives. Infection was significantly more frequent with insulin containing *m*-cresol than with insulins containing methyl-*p*-benzoate.

One of the complications of intensive insulin therapy is deterioriation of retinopathy (23, 24, 25). Two patients were described (26[C]) in whom HbA_1 decreased during treatment with CSII from 14.3 and 17.5%, respectively, to 5.7 and 7.5%. In the first 5–7 months proliferative retinopathy increased dramatically and coagulation was considered. The condition of the eyes, however, improved and during a following period of 2 and 5 years, respectively, only mild background retinopathy was found.

Another 'complication' of intensive therapy may be weight gain. In the DCCT (Diabetes Control and Complications Trial) study (27) a significantly great weight gain was recorded in the intensive treatment regimen groups (5.1 ± 4.6 kg) as compared to the standard treatment group (2.4 ± 3.7 kg, $P < 0.001$) (28).

Blood glucose meter

The increasing availability of various blood glucose meters and their increasing use has led to studies of the reliability of the various strips and meters when used by patients. There seems to be a relation between the number of actions to be performed by the patient and the accuracy of the meter (29). For a test of the various systems used the reader is referred to a report in the journal *Health Devices* (30).

ORAL HYPOGLYCEMIC DRUGS *(SED-11, 893; SEDA-13, 383)*

Pharmaceutical marketing research data from the United States on the use of oral hypoglycemic drugs have been analyzed to determine trends in the use of oral hypoglycemics over the period 1964–1986 (31[R]). The relevance of such figures to the interpretation of population data on adverse effects is obvious. Figures were derived from three pharmaceutical marketing research databases. Only one of the bases had data available as far back as 1964, but this base has changed its methodology twice. The other bases were used for the periods 1974–1986 and 1982–1986. In 1964 tolbutamide, chlorpropamide, acetohexamide, tolazamide (1966) and phenformin were in use. The so-called second-generation sulfonylureas (glyburide (glibenclamide) and glipizide) were approved in the United States only in 1984. Phenformin was withdrawn in 1977. The UGDP study (see SEDA-4, 301 and preceding Annuals) was published in 1970 and has been discussed for about 10 years, as reviewed in early Annuals. The highest prescription rate was in 1973. The use of these products then decreased until 1979 and the figures for 1986 were again comparable to those of 1974. The market share of tolbutamide had dropped from 75% in 1964 to 35% in 1973; by 1986 its share was only 10%. Chlorpropamide (which has most side effects) increased to 53% in 1981–1983 but fell back to 33% in 1986. At the end of 1986 glyburide had 29% and glipizide 12% of the market. Phenformin accounted for 9% of the dispensed agents in 1964 and at its peak in 1973 it comprised about almost 22% of the market. 56% of the drugs were used by people over 65 years, 14% were 60–64 years old and only 3% were used by people under 39 years.

The data are based on outpatient use only; hospital use is thus not included. One of the systems was based on data from community physicians only and did not include hospital-based physicians. The prescription attitude and availability of specific drugs in the United States naturally differs from other countries, but the trends are important for the student of adverse reactions.

Hypoglycemia remains a life-threatening side effect of sulfonylureas; its incidence and severity may however vary regionally. In a recent Japanese paper on the side effects of these products (32[r]) it was reported that of 494 cases of severe hypoglycemia due to sulfonylureas in Japan, 49 patients died and 45 patients suffered sequelae. In a study by Jennings et al, 219 patients aged 40–65 years treated with oral hypoglycemics (33) were interviewed as regards hypoglycemic symptoms experienced during the previous 6 months: 20.2% of 203 patients treated with sulfonylureas had experienced (major) symptoms. None of the 16 patients on metformin showed these symptoms. Mean HbA_1 and postprandial blood glucose were significantly lower in patients with symptoms. The prevalence was higher for glyburide then for gliclazide or chlorpropamide and was also higher when medications were taken that potentiated the sulfonylurea effect, notably the *sulfonamides*.

This latter interaction is illustrated by a report on hypoglycemic complications of sulfonamides making reference to 4 cases who were treated with these drugs for *Pneumocystis carinii* pneumonia (34[C]). One of the patients died during a hypoglycemic episode. The patient had no diabetes. Sulfonamides are regularly used for urinary tract infections frequently seen in older diabetics treated with oral hypoglycemic agents.

Glibenclamide *(SED-11, 898; SEDA-13, 384)*

Five cases of *hypoglycemia* (4 of them fatal) were reported in patients with impaired renal function using glibenclamide (35[C]).

Chlorpropamide *(SED-11, 898; SEDA-13, 384)*

Hypoglycemia sustained for 36 hours emerged when during a period of 4 days 3 tablets of chlorpropamide (diabinese) were taken (36[C]) from a bottle labeled 'acetozolamide' (diamox). The container had been filled with the wrong tablets in the pharmacy.

Metformin *(SED-1, 899; SEDA-13, 384)*

Indications for the existence of two compartments in the body for metformin can be derived (37[C]) from a report on a patient who was treated with 3 tablets of glicazide, 3 tablets of metformin retard and 2 tablets of methyldopa.

When she broke her leg she was operated and hospitalized; the same therapy was continued. When she became somnolent and hypotensive on the 5th day, she was transferred to the reanimation department. There she was found to be acidotic (pH 7.01), hypoglycemic (glucose 0.6 mmol/l), dehydrated and to have renal insufficiency (creatinine 703 μmol/l). The plasma- and the globulin-bound concentration of metformin was 68 and 29.7 mg/l, respectively (normal during metformin therapy, 0.56 and 0.81 mg/l). Notwithstanding alkalinization, rehydration and glucose infusion the metformin level remained elevated (28 mg/l). After hemodialysis she improved clinically, but the metformin levels remained elevated. She needed 5 days of 4 h of dialysis before her clinical values were normalized. High concentrations of metformin were found in the erythrocytes. They contributed to the slow decrease of serum values.

Aldose reductase inhibitors *(SED-11, 900; SEDA-12, 362; SEDA-13, 362)*

In a study on sorbinil, an aldose reductase inhibitor, for diabetic neuropathy 2 patients showed *hypersensitivity reactions* (38). The symptoms disappeared after the drug was discontinued. Four of the 31 patients developed a foot ulcer during the sorbinil trial.

In a short review (39[r]) on aldose reductase inhibitors the most significant side effects were hypersensitivity reactions (fever with myalgia, lymphadenopathy and a maculopapular rash on trunk and face associated with transient neutropenia, thrombocytopenia and elevated liver enzymes) (compare SEDA-12, 362; SEDA-11, 900). This syndrome has been reported in 11% of patients using sorbinil (40). More serious dermatological effects such as epidermic necrolysis and severe thrombocytopenia and leukopenia may develop when the drug is continued (41). For tolrestat no significant side effects were reported, but the period of investigation is shorter and the number of publications is less. A study in our own clinic revealed that of 38 patients who used tolrestat for 6 months or 1 year, one patient developed transient liver enzyme elevations immediately after when the period in which he used tolrestat ended.

REFERENCES

1. Zinman B (1989) The physiologic replacement of insulin, an elusive goal. *N. Engl. J. Med., 321*, 363.
2. Bergada I, Suissa S, Dufresne J, Schiffrin A (1989) Severe hypoglycemia in IDDM children. *Diabetes Care, 12*, 239.
3. Bendtson I, Kverneland A, Pramming S, Binder C (1988) Incidence of nocturnal hypoglycaemia in insulin-dependent diabetic patients on intensive therapy. *Acta Med. Scand., 223*, 543.
4. Perriello G, De Feo P, Torlone E et al (1988) The effect of asymptomatic nocturnal hypoglycemia on glycemic control in diabetes mellitus. *N. Engl. J. Med., 319*, 1233.
5. Tindall H, Bodansky HJ, Stickland M, Wales JK (1988) A strategy for selection of elderly type 2 diabetic patients for insulin therapy, and a comparison of two insulin preparations. *Diabetic Med., 5*, 533.
6. Berger W (1988) Insulin therapy in the elderly type 2 diabetic patient. *Diabetes Res. Clin. Pract., Suppl.*, 24.
7. Turner TA, O'Mullane NM, Sivener A et al (1988) Switching to human insulin. *Lancet, 2*, 1150.
8. Laron Z (1989) Hypoglycaemia in newly diagnosed diabetic children and adolescents – comparison between human and porcine insulin. *Diabetologia, 32*, 454.
9. Bhatnagar D (1988) Diagnosis of factitious hypoglycaemia. *Br. J. Hosp. Med., 40*, 140.
10. Plantin P, Sassolas B, Guillet MH et al (1988) Accidents cutanés allergiques aux insulines. *Ann. Dermatol. Vénéréol., 115*, 813.
11. Wintermantel C, Fischer N, Müller PH et al (1988) Anaphylaktische Reaktion auf Humaninsulin. *Dtsch. Med. Wochenschr., 113*, 1142.
12. Bruni B, Barolo P, Blatto A et al (1988) Treatment of allergy to heterologous monocomponent insulin with human semisynthetic insulin. *Diabetes Care, 11*, 59.
13. Loeb JA, Herold KC, Barton KP et al (1989) Systematic approach to diagnosis and management of biphasic insulin allergy with local anti-inflammatory agents. *Diabetes Care, 12*, 421.
14. Oswald-Mammosser M, Dietemann-Molard A, Oswald T et al (1988) Allergie à la protamine. *Rev. Fr. Allergol., 28*, 173.
15. Dische FE, Wernstedt C, Westermark GT et al (1988) Insulin as an amyloid-fibril protein at sites of repeated insulin injections in a diabetic patient. *Diabetologia, 31*, 158.
16. Jowett NI, McNally PG (1988) Lipoatrophy with highly purified insulins and treatment with recombinant human insulin. *Pract. Diabetes, 5*, 130.
17. Benson EA, Benson Jr JW, Fredlund PN et al (1988) Flocculation and loss of potency of human NPH insulin. *Diabetes Care, 11*, 563.
18. Perriello G, Torlone E, Di Santo S et al (1988) Effect of storage temperature of insulin on pharmacokinetics and pharmacodynamics of insulin mixtures injected subcutaneously in subjects with type I (insulin-dependent) diabetes mellitus. *Diabetologia, 31*, 811.
19. Klauser R, Schernthaner G, Prager R (1988) Mixtures of human intermediate and human regular insulin in type I diabetic patients. *Diabetes Res. Clin. Pract., 5*, 185.
20. Berger M, Cueppers HJ, Hegner H et al (1982) Absorption kinetics and biologic effects of subcutaneously injected insulin preparations. *Diabetes Care, 5*, 77.
21. Colagiuri S, Villalobos S (1986) Assessing effect of mixing insulins by glucose clamp technique in subjects with diabetes mellitus. *Diabetes Care, 9*, 579.
22. Van Faassen I, Razenberg PPA, Simmoons-Smit AM, Van der Veen EA (1989) Carriage of *Staphylococcus aureus* and inflamed infusion sites with insulin-pump therapy. *Diabetes Care, 12*, 153.
23. Van Ballegooie E, Hooymans JMM, Timmerman Z et al (1984) Rapid deterioration of diabetic retinopathy during treatment with continuous subcutaneous insulin infusion. *Diabetes Care, 7*, 236.
24. Lauritzen T, Frost-Larsen K, Larsen H-W et al (1983) Effect of 1 year of near-normal blood glucose levels on retinopathy in insulin-dependent diabetics. *Lancet, 1*, 200.
25. The Kroc Collaborative Study Group (1984) Blood glucose control and the evolution of diabetic retinopathy and albuminuria. *N. Engl. J. Med., 311*, 365.
26. Rosenlund EF, Haakens K, Brinchmann-Han-

sen O et al (1988) Transient proliferative diabetic retinopathy during intensified insulin treatment. *Am. J. Ophthalmol., 105*, 618.
27. The DCCT Research Group (1987) Diabetes Control and Complications Trial (DCCT): results of feasibility study. *Diabetes Care, 10*, 1.
28. The DCCT Research Group (1988) Weight gain associated with intensive therapy in the diabetes control and complications trial. *Diabetes Care, 11*, 567–573.
29. Jovanovic-Peterson L, Peterson CM, Dudley JD et al (1988) Identifying sources of error in self-monitoring of blood glucose. *Diabetes Care, 11*, 791.
30. Anonymous (1988) Blood glucose monitors. *Health Devices, 17*, 253.
31. Kennedy DL, Piper JM, Baum C (1988) Trends in use of oral hypoglycemic agents 1964–1986. *Diabetes Care, 11*, 558.
32. Hirata Y (1988) Cautions for the use of oral hypoglycemic agents. *Asian Med. J., 31*, 129.
33. Jennings AM, Wilson RM, Ward JD (1989) Symptomatic hypoglycemia in NIDDM patients treated with oral hypoglycemic agents. *Diabetes Care, 12*, 203.
34. Ryan DW, Oyston J (1988) Sulphonylureas and hypoglycaemia. *Br. Med. J.*, 296, 1328.
35. Kennedy TD, Keat AC, Chester M et al (1988) Predisposing factors in fatal glibenclamide induced hypoglycaemia. *Pract. Diabetes, 5*, 217.
36. Gordon MR, Flockhart D, Zawadzki JK et al (1988) Hypoglycemia due to inadvertent dispensing of chlorpropamide. *Am. J. Med., 85*, 271.
37. Lacroix C, Hermelin A, Gerson M et al (1988) Acidose lactique imputable à la metformine: intêrèt des taux intraérythrocytaires. *Presse Méd., 17*, 1158.
38. O'Hare JP, Morgan MH, Alden P et al (1988) Aldose reductase inhibition in diabetic neuropathy: clinical and neurophysiological studies of one year's treatment with sorbinil. *Diabetic Med., 5*, 537.
39. Falbe WJ, Bess DT (1988) Aldose reductase inhibitors for complications of diabetes mellitus. *Drug Intell. Clin. Pharm., 22*, 408.
40. Pitts NE, Gunderson K, Mehta DJ et al (1986) Aldose reductase inhibitors in clinical practice: preliminary studies on diabetic neuropathy and retinopathy. *Drugs, 32, Suppl. 2*, 30.
41. Jaspan JB, Towle L, Maselli R, Herold K (1986) Clinical studies with an aldose reductase inhibitor in the autonomic and somatic neuropathies of diabetes. *Metabolism, 35, Suppl. 1*, 83.

R. Bouillon and F.A. Van Assche

45 Miscellaneous hormones and prostaglandins

MISCELLANEOUS HORMONES

Calcitonin *(SED-11, 903; SEDA-12, 364; SEDA-13, 386)*

Calcitonin is a well-validated drug in the treatment of (severe) Paget's disease. When given intravenously, its effect on bone remodeling is rapid since within 24 hours a marked decrease in serum osteocalcin, a biochemical marker of bone formation, can be observed (1[c]). Intranasal administrations of synthetic salmon calcitonin, a route which is generally considered to improve tolerance, was studied in 17 patients with Paget's disease over a period of 1 year. Biochemical, clinical and radiological improvement was obvious whereas none of the usual side effects of calcitonin were observed. Local tolerance was also excellent (2[C]). Others, however, found neutralizing anti-salmon calcitonin *antibodies* in patients treated with nasal calcitonin after previous exposure to subcutaneous or intramuscular calcitonin (3[c]). Intramuscular injection of porcine calcitonin solubilized in gelatin retards the absorption as compared to the same drug in physiological saline, but the clinical advantage is not obvious (4[c]).

An excellent review on the clinical pharmacology of human calcitonin was published by an experienced researcher (5[R]), describing both its indications and side effects. Most of these side effects have been described previously (SED-11, 903), but this author points out that their incidence can be decreased by subcutaneous rather than intramuscular injection (especially when given at bedtime) and probably even better by nasal application. The induction of *secondary hyperparathyroidism* is exceptional, but bone biopsies in non-affected areas nevertheless show signs of *increased bone turnover* (5[c]). Systemic and intrathecal administration of calcitonin can have analgesic effects. Three cases with long-standing pain due to a non-malignant disease were treated successfully with continuous intrathecal calcitonin therapy without significant side effects (6[c]).

To treat or prevent postmenopausal osteoporosis, a daily dose of 32 IU of salmon calcitonin was significantly more effective than lower doses or oral calcium carbonate (7[c]). Mild or minor *gastrointestinal and vasomotor side effects* occurred in about 1 out of 4 patients, but cutaneous *rash* or *local pain* were more exceptional.

Parathyroid hormones (PTH) analogs *(SED-11, 903)*

The availability of synthetic human PTH (1–34) has stimulated further research into the best means of using it as a diagnostic test for the diagnosis of various types of hypoparathyroidism. For this purpose hPTH (1–34), 5 U/kg body wt. (max. 200 U), is infused intravenously over 10 min and blood and urine are collected before and after the injection to calculate phosphate and cAMP metabolism. No adverse reactions were observed during 30 such infusions (8[c], 9[c]). Others have confirmed this observation (10[c]), but some found 100 U (30 μg) to be a sufficient dose. Again no side effects were reported (11[c]).

Somatotrophin (human growth hormone; hGH) *(SED-11, 903; SEDA-12, 369; SEDA-13, 387)*

Growth hormone, whether endogenously produced (12[c], 13[c]) or injected as biosynthetic hGH (14[c]), has a short half-life (about 20 min in man). Its metabolic clearance rate evaluated

(Biomedical Division)
Side Effects of Drugs Annual 14
M.N.G. Dukes and L. Beeley, editors

in Rhesus monkeys, however, increases in obesity, helping to explain the low GH concentrations in obese patients (14[c]).

An excellent review by Brook has discussed the clinical treatment of growth deficiency (15[R]). The use of GH in children who are considered to be suffering from somewhat arbitrarily defined GH deficiency is challenged since it is evident that GH administration will change the rate of increase in height according to the dose of GH given (15[R]). The recommended dose would be in the range of 15–20 U/m^2/wk divided into daily subcutaneous injections. Moreover, the author supports previous findings as to the greater effect of pulsatile GH administration (15[R]), though new data fail to support this idea. Indeed, in a study by Smith et al the rate of growth of 4 children with GH deficiency was no better after pulsatile GH administration (3 boluses per night) than after a single daily evening injection (16[C]). A re-analysis of the dose–response of biosynthetic GH revealed that 2 IU/d is probably too low a dose to achieve optimal effects since mean daily IGF_1 concentrations only attained the normal range after giving 4 or 6 IU/d (17[C]). *Antibody* production against exogenous biosynthetic GH is receiving continuous attention. The greatest problem with neutralizing antibodies (which can block the growth-promoting effects) is experienced in patients with GH deficiency due to gene deletion (15[R]). Recombinant GH seems to be more immunogenic than pituitary preparations. Free GH concentrations can be measured in patients with GH antibodies and in such treated patients this concentration better reflects growth rate than do total GH concentrations (18[c]).

New indications for GH therapy now certainly include Turner's syndrome since GH therapy increases the pre-treatment growth rate by more than 2 cm/yr in 50% of patients treated with 0.5 U/kg/wk and in more than 80% if the dose is 1 U/kg/wk. Since this occurs without acceleration of bone age, a real increase in final height is to be expected. Antibodies were found in 71% and 11% of patients treated with methionyl-hGH and methionyl-free hGH respectively (19[c]). Addition of a low dose of ethinylestradiol to the GH treatment of girls with Turner's syndrome did not accelerate their growth rate (20[c]).

The use of GH in other children with short stature has been reviewed (21[R]); despite the therapeutic opportunities resulting from the greater availability of biosynthetic GH clinicians should continue to be cautious in widening its field of use, especially in view of its possible major side effects (see below). GH also has lipolytic and protein anabolic properties, which would favor its use for obese patients. GH indeed promoted nitrogen retention during caloric restriction, but this effect waned off after 5 weeks. Moreover, no increased loss of fat tissue was observed during the 5-week treatment period (22[C]). Weight and muscle loss on elderly adults could however be reversed by low-dose GH therapy provided there was adequate protein and caloric intake; elderly patients with an adequate diet showed improved nitrogen retention when GH was given. This occurred without significant disturbances in carbohydrate metabolism. This approach certainly deserves further study in catabolic diseases (23[C]).

Prion contamination The two most frightening complications of GH therapy are the contamination of prions in pituitary GH preparations and the possible association of leukemia and GH therapy (SED-11, 903; SEDA-13, 388). A very detailed overview of the events leading to the detection of the association between pituitary GH therapy and Creutzfeldt-Jakob disease was published in 1988 and is recommended reading for everyone involved in the dilemma of determining how best to react to the first sign of a possible causal relationship between drug therapy and unusual diseases (24[R]). Indeed, after the initial 3 American cases and 1 British case of this fatal neurological complication (SED-11, 903; SEDA-11, 371) no new cases were for a time found, whereas several other (probably unrelated) neurological diseases were observed (SEDA-12, 369). Recently, however, 3 additional cases have been clearly identified: a 32-year-old patient from New Zealand (25[C]) and a 37-year-old man from the U.S.A. (26[C]) (who both died from Creutzfeldt-Jakob disease) as well as a 16-year-old girl who showed clear focal signs of Creutzfeldt-Jakob disease on brain autopsy after dying from a non-related infectious disease (27[C]). Since the incidence of deaths in the U.S.A. believed to be ascribable to this infectious neurological disease may lie between 1:10 000 and 1:1 000, it is unquestionable that many batches of pituitary GH have been contaminated with the infectious prions. The proportion of dangerous batches remaining after GH purification is not yet clearly determined because of the long incubation period of the disease (as studied in primates infected with several GH batches) and it may well take another 2 years before one will know sufficient to provide adequate counselling to all patients treated with pituitary GH. A careful re-analysis of the original pituitaries used for the various batches of pituitary GH involved in the reported cases revealed that one batch of glands (but not a single batch of final GH) could have been responsible for all U.S. cases; this work is however unable to explain the New Zealand and British cases (24[R]). Although several new cases might be expected to be detected in the coming decades, no real endemic among recipients is to be feared (24[R]). Methods to reduce prion contamination 10^5- to 10^6-fold have now been described (28[c]), though their practical use in GH therapy is doubtful since biosynthetic GH has now nearly replaced human pituitary-extracted hormone worldwide. In the meantime, it is astonishing that no studies to follow up patients treated with older pituitary extracts (for diabetes insipidus or for induction of ovulation) have apparently been started or reported! Moreover, the disease might be an occupational hazard for people working as neuropathologists as well as the technicians or morticians in contact with cases; the disease has been described in a 62-year-old woman who had worked as a neuropathology histopathology technician for 22 years (29[c]).

Leukemia No new cases of leukemia related to GH therapy have been reported (SEDA-13, 388) and at a May 1988 meeting in Canada no cases of leukemia were reported among 1047 Canadian children who had previously been treated with GH. None of the 6 children who had leukemia before GH therapy relapsed during or after this therapy (30[R]). It is however advisable that all cases of leukemia as well as neurological diseases be centrally reported to facilitate further evaluation of the risk involved in this therapy.

Thyroid effects Besides the above-mentioned side effects of GH therapy, thyroid dysfunction has also been described; the incidence reported is extraordinarily variable (from less than 1% to 100% of patients!). This can be partly explained by the apparently physiological stimulant effect of GH on the conversion of thyroxine T3 (31[c]) and partly by unmasking previously existing partial TSH deficiency (32[R]).

Corticotrophin-releasing hormone (CRH)
(SED-11, 905; SEDA-12, 364; SEDA-13, 394)

CRH is a natural hypothalamic peptide regulating pituitary ACTH secretion and can be used diagnostically. Whereas a high-dose dexamethasone suppression test alone is insufficiently specific for differentiating between the several types of Cushing's disease, much better differentiation can be attained by combining it with a diagnostic CRH test (33[C]). For this purpose, ovine CRH (100 μg) is rapidly injected intravenously and ACTH and cortisol values are measured over the following 2 hours. No serious side effects have been reported. Similar conclusions have been reached in a detailed review of CRH (34[R]).

Growth-hormone-releasing hormone (GHRH)
(SED-11, 904; SEDA-12, 367; SEDA-13, 390)

The use of GHRH as a diagnostic tool for the exploration of GH secretion in several diseases revealed an exaggerated secretion of GH after intravenous GHRH injection in Type I diabetes (35[c]) but a decreased secretion in obese Type II diabetes (36[c]). In old age, however, a marked decrease in GHRH-induced GH secretion is observed, both in postmenopausal women (37[c]) and in elderly men (38[c]). In early-onset senile dementia (Alzheimer's disease), a higher GHRH-induced GH secretion was observed (38[c]). In all these studies about 100 μg of synthetic GHRH was injected intravenously without significant side effects, even when the injection was repeated over a period of 8 days (37[c]). The GHRH test is, however, not able to detect GH deficiency in a single test and a full endocrinological evaluation to substantiate this diagnosis remains necessary (39[c]). Continuous infusions of GHRH analogs in normal adults show no evidence of desensitization or of depletion of the releasable GH pool, and prolonged treatment with depot preparations of GHRH therefore appears promising (40[c]).

No systemic side effects were reported after 8 days of infusions, but *stinging* and *lumps at the infusion sites* were described. GHRH antagonists, by contrast, are able to block episodic GH secretion in immature animals and may therefore find applications in diseases associated with excess GH secretion (41[c]).

Protirelin (thyrotrophin-releasing hormone; TRH) *(SED-11, 905; SEDA-12, 367; SEDA-13, 390)*

Prolonged intrathecal infusions of TRH may improve the natural history of certain degenerative neurological diseases (SEDA-13, 391) and further positive although preliminary results are reported (42[c]). Infusion of the drug was safe and well tolerated.

Although TRH injection for measuring TSH secretion is usually a safe procedure and performed on a large scale, adverse *cardiovascular responses* have been observed before (SEDA-12, 367; SEDA-13, 390) and are again reported: in 20 patients with various cardiac diseases, a significant *increase in both systolic (+22 mmHg) and diastolic (+17 mmHg) blood pressure* was recorded within minutes after the intravenous injection of 200 μg of TRH (43[C]). In 9 patients the pressor effect lasted for 5–20 min and the maximum blood pressure rose to 220/145 mmHg. Cautious use of this test in hypertensive patients is therefore necessary.

Somatostatin and analogs *(SED-11, 904; SEDA-12, 368; SEDA-13, 390)*

Surgical removal of the pituitary adenoma responsible for the syndrome of acromegaly is often unsatisfactory even when followed by pituitary irradiation. Only certain pituitary growth-hormone-secreting adenomas are responsive to bromocriptine treatment so that a new growth-hormone-inhibitory drug is more than welcome for the treatment of acromegaly.

Somatostatin and more especially its long-lasting analog, octreotide, has been studied extensively for the treatment of acromegaly. In a series of 8 studies (44[C]–46[C], 47[R], 48[r], 49[r], 50[R], 51[C]) which describe a total of 324 patients a normalization of the growth hormone level (< 5 ng/ml) was seen in 42–80% of all patients. A significant decrease in the GH levels was observed in 74% of the patients, the proportion varying in individual reports between 44 and 87%. Shrinkage of the pituitary adenoma was observed in 18–50% of the patients. In one study of 10 patients, a 50% decrease in suprasellar expansion and 30% disappearance of (or significant decrease in) sinus cavernosus invasion was described (44[C]).

Histologically, a decrease in cell volume and perivascular fibrosis are found (44[C]). The decreased serum concentrations of growth hormone and insulin-like growth factor result in an improvement of clinical symptoms (soft tissue swellings, paresthesia, headache, asthenia and excessive sweating (50[R]). Numerous but mostly mild and transient side effects have been described and are similar to those observed during octreotide therapy for other diseases (Table 1). The most important side effects include a *decrease in postprandial insulin secretion* resulting in impairment of glucose tolerance or diabetes in some patients and decreased gallbladder contraction, thus increasing the risk of gall stone formation (47[R], 52[C]). Mild *gastrointestinal complaints* (cramps, diarrhea) are quite common during the first few days of treatment. The overall long-term effect and safety of somatostatin therapy for acromegaly has not yet been fully evaluated, but the drug is certainly a valuable acquisition for patients with persisting active disease despite previous surgery and radiotherapy. Moreover, it might be beneficial in reducing the adenoma volume before surgery (47[R], 49[r], 50[R]).

Growth hormone secretion is frequently abnormal in diabetic patients (especially in type 1 diabetes) and may aggravate insulin resistance and/or ketogenesis. Moreover, growth hormone and IGF-1 excess have been linked to diabetic retinopathy. Treatment of patients with type 1 diabetes with octreotide reduced the postprandial hyperglycemia and also insulin requirements, especially during the night, resulting in *nocturnal hypoglycemia* (53[C]). No beneficial effect on the dawn phenomenon was observed as the insulin requirement still increased before breakfast. Ketogenesis was however impaired or delayed (47[R]).

In type 2 diabetes, both insulin and glucagon levels were decreased by octreotide treatment, leaving glucose levels either unchanged or slightly elevated. The growth hormone levels were insufficiently suppressed and the side ef-

Table 1. *Side effects after Sandostatin (%)*

	Patients with gastrointestinal tumors ($n=196$)	Healthy volunteers ($n=264$)	Total
Abdominal discomfort	8	62	70
Nausea	17	51	68
Diarrhea	12	47	59
Injection site pain	16	25	41
Loose stools	6	31	37
Fatty stools	7	19	26
Headache	3	22	25
Dizziness	3	21	24
Flushing	1	21	22
Vomiting	5	1	6
Flatulence	1	5	6
Other	31	43	74
Total	110	348	458
%	34	50	43

fects on glycemic regulation argue against a clinical role for this somatostatin analog in diabetes mellitus (53[C]).

Somatostatin analogs have also been successfully used in several other types of excessive hormone secretion. One report describes the control of hyperthyroidism in 5 patients with excessive TSH secretion due to inappropriate TSH secretion of neoplastic origin (54[C]). Another case-report described the suppression of ectopic adrenocorticotrophin secretion with normalization of urinary cortisol excretion after 2 days of treatment but without control of tumor progression (55[C]).

The therapeutic characteristics of somatostatin in gastroentero-pancreatic tumors have been set out in a company report summarizing work in 173 patients (56[R]). After 1 year of treatment, 85 patients with a carcinoid syndrome experienced an 86% improvement in or reduction of diarrhea, (worsening in 8%) and a 93% improvement in flushing after. An improvement in the biochemical markers of the carcinoid syndrome was observed in 58% of the octreotide-treated patients (56[R]). In only 2 patients (2%) was a decrease in tumor size found.

After 12 months of treatment with octreotide 24 out of 25 patients with a VIPoma reported an improvement in their severe diarrhea, and withdrawal of parenteral supplements was possible in 87% of the patients who had needed this substitution before somatostatin therapy (56[R]). Effects in 16 patients with glucagonoma comprised improvement or reduction of migratory erythema after 2 weeks (in 55%), improvement in diarrhea in 33% and resolution of diarrhea in 66%, but little or no effect on plasma glucagon levels in 4 patients with diabetes mellitus. In patients with gastrinoma a similar improvement in diarrhea was observed in 42% of 26 patients after 3 months of therapy (56[R]). 50% of the patients with abdominal pain had improvement or resolution of their complaints. Suppression of the gastrin level was found in 57%, unchanged or variable levels in 12% and an elevation in 27%. About half of the insulinoma patients (56[R]) had an improvement of hypoglycemia; 75% of GRFoma patients (56[R]) showed a symptomatic improvement and 100% of PPoma patients (56[R]) an improvement of diarrhea and a decrease of PP. Side effects were comparable in all studies (Table 1).

Gonadorelin (gonadotrophin-releasing hormone; GnRH) *(SED-11, 906; SEDA-12, 365; SEDA-13, 391)*

Pulsatile administration of GnRH is used to stimulate the pituitary gonadal axis, in order to induce puberty and fertility. The subcutaneous (and sometimes intravenous) route of application is necessary.

In men with idiopathic hypogonadotrophic hypogonadism, pulsatile subcutaneous GnRH treatment can induce spermatogenesis, but the success rate after 6 months of treatment does not exceed 50% (57[R]). The relative merits of GnRH over human chorionic gonadotrophin (hCG) remain to be established, though a case resistant to hCG and responsive to GnRH has been reported (58[c]). Allergic reactions and development of antibodies to GnRH are rare. Recently, however, 2 serious allergic reactions, one of them anaphylactic, were reported, following standard testing with a 100 μg intravenous dose of GnRH after long-term low-dose subcutaneous pulsatile GnRH administration, during which only minor complaints of hypersensitivity or none had been noted (59[c]).

Cases of infertility and amenorrhea which are due to isolated gonadotrophin deficiency, Kallman's syndrome or weight loss which are generally 'hypothalamic' in origin are best treated with pulsatile GnRH (57[R]). Ovulation occurs in about 90% of treatment cycles and cumulative pregnancy rates up to 80% have been reported (60[R]). Treatment is well tolerated and without serious complications: *multiple pregnancies* are few in comparison to those following gonadotrophin treatment regimens (57[R]). In patients with polycystic ovarian disease, in whom pulsatile GnRH is usually administered intravenously, lower success rates were report ed (40% ovulation) and multiple pregnancies seem to be more common (61[c], 62[c]). To prevent hyperstimulation the use of lower GnRH dosages and avoidance of hCG have been recommended. This approach does not, however, totally eliminate the problem since a case of triple pregnancy after low-dose pulsatile GnRH (5 μg/h i.v.) has been described (63[c]). The authors suggest that the pituitary gonadotrophin reserve and/or sensitivity to GnRH are increased in polycystic ovarian disease.

Gonadorelin (gonadotrophin-releasing hormone; GnRH) and analogs *(SED-11, 906; SEDA-12, 365; SEDA-13, 391)*

Several LHRH analogs mimic the actions of natural LHRH, but they are considerably more potent and have a longer half-life. As such, nafarelin has been used to evaluate pituitary and gonadal secretion in the polycystic ovary syndrome (64[c]). Chronic administration of synthetic analogs of LHRH results in a depletion of pituitary luteinizing hormone followed by downregulation of LHRH receptors. As a result the pituitary becomes refractory or insensitive to further LHRH stimulation, resulting in low gonadotrophin levels and a (reversible) suppression of the pituitary gonadal axis.

There is a tendency to replace the subcutaneous administration of LHRH analogs by the intranasal route, but depot preparations with permanent release (applied subcutaneously or intramuscularly) are now considered to be the treatment of choice as they seem to induce a steadier castrate level of testosterone or estradiol and prove superior with regard to cost, effectiveness and patient compliance.

Precocious puberty of central origin can be effectively suppressed by LHRH analogs. Different treatment regimens have been employed and have proved equally effective; they comprise the use of buserelin intranasally (maximum absorption 6%) with or without initial subcutaneous treatment (65[c], 66[c]), high-dose nafarelin intranasally (67[c]) or the more potent (D-Trp^6)GnRH analog (68[c]). The only local adverse effect was a sensation of *fullness in the nose*, but this was noted only in a few children and lasted only for a few minutes. An increased *incidence of inflammatory cells in the vaginal smears* was observed, but none of the children had signs or symptoms of infection. Systemic side effects were absent. During GnRH analog therapy a decrease in physiological GH secretion and a concomitant growth deceleration has been described, probably due to a decrease in sex-steroid secretion. Since this is combined with slowing of the rate of epiphyseal maturation, no alteration in the final height prognosis occurs (68[c]).

Nafarelin was also used as a nasal spray in the treatment of hirsutism in 6 women with excess ovarian androgen production (69[c]). Hirsutism scores improved in 4 of the 6 patients during the 6 months of treatment. Androgen and estrogen production was effectively suppressed and all patients became anovulatory and amenorrheic while taking the drug. Most had hot flushes, but none discontinued the medication. The 2 patients who were eumenorrheic and one who was oligomenorrheic before treatment had menses during the 2-month follow-up afterwards. Two other oligomenorrheic patients did not.

In a recent controlled trial the association of buserelin (6 times 100 μg intranasally) with HMG has been shown to improve considerably the embryological and clinical outcomes in patients in whom the standard treatment with clomiphene and HMG had failed to induce folliculogenesis (70[c]). The pregnancy rate per embryo transfer was 16% (0% in the control group), a rate similar to that in their total group of in vitro fertilizations. Side effects were not mentioned.

Numerous clinical studies, investigating various analogs administered by different routes and at different dosages, have suggested that GnRH agonists are efficacious in the treatment of endometriosis (71[R]). All patients reported progressive pain relief and in all studies a marked regression of the disease was observed at follow-up laparoscopy, independent of the level of ovarian suppression. The frequency of recurrence of pain symptoms at the end of treatment is often high and the data on recovery of fertility are conflicting (varying from 0–60%). It is therefore not yet clear whether these analogs are superior to the other drugs used in the treatment of this disease. Their greatest advantage is their safety and good tolerance. The most frequent side effects are symptoms of *hypoestrogenism* (hot flushes in almost all patients, and, less frequently, vaginal dryness, decreased libido and breast discomfort), initial headache and bleeding (corresponding to the fall in estrogen levels or due to insufficient or unstable inhibition of estradiol levels). Blood lipids do not appear to be negatively influenced, but *osteoporosis* could be a potential serious effect. In a recent clinical study (13 premenopausal women with endometriosis) use of intranasal buserelin 400 μg 3 times daily for 6 months resulted in a significant loss of lumbar vertebral trabecular bone density of 5.9% and a marginally significant reduction of 0.9% in the mean cortical bone mineral content of the femur (72[c]). Six months after treatment, however, the bone density had returned to normal. The authors suggest that until more is known about the effects on bone loss of longer or repeated therapy courses, GnRH analogs should be used with discretion in women considered to be at high risk for osteopenia.

Advanced premenopausal breast cancer can also be treated with GnRH analogs (57[R]). In a trial with the D-Ser (tBu) 6-Aza–Gly^{10} analog (goserelin or Zoladex) the daily subcutaneous injection of 500 or 1000 μg was compared to a monthly subcutaneous depot preparation of 3.6 mg (73[c]). Suppression of both pituitary and ovarian hormones was maintained in $\pm 90\%$ of patients in both groups. Of the 5 patients with incomplete ovarian suppression, one nevertheless showed objective signs of response during the treatment indicating a direct anti-tumoral effect. This direct inhibitory effect was previously demonstrated in the MCF-7 breast tumor line (74[c]). Overall 31% of the 55 patients showed an objective response. Side effects were, as expected, related to hypogonadism: hot flushes in most patients, nausea in some. All patients with successful suppression had ceased to menstruate within 2 months of initiation of therapy.

More recently, buserelin has been used with some success in the treatment of advanced male breast cancer (75[c]). Intranasal administration of a daily dose of 1.2 mg seemed sufficient to decrease serum testosterone concentrations to castration levels within 3 weeks. The subsequent decrease in peripheral aromatization is reflected by a decrease in estradiol-17β levels. This deprivation of estrogens might partly explain the efficacy of buserelin in male breast cancer. The anti-tumor effect of buserelin alone (5 patients) at the dosage used was inferior to the results obtained by surgical castration. In 4 of these patients an *intensification of bone pain* occurred during the first week of therapy, which could be avoided by the addition of flutamide (a non-steroidal antiandrogen) at the beginning of treatment. Other side effects such as mild hot flushes, decrease or loss of libido and impotence were well tolerated.

Many clinical trials of long-acting GnRH analogs in metastatic prostatic cancer have been performed. The initial response rate of about 70% and the duration of the response is similar to that achieved by other treatments, i.e. orchidectomy or diethylstilbestrol (57[R]). Survival does no improve with either therapy. The advantage over estrogens is primarily related to a lower incidence of cardiovascular toxicity (salt and fluid retention, myocardial ischemia, thromboembolism) and gynecomastia (76[R]). Serum lipid concentrations remain virtually unchanged during GnRH therapy (associated with an antiandrogen), whereas estrogen therapy induced a VLDL-hypertriglyceridemia and orchidectomy was associated with a significant increase in total and LDL-cholesterol (77[c]). There is, however, no definite medical advantage over orchidectomy and one has to weigh the higher financial cost of GnRH against the greater adverse psychological impact of orchidectomy.

To date, some 4000 patients with advanced prostatic cancer have been treated with goserelin (Zoladex) in various European clinical trials of whom at least 3500 have received the subcutaneous depot form, i.e. a biodegradable slow-release implant of 3.6 mg once every 28 days (78[c]–88[c]). The objective response rate was 70–80%. Besides *hot flushes* and *impotence* in the majority of patients with *gynecomastia* and *breast tenderness* in some, the depot treatment was well tolerated. Sporadic *local reactions* (bruising or erythema) were related to the trauma of the subcutaneous injection and not to the presence of the depot. Less than 2% of patients had mild or moderate *skin eruptions*, most commonly generalized maculopapular rashes, which resolved (12 of 14 patients) despite continuation of Zoladex. A *worsening of signs and symptoms of the disease* during the first month of therapy, probably due to the initial stimulation of gonadotrophins and hence of testosterone production, has been noted in a small proportion of patients. In a comparative study of 800 patients randomly allocated to Zoladex versus standard therapy or LHRH analog combined with an antiandrogen, a temporary *increase in bone pain*, was the only flare-up sign statistically more frequent in the Zoladex-treated group (4.25% vs 1.5%) (88[c]). The development of ureteric obstruction or spinal cord compression during the first month did not differ between the two groups. It is advocated, however, that the use of an LHRH analog in patients at risk for these complications should be carefully considered and the patients closely monitored.

Another analog, D-Trp[6]–LHRH, was administered in one study by daily subcutaneous injection (89[c]). The overall rate of complete or partial reduction of prostatic enlargement was 44% after 3 months. A major improvement in bone scans was observed in 37% after 6 months. The same analog was also used in an intramuscular depot form, employing a dose of 3.2 mg every 4 or 5 weeks (90[c], 91[c]). The remission rate according to the U.S. National Prostatic Cancer Treatment Group Criteria was 70–80%. No flare-up symptoms were reported nor were side effects other than impotence and hot flushes.

Buserelin given subcutaneously or intranasally (series of 24 by prostatic cancer cases) (500 μg s.c. for an initial period of 7 days and afterwards either 200 μg s.c. once daily or 400 μg intranasally t.d.) was followed by partial remission according to U.S. criteria, in 54% of patients (92[c]). One-third of the patients had a transient *increase in testosterone*, of more than 25%, though only one of these exhibited a treatment flare-up of symptoms. More recently, a 2-monthly depot preparation of 6.8 mg buserelin has been synthesized, which is as effective as the conventional therapies (93[c]). In conclusion, GnRH analogs seem to be safe, well-tolerated and effective drugs for the treatment of prostatic cancer. Questions as to the clinical significance of the initial flare-up phenomenon and the influence of 'GnRH non-suppressible' androgens from the adrenals are, however, not yet definitely resolved.

Evidence is growing that the association of an antiandrogen might be beneficial. Nilutamide (300 mg daily by mouth) has very recently been shown to be effective in preventing the adverse consequences of the initial buserelin-induced transient increase in plasma testosterone levels. Compared to buserelin alone (500 μg s.c. daily), there was a significant reduction in bone pain and a prevention of the rise in the level of plasma prostatic acid phosphatase (94[c]). A larger (603 patients) randomized double-blind trial has demonstrated that the combined treatment of another non-steroidal antiandrogen (flutamide) and the GnRH analog, leuprolide, is superior in terms of progression-free survival (16.5 vs. 13.9 months) and overall survival (mean length of survival 35.6 vs. 28.3 months) (95[c]). One case is reported of *pulmonary fibrosis* following combination therapy of buserelin and a true non-steroidal antiandrogen (nilutamide) with spontaneous regression of the clinical and radiological findings after withdrawal of the LHRH analog (96[c]). Since the complication is very unexpected with buserelin alone, the possibility that the combination was responsible must nevertheless be considered.

These results support the use of 'complete androgen blockade' for the treatment of metastatic cancer of the prostate, as previously reported in an uncontrolled study; the remarkably better results, however, still await confirmation (97[c]).

Vasopressin and analogs *(SED-11, 905; SEDA-12, 371; SEDA-13, 387)*

The vasopressin analog DDAVP (SED-11, 905) is widely used as a treatment for central diabetes insipidus and real side effects are rare. The drug also has hemostatic properties because of its ability to raise plasma levels of Von Willebrand factor antigen 2–4-fold. It can therefore replace cryoprecipitate in some patients with congenital or acquired deficiency of this factor (98[C]). Not all patients, however, respond equally well and preoperative testing is thus necessary (98[C], 99[c], 100[r], 101[R]). Moreover, DDAVP may increase *platelet aggregation* and the risk of *thrombocytopenia* (99[C]). Mild transient *flushing* was seen in half the patiens, but no other side effects were observed (98[c]). Serious reactions were however observed in a 21-month-old girl with tetralogy of Fallot when she was treated with desmopressin (DDAVP) 0.3 μg/kg to improve her bleeding time in preparation for surgical intervention. The child developed marked *cyanosis* and *dyspnea* necessitating resuscitation (102[c]). The authors ascribe these side effects to the vasodilator effects of this dose of DDAVP resulting in increased right-to-left shunting of blood during the infusion. *Cerebral thrombosis* was reported in a 93-year-old patient during DDAVP infusion, given in an effort to correct his prolonged bleeding time during cystoscopy (103[c]). Caution is thus warranted in the use of DDAVP in patients with atherosclerosis. Even patients with kidney resistance to vasopressin still demonstrate the coagulation effect of DDAVP administration (104[c]).

Acute DDAVP administration can also be used as a test to investigate tissue plasminogen activator activity and therefore to define patients at increased risk for thrombosis (105[c]). Intravenous use of DDAVP causes mild vasodilatation and flushing in all patients with earache, palpitations or watery eyes in some (105[c]). Intranasal application is much better tolerated (flushing and watery eyes only).

Antibodies to vasopressin are frequently observed in patients after prolonged treatment with lysine or arginin vasopressin, at least when sensitive radioimmunoassay techniques are used (106[C]). The vasopressin efficacy decreases in patients with drug-induced antibodies, but they still retain normal sensitivity to DDAVP (106[C]). Allergic reactions were quite frequent so long as pituitary extracts were used for treatment of diabetes insipidus, but a case of exogenous-allergic alveolitis is now reported in such a patient after nasal treatment with synthetic DDAVP. After starting steroid therapy and switching to intramuscular injection of vasopressin tannate, clinical and radiological improvement was rapidly observed (107[c]). Continuous intravenous infusion of vasopressin or its synthetic analog, terlipressin, can be used to control serious acute bleeding from esophageal varices (SED-11, 905) and combination with nitroglycerin can decrease its systemic side effects (108[R]). Similar results are now also reported in children, in whom bleeding could be controlled in 9 of 17 bleeding episodes (109[c]). Complications were only observed when more than 0.01 U/kg/min was given. These complications included *electrolyte abnormalities, fluid overload, hypertension* and *cardiac dysrhythmias*. Since more than 0.01 U/kg/min of vasopressin was not more effective in bleeding control than lower doses, such higher dosage should be avoided (109[C]).

Oxytocin *(SED-11, 906; SEDA-12, 364; SEDA-13, 394)*

Oxytocin is frequently used to induce or advance labor. Although its correct use is considered safe, accidents and side effects are still reported.

During pregnancy intravenous oxytocin is rapidly inactivated by oxytocinase. Acute *water intoxication* seems to be related to the antidiuretic effect of the drug (about 100 times less than the antidiuretic effect of ADH), aggravated by the volume of fluid necessary for administration. Acute water intoxication can lead to cerebral edema, manifested as a decreased level of consciousness, convulsions and even death. Less than 50 cases have been reported in the literature, almost always when oxytocin is used for abortion.

In order to avoid hyponatremia, oxytocin should be given with fluid containing electrolyte such as normal saline or Hartman's solution. A comparison of hyponatremic and normonatremic cord blood showed no significant difference in serum bilirubin levels on red cell counts, but hyponatremic infants were more prone to develop neonatal jaundice.

With large doses, a transient *decrease in systolic and diastolic blood pressure* due to a direct relaxing effect on vascular smooth muscle can occur; this is especially dangerous in hypovolemic patients or those with cardiac disease with limited cardiac output.

Allergic anaphylactoid reactions are extremely rare, but the possibility must be kept in mind by those involved in obstetric practice. Adrenaline appears to be more effective in improving the severe hypotension than ephedrine.

A further case of oxytocin-induced *rupture of an unscarred uterus* during the second trimester has been mentioned by Jan E. Dickinson (personal communication).

PROSTAGLANDINS (PG) *(SED-11, 910; SEDA-12, 372; SEDA-13, 395)*

Prostaglandins in cardiovascular disease *(SED-11, 912; SEDA-12, 372; SEDA-13, 395)*

PGE_1 and PGE_2 are effective in many cases of congenital cardiac malformations with reduced pulmonary blood flow. They are effective in maintaining patency of the ductus arteriosus. Infusions have been successfully used in infants with simple transposition and severe hypoxemia, both before and after cardiac catheterization and after atrial septotomy.

The most frequent side effects during prolonged treatment are *diarrhea, necrotizing enterocolitis, hypotension* and *cortical hyperostosis*. Severe complications such as *apnea* and *muscle twitching* are only observed during intravenous administration.

PGE_1 infusion did not perform better than placebo in patients with Raynaud's syndrome and failed to promote ischemic skin ulcer healing. Moreover, marked side effects were observed including *flushing, headache, peripheral edema, inflammation* and *pain at the injection site* (110[c]). On the other hand, dermal application of PGE_2 for 6 weeks resulted in both subjective and objective improvement in patients with Raynaud's syndrome and produced only minor side effects.

PGE_1 significantly reduces right ventricular pulmonary afterload in patients with pulmonary hypertension due to chronic obstructive pulmonary disease (111[c]). It is a promising agent for the treatment of adult respiratory distress syndrome because it has no serious side effects and does not increase the susceptibility to infection. PGE_1 does not alter liver function (112[c]).

Prostaglandins in gastrointestinal disease *(SEDA-12, 372; SEDA-13, 395)*

Prostaglandins of the E-type possess antiulcer activity in the upper gastrointestinal tract. They inhibit gastric acid secretion and, at non-antisecretory doses, still protect the mucosa against a variety of noxious agents, e.g. nonsteroidal anti-inflammatory drugs, smoking, alcohol and chemotherapy.

Some synthetic analogs are under study in the hope of attaining greater specificity, increased potency and longer duration of action; they include enprostil (anti-gastrin effect) and misoprostol (a 15-deoxy-16-hydroxy-16-methyl-PGE_1 methylester).

The cure rate for gastric and duodenal ulcers varies between 60 and 70% after 4 weeks treatment and this is comparable to the results of treatment with H_2-receptor antagonists (ranitidine, cimetidine). Healing of a significant proportion of duodenal ulcers refractory to H_2-receptor antagonists has been described (113[c]–115[c]).

Diarrhea (between 4 and 38%), *abdominal pain* or *cramp flatulence* and *nausea or vomiting* account for most of the side effects reported. No biochemical or hematological side effects were noted.

Until the propensity of the PG analogs to cause abortifacient effects has been clarified, they are contraindicated in women of childbearing-age unless they are taking adequate contraceptive measures.

Topical administration of PGE_2 appears to be useful for treatment of chemotherapy-associated oral mucosal lesions of patients with hematological malignancies.

Clinical use of prostacyclin (PGI_2) and analogs *(SEDA-13, 396)*

PGI_2 is a vasodilator and inhibits platelet aggregation. Its use was suggested for the treatment of conditions associated with a significant rise in vascular resistance (advanced obliterative arteriosclerosis, Raynaud's syndrome) or an increase in platelet activation (extracorporeal circulation). Although benefit has been reported in Raynaud's disease, prostacyclin infusion in men with persistent pain associated with Peyronie's disease was of little value but produced marked side effects *(bradycardia* and *hypotension, nausea, flushing*) (116[c]).

Whereas PGI_2 is chemically instable, its synthetic analog iloprost is stable in solution and orally active. The hemodynamic effects include a decrease in total peripheral and pulmonary resistance, a decrease in mean arterial pressure and an increase in heart rate. It is also natriuretic, a predominantly tubular effect (117[c]).

Prostaglandins in urology

A single dose of intracorporeally applied PGE_1 is more effective and has fewer side effects than papaverine and phentolamine in inducing artificial penile erection for diagnostic or therapeutic procedures in cases of erectile dysfunction. The only side effect reported was a *burning sensation* (75%) (118[c]).

Massive diffuse hemorrhage due to cyclophosphamide-induced or radiation cystitis has been treated successfully with PGE_2 and (15S)-15-methyl-$PGF_{2\alpha}$ intravesically. *Febrile reactions* and severe *bladder spasm* are dose-dependent (119[c]).

Prostaglandins in obstetrics *(SED-11, 910; SEDA-12, 373; SEDA-13, 396)*

One of the most important therapeutic indications of prostaglandins remains the induction of first and second trimester abortion. The natural prostaglandins PGE_2 and PGF_2 shorten and dilate the cervix and provoke contractions of the myometrium at any phase of pregnancy. Unfortunately, they have some strong side effects such as nausea, vomiting, diarrhea and pain. The use of analogs permits one to lower the dose and to reduce the side effects. Since they are not broken down by 17-hydroxy-prostaglandin-dehydrogenase, their biological activity is much higher than that of natural prostaglandins.

Intravenously administered prostaglandins are used for induction of labor in cases of abortion and intrauterine fetal death. The success rate of this therapy, when monitored well, is high. Sulprostone (16-phenoxy-ω-17,18,19,20-tetranor-PGE_2-methylsulfanylamide) is especially effective.

Intramuscular administration of $PG(F_2)$ for second trimester abortion is rare. Cases of *posterior cervical rupture have however been described* (120[c]).

Vaginally applied gemeprost (16,16-dimethyl-*trans*^{2}-PGE_1-methylester) is effective in inducing first and second trimester abortion and in evacuation of the uterus in cases of intrauterine fetal death or hydatiform mole. There are fewer side effects (pyrexia, vomiting, diarrhea about 20%). Administration of gemeprost 4 hours before vacuum aspiration is easier and better accepted by the patient than intramuscular injection of sulprostone some 16 hours before the procedure. A dangerous *rise in blood pressure* occurred in a few cases in which fetal death was associated with unresolved pre-eclampsia. The presence of *pain* correlates well with efficacy. Analgesics may be necessary (10%).

The use of PGE_2 for cervical ripening and induction of labor is becoming more common. Local application in a viscous gel, vaginal tablets or pessaries has fewer side effects than intravenous administration. One case of neonatal respiratory distress is reported, due to the aspiration of a vaginal PG tablet with mechanical obstruction of the airways. The total dose of oxytocin needed to induce labor is significantly lower after cervical priming. As compared to early amniotomy, PGE_2 tablets are an efficacious, low-risk and comfortable alternative.

Intensive monitoring of uterine activity and fetal condition is essential since the rate of absorption of PGE_2 after vaginal insertion is unpredictable. Early rupture of the membranes should be considered after the onset of uterine contractions to reduce the risk of amniotic fluid infusion if absorption is rapid. Uterine hyperstimulation can lead to *uterine rupture*, even in previously unscarred uteri (121[c]). This can be prevented by using a lower dose (<5 mg). In the event of uterine hyperactivity, terbutaline may prove effective in reducing contractions. Severe fetal heart rate decelerations are reported, so special caution is indicated in patients at risk for placental insufficiency. *Contraindications* to the use of PG are asthma and severe liver, kidney, lung and heart diseases.

Postpartum hemorrhage secondary to uterine atony has been treated successfully with 15-methyl $PGF_{2\alpha}$. However, marked transient *maternal arterial oxygen desaturation*, possibly due to an increase in the intrapulmonary shunt, was observed (122[c]).

Oral PGE_2 (from day 3 or 4 for 24 h) is as effective as bromocriptine in suppressing lactation and there is less 'rebound' breast tenderness (123[c]). Management of ectopic pregnancy by intratubal and intraovarian injections of $PGF_{2\alpha}$ has been reported (124[c]).

Prostaglandins in ophthalmology

Topical PGE_2 and $PGF_{2\alpha}$ significantly reduce intraocular pressure for at least 24 hours and deserve further study as hypotensive agents for glaucoma. Transient ocular side effects include *reddened skin of the lower lid*, mild *eye-ache*, intermittent *photophobia* and *headache* (125[c], 126[c]).

REFERENCES

1. Mulder H, Schop C, Koster JC (1989) Influence of pharmacological doses of calcitonin on serum osteocalcin concentration in patients with Paget's disease of the bone. *Acta Endocrinol., 120*, 721.
2. Reginster JY, Jeugmans-Huynen AM, Albert A et al (1988) One year's treatment of Paget's disease of bone by synthetic salmon calcitonin as a nasal spray. *J. Bone Miner. Res., 3*, 249.
3. Levy F, Muff R, Dotti-Sigrist S et al (1988) Formation of neutralizing antibodies during intranasal synthetic salmon calcitonin treatment of Paget's disease. *J. Clin. Endocrinol. Metab., 67*, 541.
4. Brooks SG, Butterworth KR, Christie RB, Fox J (1988) Comparison of the pharmacokinetics of porcine calcitonin in saline and in gelatin diluents in healthy volunteers. *Eur. J. Drug Metab. Pharmacokinet., 13*, 91.
5. Meunier PJ (1985) Pharmacologie clinique de la calcitonine synthétique humaine. *Rhumatologie, 15*, 47.
6. Lutze M, Weigel K, Brock M (1988) Zur Problematik der intrathekalen Application von Calcitonin in der Schmerztherapie. *Intensivmedizin, 25*, 278.
7. Gnudi S, Mongiorgi R, Moroni A, Bertocchi G (1988) Densitometric analysis in in vivo evaluation of synthetic salmon calcitonin activity. *J. Clin. Pharmacol. Ther., 13*, 125.
8. Mallette LE (1988) Synthetic human parathyroid hormone 1–34 fragment for diagnostic testing. *Ann. Intern. Med., 109*, 800.
9. Mallette LE, Kirkland JL, Gagel RF et al (1988) Synthetic human parathyroid hormone-(1–34) for the study of pseudohypoparathyroidism. *J. Clin. Endocrinol. Metab., 67*, 964.
10. Furlong TJ, Seshadri MS, Wilkinson MR et al (1986) Clinical experiences with human parathyroid hormone 1–34. *Aust. NZ J. Med., 16*, 794.
11. Yamamoto M, Furukawa Y, Konagaya Y et al (1989) Human PTH (1–34) infusion test in differential diagnosis of various types of hypoparathyroidism: an attempt to establish standard clinical test. *Bone Miner., 6*, 199.
12. Jørgensen JOL, Flyvbjerg A, Christiansen JS (1989) The metabolic clearance rate, serum half-time and apparent distribution space of authentic biosynthetic human growth hormone in growth hormone-deficient patients. *Acta Endocrinol., 120* 8.
13. Faria ACS, Veldhuis JD, Thorner MO, Vance ML (1989) Half-time of endogenous growth hormone (GH) disappearance in normal man after stimulation of GH secretion by GH-releasing hormone and suppression with somatostatin. *J. Clin. Endocrinol. Metab., 68*, 535.
14. Dubey AK, Hanukoglu A, Hansen BC, Kowarski AA (1988) Metabolic clearance rates of synthetic human growth hormone in lean and obsese male Rhesus monkeys. *J. Clin. Endocrinol. Metab., 67*, 1064.
15. Brook CGD (1988) Treatment of growth deficiency. *Clin. Endocrinol., 30*, 197.
16. Smith PJ, Pringle PJ, Brook CGD (1987) Single dose and pulsatile treatment with human growth hormone in growth hormone deficiency. *Arch. Dis. Child., 62*, 849.
17. Jørgensen JOL, Flyvbjerg A, Lauritzen T et al (1988) Dose–response studies with biosynthetic human growth hormone (GH) in GH-deficient patients. *J. Clin. Endocrinol. Metab., 67*, 36.
18. Demura R, Ishiwatari N, Nomura T et al (1989) Measurement of plasma free and total growth hormone concentrations in patients with growth hormone antibodies developed in response to therapy. *Acta Endocrinol., 120*, 161.
19. Takano K, Shizume K, Hibi I et al (1989) Turner's syndrome: treatment of 203 patients with recombinant human growth hormone for one year. *Acta Endocrinol., 120*, 559.
20. Ross JL, Cassorla F, Carpenter G et al (1988) The effect of short term treatment with growth hormone and ethinyl estradiol on lower leg growth rate in girls with Turner's syndrome. *J. Clin. Endocrinol., Metab., 67*, 515.
21. Knudtzon J, Aarskog D (1987) Growth hormone therapy in short stature. *Pediatrician, 14*, 172.
22. Snyder DK, Clemmons DR, Underwood LE (1988) Treatment of obese, diet-restricted subjects with growth hormone for 11 weeks: effects on ana-

bolism, lipolysis and body composition. *J. Clin. Endocrinol. Metab.*, *67*, 54.
23. Binnerts A, Wilson JHP, Lamberts SWJ (1988) The effects of human growth hormone administration in elderly adults with recent weight loss. *J. Clin. Endocrinol. Metab.*, *67*, 1312.
24. Brown P (1988) Human growth hormone therapy and Creutzfeldt-Jakob disease: a drama in three acts. *Pediatrics*, *81*, 85.
25. Croxson MS, Brown P, Synek BJL et al (1988) A new case of Creutzfeldt-Jakob disease associated with human growth hormone therapy in New Zealand. *Neurology*, *38*, 1128.
26. Marzewski DJ, Towfighi J, Harrington MG et al (1988) Creuzfeldt-Jacob disease following pituitary-derived human growth hormone therapy: a new American case. *Neurology*, *38*, 1131.
27. New MI, Brown P, Temeck JW et al (1988) Preclinical Creutzfeldt-Jakob disease discovered at autopsy in a human growth hormone recipient. *Neurology*, *38*, 1133.
28. Pocchiari M, Macchi G, Peano S, Conz A (1988) Can potential hazard of Creutzfeldt–Jakob disease infectivity be reduced in the production of human growth hormone? Inactivation experiments with the 263K strain of scrapie. *Arch. Virol.*, *98*, 131.
29. Miller DC (1988) Creutzfeldt-Jakob disease in histopathology technicians. *N. Engl. J. Med.*, *318*, 853.
30. Dean HJ (1988) Growth hormone treatment and leukemia. *Can. Med. Assoc. J.*, *139*, 877.
31. Grunfeld C, Sherman BM, Cavalieri RR (1988) The acute effects of human growth hormone administration on thyroid function in normal men. *J. Clin. Endocrinol. Metab.*, *67*, 1111.
32. Drayer NM (1988) Neveneffecten van groeihormoonbehandeling. *Tijdschr. Kindergeneeskd.*, *56*, *Suppl. I*, 40.
33. Grossman AB, Howlett TA, Perry L et al (1988) CRF in the differential diagnosis of Cushing's syndrome: a comparison with the dexamethasone suppression test. *Clin. Endocrinol.*, *29*, 167.
34. Taylor AL, Fishman LM (1988) Corticotropin-releasing hormone. *N. Engl. J. Med.*, *319*, 213.
35. Krassowski J, Felber JP, Rogala H et al (1988) Exaggerated growth hormone response to growth hormone-releasing hormone in type I diabetes-mellitus. *Acta Endocrinol.*, *117*, 225.
36. Kopelman PG, Mason AC, Noonan K, Monson JP (1988) Growth hormone response to growth hormone releasing factor in diabetic men. *Clin. Endocrinol.*, *28*, 33.
37. Franchimont P, Urbain-Choffray, D., Lambelin P et al (1989) Effects of repetitive administration of growth hormone-releasing hormone on growth hormone secretion, insulin-like growth factor I, and bone metabolism in postemenopausal women. *Acta Endocrinol.*, *120*, 121.
38. Cacabelos R, Niigawa H, Ikemura Y et al (1988) GHRH-induced GH response in patients with senile dementia of the Alzheimer type. *Acta Endocrinol.*, *117*, 295.
39. Butenandt O (1989) Diagnostic value of growth hormone-releasing hormone tests in short children. *Acta Pediatr. Scand.*, *Suppl.*, *349*, 93.
40. Brain C, Hindmarsh PC, Brook CGD, Matthews DR (1988) Continuous subcutaneous growth hormone releasing factor analogue augments growth hormone secretion in normal male subjects with no desensitization of the somatotroph. *Clin. Endocrinol.*, *28*, 543.
41. Lumpkin MD, Mulroney SE, Haramati A (1989) Inhibition of pulsatile growth hormone (GH) secretion and somatic growth in immature rats with a synthetic GH-releasing factor antagonist. *Endocrinology*, *124*, 1154.
42. Munsat TL, Taft J, Kasdon D, Jackson IMD (1988) Prolonged intrathecal infusion of thyrotropin releasing hormone in amyotrophic lateral sclerosis. *Ann. NY Acad. Sci.*, *531P*, 187.
43. Sobel RJ, Ariad S (1987) Adverse cardiovascular responses to thyrotropin-releasing hormone (200 μg) in cardiac ptients. *Isr. J. Med. Sci.*, *23*, 1107.
44. Barkan AL, Lloyd RV, Chandler WF et al (1988) Preoperative treatment of acromegaly with long-acting somatostatin analog SMS 201-995: shrinkage of invasive pituitary macroadenomas and improved surgical remission rate. *J. Clin. Endocrinol. Metab.*, *67*, 1040.
45. Quabbe HJ, Plöckinger U (1989) Dose–response study and long term effect of the somatostatin analog octreotide in patients with therapy-resistant acromegaly. *J. Clin. Endocrinol. Metab.*, *68*, 873.
46. Tauber JP, Babin T, Tauber MT et al (1989) Long-term effects of continuous subcutaneous infusion of the somatostatin analog octreotide in the treatment of acromegaly. *J. Clin. Endocrinol. Metab.*, *68*, 917.
47. Lamberts SWJ (1988) Therapeutic effects of somatostatin analogs. *ISI Atlas of Science. Pharmacology*, *Vol. 2*, p. 179.
48. Lamberts SWJ, Klijn JG, Van Vroonhoven CC et al (1986) The sensitivity of growth hormone and prolactin secretion to the somatostatin analogue SMS 201-995 in patients with prolactinomas and acromegaly. *J. Clin. Endocrinol.*, *25*, 201.
49. Lamberts SWJ, Uitterlinden P, Verleun T (1987) Relationship between growth hormone and somatomedin-C levels in untreated acromegaly, after surgery and radiotherapy and during medical therapy with sandostatin (SMS 201-995). *Eur. J. Clin. Invest.*, *17*, 354.
50. Harris A: Nieuwe therapeutische perspectieven voor sandostatine. [Company information]
51. Lamberts SWJ, Uitterlinden P, Schuijff PC, Klijn JGM (1988) Therapy of acromegaly with sandostatin: the predictive value of an acute test, the

value of serum somatomedin-C measurements in dose adjustment and the definition of a biochemical 'cure'. *Clin. Endocrinol., 29*, 411.
52. Candrina R, Gussago A, Giustina G (1988) Effect of a new long-acting somatostatin analogue (SMS 201-995) on glycemic and hormonal response to a mixed meal in acromegalic patients. *J. Endocrinol. Invest., 11*, 21.
53. Davies RR, Turner SJ, Alberti KGMM, Johnston DG (1989) Somatostatin analogues in diabetes mellitus. *Diabetic Med., 6*, 103.
54. Beck-Peccoz P, Mariotti S, Guillausseau PJ et al (1989) Treatment of hyperthyroidism due to inappropriate secretion of thyrotropin with the somatostatin analog SMS 201-995. *J. Clin. Endocrinol. Metab., 68*, 208.
55. Bertagna X, Caine C, Escourdle H et al (1989) Suppression of ectopic adrenocorticotropin secretion by the long-acting somatostatin analogue octreotide. *J. Clin. Endocrinol. Metab., 68*, 988.
56. Sandostatin in GEP endocrine tumours: therapeutic characteristics. [Company information]
57. Clayton RN (1987) Gonadotropin releasing hormone: from physiology to pharmacology. *Clin. Endocrinol., 26*, 361.
58. Donald RA, Wheller M, Sonksen P, Lowy C (1983) Hypogonadotrophic hypogonadism resistant to hCG and responsive to LHRH: report of a case: *Clin. Endocrinol., 18*, 385.
59. Popovic V, Miloseciv Z, Djukanovic R et al (1988) Hypersensitivity reaction with intravenous GnRH after pulsatile subcutaneous GnRH treatment in male hypogonadotrophic hypogonadism. *Postgrad. Med. J., 64*, 245.
60. Ross LD, Robertson G, Milton PJ, Blows R (1985) The induction of ovulation using pulsatile luteinising hormone-releasing hormone in clinical practice. *Br. J. Obstet. Gynaecol., 92*, 815.
61. Bogchelman D, Lappöhn RE, Janssens J (1982) Triplet pregnancy after pulsatile administration of gonadotropin releasing hormone. *Lancet, 2*, 45.
62. Heineman MJ, Bouckaert PXJM, Schellekens LA (1984) A quadruplet pregnancy following ovulation induction with pulsatile LH-RH. *Fertil Steril., 42*, 300.
63. Filicori M, Michellacci L, Ferrari P et al (1986) Triplet pregnancy after low-dose pulsatile gonadotropin-releasing hormone in polycystic ovarian disease. *Am. J. Obstet. Gynecol., 155*, 768.
64. Barnes RB, Rosenfield RL, Burstein S, Ehrmann DA (1989) Pituitary-ovarian responses to nafarelin testing in the polycystic ovary syndrome. *N. Engl. J. Med., 320*, 559.
65. Luder AS, Holland FJ, Costigan DC et al (1984) Intranasal and subcutaneous treatment of central precocious puberty in both sexes with a long-acting analogue of LHRH. *J. Clin. Endocrinol., 58*, 966.
66. Holland FJ, Fishman L, Costigan DC et al (1986) Pharmacokinetic characterization of the gonadotropin-releasing hormone analogue D-Ser(T-BU)-^{6}EA-^{10}LH-RH (buserelin) after subcutaneous and intranasal administration in children with central precocious puberty. *J. Clin. Endocrinol., 63*, 1065.
67. Tsu-Hui Lin, Le Page ME, Henzl M, Kirkland JL (1986) Intranasal nafarelin. An LH-RH analogue treatment of gonadotropin-dependent precocious puberty. *J. Pediatr., 109*, 954.
68. Stanhope R, Pringle PJ, Brook CGD (1988) Growth, growth hormone and sex steroid secretion in girls with central precocious puberty treated with a gonadotropin releasing hormone (GnRH) analogue. *Acta Paediatr. Scand., 77*, 525.
69. Andreyko JL, Monrue SE, Jaffe RB (1986) Treatment of hirsutism with a gonadotropin-releasing hormone agonist (nafarelin). *J. Clin. Endocrinol., 63*, 854.
70. MacLachlan V, Besanko M, O'Shea F et al (1980) A controlled study of luteinizing hormone-releasing hormone agonist (buserelin) for the induction of folliculogenesis before in vitro fertilization. *N. Engl. J. Med., 320*, 1233.
71. Fedele L, Bianchi S, Arcaini L et al (1988) GnRH agonists in the treatment of endometriosis. *Acta Eur. Fertil., 19*, 5.
72. Matta WH, Shaw RW, Hesp R, Evans R (1988) Reversible trabecular bone density loss following induced hypo-oestrogenism with the GnRH analogue buserelin in premenopausal women. *Clin. Endocrinol., 29*, 45.
73. Williams MK, Walker KJ, Turkes A et al (1986) The use of an LH-RH agonist (ICI-118630, Zoladex) in advanced premenopausal breast cancer. *Br. J. Cancer, 53*, 629.
74. Miller WR, Scott WN, Morris R et al (1985) Growth of human breast cancer inhibited by a LH-RH agonist. *Nature 313*, 231.
75. Doberauer C, Niederle N, Schmidt CG (1988) Advanced male breast cancer treatment with the LH-RH analogue buserelin alone or in combination with the antiandrogen flutamide. *Cancer, 62*, 474.
76. Eisenberger MA, O'Dwyer PJ, Friedman MA (1986) Gonadotropin hormone-releasing hormone analogues: a new therapeutic approach for prostatic carcinoma. *J. Clin. Oncol., 4*, 414.
77. Moorjani S, Dupont A, Labrie F et al (1988) Changes in plasma lipoproteins during various androgen suppression therapies in men with prostatic carcinoma: effects of orchiectomy, estrogen, and combination treatment with luteinizing hormone-releasing hormone agonist and flutamide. *J. Clin. Endocrinol. Metab., 66*, 314.
78. Perren TJ, Clayton RN, Blackledge G et al (1986) Pharmacokinetic and endocrinological parameters of a slow-release depot preparation of the GnRH analogue ICI-118630 (Zoladex) compared with a subcutaneous bolus and continuous subcu-

taneous infusion of the same drug in patients with prostatic cancer. *Cancer Chemother. Pharmacol.*, *18*, 39.

79. Van Cangh PJ, Opsomer RJ (1986) Treatment of advanced carcinoma of the prostate with a depot luteinizing hormone-releasing hormone analogue (ICI-118630). *J. Urol.*, *137*, 61.

80. Litjens TTJ, Del Moral PF, Van Laarhoven JPRM et al (1986) Behandeling van gevorderd prostaatcarcinoom met een depotvorm van LH-RH analogen: eerste endocrinologische en klinische resultaten. *Ned. Tijdschr. Geneeskd.*, *130*, 787.

81. Robinson MRG (1987) The preliminary clinical evaluation of Zoladex® depot injection in the management of carcinoma of the prostate. In: Motta M, Serio M (Eds.), *Hormonal Therapy of Prostatic Diseases: Basic and Clinical Aspects. International Symposium on the European Experience with an LHRH Analogue, Milan, Italy*, p. 12.

82. Bianco AR, Iaffaioli PV, Albano D et al (1987) Treatment of advanced prostatic carcinoma with the LHRH agonist Zoladex®: results of a multicentre phase II study. In: Motta M, Serio M (Eds.), *Hormonal Therapy of Prostatic Diseases: Basic and Clinical Aspects. International Symposium on the European Experience with an LHRH Analogue, Milan, Italy*, p. 18.

83. Turkes AO, Peeling WB, Griffiths K (1987) Management of patients with advanced carcinoma of the prostate: a randomized phase III trial of Zoladex® against castration by the British Prostate Group. In: Motta M, Serio M (Eds.), *Hormonal Therapy of Prostatic Diseases: Basic and Clinical Aspects. International Symposium on the European Experience with an LHRH Analogue, Milan, Italy*, p. 29.

84. Lunglmayr G, Girsch E, Bieglmayr (1987) Acceptance of orchidectomy versus GnRH agonist therapy in the management of advanced carcinoma of the prostate. In: Motta M, Serio M (Eds.), *Hormonal Therapy of Prostatic Diseases: Basic and Clinical Aspects. International Symposium on the European Experience with an LHRH Analogue, Milan, Italy*, p. 40.

85. Pagano F, Prayer T, Zattoni F (1987) Treatment of advanced prostatic cancer with the LHRH agonist Zoladex®. In: Motta M, Serio M (Eds.), *Hormonal Therapy of Prostatic Diseases: Basic and Clinical Aspects. International Symposium on the European Experience with an LHRH Analogue, Milan, Italy*, p. 58.

86. Di Silverio F, Tenaglia R, Biggio A, Sciarra F (1987) Treatment of advanced prostatic carcinoma with LHRH agonist alone or combined with cyproterone acetate. In: Motta M, Serio M (Eds.), *Hormonal Therapy of Prostatic Diseases: Basic and Clinical Aspects. International Symposium on the European Experience with an LHRH Analogue, Milan, Italy*, p. 72.

87. Denis L, Mahler C (1987) LHRH agonist combination treatment. In: Motta M, Serio M (Eds.), *Hormonal Therapy of Prostatic Diseases: Basic and Clinical Aspects. International Symposium on the European Experience with an LHRH Analogue, Milan, Italy*, p. 85.

88. Milsted RAV (1987) A review of the international experience with the LHRH agonist Zoladex® in prostatic carcinoma. In: Motta M, Serio M (Eds.), *Hormonal Therapy of Prostatic Diseases: Basic and Clinical Aspects. International Symposium on the European Experience with an LHRH Analogue, Milan, Italy*, p. 47.

89. Mathé G, Schally AV, Comaru-Schally AM et al (1986) Phase II trial with D-Trp-6-LH-RH in prostatic carcinoma: comparison with other hormonal agents. *Prostate*, *9*, 327.

90. Papadopoulos I, Kleinschmidt K, Weissbach L (1986) Behandlung des fortgeschrittenen Prostatakarzinoms mit der Depotform eines LHRH-Analogons (Decapeptyl). *Aktuel. Urol.*, *17*, 315.

91. Wenderoth UK, Spindler HW, Jacobi GH (1986) Fünfwöchentliche intramuskuläre Applikation des Gn-RH-Analogs Decapeptyl-Depot bei fortgeschrittenen Prostatakarzinom. *Aktuel. Urol.*, *17*, 320.

92. Presant CA, Soloway MS, Klioze SS et al (1985) Buserelin as primary therapy in advanced prostatic carcinoma. *Cancer*, *56*, 2416.

93. Waxman JH, Sandow J, Abel P et al (1989) Two-monthly depot gonadotropin releasing hormone agonist (buserelin) for treatment of prostatic cancer. *Acta Endocrinol.*, *120*, 315.

94. Kuhn JM, Billeband T et al (1989) Prevention of the transient adverse effects of a gonadotropin-releasing hormone analogue (buserelin) in metastatic prostatic carcinoma by administration of an antiandrogen (nilutamide). *N. Engl. J. Med.*, *321*, 413.

95. Crawford ED, Eisenbüger MA et al (1989) A controlled trail of leuprolide with and without flutamide in prostatic carcinoma. *N. Engl. J. Med.*, *321*, 419.

96. Seigneur J, Trechot P (1988) Pulmonary complications of hormone treatment in prostate carcinoma. *Chest*, *93*, 1106.

97. Labrie F, Dupont A, Belanger A et al (1986) Treatment of prostate cancer with gonadotropin-releasing hormone agonists. *Endocr. Rev.*, *7*, 67.

98. Nieuwenhuis HK, Sixma JJ (1988) 1-Desamino-8-D-arginine vasopressin (desmopressin) shortens the bleeding time in storage pool deficiency. *Ann. Intern. Med.*, *108*, 65.

99. Kyrle PA, Niessner H, Dent J et al (1988) IIB von Willebrand's disease: pathogenetic and therapeutic studies. *Br. J. Haematol.*, *69*, 55.

100. Sas S, Baele G, Van Hove W (1988) Het vasopressine analoog DDAVP: een synthetisch vasopressine analoog, als therapeutische aanwinst bij de behandeling van hemofilie A en de ziekte van von Willebrand. *Tijdschr. Geneeskd.*, *44*, 1477.

101. Mannucci PM, Altieri D, Faioni E (1987) Vasopressin analogues: their role in disorders of hemostasis. *Ann. NY Acad. Sci., 509*, 71.
102. Israels SJ, Kobrinsky NL (1989) Serious reaction to desmopressin in a child with cyanotic heart disease. *N. Engl. J. Med., 320*, 1563.
103. Byrnes JJ, Larcada A, Moake JL (1988) Thrombosis following desmopressin for uremic bleeding. *Am. J. Hematol., 28*, 63.
104. Brenner B, Seligsohn U, Hochberg Z (1988) Normal response of factor VIII and von Willebrand factor to 1-desamino-8-D-arginin vasopressin in nephrogenic diabetes insipidus. *J. Clin. Endocrinol. Metab., 67*, 191.
105. Sultan Y, Harris A, Strauch G et al (1988) A dynamic test to investigate potential tissue plasminogen activator activity: comparison of deamino-8-D-arginin vasopressin with venous occlusion in normal subjects and patients. *J. Lab. Clin. Med., 111*, 645.
106. Vokes TJ, Gaskill MB, Robertson GL (1988) Antibodies to vasopressin in patients with diabetes insipidus: implications for diagnosis and therapy. *Ann. Intern. Med., 108*, 190.
107. Krumhaar D, Urban M, Stempinski E, Otto H (1988) Die sogenannte Hypophysenschnupferlunge. *Dtsch. Med. Wochenschr., 113*, 857.
108. Terblanche J, Burroughs AK, Hobbs KEF (1989) Controversies in the management of bleeding esophageal varices (I). *N. Engl. J. Med., 320*, 1393.
109. Tuggle DW, Bennett KG, Scott J, Tunell WP (1988) Intravenous vasopressin and gastrointestinal hemorrhage in children. *J. Pediatr. Surg., 23*, 627.
110. Nakata Y, Sakurai T, Yamada I (1988) Long-term intra-arterial infusion therapy with prostaglandin E_1 in patients with ischemic ulcer of the extremities. *Vasc. Surg. 22*, 160.
111. Gassner A, Sommer G, Fridrich L et al (1988) Der Einfluss von Prostaglandin E_1 (Alprostadil) auf die pulmonale Hypertonie bei Patienten mit chronisch obstructiven Atemwegserkrankungen (COPD). *Prax. Klin. Pneumol., 42*, 521.
112. Sinzinger H, Fitscha P (1988) Leberfunktionsparameter und Fibrinogen bei i.a. und i.v. PG E_1-infusion. *Wien. Klin. Wochenschr., 14*, 488.
113. Goldin E, Fich A, Eliakim R et al (1988) Comparison of misoprostol and ranitidine in the treatment of duodenal ulcer. *Isr. J. Med. Sci., 24*, 282.
114. Wilson DE (1988) Misoprostol and gastroduodenal mucosal protection (cytoprotection). *Postgrad. Med. J., 64, Suppl. I*, 7.
115. Watkinson G, Hopkins A, Akbar FA (1988) The therapeutic efficacy of misoprostol in peptic ulcer disease. *Postgrad. Med. J., 64, Suppl. I*, 60.
116. Strachan JR, Pryor JP (1988) Prostacyclin in the treatment of painful Peyronie's disease. *Br. J. Urol., 61*, 516.
117. Angeli P, Gatta A, Caregaro L (1988) Effects of iloprost, a prostacyclin analog derivative, on renal plasma flow, renal function and renin–aldosterone system in humans. *Clin. Pharmacol. Ther., 44*, 211.
118. Waldhauser M, Schramek P (1988) Efficiency and side effects of prostaglandin E_1 in the treatment of erectile dysfunction. *J. Urol. 140*, 525.
119. Hemal AK, Vaidyanathan S, Sankaranarayanan et al (1988) Control of massive vesical hemorrhage due to radiation cystitis with intravesical instillation of 15(*S*)-15-methyl-prostaglandin F_2-alpha. *Int. J. Clin. Pharmacol., 26*, 477.
120. Intaraprasert S, Sugkraroek P (1988) Clinical trials of intramuscular sulprostone for second trimester abortion, *J. Med. Assoc. Thailand, 71, Suppl. I*, 58.
121. Thavarasah AS, Siva Achanna K (1988) Uterine rupture with the use of Cervagem (prostaglandin E_1) for induction of labour on account of intrauterine death. *Singapore Med. J., 29*, 351.
122. Hankins GDV, Berryman GK, Scott RT et al (1988) Maternal arterial desaturation with 15-methyl prostaglandin F_2-alpha for uterine atony. *Obstet. Gynecol., 72*, 362.
123. England MJ, Tjallinks A, Hofmeyr J et al (1988) Suppression of lactation: a comparison of bromocriptine and prostaglandin E_2. *J. Reprod. Med. 33*, 630.
124. Egarter CH, Husslein P (1988) Treatment of tubal pregnancy by prostaglandins. *Lancet, 14.1(8594)*, 1104.
125. Flach AJ, Eliason JA (1988) Topical prostaglandin E_2 effects on normal human intraocular pressure. *J. Ocular Pharmacol., 4*, 13.
126. Lee PY, Shao H, Xu L et al (1988) The effect of prostaglandin F_2-alpha on intraocular pressure in normotensive human subjects. *Invest. Ophthalmol., 29*, 1474.

O.R. Ødegaard

46 Drugs affecting lipid metabolism

The close relationship between the level of plasma cholesterol and the incidence of coronary heart disease leaves little doubt about the benefit of reducing hyperlipidemia towards lower values, to reduce the risk of coronary heart disease (1[R]). Dietary intervention has provided experimental evidence confirming this view (2[C]), and most health authorities advise such patients to reduce their intake of saturated fat, to reduce overweight, and to stop smoking (3[R]). When these measures fail, the decision to start pharmacological treatment must be based on the risk situation in the individual patient. The indication for treatment is often considered as stronger in younger than in older persons with the same risk profile. The recent discovery of the HMG coenzyme A reductase inhibitors has led to vigorous promotion of the various hypocholesterolemic drugs.

It is important to bear in mind that dietary treatment is still the cornerstone of therapy. None of the drug trials performed up to now has shown a reduced total mortality in the treated groups, and there is considerable uncertainty about possible long-term adverse effects.

CLOFIBRATE AND CONGENERS *(SED-11, 916; SEDA-12, 378; SEDA-13, 403)*

Clofibrate *(SED-11, 916; SEDA-12, 378; SEDA-13, 403)*

The side effects of clofibrate have been extensively reviewed in earlier volumes. It lowers serum triglyceride concentration and LDL cholesterol, but an increased mortality from *malignant* and *gastrointestinal disease*, and a higher rate of cholecystectomy for *gallstones* has been observed during clofibrate treatment (4[C]). The occurrence of myositis in some patients during clofibrate therapy is well known, and is more common in patients with impaired renal function. The U.S. Food and Drug Administration has limited the indications for long-term use of clofibrate to Type III hyperlipidemia, and for Type IV hyperlipidemia only if other drugs have failed, or are not tolerated (5[r]).

Gemfibrozil *(SED-11, 921; SEDA-12, 378; SEDA-13, 404)*

In the Helsinki Heart Study, a 34% reduction in the incidence of coronary heart disease was observed in dyslipidemic men treated with gemfibrozil (6[C]). The total mortality, however, was not influenced. There were 31 cancers in the gemfibrozil group and 26 in the placebo group. This difference is not significant. In the subgroup analysis, there were 5 basal-cell carcinomas in the gemfibrozil group, and none in the placebo group, a difference which is of borderline significance. A significantly higher number of *gastrointestinal* operations was performed in the gemfibrozil group (81 versus 53 in the placebo group).

The number of gallstone operations was 18 in the gemfibrozil group, versus 12 in the placebo group. This difference was not significant. Like clofibrate, gemfibrozil can potentiate the effect of oral anticoagulants, and increase biliary cholesterol saturation. At present, it seems that the adverse reactions and interactions recorded closely resemble those of clofibrate.

(Biomedical Division)
Side Effects of Drugs Annual 14
M.N.G. Dukes and L. Beeley, editors

HMG COENZYME-A REDUCTASE INHIBITORS *(SED-11, 924; SEDA-12, 378; SEDA-13, 404)*

Lovastatin (MK-803, Mevinolin, Mevacor) *(SED-11, 924; SEDA-12, 378; SEDA-13, 404)*
Mevastatin (ML-2368, Compactin) *(SEDA-12, 404)*
Pravastatin (CS 514, SQ031 000, Eptastatin)
Simvastatin (MK-733, Synvinolin, Zocor)

Of these compounds lovastatin is the most extensively studied. In a recent 12-week study (7[C]) a dose of 20 or 40 mg, twice daily, was more effective in lowering elevated total and LDL-cholesterol than 12 g of cholestyramine twice daily. HDL-cholesterol concentrations generally increase or remain the same. In short-term studies, lovastatin is usually better tolerated than other lipid-lowering drugs, but serious side effects can occur even after a short time on treatment.

One patient developed nausea, fatigue and pain in the thighs on day 28 of lovastatin therapy, with a creatine kinase value of 10 000 U/l, an aspartate aminotransferase value of 460 U/l and an alanine aminotransferase level of 380 U/l. Her symptoms disappeared within 1 week of not taking lovastatin, and she was considered to have a drug-induced *myopathy*.

In a recent overview of the long-term safety of lovastatin and simvastatin, including 744 patients taking one of these drugs for 3 years, 2.2% withdrew because of drug-attributable adverse events. Raised transaminase levels were observed in 1.3%. The reasons for the *hepatic effects* are at present unknown, but they may be aggravated by concomitant alcohol consumption. Of all patients taking lovastatin in clinical trials, myopathy occurred in 0.5% and a few cases progressed to rhabdomyolysis and renal failure (8[c]). It is therefore recommended that treatment is stopped in patients with serious infections, and in conditions which may lead to hypotension and impaired renal function, e.g. surgical trauma. Concern about cataract formation after short-term use of lovastatin treatment has recently diminished, and some authors consider that their is no need for concern (9[r]). Nevertheless, the manufacturers still recommend initial and periodic ophthalmological examinations to check for cataract development. In an unpublished Japanese study, it was found that compactin induced lymphomas in dogs (10[r]). At present, nothing similar has been observed in patients, but the risk cannot be excluded until long-term experience with this group of drugs is available.

Interactions *Ciclosporin* has been reported to increase the plasma concentration of lovastatin, and to increase the risk of myopathy. Rhabdomyolysis has also been observed in association with *erythromycin* treatment. Lovastasin may prolong the prothrombin time in patients on *dicoumarol*.

NICOTINIC ACID DERIVATIVES *(SED-11, 923; SEDA-13, 405)*

Niceritrol (pentaerythrityl tetranicotinate)

This nicotinic acid derivative has been given to 25 hypercholesterolemic patients in a dose of 750 mg/d increased at weekly intervals over 4 weeks to the maximum tolerated dose up to 3 g/d, and continued for a further 8 weeks. All patients reported *flushing* and some had *gastrointestinal symptoms*. Three of the patients dropped out at an early stage because of severe flushing, skin rash and diarrhea. Six patients complained of nausea, and 2 of vomiting (11[C]).

MISCELLANEOUS DRUGS

Probucol *(SED-11, 924)*

Probucol has been shown to produce QT prolongation in man. More recent studies suggested that the QT/QS2 relation is a stronger indicator of risk for sudden death than the QT corrected for heart rate. Recently, the QT, QTc and QS2 intervals were measured before and after 3 months treatment with 1 g probucol daily. Both *QT and QTc intervals increased* significantly, whereas no significant changes were observed between the pre- and post-treatment QT/QS2 ratio. The authors consider that these results might help explain why prolongation of the QTc interval does not seem to result in serious arrhythmias (12[C]).

Activated charcoal

Activated charcoal was recently given as a suspension in water at a dose of 8 g 3 times daily for 4 weeks. The serum concentration of total cholesterol was reduced by 27%. The effect was accompanied by a moderate elevation in serum squalene and desmosterol concentration and by a a marked increase in serum lathosterol and Δ^8-lathosterol concentrations. The authors interpretation of these observations is that treatment with activated charcoal increases cholesterol synthesis by interfering with the enterohepatic circulation of bile acids (13^{C}). Nothing is known about the possible side effects of long-term intake of activated charcoal.

REFERENCES

1. Keys A (1980) *Seven Countries. Death and Coronary Heart Disease*. Harward University Press, Cambridge, MS.
2. Hjermann I, Velve Byre K, Holme I et al (1981) Effect of diet and smoking intervention on the incidence of coronary heart disease. *Lancet, 2,* 1303.
3. Anonymous (1989) *Treatment of Hyperlipidemia (Proceedings of Workshop)*. National Board of Health and Welfare, Drug Information Committee, Sweden.
4. Committee of Principal Investigators (1978) A cooperative trial in the primary prevention of ischaemic heart disease using clofibrate. *Br. Heart J., 40,* 1069.
5. Detullo PL, Wong H (1988) Treatment of Type IV hyperlipidemias. *Drug Intell. Clin. Pharm., 22,* 237.
6. Manninen V, Elo MO, Frick MH et al (1988) Lipid alterations and decline in the incidence of coronary heart disease in the Helsinki Heart Study. *J. Am. Med. Assoc., 260,* 641.
7. Lovastasin Study Group III (1988) A multicenter comparison of lovastatin and cholestyramine for severe primary hypercholesterolemia. J. Am. Med. Assoc., 260, 359.
8. Bilheimer DW (1989) An overview: longterm clinical tolerability of lovastatin and simvastatin. In: *Abstracts, International Atherosclerosis Congress, Vienna, 1988.*
9. Schechter RJ (1988) Unnecessary alarm about lovastatin and cataracts. *J. Cataract Refract, Surg., 14,* 581.
10. Anonymous (1988) Choice of cholesterol-lowering drugs. *Med. Lett. Drugs Ther., 30,* 81.
11. Curtis LD, Reckless JPD, Winder AF et al (1988) Clinical and laboratory responses to niceritrol in the treatment of hypercholesterolaemia. *Postgrad. Med. J., 64,* 672.
12. Romics L, Littmann L, Laszlo Z et al (1988) The effects of probucol on QT/QS2 relation and systolic time intervals. *Int. J. Cardiol., 19,* 303.
13. Neuvonen PJ, Kuusisto P, Manninen V et al (1989) The mechanism of the hypocholesterolaemic effect of activated charcoal. *Eur. J. Clin. Invest., 19,* 251.

Nigel Bailey and George Blackledge

47

Cytostatics and immunosuppressive drugs

CARDIOVASCULAR TOXICITY *(SED-12, 934; SEDA-12, 380; SEDA-13, 407)*

Amsacrine (m-AMSA) Cardiac arrhythmias have been documented after amsacrine therapy and have been related to demonstrable hypokalemia. Pre-existing supraventricular arrhythmias or ventricular ectopy are not absolute contraindications to its use (1[c]).

Doxorubicin (adriamycin) This anthracycline has been well documented to cause cardiotoxicity both acutely in the form of arrhythmias (2[R]) and in the long term as a dose-related cardiomyopathy. Several studies have concerned early detection of such adverse effects using electrocardiography, echocardiography (3[c]) (4[c]) or serial radionuclide angiography (5[R]). None of these is particularly sensitive. Endomyocardial sampling (6[cr]) is probably the most reliable, but its invasive nature precludes widespread use.

Work continues to find a protective agent to use with doxorubicin. The bispiperazinedione ICRF-187 has been shown to diminish the cardiotoxic effect of doxorubicin in a randomized trial (7[R]). It is not, however, completely protective. Further trials are needed for confirmation of this effect.

Anesthesia is difficult in patients with cumulative cardiotoxicity and has proved fatal on occasions (8[cr]). Heart transplantation has been successfully undertaken in patients developing progressive late cardiomyopathy with no evidence of recurrent disease (9[c]).

Epirubicin Epirubicin has been well documented to cause less toxicity compared with doxorubicin (2[r]). This is most likely to be due to more rapid clearance and elimination of the drug rather than a different mode of action (10[r]).

Esorubicin This doxorubicin derivative when given by 48-hour infusion has dose-limiting non-hematological toxicity of mucositis. This method of administration does not appear to protect against cardiotoxicity (11[r]). A recent fatal case of dilated cardiomyopathy secondary to esorubicin (740 mg/m^2) may well have been precipitated by prior transfusion of 3 units of blood (12[R]). Previous reports of altered ejection fraction have been rare although a much lower total dose has usually been employed.

5-Fluorouracil (5-FU) The number of reports of 5-FU-induced cardiac toxicity manifest as *constrictive anginal chest pain* during infusion is rapidly increasing. Non-specific ST-T ECG changes are seen. This seems sporadic and outcome is favorable if the drug is stopped. Reintroduction of the drug has been associated with occasional fatal outcome and is not recommended (13[c]). Sudden deaths due to presumed ventricular fibrillation have been recorded (14[c], 15[c]).

The onset of an *acute dilated cardiomyopathy* with left ventricular dysfunction temporally related to 5-FU and cisplatin infusion and with subsequent complete recovery has been tentatively linked to the 5-FU (16[c]). Similar events are reported (17[c], 18[c]). Chaudary et al (17[c]) postulate a direct effect of uncoupling electromechanical myocardial function possibly at the level of ATP generation. The precise mechanism for 5-FU cardiotoxicity is unknown.

Suggested mechanisms include: (a) an immunoallergic reaction following sensitization by a complex of 5-FU and cardiac cells; (b) vasospasm secondary to either 5-FU or released products; (c) a direct toxic effect on the myocardium. Most reports specifically related to chest pain favor the vasospastic hypothesis

Side Effects of Drugs Annual 14
M.N.G. Dukes and L. Beeley, editors

(19[c]). Synergistic toxicity secondary to cisplatin administration is possible.

Interferon First reports of interferon causing *congestive heart failure* occurred in 1982. A recent case of a 70-year-old man who died suddenly after the first injection of interferon 5×10^6 IU/M^2 may have been related to the initial febrile reaction (20[c]). Autopsy, however, demonstrated diffuse parenchymal leukemic infiltration, degenerative cardiomyopathy and pulmonary edema. A similar case-report (21[C]) showed improvement of cardiac function following cessation of interferon therapy. However, it was clearly stated that a viral myocarditis could not be excluded as causative.

Mitomycin (mitomycin C) A study suggesting that mitomycin is synergistic with doxorubicin in causing cardiotoxicity can be criticized on several issues: low numbers of patients (one 73-year-old patient affected out of 37 evaluable), no histological evidence of cardiac damage and poor predicitive diagnostic tests of cardiac damage (22[c]). The true incidence of mitomycin cardiotoxicity is likely to be low.

Mitoxantrone (mitozantrone) Anthracyclines have the ability inherent in the quinone structure to form free-radical semiquinones which directly interact with oxygen causing peroxidation of the lipid membranes of the heart. This reaction has not, however, been demonstated with mitoxantrone and the mechanism is unknown. The South West Oncology Group (23[CR]) reported data on 801 patients treated with mitoxantrone: 1.5% developed congestive cardiac failure, 1.5% had a decrease in left ventricular ejection fraction (LVEF) and 0.25% had a myocardial infarction.

Predisposing factors to such effects include increasing age, prior anthracycline therapy, previous cardiovascular disease, mediastinal radiotherapy and a cumulative dose > 120 mg/m^2.

A study from Scotland found evidence of abnormalities of LVEF in 46% of patient's ($n = 14$) treated with mitoxantrone (14 mg/m^2) together with vincristine and prednisolone (24[C]). Patients with pre-existing history of cardiac disease or previous anthracycline exposure were excluded. Only 1 patient developed evidence of clinically overt congestive cardiac failure. Other reports have demonstrated less cardiotoxicity compared to the parent compound, doxorubicin (2[r], 25[r]).

Thrombosis An increased incidence of *thrombotic episodes* has been documented after chemotherapeutic treatment of breast cancer and lymphoma (26[R], 27[R]). Goodnough et al (28[c]) failed to show an increased risk in breast cancer with hormonal therapy alone, suggesting that the effect is related to the chemotherapy itself. An alternative explanation is lysis of tumor cells producing a procoagulant.

Vascular The incidence of *Raynaud's phenomenon* has doubled since the addition of cisplatin to vinblastine and bleomycin (PVB) in the treatment of testicular cancer and has been reported in up to 49% of patients (29[CR], 30[r]). Hypomagnesemia provoking arterial spasm has been suggested as causative, but the exact mechanism is unknown (see also under 5-FU also). Dose is an unimportant variable in this regard (31[r]).

Evidence is also mounting for a direct relationship between cisplatin and major vascular events such as *myocardial infarction* (32[c]) *angina pectoris, coronary heart disease and arterial occlusive events* (31[cr]).

A report of a 22-year-old receiving PVB wno subsequently developed *severe encephalopathy* with grand mal seizures and visual disturbance has been tentatively linked to vascular toxicity (33[c]). An association with arrhythmias is unproven (34[c]).

PULMONARY TOXICITY *(SED-11, 937; SEDA-13, 408)*

Bleomycin Diffuse interstitial *pneumonitis* has been well documented with bleomycin with a significant mortality. The mechanism by which it occurs, however, is unknown.

Lipid peroxidation of cell membranes has been suggested, but recent work has failed to support this hypothesis (35[r]). Others have postulated a role of angiotensin-converting enzyme in the production of lung damage (36[r]), but the data remain conflicting.

The logical development of short-course weekly alternating chemotherapy regimes for the lymphomas has proceeded throughout the world in the past decade. In an effort to diminish myelosuppression, vincristine and bleomycin have been incorporated with greater frequency in such regimes. It is therefore not surprising that toxicities are altered from those previously encountered. Less myelosuppression and gastrointestinal toxicity is seen at the expense of an increased occurrence of lung toxicity (37[c]). This may occur even at low cumulative bleomycin doses during concurrent treatment with cyclophosphamide which can independently cause pulmonary toxicity. Quigley's series of 19 patients (37[c]) revealed an unacceptably high incidence of fatal pulmonary toxicity (26%) and warrants caution in the use of such chemotherapy combinations.

Busulfan Vergnon described 3 cases of busulfan-induced interstitial pneumonitis (38[c]). All 3 had circulating immune complexes and alveolitis and histology demonstrated consistent abnormalities of Type I pneumocytes and rarefaction of Type II pneumocytes.

Cyclophosphamide A recent literature review found 29 cases of cyclophosphamide induced pneumonitis (39[c]). Considering the widespread usage of this drug over many years, this remains a very rare adverse effect.

Methotrexate Acute life-threatening pneumonitis confirmed by transbronchial biopsy has been reported following a dose of only 12.5 mg methotrexate in the treatment of rheumatoid arthritis (41[c]). The possibility of an increased susceptibility to methotrexate pneumonitis of rheumatoid patients has been postulated and pneumonitis may become clinically apparent in patients with undetected preexisting rheumatoid lung dysfunction. Of note, no correlations between HLA phenotypes and toxicity of the drug have been found (42[r]).

Mitomycin (mitomycin C) Biopsy-proven mitomycin pneumonitis occurred in 5 of 44 patients treated with this drug and weekly low-dose doxorubicin (20 mg) (40[c]). Patients developed pulmonary infiltrates, progressive dyspnea and hypoxia and improved on steroids. The mean total dose of mitomycin used in these 5 patients was 89 mg.

NEUROTOXICITY (*SED-11, 939; SEDA-12, 381; SEDA-13, 409)*

L-Asparaginase *Thrombosis and hemorrhage* are well-recognized complications in 1–2% of patients receiving L-asparaginase therapy. This is due to the toxic effect of coagulopathy which has been variously attributed to decreased levels of fibrinogen (43[r]), Factor IX, Factor XI, Factor VIII complex, antithrombin III and plasminogen. In a review of 28 CNS thrombotic or hemorrhagic events and 8 peripheral thromboses related to L-asparaginase the median time from initial treatment to adverse reaction was 16–17 days (44[r]). Most patients recovered completely, although 5 cases had residual neurological deficits and 1 patient died with a superior sagittal sinus thrombosis.

Cisplatin (CDDP) Cisplatin causes a well-recognized reversible *sensory peripheral neuropathy* commencing with depressed deep tendon reflexes and loss of vibration sense (45[c]) and progressing to a sensory ataxia. This may be age related as the use of high-dose cisplatin in children with neuroblastoma has not been associated with peripheral neuropathy (46[c]). Motor nerves are spared (47[r]).

Protection from neuropathy has been reported with concurrent administration of WR-2721, an investigational radioprotective compound (48[CR]).

Walker and co-workers record 5 cases of cerebral herniation following cisplatin therapy (49[C]). All cases, however, had evidence of intracerebral tumor with mass effect and the herniation of the brain was thought to be multifactorial rather than directly related to cisplatin treatment.

Hypomagnesemia secondary to cisplatin administration may be severe enough to present as *generalized seizures* (50[R]). It more commonly presents with muscular weakness, tremulousness, peripheral paraesthesiae, tetany and personality changes. It is both dose- and schedule-dependent. Loss of magnesium may be prevented by prophylactic magnesium infusion prior to and during cisplatin administration (51[c]), but this is not universally recommended (50[r]) because of the risk of acute uremia.

High-dose cisplatin (CDDP) Use of aggressive hydration, hypertonic saline, sodium thiosulfate and dose-scheduling has led to diminution of dose-limiting nephrotoxicity and thus the evolution of high-dose cisplatin (defined as >200 mg/m^2/course). At such a dose toxicities are predominantly severe neurotoxicity in the form of *chronic peripheral neuropathy, ototoxicity* and myelosuppression. There is some evidence that these effects can be reduced by lengthening the infusion time of the cisplatin (46[c]).

Etoposide *Acute neurologic dysfunction* with exacerbation of pre-existing neurological deficits has been reported following treatment with high-dose (>800 mg/m^2/d $\times$ 3) etoposide and autologous bone marrow transplantation (52[C]). This tended to occur 9–10 days after treatment initiation and abated without sequelae following prompt steroid therapy. Changes in intracranial pressure have been proposed as causative of this acute dysfunction.

Ifosfamide *Severe encephalopathy* has been seen in children treated with ifosfamide (1.8 g/m^2) alone. No predisposing risk factors such as impaired renal function or lowered albumin were present. EEG abnormalities and seizures were reversible despite prolonged coma (53[c]).

Interferon Neurotoxicity affecting psychic and motor functions has been reported in patients receiving high-dose interferon. These are usually reversible when therapy is discontinued. A Finnish report of a 7-year-old boy receiving human leukocyte interferon at a dose varying from 2×10^6 IU on alternate days to 3×10^6 IU daily for juvenile laryngeal papillomatosis documents the development of a spastic diplegia after 7 months of treatment (54[C]). This neurological sequela persisted following treatment cessation.

High-dose methotrexate Of particular concern are autopsy or biopsy verified reports of *necrotizing leukoencephalopathy* (55[c], 56[c]). Serial EEGs may predict such an outcome with the development of a/s ratio showing slowing activity upon administration of high-dose methotrexate which becomes irreversible. Necropsy has demonstrated widespread necrosis and spongiosis in the cerebral and cerebellar white matter in such cases (55[c]).

A recent report of a 7-year-old child treated with intrathecal methotrexate (228 mg total dose) for acute lymphocytic leukemia demonstrated a rim-enhancing mass lesion on CT scanning in the left frontal lobe associated with a right paraparesis (56[c]). This mimicked a cerebral abcess. However, no pus was obtained on multiple needle aspirates. The lesion resolved spontaneously with complete clinical recovery. Although intracerebral calcification and hypodense areas have been previously reported in methotrexate leukoencephalopathy, only 1 previous case of a rim-enhancing mass has been described.

Mitoxantrone (mitozantrone) Intrathecal use of mitoxantrone has not been recommended following a report of 1 patient who became *paraplegic* after intrathecal mitoxantrone given for resistant CNS leukemia (57[c]).

Vincristine Pre-existing neurological disease may predispose to severe vincristine neuropathy (58[R], 59[r]) and a diagnosis of Charcot-Marie-Tooth (CMT) disease is a suggested contraindication to its use (58[C]). Four cases of vincristine-induced neuropathy in patients with CMT have been described, one being fatal and the remainder causing *severe quadriplegia* with recovery. A similar abnormal sensitivity to development of vincristine neuropathy was seen in a patient with pre-existing Friedreich's ataxia (59[r]).

No such pre-existing neurological disease was seen in an 8-year-old child with acute lymphoblastic leukemia who developed recurring generalized seizures 36 hours after her 2nd weekly dose of conventional vincristine therapy (1.5 mg/m^2). Seizures continued for 5 days despite anticonvulsants. CT scans demonstrated temporary bilateral lucencies throughout the brain and a subsequent open brain biopsy revealed axonal disruption similar to that seen in animal models of vincristine toxicity. Cessation of the drug resulted in complete clinical recovery (60[CR]).

Scheduling of vincristine by 5-day infusion may allow the dose-limiting toxicity of marked paraesthesiae, paralytic ileus and grand-mal seizures to be overcome (60[r]). In a study of 7 patients treated this way (median age 7 years), *limb and jaw muscle pain* starting at days 3–5 of the infusion and needing opiate analgesia was the most marked toxicity (61[c]). This has been clearly described in dose escalation studies in adults and in subsequent clinical studies. In contrast, abdominal pain and paralytic ileus was less than expected and peripheral neuropathy was not a problem.

An alternative approach to minimizing neurotoxicity has been the concurrent administration of 'protective agents'. Initial work in a murine model identified glutamic acid as a promising agent.

In a prospective double-blind trial with placebo controls conducted by the Piedmont Oncology Association concurrent administration of 500 mg of oral glutamic acid thrice daily resulted in a significant subjective and objective diminution in the incidence of vincristine-induced neurotoxicity (62[C]). However, there were no differences in constipation, weakness or loss of knee reflexes. Unlike previous trials from the 1960s severe gastrointestinal side effects were not seen, probably due to the much smaller doses used. The mechanism for this protective effect is unknown. Caution must also be exercised as in this trial the chemotherapy was used in an adjuvant setting. Further work is needed to demonstrate that the efficacy of vincristine is unaltered by glutamic acid administration.

HEMATOLOGICAL TOXICITY *(SEDA-13, 416)*

Busulfan There has been one report of an *acquired sideroblastic anemia* which resolved following withdrawal of busulfan therapy in a patient with chronic myeloid leukemia (CML) (63[c]). Previous reports have tended to favor a myeloblastic transformation of the CML, but this case was entirely reversible.

High-dose methotrexate Interaction with other drugs, renal impairment or an idiosyncratic response may be the mechanism responsible for cases of pancytopenia occurring (64[r]) sporadically with high-dose methotrexate. A report of fatal *pancytopenia* with methotrexate given intramuscularly together with the administration of glafenine suggests that competitive protein binding led to methotrexate potentiation (65[c]).

Mitoxantrone (mitozantrone) Escalating doses of mitoxantrone cause prolonged myelosuppression. A report of a 73-year-old lady inadvertently receiving 275 mg of mitoxantrone together with 300 mg cyclophosphamide and 1.5 mg vincristine documents her survival following intensive supportive treatment (66[c]). During the infusion she developed shaking chills, nausea and vomiting. Subsequently her urine became green. Bone marrow suppression persisted for 20 days. There were no signs of stomatitis, mucositis or diarrhea. After bone marrow recovery, left ventricular ejection fraction (LVEF) was 76%, demonstrating no evidence of cardiac decompensation after such a massive dose.

HEPATOTOXICITY *(SED-11, 245; SEDA-12, 386; SEDA-13, 414)*

Busulfan The alkylating agent busulfan has also recently been reported to cause hepatitis, however, other causes including disease involvement of the liver could not be totally excluded (67[r]).

Cyclophosphamide Cyclophosphamide causes dose-dependent hepatic injury which is probably due to impaired metabolism of the metabolite, acrolein (68[r]). Clinically this presents as raised serum aminotransferase levels (69[c]) and maybe precipitated by prior exposure to azathioprine.

Dacarbazine (DTIC) Likewise single-dose dactinomycin (70[C]) and DTIC (71[C], 72[c]) have been reported to be hepatotoxic, presenting as *acute liver necrosis* with hepatic venous thrombosis which is often fatal.

Methotrexate Elevated AST levels are common in patients on long-term methotrexate therapy. These may be indicative of liver fibrosis or cirrhosis, and liver biopsy is the most reliable way of documenting liver damage. This procedure is however invasive and carries a mortality rate, albeit a low one. An attempt to find non-invasive methods of evaluating liver damage has led to measurement of the serum amino-terminal propeptide of Type III procollagen (PIII NP). Risteli and co-workers have described a correlation between high levels of PIII NP and positive fibrotic liver biopsies (73[r]). Of note, no patient with a normal PIII

NP level had an abnormal biopsy. This assay has thus been suggested as a preliminary test to avoid unnecessary liver biopsies. It was emphasized that PIII NP is not specific for liver fibrogenesis.

Thiopurines The thiopurines (azathiaprine, 6-mercaptopurine and 6-thiouracil) are implicated in the liver vascular disorders, peliosis hepatis (74[c]) and hepatic veno-occlusive disease. Azathioprine has been implicated in the development of nodular regenerative hyperplasia of the liver (75[c]). It is conceivable that this hepatic injury may precede veno-occlusive disease.

GASTROINTESTINAL TOXICITY *(SED-11, 948; SEDA-13, 415)*

Oral Cytotoxic chemotherapy is toxic to the mucosal surfaces. A study from Sweden found no evidence of a change in the oral microflora of patients receiving chemotherapy when compared with hospitalized controls or pre-treatment patients (76[c]). Although there were increased numbers of enterobacteria compared with non-hospitalized patients, there was no direct association with chemotherapeutic therapy.

Antiemetics Efforts have been made to improve patients acceptance of chemotherapy, in particular with better control of nausea and vomiting. Comparisons have been made between metoclopramide and steroids as antiemetics. Metoclopramide causes *extrapyramidal side effects* especially in patients under 30 years of age. A dose of <20 mg every 6 hours for 7 days has been reported as the maximum tolerated dose in this age group when used prophylactically to reduce late cisplatin-induced vomiting (77[c]). However, this trial was terminated when 3 of 5 patients failed to complete a week's course of 20 mg metoclopramide q.d.s. There seems to be a cumulative effect with oral dosage. In older patients agitated depression is the dose-limiting toxicity.

Glucagon, a physiological hormone given at 1 mg intravenous bolus, prevents upper gastrointestinal peristalsis and has been suggested as an antiemetic (78[c]). Randomized trials are awaited. Similarly trials of the new 5-HT3 antagonists are currently underway and will be increasingly reported in the forthcoming year.

High-dose methotrexate High-dose methotrexate has been advocated for osteosarcoma, childhood acute lymphocytic leukemia, gliomas, lymphoma and melanoma (79[c]). Side effects of myelosuppression, hepatic dysfunction and mucocutaneous damage are all predictable. Side effects of mucositis and skin rashes are reduced by administration of citrovorum factor (80[c]).

PVB (cisplatin/vinblastine/bleomycin) *Acute pancreatitis* is rare following chemotherapy. It has usually been reported after use of L-asparaginase or cytarabine. Socinski and Garnick report 2 cases following PVB chemotherapy. Whether the combination itself or one of the agents alone is implicated is unknown (81[c]).

NEPHROTOXICITY AND OTHER URINARY SYSTEM TOXICITY *(SED-11, 949; SEDA-12, 384; SEDA-13, 412)*

Carboplatin Carboplatin is a second-generation platinum analog with dose-limiting myelosuppression. When used at doses causing similar hematological toxicity to cisplatin, it has negligible renal, neurological and auditory toxicity (82[r]–85[r]). In combination with other agents the maximum tolerated dose is reduced because of myelosuppression (86[r]).

It may therefore be given on an outpatient basis. If the dose is escalated, however, as in the treatment of acute non-lymphocytic leukemia where a dose of 200–300 mg/m^2 daily for 5 days is employed, then significant, high-tone hearing loss and renal impairment are seen. This was evident in a study from the NCl (87[r]). All but one patient developing such side effects had received concomitant aminoglycoside antibiotics.

Measurement of pre- and post-treatment urinary protein enzyme excretion (alkaline phosphatase, lactate dehydrogenase, and *N*-acetylglucosaminidase) have not shown significant differences (88[r]). This work confirms previous reports suggesting the lack of nephotoxicity of carboplatin as assessed by such biochemical parameters.

Cisplatin (CDDP) Cisplatin is *nephrotoxic* and the nephrotoxicity is often dose-limiting (89[R]). This is predominantly due to proximal tubular dysfunction (90[r]) and is clearly minimized with adequate hydration which decreases drug exposure in the renal tubules. Impairment of renal function may be manifest for at least 6 months after termination of treatment.

Sodium thiosulfate likewise protects against nephrotoxicity by reacting with cisplatin covalently in the renal tubules. Other agents studied as protectors include probenecid, orgotein, fosfomycin (91[c]) and amifostine (WR-2721), an anthiol. The beneficial role of furosemide remains controversial.

Nephrotoxicity may be detected by a rise in serum urea or creatinine or a fall in creatinine clearance. Tubular dysfunction may be manifest by a fall in serum levels of sodium (92[R]), potassium, magnesium (93[r]) and phosphorus.

Hyponatremia has been reported to occur secondary to renal sodium loss (92[R]), although others have demonstrated inappropriate ADH secretion to be partially responsible (90[r]).

Renal magnesium wasting is the major mechanism responsible for the hypomagnesemia associated with cisplatin administration (50[r]) and has been described together with enhanced tubular reabsorption of calcium causing hypocalciuria (93[r]). This dissociation of renal calcium and magnesium handling is similar to that seen in Bartter's syndrome. The site of the renal tubular defect in these conditions is uncertain, but evidence suggests that the renal tubular active-transport systems are disrupted.

Recent attention has turned to the early detection of renal impairment. Urine to plasma β-microglobulin ratio, *N*-acetyl-β-glucosaminidase (NAG) and leucine aminopeptidase (LAP) measured in urine (94[r]) and serum α_1-microglobulin (95[r]) have all been proposed as indicators of early tubular dysfunction following cisplatin administration. However, their value in clinical decisions is limited.

It has been suggested in a murine model that coadministration of diethyldithiocarbamate (DDTC) with high-dose platinum compounds results in protection from hematological, renal and gastrointestinal side effects. A recent trial, however, failed to confirm this (96[r]). Also the specific side effects of DDTC, namely anxiety, feelings of apprehension and autonomic effects, were so severe that it was concluded this drug was of no clinical benefit.

High-dose methotrexate (HD-MTX) Renal toxicity is seen with HD-MTX. This is more likely to occur with concomitant administration of other nephrotoxic agents such as aminoglycosides, cephalosporins, non-steroidal anti-inflammatory agents or diuretics (97[R]).

The pathogenesis is unclear but is believed to be secondary to crystallization of methotrexate within the renal tubules. Adequate hydration and urinary alkalinization are important to minimize this effect (98[r]). Urinary β_2-microglobulin has been suggested as a useful marker of impaired excretion of high-dose methotrexate (99[r]).

With high serum drug levels rescue with leucovorin may prevent renal failure. Methotrexate levels are only transiently lowered with hemoperfusion and unaffected by peritoneal dialysis should acute renal failure supervene. Two reports have demonstrated sustained lowering of drug levels and recovery of renal function following charcoal hemoperfusion with sequential hemodialysis (100[c], 101[c]).

Procarbazine coadministration as seen in the treatment of medulloblastomas appears to increase susceptibility to this renal effect. It has been suggested that delay of administration of HD-MTX until 72 hours after completion of procarbazine therapy decreases the risk of renal toxicity (102[c]).

Interferon Cox and co-workers treated 24 patients with myeloma with human lymphoblastoid interferon at 15 MU/m_2 twice weekly. Two patients developed *acute renal failure* (103[c]). One had pre-existing heavy proteinuria and recovered normal renal function after dialysis, the other died of superimposed pneumonia. Renal complications have been previously reported in interferon-treated myeloma; the mechanism is not clear. Work on a mouse model has suggested glomerular damage is implicated in interferon nephritis (103[r]).

Mitomycin (mytomycin C) *Hemolytic uremic syndrome* has been previously described in over 50 cases with mitomycin therapy (104[R]). It presents with a Coombs-negative microangiopathic hemolytic anemia, thrombocytopenia and renal failure and is often fatal. The suspected pathology is vascular endothelial damage. This occurs from 4–7 months after commencement of chemotherapy. Of interest, blood transfusions induce clinical deterioration in those affected (105[r]). Treatment with hemodialysis and use of immunosuppressive drugs is not always successful.

Histology of the kidney in this syndrome shows mesangial proliferative glomerulonephritis with partial thickening and/or splitting of the basement membrane. Electron microscopy demonstrates accumulation of non-homogenous material in subendothelial spaces. Neither immunoglobulin nor complement deposition was seen (106[r]) in this study.

SKIN TOXICITY *(SED-11, 949; SEDA-13, 417)*

Bleomycin Topical bleomycin (0.5–1%) once daily may cause mild and transient erythema associated with the sensation of skin burning. Occlusive dressings increase the severity and incidence of this effect.

A case-report of *pigmented abdominal striae* following intense pruritus in a 65-year-old man with Hodgkin's disease has been suggested as secondary to a cumulative bleomycin dose of 112 mg. Biopsy of the lesion demonstrated melanotic hyperpigmentation only (107[c]).

Cytosine arabinoside/5-fluorouracil (5-FU) Acute painful swollen erythematous hands and soles, self-limiting in nature, have been reported following conventional induction therapy for acute myelogenous leukemia (108[Cr]). Histology lacks diagnostic specificity. This effect has been attributed to cytosine and has also been well documented with protracted (5-FU) infusion (109[c]). Some authors use the term palmar-plantar erythrodysesthesia for this syndrome. 5-FU also commonly causes other mucocutaneous complications such as *hyperpigmentation and multiple pigmented macules* (110[c]).

Methotrexate Reactivation of sunburn has been reported following intermediate-dose methotrexate (111[c]). It was not prevented by concurrent leucovorin administration.

Mitomycin (mitomycin C) Extravasation of this drug may cause painful ulceration necessitating surgical debridement. A recent report suggests a diminution of pain and necrosis with local injection of pyridoxine (112[c]). Carboplatin is also a vesicant agent and extravasation may require skin grafting (113[c]).

Mitoxantrone (mitozantrone) Mitoxantrone can cause *urine and sclera to turn blue or blue green* (66[c], 114[c]). There has been one report of hidradenitis associated with mitoxantrone (115). In this case a 59-year-old female treated with cyclophosphamide and mitoxantrone developed multiple reddish pustules and papules on her lymphedematous arm. Biopsy demonstrated a granulocytic infiltrate around the acrosyringial part of the sweat gland duct. These lesions resolved on changing to cyclophosphamide, methotrexate and 5-fluorouracil chemotherapy.

Painful onycholysis has occurred in those treated with mitoxantrone. Blue discoloration of nails has been reported (116[c]) and reversible loss of fingernails (117[c]).

OCULAR TOXICITY *(SED-11, 950)*

Interferon In a report of 57 patients treated with interferon for renal cell carcinoma 2 patients developed *multiple retinal exudates* associated with visual disturbance (previously unreported). Both patients were concurrently receiving vinblastine. Thus the exact role of interferon is unknown (118[cr]).

Vinca alkaloids Peripheral neuropathy and cranial nerve palsies are common with the Vinca alkaloids *Optic neuropathy* following a single small dose of vincristine has never been previously reported until Teichmann and Dabbagh reported a case (119[R]). This occurred in an 11-year-old Saudi girl who presented with a spinal astrocytoma. She was initially treated with radiotherapy, but 4 months later relapsed. She was then treated with a single injection of vincristine (1.275 mg), CCNU (80 mg) and procarbazine (80 mg). Six weeks later visual acuity was reduced to hand-movements with bilateral large central scotomas. This deteriorated over the succeeding 7 months before the patient died. There was no evidence on CT or MRI scans of optic nerve compression or intracranial disease. Unlike previous reports, the dose of vincristine was small (1.275 mg) and the latency period before onset of visual loss short (6–8 weeks). Most previously reported cases have had multiple injections of vincristine and the latency period has been greater than 3 months.

Studies on monkeys have demonstrated visual loss and optic atrophy with intravitreous injection of vincristine. Clinical reports of post-vincristine optic atrophy are fortunately rare; however, most reported cases are irreversible and the majority progresses to permanent blindness. Most cases have a coexistent peripheral neuropathy. It is conceivable that some patients are more sensitive and thus predisposed to vincristine-induced optic atrophy than others (61[cr]).

OTOTOXICITY *(SED-11, 952; SEDA-12, 387)*

Cisplatin (CDDP) High-tone hearing loss is consistent in patients receiving cisplatin. Progressive loss occurs with repeated administration of the drug until a threshold plateau is reached at the 3000–8000 Hz range (120[c]). This is directly related to organ of Corti damage. The ototoxicity is bilateral, symmetrical, progressive and irreversible. In this study following one course of cisplatin (150–225 mg/m^2) the mean hearing loss recorded was 27 dB at 8000 Hz, 21 dB at 6000 Hz, and 11 dB at 4000 Hz. The development of hearing loss is independent of pre-treatment hearing function (121[c]).

REPRODUCTIVE AND SEXUAL TOXICITY *(SED-11, 952; SEDA-13, 419)*

Cyclophosphamide Ovarian function may recover occasionally with successful pregnancies up to 7 years after treatment with cyclophosphamide and bone marrow transplant (122[R]). No specific factors were found to correlate with recovery of normal ovarian function. Recovery was very rare, however, if the patient had concurrent total body irradiation.

For further information on the effects of chemotherapy on the reproductive system, the reader is refered to a review by Gradishar and Schilsky (123[R]).

Nitrosoureas A study of boys treated with carmustine (BCNU) or lomustine (CCNU) alone or in combination with procarbazine and vincristine, for brain tumors demonstrated 20 cases of *persistent testicular damage* out of 21 cases studied (124[c]). From assessment of testicular size it seems likely that the majority of these boys remains infertile. This study supports the hypothesis that germinal epithelium is more susceptible than the Leydig cells to cytotoxic-induced damage.

PVB (cisplatin/vinblastine/bleomycin) *Sexual function* may be compromised in men following treatment with PVB chemotherapy. In a study of 54 patients 54% experienced disorders of sexual function 2 years after completion of treatment (125[R]). *Ejaculatory dysfunction* was tentatively linked to chemotherapy in 30% of those affected. *Diminished libido*, although usually reversible, was found in 75% at the time of receiving chemotherapy.

TERATOGENESIS *(SED-11, 953; SEDA-13, 418)*

Cyclophosphamide Cyclophosphamide is teratogenic. Exposure to the drug in the first trimester has been associated with anomalies of the extremities (126[c]), cleft palate, low-set ears and multiple eye abnormalities (117[c]).

CARCINOGENICITY *(SED-11, 929; SEDA-13, 418)*

The carcinogenic potential of cytotoxic agents has become an important consideration due predominantly to the success of these drugs in prolongation of life.

Alkylating agents have been positively implicated in the causation of secondary tumors, including acute myeloid leukemias (AML), myelodysplatic syndromes (128[R]) and solid tumors (129[c], 130[c]), and series have been reported following the treatment of Hodgkin's disease (HD) (131[c], 132[CR]), ovarian cancer (133[c], 134[c]) and gastric cancer (128[R]). Survival from the time of diagnosis of secondary malignancies is usually very brief (128[R]).

Van der Velden and colleagues in a multicenter case-controlled study found the incidence of AML in treated HD to be 64 times higher than in the general population, the risk being greater for males. They also demonstrated significant associations between the use of extensive radiotherapy, vincristine/procarbazine, splenectomy and the dose of mechlorethamine and the development of AML (132[CR]).

The increased risk is believed to be secondary to the increased occurrence of chromosomal aberrations or genomic instability (135[R]) in alkylating-agent-treated patients. Some authors have however failed to show an increase in aberrations in those with secondary tumors over and above those without (134[R]).

Azathioprine Azathioprine is a thiopurine immunosuppressive in widespread use. Often it has been difficult to demonstrate an increased incidence of secondary tumors (136[c]) over and above that of matched controls, yet sporadic reports of malignancies continue to be published. Skin (predominantly squamous-cell carcinomas) and lip cancers, Kaposi's sarcoma, and carcinoma of the cervix and anus are undoubtably much commoner following azathioprine therapy than in the general population (137[r]).

Carboplatin Carboplatin has the ability to induce sister chromatid exchange both in vitro and in vivo. This effect is dose-dependent and is a manifestation of DNA damage. Similarly chromosome aberrations such as gaps or breaks are induced by carboplatin. However, a recent study suggests that such potentially carcinogenic effects are considerably less than that seen with cisplatin (138[r]).

Ciclosporin (cyclosporin) There is a disproportionately high incidence of lymphomas, Kaposi's sarcoma (139[c]) and renal carcinoma in ciclosporin-treated patients (137[c], 140[c], 141[c]). Of particular interest is a report of complete regression of Kaposi's sarcoma following cessation of ciclosporin (142[c]). Fukuda and colleagues have noted a serum ciclosporin level related increase in chromosomal abnormalities in patients receiving ciclosporin following kidney transplantation (143[c]). This may be responsible for the excess numbers seen.

Cisplatin (CDDP) There is little convincing evidence of an increased risk of hematological malignancies following cisplatin therapy with vinblastine and bleomycin for testicular cancer (29[c], 30[c]). Most reported cases have received combined radiotherapy and chemotherapy, making it difficult to evaluate the contribution of the chemotherapy.

MISCELLANEOUS

Anaphylaxis *(SED-11, 928)* In a study of 46 patients treated for non-Hodgkin's lymphoma with **ifosfamide** one patient developed an anaphylactic-type reaction with acute wheeze and stridor on the 2nd day of the 4th course. Following treatment with diphenhydramine these symptoms resolved in 2 minutes. No further challenge with ifosfamide was performed (144[c]). This has not been previously reported.

There has been one report of acute anaphylaxis following a test repeat dose of **dacarbazine**. This has not been previously documented (145[c]).

Fever A report from Japan of fever $>38°C$ in 9 of 31 children receiving maintenance **vincristine** chemotherapy for either leukemia or lymphoma has proposed an allergic mechanism. Concurrent corticosteroid as part of the regime seems protective. Younger children are at greater risk and peak temperatures occur within 24 hours of vincristine administration. The pyrexia may last from 6 hours to 4 days and is self-limiting (146[C]).

Sixty milligrams of intrapleural **bleomycin** caused a fever $>39°C$ in 2 of 21 patients (147[c]) treated for malignant pleural effusion. This subsided without treatment and was not associated with any local discomfort.

Anthracyclines **Idarubicin** (4-demethoxydaunorubicin) is an anthracycline analog which is active orally. It is believed to have less cardiotoxicity than the parent compound (148[c], 149[c]). Bone marrow suppression at 60 mg/m^2 orally every 3 weeks was the dose-limiting toxicity in adults (150[c]) and gastrointestinal complications were dose-limiting at 40 $mg/m^2/d \times 3$ in children treated for relapsed acute non-lymphocytic leukemia (151[c]). Prior radiation may well exacerbate these adverse effects as noted with other anthracyclines.

Administration of idarubicin orally does seem to induce a *higher incidence of nausea and vomiting*, albeit mild, than intravenous administration (149[c], 152[c], 153[c]). Alopecia is mild (149[c]).

Low-dose methotrexate A wealth of literature has emerged in the past year on the oral use of methotrexate, for non-oncological disorders such as rheumatoid arthritis (42[c], 80[c], 154[c]–157[c]), psoriasis and systemic lupus erythematosus (158[c]). The drug is usually administered in a low dose of 7.5–15 mg weekly. Side effects of pancytopenia, gastrointestinal toxicity, skin rash, headache, mucositis, hepatotoxicity and pulmonary toxic effects have all been reported at this low dose (42[c], 159[c]) and are usually mild. These effects remain constant with prolonged use (mean 53 months) (42[c]). A double-blind randomized cross-over trial comparing placebo with leucovorin failed to demonstrate any diminution of nausea with the latter (160[c]). However, the *altered taste sensation* related to methotrexate may be restored by pharmacological doses of leucovorin (161[c]).

ALTERNATIVE MODES OF CHEMOTHERAPY ADMINISTRATION

Hepatic artery chemotherapy

Selective hepatic arterial infusion of chemotherapy using totally implantable reservoirs has been advocated for the treatment of primary and metastatic liver tumors particularly in the United States and Japan. Cisplatin, mitomycin, doxorubicin, 5-fluorodeoxyuridine (FUDR) and 5-fluorouracil have all been administered this way. Technical problems have occurred with sepsis, catheter dislodgement and inability to perfuse the liver as well as 'local toxicity' of continuous infusion (see below).

An *erythematous blistering skin rash* corresponding to the distribution of the selected artery has occurred with 5-fluorouracil use and usually subsides 1–2 months after stopping treatment leaving residual pigmentation (162[c], 163[c]). *Persistent neck and shoulder pain* has been reported (164[c]) and was abolished by the injection of long-acting local anesthetic through the hepatic artery infusion catheter. It was thought this pain was referred from the diaphragm.

Goldin and colleagues report 4 cases of *giant duodenal ulcer* (>2.5 cm diameter) secondary to hepatic intra-arterial chemotherapy and ligation of the gastroduodenal and right gastric arteries (165[c]). The drugs used were infusional floxuridine (FUDR) and intermittent bolus mitomycin. The interval between initial chemotherapy administration and development of symptoms ranged from 5 to 7 months. Two of these patients died from severe gastointestinal hemorrhage which was the predominant presenting symptom. Pre-treatment endoscopy was recommended by the authors. Others have reported similar cases (166[c], 167[c]). *Cholestatic jaundice* is also a particular complication of hepatic intra-arterial chemotherapy. This may respond to corticosteroids (168[c]). Pre-existing cirrhosis is a discriminatory poor prognostic factor for the development of intra-arterial chemotherapy-induced hepatic failure (167[cr]).

Cisplatin (CDDP)

Intra-arterial Administration of cisplatin by intra-arterial carotid infusion with plasma removal of the drug by plasmapheresis has been reported as successful in minimizing systemic side effects whilst maintaining efficacy (169[c]). At a dose of 100 mg/m^2 given over 30–60 min weekly pain along the arterial distribution is the predominant rate-limiting factor. *Ipsilateral hemialopecia, transient facial palsy and blurred vision* are adverse effects unique to this route of administration (170[c]). Further trials using such an approach are awaited.

Limb perfusion Cisplatin given by regional limb perfusion has been advocated for melanoma and soft tissue sarcoma of the extremities. Compartment syndrome necessitating fasciotomies with permanent loss of dorsiflexion has been described following this procedure (171[c]). Local adverse effects also include cellulitis and wound infections and are likely to be secondary to the technique of limb perfusion rather than the drug itself.

Local Direct intrapericardial instillation of cisplatin (10 mg in 20 ml saline) daily for 5 days for malignant pericardial effusion is well tolerated with only mild nausea (172[c]). Constrictive pericarditis is not produced.

Intravesical Allergic reactions including rash, pruritus, dyspnea and anaphylaxis have been reported in Spain secondary to intravesical cisplatin chemotherapy (173[c], 174[c]).

Intraperitoneal therapy

Doxorubicin microspheres A novel approach to the administration of chemotherapy has been the incorporation of drug into albumen microspheres. When used with doxorubicin in intra-arterial injection, local side effects of pain, skin rash and blistering occurred (175[c]).

Mytomycin (mitomycin C) Intraperitoneal mitomycin therapy has been advocated for salvage treatment in relapsed gynecological malignancies involving the abdomen. Mitomycin given this way produces dose-limiting *chemical peritonitis*. This is cumulative and limits therapy to 3–4 seperate monthly instillations of 2 liters of fluid containing 10 mg/m^2 mitomycin (176[c]). Systemic toxicity is thereby restricted to mild myelosuppression usually in the form of thrombocytopenia. This is not seen, however, when mitomycin is used intravesically at a dose of 40 mg in 40 ml for both prophylactic and definitive treatment of superficial bladder cancer. This lack of systemic effect is thought to be due to low absorption of the drug into the general circulation (177[cr]). Local effects of contact exanthema of the bladder and chemical cystitis are mild at this dose (177[cr], 178[c]).

Mitoxantrone (mitozantrone) Intraperitoneal mitoxantrone is well tolerated up to doses of 30 mg/m^2. At 35–40 mg/m^2 (179[c]) 1 patient out of 4 treated developed *chemoperitonitis* but none of 15 others treated at <30 mg/m^2 developed this complication. Systemic absorption is demonstrated by the occurrence of neutropenia in 4 cycles (WHO Grades 1–4) out of 6 given at the higher dosage. This is despite a marked pharmacological peritoneal advantage of the intraperitoneal route over intravenous administration. The authors concluded the optimal intraperitoneal dose to be 30 mg/m^2. A Phase I trial by Alberts and colleagues demonstrated a similar maximum tolerated dose of 38 mg/m^2 (180[c]) with abdominal pain and leukopenia again proving dose-limiting.

BIOLOGICAL RESPONSE MODIFIERS

Interferon-α *Fever, fatigue, anorexia, subsequent weight loss and general malaise* are all non-specific common 'flu'-like symptoms associated with interferon-α therapy (119[c], 181[c]–184[c]) Myelosuppression usually of no clinical significance (185[c]), gastrointestinal effects and elevation of liver enzymes are similarly all well reported (186[c]). Most effects are dose-related, tachyphylaxis occurs (187[c]) and control of adverse effects is easy with dose manipulation (183[c]). However, such adverse effects may seriously impair quality of life and lead to patients abandoning therapy (188[c]).

Clinical hypothyroidism preceded by the appearance of thyroid autoantibodies has been reported in patients receiving daily long-term interferon. Fentiman and colleagues have refuted the hypothesis that this is directly related to aberrant induction of Class II HLA expression and has suggested that the development of autoimmunity may be related to contaminants of the interferon-α preparation (189[r]). No consensus has yet been achieved.

Interferon-β Interferon-β has unique effects on cell differentiation, oncogene expression and cell proliferation. In a Phase I trial administering interferon on a 14-day intravenous bolus regime the maximum tolerated dose was 30×10^6 units at which Grade III hematological (both *neutropenia and thrombocytopenia*) toxicity is seen (187[c]).

Interferon-γ In a Phase I trial of interferon-γ dose-limiting toxicities were *malaise and orthostatic hypotension*. Similar acute adverse effects were seen to those of other interferon species. The maximum tolerated dose was 500–1000 μg/m^2/d when given for 10 days over a 2-week period (190[c]). No significant difference was observed when intravenous, intramuscular or subcutaneous routes were used.

Interleukin-2 Interleukin-2 (IL-2) is a lymphokine produced by lymphocytes currently being tested in renal cell carcinoma and melanoma. The major toxicity seen is hypotension. Fever, chills, malaise, nausea, diarrhea, headache, rash, fluid retention and myalgia are common (191[c]). Mild liver dysfunction, hypophosphatemia, hypomagnesemia and eosinophilia are the most common laboratory abnormalities (192[c], 193[c]). The development of pulmonary edema as part of the so-called *capillary leak syndrome* is of particular concern.

Renal toxicity with hypotension is often

dose-limiting with IL-2. It is manifest by uremia, oliguria fluid retention and avid tubular sodium reabsorption (193[c]). No evidence of tubular dysfunction has been found.

Tumor necrosis factor Tumor necrosis factor is naturally produced by the cells of the macrophage/monocyte system. When given by intravenous infusion, it causes similar symptoms to those of interleukin-2 by producing a capillary leak syndrome (194[c]). Thus, dose-limiting effects again are *severe hypotension, fluid retention, diarrhea, fatigue and confusion.*

OTHER DRUGS

Ciclosporin (cyclosporin A) Ciclosporin is a potent immunosuppressive agent. It is universally accepted as first-line anti-rejection therapy following renal transplantation and is commonly used in other organ transplantations. Others have advocated it in such diverse chronic diseases as diabetes mellitus, rheumatoid arthritis, psoriasis, inflammatory bowel disease, multiple sclerosis, nephrotic syndrome, myasthenia gravis, uveitis, HIV infection and alopecia arreata. The principal adverse effects are listed in Table 1. Unlike azathioprine, it does not depress the bone marrow.

Table 1. *Principal adverse effects of ciclosporin*

Effect	Reference
Nephrotoxicity Acute Chronic	195[c]–199[c]
Hypertension This is not confined to renal transplants	198[R], 199[R]
Secondary malignancies	141[c], 140[R], 137[c]
Erythrocytosis*	200[R], 201[c], 202[r], 203[c]
Thrombocytosis	204[r]
Hepatotoxicity	205[cr]
Hirsutism	206[c]
Gingival hyperplasia	139[c], 206[c]
Neurotoxicity	207[c]
Hypertriglyceridemia	208[c]

*The etiology of this effect is probably multifactorial. Some authors dispute a true increase in red cell volume. The role of ciclosporin in causation continues to be disputed.

Cyclophosphamide Cyclophosphamide is a well-known cause of *hemorrhagic cystitis* being first reported in 1959. It also causes *bladder fibrosis, hydronephrosis, vesicoureteral reflux* (209[c]) and *secondary urothelial malignancies.*

Cytarabine (ARA-C) There is currently considerable work on the use of high-dose (3 g/m^2 b.d.) ara-C in acute myeloid leukemia, particularly in combination with other agents (210[c]–214[c]). Aside from predictable adverse effects other reported side effects seen include *cerebellar neurotoxicity, progressive hepatic failure and adult respiratory distress syndrome* (212[c], 214[c]).

Ifosfamide Ifosfamide is a structural isomer of cyclophosphamide and side effects of myelosuppression, nausea, vomiting, alopecia, encephalopathy and of course *hemorrhagic cystitis* have all been well documented (53[c], 144[c], 215[c], 216[c]). Reduction in the severity of these effects has been described by administering a high fluid intake, urine alkalinization, use of mesna as a uroprotector and dose-fractionation.

Iproplatin This is a second-generation platinum compound. It has a similar toxicity profile to that of carboplatin (88[r]), although it has been shown to cause more diarrhea and thrombocytopenia when used in combination with cyclophosphamide (85[c]).

NEW DRUGS AND INVESTIGATIONAL SUBSTANCES

Acivicin This is an inhibitor of glutamine-dependent enzymes. It is a fermentation product of *Streptomyces sviceus*. The principal side effect is *neurotoxicity*, the severity of which is dose-dependent. At low dose, nightmares, confusion and headaches occur, with dysphasia, hallucinations and ataxia occurring at higher dose (e.g. 11 $mg/m^2/d \times 7$) (217[c]). Disorientation, depression, paranoia, amnesia, muscle twitching, mood changes and coma have been reported (218[c]). The etiology of acivicin-induced neurotoxicity is unclear.

Aminothiadiazole (ADTA) ADTA was first examined for its carcinostatic effects in 1955. It has now been demonstrated that its toxicity is secondary to a competitive antagonism of nicotinamide (219[c]). Clinical studies have identified dose-limiting effects of *mucosal toxicity*, predominantly oral (218[c]). Hyperuricemia occurs at even the lowest doses and allopurinol is advised throughout ADTA therapy.

AZQ This compound is an aziridinylbenzoquinone with characteristics suggesting good CNS penetration. The murder of a pet canary following a fit of rage in a patient experiencing a psychotic personality change may be temporally related to AZQ, although the patient was on concurrent steroid medication (220[c]).

Carmofur A reversible leukoencephalopathy with *dysarthria, muscular weakness and rigidity and involuntary movement* has been reported following carmofur administration (221[c]). Brain CT scan demonstrated periventricular lucency.

Carbetimer This is a low-molecular-weight polyelectrolyte. It is thought to have an immunomodulatory effect as it has been demonstrated to increase peripheral T-helper cells. One Phase I trial recommended a dose of 6500 mg/m^2 every 28 days for Phase II studies (222[c]). No myelosuppression of note was seen. Interestingly the dose-limiting toxicity was that of *hypercalcemia*. This tended to occur later than 10 days after treatment.

Another Phase I trial demonstrated limiting toxicity of *ocular symptoms* of flashing lights accompanied by modest fall in blood pressure at 16 690 $mg/m^2/1$ h. Pain at the injection site was limited to those receiving high doses over 1 hour. Prolonging the infusion to 2 hours resolved this effect, 12 550 $mg/m^2/2$ h was the suggested dose for Phase II trials (223[c]). Urinary phosphate and cAMP were significantly elevated at 24 hours post-treatment. These results suggest that carbetimer modulates the secretion or the action of parathyroid hormone. Further studies are likely. *Reversible mild proteinuria and hematuria* were also observed.

CI-921 This is a derivative of amsacrine which is more active than the parent compound against animal model tumors. A Phase I trial demonstrated the MTD to be 648 mg/m^2 at which dose *neutropenia, thrombophlebitis and oral toxicity* were common (224[c]). The drug does not seem to be vesicant.

CO17-1A This is murine monoclonal antibody which binds to a cell surface glycoprotein expressed preferentially by adenocarcinomas of the gastrointestinal tract. This agent enhances antibody-dependent cellular cytotoxicity by monocytes and lymphocytes and has no specific adverse reactions (225[c]). Interferon-γ at low dose ($< 1.0 \times 10^6$ $IU/m^2/d$) potentiates this mechanism. Phase I trials using escalating doses of CO17-1A to determine the maximal tolerated dose and dose-limiting toxicities are required.

10-EDAM This is a methotrexate derivative. Toxicity is qualitatively similar to that of the parent drug, oral *mucositis* being dose-limiting (226[c]). Skin rash is a dose-related effect.

Elliptinium acetate When administered on a weekly schedule this intercalating agent may cause *intravascular hemolysis*. This occurs secondary to the formation of anti-elliptinium antibodies and may be avoided by screening for these antibodies (227).

Flavone acetic acid (FAA) Flavanoids occur naturally in all plant cells. FAA is a synthetic flavanoid with anti-tumor effects demonstrated in animals. Phase I trials have demonstrated dose-limiting sporadic *reversible hypotension, generalized fatigue and asthenia*. Myelosuppression and alopecia were not seen. In one such trial (228[c]) a patient had a sudden cardiac arrest and died 1 hour after infusion of his second dose (3000 mg/m^2) of FAA. Autopsy demonstrated no evidence of cardiac disease and the event may be causally related to drug administration. Of less importance is the development of dose-related diarrhea starting 1 hour into the FAA infusion and lasting up to 2 days.

Fludarabine phosphate This is a derivative of ara-A which is relatively resistant to deamination to inactive metabolites. *Myelosuppression is dose-limiting* (229[c]). Delayed neurotoxicity can occur following high doses.

Harringtonine This is an alkaloid derived

from the South China tree, *Cephalotaxus hainanensis*. In vitro work has suggested it may have a role in differentiaton of leukemia cells. Other authors have claimed its effect is purely cytotoxic. *Pancytopenia* is common. Non-specific reversible ECG changes and tachycardia have been reported with its administration (230[c], 231[c]).

Isotretinoin This is a synthetic analog of vitamin A. It is postulated to work by increasing epidermal growth factor (EGF) receptors. EGF has been shown to modulate cell proliferation possibly through protein kinase-C. Toxic retinoid effects consist primarily of *mucocutaneous effects* (232[c]). Recent studies have demonstrated markedly reduced toxicity by combining retinoids with vitamin E.

MDMS Methylene dimethane sulfonate (MDMS) is the first member of dimethane sulfonic acid esters. It acts as an alkylating agent. *Alopecia, nausea, vomiting and dose-limiting cumulative thrombocytopenia* occur at a dose of 125 mg/m^2 given every 35 days (233[c]).

Misonidazole This was the first in a series of hypoxic cell radiosensitizers which is currently being evaluated also as a chemosensitizer in vivo (234[c]). The precise mechanism of chemosensitization is unknown. It does not have antitumor activity alone. It causes a dose-limiting *peripheral neuropathy* and other less neurotoxic agents are being developed.

Mitoquidone (MTQ) This drug is the first of a novel group of pentacylic pyrroloquinones. Further analogs are likely. Preclinical studies demonstrated no appreciable neutropenia. The most frequently encountered adverse effects were nausea and vomiting (not dose-related) and dyspnea. In a Phase I trial 10 patients developed *sudden onset dyspnea* (25% incidence), 8 experiencing concurrent chest pain (235[c]). Two of these patients had a proven pulmonary embolism. Three patients died unexpectedly suddenly, but there was no evidence at autopsy that these deaths were treatment-related. The high incidence of *pulmonary complications* is possibly due to the microcrystalline suspension formulation of the drug.

Muroctasin This agent is a muramyl dipeptide derivative (MDP-Lys (L18)) which has non-specific host defence mechanism stimulating properties. It has been demonstrated to enhance serum colony stimulating factor (CSF) activity in mice and has been advocated as a means of recovery from chemotherapy-induced neutropenia. The most common side effects was *fever*, which was dose-dependent, more pronounced with alternate-day subcutaneous dosing, and generally well controlled with antipyretics. *Injection site reactions* were seen and were mild (236[c]). Fever may be secondary to interleukin 1 (IL-1) production.

PCNU This is an intravenous lipid soluble nitrosourea. Severe life-threatening *hematological toxicities* (cumulative) have been documented (237[c]). Development of acute leukemia and secondary cancers following chemotherapy, especially with alkylating agents and nitrosoureas, has become an increasingly common late complication. The first report of *secondary leukemia* following treatment with this new nitrosourea is therefore not surprising (238[c]). A disturbing point in this case however was the short latency period of only 9 months.

PLAC (N^4-palmitoyl-1-β-D-arabinofuranosyl cytosine) This is an orally administered ara-C analog. Myelosuppression, nausea, vomiting and diarrhea have been seen (239[c]).

Spirogermanium This drug is an azaspirane. Phase I trials have demonstrated neurotoxicity as the major side effect. A Phase II trial confirmed this with additional *hepatic toxicity* manifest as progressive increase in liver enzymes (240[c]). It was unclear whether the 2 deaths reported (1 acute respiratory and 1 acute renal failure) were related to the drug.

Trimetrexate This compound is active in head and neck, breast and non-small-cell lung cancers (241[c]). It is a lipid-soluble dihydrofolate reductase inhibitor. It has a similar toxicity profile to that of methotrexate, dose-limiting effects being myelosuppression (nadir counts occurring at a median of 12 days) and mucositis. Like methotrexate there is a wide variability in myelosuppressive effect seen in individual patients (242[c], 243[c]). No cumulative effect is seen (244[c], 245[c]). Several Phase I trials have been done with a maximum tolerated dose of

10.5–15 mg/m²/d for 5 days. There is some evidence that it may be effective against methotrexate-resistant cells (246[c]) possibly due to differing mechanisms for cellular transport for the two drugs.

Non-hematological toxicity includes mild nausea and vomiting and a rash which tends to occur in sun-exposed areas on the 5th day following treatment (247[c]).

UFT This is an oral compound containing 80% futraful, which is gradually converted to 5-FU in the liver, and 20% uracil, which enhances tumor tissue toxicity. *Gastrointestinal side effects* including anorexia, nausea, vomiting and diarrhea are prominent. Hematological toxicity is rare (<10%) (248[c]). *Pigmentation and neurological adverse effects* have been reported.

REFERENCES

1. Puccio C, Feldman E, Arlin Z (1988) Amsacrine is safe in patients with ventricular ectopy. *Am. J. Hematol., 28,* 197.
2. Okuma K, Ariyoshi Y, Ota K (1988) Clinical study of acute cardiotoxicity of anti-cancer agents—analysis using Holter ECG monitoring. *Jpn. J. Cancer Chemother, 15,* 1893.
3. Solymar L, Marky I, Mellander L, Sabel K (1988) Echocardiographic findings in children treated for malignancy with chemotherapy including adriamycin. *Pediatr. Hematol. Oncol., 5,* 209.
4. Nakamura K, Miyake T, Kawamura T, Maekawa I (1988) Prospective monitoring of adriamycin cardiotoxicity with systolic time intervals. *J. Jpn. Soc. Cancer Ther., 23,* 1633.
5. Dey HM, Kassamali H (1988) Radionuclide evaluation of doxorubicin cardiotoxicity: the need for cautious interpretation. *Clin. Nuclear Med., 13,* 565.
6. Rowan R, Masek M, Billingham M (1988) Ultrastructural morphometric analysis of endomyocardial biopsies. *Am. J. Cardiol. Pathol., 2,* 137.
7. Speyer J, Green M, Kramer E et al (1988) Protective effect of the bisiperazinedione ICRF-187 against doxorubicin-induced cardiac toxicity in women with advanced breast cancer. *N. Engl. J. Med., 319,* 745.
8. McQuillan P, Morgan B, Ramwell J (1988) Adriamycin cardiomyopathy. *Anaesthesia, 43,* 301.
9. Goenen M, Baele P, Lintermans J et al (1988) Orthotopic heart transplantation eleven years after left pneumonectomy. *J. Heart Transplant., 7,* 309.
10. Camaggi C, Comparsi R, Strocchi E et al (1988) Epirubicin and doxorubicin comparative metabolism and pharmacokinetics. *Cancer Chemother. Pharmacol., 21,* 221.
11. Kreis W, Rottach C, Budman DR et al (1988) Pharmokinetics and Phase I evaluation of esorubicin (4′-deoxydoxorubicin) by continuous infusion over forty-eight hours in patients with leukemia. *Cancer Res., 48,* 5580.
12. Diehl LF, Banks A, Carter W et al (1988) Fatal esorubicin-induced cardiomyopathy: report of a case and review of the literature. *Cancer Chemother, Pharmacol., 21,* 347.
13. Clavel M, Simeone P, Grivet B (1988) Toxicité cardiaque du 5-fluorouracile. *Presse Méd., 17,* 1675.
14. Eskilsson J, Albertsson M, Mercke C (1988) Adverse cardiac effects during induction chemotherapy treatment with cis-platin and 5-fluorouracil. *Radiother. Oncol., 13,* 41.
15. Mortimer J, Higano C (1988) Continuous infusion 5-fluorouracil and folinic acid in disseminated colorectal cancer. *Cancer Invest., 6,* 129.
16. Coronel B, Madonna O, Mercatello A et al (1988) Myocardiotoxicity of 5-fluorouracil. *Intensive Care Med., 14,* 429.
17. Chaudary S, Thomas Song S, Jaski B (1988) Profound, yet reversible heart failure secondary to 5-fluorouracil. *Am. Med., 85,* 454.
18. Jakubowski A, Kemeny N (1988) Hypotension as a manifestation of cardiotoxicity in three patients receiving cisplatin and 5-fluorouracil. *Cancer, 62,* 266.
19. Kleiman N, Lehane D, Geyer C et al (1987) Prinzmetal's angina during 5-fluorouracil chemotherapy. *Am. J. Med., 82,* 566.
20. Alimena G, Morra E, Lazzarino M et al (1988) Interferon alpha-2b as therapy for Ph′-positive chronic myelogenous leukemia: a study of 82 patients treated with intermittent or daily administration. *Blood, 72,* 642.
21. Simone G, Iaffaioli V, Mura G et al (1988) Reversible heart failure in a non-Hodgkin's lymphoma patient being treated with alpha-interferon. *Curr. Ther. Res., 44,* 78.
22. Verweij J, Funke-Kupper A, Teule G, (1988) A prospective study on the dose dependency of cardiotoxicity induced by mitomycin-C. *Med. Oncol. Tumour Pharmacother., 5,* 159.
23. South West Oncology Group (1987) *Cancer Treat. Rep., 71,* 609.
24. Cassidy J, Merrick M (1988) Cardiotoxicity of mitoxantrone assessed by stress and resting nuclear ventriculography. *Eur. J. Clin. Oncol., 24,* 935.
25. Brusamolino E, Bertini M, Guidi S et al (1988) CHOP vs CNOP (N = mitoxantrone) in non-Hodgkins's lymphoma: an interim report comparing efficacy and toxicity. *Haematologica, 73,* 217.
26. Glenn L, Armitage J, Goldsmith J et al (1988)

Pulmonary emboli in patients receiving chemotherapy for non-Hodgkin's lymphoma. *Chest, 94,* 589.
27. Cantwell B, Carmichael J, Ghani S (1988) Thromboses and thromboemboli in patients with lymphoma during cytotoxic chemotherapy. *Br. Med. J., 297,* 179.
28. Goodnough L, Pearson O (1988) Adjuvant therapy for breast cancer. *N. Engl. J. Med., 319,* 443.
29. Roth B, Einhorn L, Greist A (1988) Long-term complications of cisplatin-based chemotherapy for testis cancer. *Semin. Oncol., 15,* 345.
30. Roth B, Greist A, Kubllis P et al (1988) Cisplatin-based combination chemotherapy for disseminated germ cell tumors: long-term follow-up. *J. Clin. Oncol., 6,* 1239.
31. Stefenelli T, Kuzmits R, Ulrich W, Glogar D (1988) Acute vascular toxicity after combination chemotherapy with cisplatin, vinblastine and bleomycin for testicular cancer. *Eur. Sox. Cardiol., 9,* 552.
32. Raghavan D (1988) Chemotherapy in the management of invasive and metastatic bladder cancer. *Eur. Urol., 14,* 21.
33. Hitchins R, Thomson D (1988) Encephalopathy following cisplatin, bleomycin and vinblastine therapy for non-seminomatous germ cell tumour of testis. *Aust. NZJ. Med., 18,* 67.
34. Tondini M, Corbellini D, Totteri A (1987) Aritmie cardiache in corso di terapia con cisplatino: presentazione di 3 nuovi casi. *Folia Oncol., 10,* 167.
35. Jenkinson S, Duncan C, Lawrence R, Collins J (1987) Lack of enhancement of bleomycin lung injury in vitamin E-deficient rats. *J. Crit. Care, 2,* 264.
36. Nussinovitch N, Peleg E, Yaron A et al (1988) Angiotensin converting enzyme in bleomycin-treated patients. *Clin. Pharmacol. Ther. Toxicol., 26,* 310.
37. Quigley M, Brada M, Heron C, Horwich A (1988) Severe lung toxicity with a weekly low-dose chemotherapy regimen in patients with non-Hodgkin's lymphoma. *Haematol. Oncol., 6,* 319.
38. Vergnon J, Boucheron S, Riffat J et al (1988) Pneumopathies interstitielles au busulfan: analyse histologique, evolutive et par lavage broncho-alvéolaire de trois observations. *Rev. Méd. Interne, 9,* 377.
39. Glatt V, Henke M, Sigmund G, Costabel U (1988) Cyclophosphamid-induzierte Pneumonitis. *Fortschr. Röntgenstr., 148,* 545.
40. Colozza M, Tonato M, Grignani F, Davis S (1988) Low-dose mitomycin and weekly low-dose doxorubicin combination chemotherapy for patients with metastatic breast carcinoma previously treated with cyclophosphamide, methotrexate, and 5-fluorouracil. *Cancer, 62,* 262.
41. Ridley M, Wolfe C, Mathews J (1988) Life threatening acute pneumonitis during low-dose methotrexate treatment for rheumatoid arthritis: a case report and review of the literature. *Ann. Rheum. Dis., 47,* 784.
42. Kremer J, Lee J (1988) A long-term prospective study of the use of methotrexate in rheumatoid arthritis. *Arthritis Rheum., 31,* 577.
43. O'Meara A, Daly M, Hallinan F (1988) Increased antithrombin III concentration in children with acute lymphatic leukaemia receiving L-asparaginase therapy. *Med. Pediatr. Oncol., 16,* 169.
44. Ott N, Ramsay N, Priest J et al (1988) Sequelae of thrombotic or hemorrhagic complications following L-asparaginase therapy for childhood lymphoblastic leukemia. *Am. J. Pediatr. Hematol. Oncol., 10,* 191.
45. Gessini L, Jandolo B, Pollera C et al (1987) Neuropatia da cisplatino: un nuovo tipo di polineuropatia assonale ascendente progressiva. *Riv. Neurobiol., 33,* 75.
46. Holleran W, De Gregorio M (1988) Evolution of high-dose cisplatin. *Invest. New Drugs, 6,* 135.
47. Riggs J, Ashraf M, Snyder R, Gutmann L (1988) Prospective nerve conduction studies in cisplantin therapy. *Ann. Neurol., 23,* 92.
48. Mollman J, Glover D, Hogan M, Furman R (1988) Cisplantin neuropathy: risk factors, prognosis, and protection by WR-2721. *Cancer, 61,* 2192.
49. Walker R, Cairncross J, Posner J (1988) Cerebral herniation in patients receiving cisplatin. *J. Neuro-Oncol., 6,* 61.
50. Bellin S, Selim M (1988) Cisplatin-induced hypomagnesemia with seizures: a case report and review of the literature. *Gynecol. Oncol., 30,* 104.
51. Kibirige M, Morris-Jones P, Addison G (1988) Prevention of cisplatin-induced hypomagnesemia. *Pediatr. Hematol. Oncol., 5,* 1.
52. Leff R, Thomspon J, Daly M et al (1988) Acute neurologic dysfunction after high-dose etoposide therapy for malignant glioma. *Cancer, 62,* 32.
53. Gieron M, Barak L, Estrada J (1988) Severe encephalopathy associated with ifosfamide administration in two children with metastatic tumors. *J. Neuro-Oncol., 6,* 29.
54. Vesikari T, Nuutila A, Cantell K (1988) Neurologic sequelae following interferon therapy of juvenile laryngeal papilloma. *Acta Paediatr. Scand., 77,* 619.
55. Fujii Y, Mizuno Y, Hongo T et al (1988) Serial spectral EEG analysis in a patient with non-Hodgkin's lymphoma complicated by leukoencephalopathy induced by high dose methotrexate. *Jpn. J. Cancer Chemother., 15,* 713.
56. Poskitt K, Steinbok P, Flodmark O (1988) Methotrexate leukoencephalopathy mimicking cerebral abcess on CT brain scan. *Child's Nerv. Syst., 4,* 119.
57. Lakhani AK, Zuiable AG, Pollard CM et al (1986) Paraplegia after intrathecal mitozantrone (Letter to Editor). *Lancet, 2,* 1393.
58. Dickerhoff R, Lindner W, Scheiber W (1988)

Severe vincristine neurotoxicity in a patient with Charcot-Marie-Tooth disease. *Pediatr. Hematol. Oncol.*, *5*, 61.
59. Thoumie P, Diverrez JP, Guidet B (1989) Polynévrite aiguë à la vincristine préscrite pour un cancer du sein chez une patiente atteinte de maladie de Friedreich. *Sem. Hôp. Paris*, *65*, 30.
60. Hurwitz R, Mahoney D, Armstrong D, Browder T (1983) Reversible encephalopathy and seizures as a result of conventional vincristine administration. *Med. Pediatr. Oncol.*, *16*, 216.
61. Pinkerton C, McDermott B, Philip T, Biron P (1988) Continuous vincristine infusion as part of a high dose chemoradiotherapy regimen: drug kinetics and toxicity. *Cancer Chemother. Pharmacol.*, *22*, 271.
62. Jackson D, Wells H, Atkins J (1988) Amelioration of vincristine neurotoxicity by glutamic acid. *Am. J. Med.*, *84*, 1016.
63. Fernandez L, Zayed E (1988) Busulfan-induced sideroblastic anemia. *Am. J. Hematol.*, *28*, 199.
64. Shupack J, Webster G (1988) Pancytopenia following low-dose oral methotrexate therapy for psoriasis. *J. Am. Med. Assoc.*, *259*, 3594.
65. Dubost J, Sauvezie B (1988) Fatal bone marrow toxicity in a patient treated with methotrexate and glafenine for rheumatoid arthritis. *Clin. Exp. Rheumatol.*, *6*, 97.
66. Koppensteiner R, Minar E (1988) Survival following an extremely high-dose of mitoxantrone in a 73 year old female with small-cell bronchial carcinoma (Letter). *J. Cancer Res. Clin. Oncol.*, *114*, 324.
67. Morris L, Guthrie T (1988) Busulfan-induced hepatitis. *Am. J. Gastroenterol.*, *83*, 682.
68. Honjo I, Suou T, Hirayama C (1988) Hepatotoxicity of cyclophosphamide in man: pharmacokinetic analysis. *Res. Commun. Chem. Pathol. Pharmacol.*, *61*, 149.
69. Shaunak S, Munro J, Weinbren K et al (1988) Cyclophosphamide-induced liver necrosis: a possible interaction with azatioprine. *Q. J. Med.*, *67*, 309.
70. Green D, Finklestein J, Norkool P, d'Angion J (1988) Severe hepatic toxicity after treatment with single-dose dactinomycin and vincristine. *Cancer*, *62*, 270.
71. Ceci G, Bella M, Melissari M et al (1988) Fatal hepatic vascular toxicity of DTIC. *Cancer*, *61*, 1988.
72. Lejeune F, Macher E, Kleeberg U et al (1988) An assessment of DTIC vs levamisole or placebo in the treatment of high risk stage I patients after surgical removal of a primary melanoma of the skin: a Phase III adjuvant study. *Eur. J. Cancer Clin. Oncol.*, *24*, 81.
73. Risteli J, Sogaard H, Oikarinen A et al (1988) Aminoterminal propeptide of type III procollagen in methotrexate-induced liver fibrosis and cirrhosis. *Br. J. Dermatol.*, *119*, 321.
74. Larrey D, Freneaux E, Berson A et al (1988) Peliosis hepatis induced by 6-thioguanine administration. *Gut*, *29*, 1265.
75. Jones M, Best P, Catto G (1988) Is nodular regenerative hyperplasia of the liver associated with azathioprine therapy after renal transplantation? *Nephrol. Dialysis Transplant.*, *3*, 331.
76. Wahlin Y, Holm A (1988) Changes in the oral microflora in patients with acute leukemia and related disorders during the period of induction therapy. *Oral Surg. Oral Med. Oral Pathol.*, *65*. 411.
77. Grunberg S, Ehler E, McDermed J, Akerley W (1988) Oral metoclopramide with or without diphenhydramine: potential for prevention of late nausea and vomiting induced by cisplatin. *J. Natl. Cancer Inst.*, *80*, 864.
78. Bindi M, Pepi F, Sebaste L et al (1988) Combination of glucagon and low-dose metoclopramide in management of cis-platin induced nausea and vomiting. *J. Natl. Cancer Inst.*, *80*, 97.
79. Qilu W, Yan S, Jichang Z et al (1988) High-dose methotrexate with citrovorum factor rescue (HD-MTX-CFR) in the treatment of malignant solid tumours: clinical analysis of 62 patients. *Chin. J. Oncol.*, *10*, 152.
80. Reggev A, Djerassi I (1988) The safety of administration of massive doses of methotrexate (50 g) with equimolar citrovorum factor rescue in adult patients. *Cancer*, *61*, 2423.
81. Socinski M, Garnick M (1988) Acute pancreatitis associated with chemotherapy for germ cell tumors in two patients. *Ann. Intern. Med.*, *108*, 567.
82. Ten Bokkel Huinink W, Van der Burg M, Van Oosterom A et al (1988) Carboplatin in combination therapy for ovarian cancer. *Cancer Treat. Rev.*, *15, Suppl. B*, 9.
83. Calvert A, Horwich A, Newlands E et al (1988) Carboplatin or cisplatin? *Lancet*, *2*, 577.
84. Conte P, Bruzzone M, Chiara S et al (1988) Carboplatin (JM 8), adriamycin and cyclophosphamide (JAC) in advanced ovarian carcinoma: a pilot study. *Tumori*, *74*, 217.
85. Anderson H, Wagstaff J, Crowther D et al (1988) Comparative toxicity of cisplatin, carboplatin (CBDCA) and iproplatin (CHIP) in combination with cyclophosphamide in patients with advanced epithelial ovarian cancer. *Eur. J. Cancer Clin. Oncol.*, *24*, 1471.
86. Tueni E, Sculier J, Klastersky J (1988) Phase I study of a carboplatin–etoposide Combination in advanced thoracic cancer. *Eur. J. Cancer Clin. Oncol.*, *24*, 963.
87. Lee E, Egorin M, Van Echo D et al (1988) Phase I and pharmacokinetic trial of carboplatin in refractory adult leukaemia. *J. Natl. Cancer Inst.*, *80*, 131.
88. Skillen A, Buamah P, Cantwell B et al (1988) Urinary protein and enzyme excretion in patients receiving chemotherapy with the cis-platinum analogs carboplatin (CBDCA, JM8) and iproplatin (CHIP, JM9). *Cancer Chemother. Pharmacol.*, *22*, 228.

89. Bergevin P (1988) Nephrotoxicity of cisplatin (*cis*-diamminedichloroplatinum(II)). *Drugs Today, 24,* 403.
90. Daugaard G, Abildgaard U, Holstein-Rathlou N et al (1988) Renal tubular function in patients treated with high-dose cisplatin. *Clin. Pharmacol. Ther., 44,* 164.
91. Saito M, Masaki T, Kato H (1988) A clinical evaluation of the protective effect of fosfomycin (FOM) against the *cis*-diamminedichloroplatinum (CDDP)-induced nephrotoxicity. *Acta Urol. Jpn., 34,* 782.
92. Mariette X, Paule B, Bennet P et al (1988) Cisplatin and hyponatremia. *Ann. Intern. Med., 108,* 770.
93. Mavichak V, Coppin C, Wong N et al (1988) Renal magnesium wasting and hypocalciuria in chronic cis-platinum nephropathy in man. *Clin. Sci., 75,* 203.
94. Suzumori K, Yasui Y, Suzumori K et al (1988) Comparison of methods for evaluating nephrotoxicity of cisplatin. *Jpn. J. Cancer Chemother., 15,* 2251.
95. Ujiie T, Maruta H, Ito N (1988) Studies on serum and urinary α-microglobulin levels as parameter of the renal function after CDDP administration. *Acta Urol. Jpn., 34,* 790.
96. Rothenberg ML, Ostchega Y, Steinberg SM et al (1988) High-dose carboplatin with diethyldithiocarbonate chemoprotection in treatment of women with relapsed ovarian cancer. *Natl. Cancer Inst., 80,* 1488.
97. Maiche A, Lappalainen K, Teerenhovi L (1988) Renal insufficiency in patients treated with high dose methotrexate. *Acta Oncol., 27,* 73.
98. Christensen M, Rivera G, Crom W et al (1988) Effect of hydration on methotrexate plasma concentrations in children with acute lymphocytic leukemia. *J. Clin. Oncol., 6,* 797.
99. Amino K, Kawaguchi N, Matsumoto S et al (1988) Urinary β_2-microglobulin as an indicator of impaired excretion of methotrexate. *Jpn. J. Cancer Chemother., 15,* 3103.
100. Molina R, Fabian C, Cowley B (1987) Use of charcoal hemoperfusion with sequential hemodialysis to reduce serum methotrexate levels in a patient with acute renal insufficiency. *Am. J. Med., 82,* 350.
101. Relling M, Bruder Stapleton F, Ochs J et al (1988) Removal of methotrexate, leucovorin, and their metabolites by combined hemodialysis and hemoperfusion. *Cancer, 62,* 884.
102. Price P, Thompson H, Bessell E, Bloom H (1988) Renal impairment following the combined use of high-dose methotrexate and procarbazine. *Cancer Chemother. Pharmacol., 21,* 265.
103. Cox E, Laszlo J, Krown S et al (1988) Phase II study of human lymphoblastoid interferon in patients with multiple myeloma. *J. Biol. Response Modif., 7,* 318.
104. Mackintosh J, Tattersal M (1988) Mitomycin-C induced hemolytic-uraemic syndrome. *Aust. NZJ. Med., 18,* 182.
105. Ries F (1988) Nephrotoxicity of chemotherapy. *Eur. J. Cancer Clin. Oncol., 21,* 951.
106. Hayano K, Fukui H, Otsuka Y, Hattori S (1988) Three cases of renal failure associated with microangiopathic hemolytic anemia after mitomycin C therapy (in Japanese). *Jpn. J. Nephrol., 7,* 835.
107. Massone L, Pestarino A, Borghi S et al (1988) Strie iperpigmentate dopo terapia con bleomicina. *G. Ital. Dermatol. Venereol., 123,* 225.
108. Shall L, Lucas G, Whittaker J, Holt P (1988) Painful red hands: a side effect of leukaemia therapy. *Br. J. Dermatol., 119,* 249.
109. Bellmunt J, Navarro M, Hidalgo R, Sole L (1988) Palmar-plantar erythrodysesthesia syndrome associated with short-term continuous infusion (5 days) of 5-fluorouracil. *Tumori, 74,* 329.
110. Cho K, Chung J, Lee A et al (1988) Pigmented macules in patients treated with systemic 5-fluorouracil. *J. Dermatol., 15,* 342.
111. Lawrenz-Wolf B, Wehinger H (1988) Zur Reaktivierung von Sonnenbranden durch Methotrexat. *Klin. Pädiatr., 200,* 335.
112. Godfrey T (1988) Mitomycin C in advanced breast cancer: an update. *Semin. Oncol., 15,* 71.
113. Eisenberger M, Sinibaldi V, Jacobs M, Gray W (1988) Simultaneous treatment with carboplatin (NSC-241-240) and radiotherapy in advanced unresectable squamous cell carcinomas of the head and neck. *Cancer Treat. Rev., 15, suppl. B,* 3.
114. Anonymous (1988) Mitoxantrone. *Med. Lett.,* 68.
115. Burg G, Bieber T, Langecker P (1988) Lokalisierte neutrophile ekkrine Hidradenitis unter Mitoxantron: eine typische Zytostatikanebenwirkung. *Hautarzt, 39,* 233.
116. Speechly-Dick ME, Owen ERTC (1988) Mitozantrone induced onycholysis. *Lancet, 1,* 113.
117. Werner Hansen S, Nissen N, Mork Hansen M et al (1988) High activity of mitoxantrone in previously untreated low-grade lymphomas. *Cancer Chemother. Pharmacol., 22,* 77.
118. Fossa SD (1988) Is interferon with or without vinblastine the 'treatment of choice' in metastatic renal cell carcinoma? The Norwegian Radium Hospital's experience. *Semin. Surg. Oncol., 4,* 178.
119. Teichmann K, Dabbagh N (1988) Severe visual loss after a single dose of vincristine in a patient with spinal cord astrocytoma. *J. Ocul. Pharm., 4,* 117.
120. Kopelman J, Budnick A, Sessions RB, Wong GY (1988) Ototoxicity of high-dose cisplatin by bolus administration in patients with advanced cancers and normal hearing. *Laryngoscope, 98,* 858.
121. Laurell G, Borg E (1988) Ototoxicity of cisplatin in gynaecological cancer patients. *Scand. Audiol., 17,* 241.

122. Sanders J, Buckner C, Amos D et al (1988) Ovarian function following marrow transplantation for aplastic anemia or leukemia. *J. Clin. Oncol., 6,* 813.
123. Gradishar W, Schilsky R (1988) Effects of cancer treatment on the reproductive system. *CRC Crit. Rev. Oncol. Hematol., 8,* 153.
124. Clayton P, Shalet S, Price D, Campbell R (1988) Testicular damage after chemotherapy for childhood brain tumors. *J. Pediatr., 112,* 922.
125. Nijman J, Koops H, Oldhoff J et al (1988) Sexual function after surgery and combination chemotherapy in men with disseminated nonseminomatous testicular cancer. *J. Surg. Oncol., 38,* 182.
126. Feliu J, Mondejar J, Martinez B et al (1988) Sarcoma de Ewing y gestación. *Med. Clín (Barc.), 91,* 25.
127. Kirshon B, Wasserstrum N, Willis R et al (1988) Teratogenic effects of first-trimester cyclophosphamide therapy. *Obstet. Gynecol., 72,* 462.
128. Bennett J, Moloney W, Greene M, Boice J (1987) Acute myeloid leukemia and other myelopathic disorders following treatment with alkylating agents. *Hematol. Pathol., 1,* 99.
129. Pedersen-Bjergaard J, Ersball J, Hansen V et al (1988) Blasenkarzinom nach Cyclophosphamid-Langzeittherapie. *Aktel. Urol., 19,* 275.
130. O'Keane J (1988) Carcinoma of the urinary bladder after treatment with cyclophosphamide (Letter to Editor). *N. Engl. J. Med., 319,* 871.
131. Mahe M, Raffi F, Rojouan J et al (1988) Cancers secondaires après maladie de Hodgkin. *Sem. Hôp. Paris, 64,* 3013.
132. Van der Velden J, Van Putten W, Guinee V et al (1988) Subsequent development of acute nonlymphocytic leukemia in patients treated for Hodgkin's disease. *Int. J. Cancer, 42,* 252.
133. Guyotat D, Coiffier B, Camos L et al (1988) Acute leukaemia following high-dose chemoradiotherapy with bone marrow rescue for ovarian teratoma. *Acta Haematol., 80,* 52.
134. Einhorn N, Eklund G, Lambert B (1988) Solid tumours and chromosome aberrations as late side effects of melphalan therapy in ovarian carcinoma. *Acta Oncol., 27,* 215.
135. Genuardi M, Zollino M, Serra A et al (1988) Long-term cytogenetic effects of antineoplastic-treatment in relation to secondary leukemia. *Cancer Genet. Cytogenet., 33,* 201.
136. Wessel G, Abendroth K, Wisheit M (1988) Malignant transformation during immunosuppressive therapy (azathioprine) of rheumatoid arthritis and systemic lupus erythematosus: a retrospective study. *Scand. J. Rheumatol., 67,* 73.
137. Penn I (1988) Immunosuppression and neoplasia cancers after cyclosporine therapy. *Transplant. Proc., 20,* 276.
138. Shinkai T, Saijo N, Eguchi K et al (1988) Cytogenetic effect of carboplatin on human lymphocytes. *Cancer Chemother. Pharmacol., 21,* 203.
139. Qunibi W, Akhtar M, Ginn E, Smith P (1988) Kaposi's sarcoma in cyclosporine-induced gingival hyperplasia. *Am. J. Kidney Dis., 11,* 349.
140. Penn I (1988) Posttransplant malignancies. *World J. Urol., 6,* 125.
141. Penn I, Brunson M (1988) Cancers after cyclosporine therapy. *Transplant. Proc., 20,* 885.
142. Pilgrim M (1988) Spontane Manifestation und Regression eines Kaposi-Sarkoms unter Cyclosporin A. *Hautarzt, 39,* 368.
143. Fukuda M, Ohmori Y, Aikawa I et al (1988) Mutagenicity of cyclosporine in vivo. *Transplant. Proc., 20,* 929.
144. Case DC, Anderson J, Ervin T, Gottlich A (1988) Phase II trial of ifosfamide and mesna in previously treated patients with non-Hodgkin's lymphoma: cancer and leukaemia group B study 8552. *Med. Pediatr. Oncol., 16,* 182.
145. Abhyankar S, Rao S, Pollio L, Miller S (1988) Anaphylactic shock due to dacarbazine (NSC-45 388). *Am. J. Dis. Child., 142,* 918.
146. Ishii E, Hara T, Mizuno Y, Ueda K (1988) Vincristine-induced fever in children with leukaemia and lymphoma (in Japanese). *Saishin Igaku, 6,* 1341.
147. Hsu NY, Chen C (1988) Intrapleural bleomycin in the management of malignant pleural effusion. *J. Surg Assoc. ROC, 21,* 302.
148. Bertelli G, Amoroso D, Pronzato P, Rosso R (1988) Idarubicin: an evaluation of cardiac toxicity in 77 patients with solid tumours. *Anticancer Res., 8,* 645.
149. Kolaric K, Potrebica V, Vukas D et al (1988) Combination chemotherapy with 5-fluorouracil, oral idarubicin, and cyclophosphamide (FIC) in metastatic breast cancer—an open Phase II study. *J. Cancer Res. Clin. Oncol., 114,* 301.
150. Erttmann R, Bode U, Erb N et al (1988) Antineoplastische Wirksamkeit und Toxizität von Idrarubicin (4-Demethoxydaunorubicin) bei rezidivierten akuten Leukämien des Kindesalters. *Klin. Pädiatr. 200,* 200.
151. Pui C, De Graaf S, Dow L et al (1988) Phase I clinical trial of orally administered 4-demethoxydaunorubicin (idarubicin) with pharmacokinetic and in vitro drug sensitivity testing in children with refractory leukemia. *Cancer Res., 48,* 5348.
152. Gillies H, Liang R, Rogers H et al (1988) Phase II trial of idarubicin in patients with advanced lymphoma. *Cancer Chemother. Pharmacol., 21,* 261.
153. Chisesi T, Capnist G, De Dominicis E, Dini E (1988) A Phase II study of idarubicin (4-demethoxydaunorubicin) in advanced myeloma. *Eur. J. Cancer Clin. Oncol., 24,* 681.
154. Chamot A, Gerster J, Van Melle G (1988) Le méthotrexate à faibles doses orales dans le traite-

ment de la polyarthrite rhumatoïde. *Schweiz. Med. Wochnschr., 118,* 1267.
155. Karger T, Rau R (1988) Behandlung der chronischen Polyarthritis mit niedrig dosiertem Methotrexat. *Dtsch. Med. Wochenschr., 113,* 839.
156. Nolla J, Roig D, Lopez J et al (1988) Metotrexato en la artritis reumatoidea. *Rev. Esp. Reumatol., 15,* 49.
157. Scott D (1988) Methotrexate and rheumatoid arthritis. *J. Clin. Pharmacol. Ther., 13,* 85.
158. Rothenberg R, Graziano F, Grandone J et al (1988) The use of methotrexate in steroid-resistant systemic lupus erythematosus. *Arthritis Rheum., 31,* 612.
159. Abel E, Farber E (1988) Pancytopenia following low-dose methotrexate therapy. *J. Am. Med. Assoc., 259,* 3612.
160. Hanrahan P, Russell A (1988) Concurrent use of folinic acid and methotrexate in rheumatoid arthritis. *J. Rheumatol., 15,* 1078.
161. Duhra P, Foulds I (1988) Methotrexate-induced impairment of taste acuity. *Clin. Exp. Dermatol., 13,* 126.
162. Suzuki K, Takeda Y, Nishio K et al (1988) Skin manifestations caused by intraarterial infusion of anti-cancer drugs (in Japanese). *Skin Res., 5,* 626.
163. Sawada T, Hojo K, YM (1988) Results of intra-arterial infusion chemotherapy in colorectal cancer patients with metastatic liver cancer. *Jpn. J. Cancer Chemother., 15,* 2437.
164. Khoury GF, Stein C, Ramming KP (1988) Neck and shoulder pain associated with hepatic arterial chemotherapy using an implantable pump. *Pain. 32,* 275.
165. Goldin E, Peretz T, Libson E (1988) Giant duodenal ulcer: the hepatic intra-arterial chemotherapy variant. *Postgrad. Med. J., 64,* 431.
166. Safi F, Roscher R, Heymer B et al (1988) Erosive Gastroduodenitis mit schweren Epitheldysplasien als Komplikation der lokoregionalen intraarteriellen Chemotherapie bei Lebermetastasen *Aktuel. Chir., 23,* 69.
167. Doci R, Bignami P, Bozzetti F et al (1988) Intrahepatic chemotherapy for unresectable hepatocellular carcinoma. *Cancer, 61,* 1983.
168. Janis L, Leming P, Leder W (1988) Nonspecific corticosteroid therapy in patients receiving intraarterial chemotherapy for hepatic metastases of colorectal origin. *Cancer Invest., 6,* 267.
169. Tateyama I, Mori T, Tominaga T et al (1988) Selective intra-arterial administration of high-dose of CDDP in combination with plasmapheresis. *J. Jpn. Soc. Cancer Ther., 23,* 889.
170. Mortimer J, Taylor M, Schulman S et al (1988) Feasibility and efficacy of weekly intraarterial cisplatin in locally advanced (Stage III and IV) head and neck cancers. *J. Clin. Oncol., 6,* 969.
171. Pommier R, Moseley H, Cohen J et al (1988) Pharmacokinetics, toxicity, and short-term results of cisplatin hyperthermic isolated limb perfusion for soft-tissue sarcoma and melanoma of the extremities. *Am. J. Surg., 155,* 667.
172. Fiorentino M, Daniele O, Morandi P et al (1988) Intrapericardial instillation of platin in malignant pericardial effusion. *Cancer, 62,* 1904.
173. Gimeno M, Orgaz R, Menor F et al (1987) Reacciones alergicas en las instilaciones intravesicales de cisplatino. *Actas Urol. Esp., XI,* 461.
174. Iborra Juan I, Monros Lliso J, Ricos Torrent J et al (1988) Estudio comparativo de 62 enfermos tratados aleatoriamente con adriamicina o cisplatino como quimioprofilaxis de su carcinoma vesical superficial. *Actas Urol. Esp., XII,* 20.
175. Asashi K, Toda K, Watanabe Y et al (1988) Intraarterial chemo-embolization with adriamycin containing albumin micro-spheres. *Jpn. J. Cancer Chemother., 15,* 2484.
176. Monk B, Surwit E, Alberts D, Graham V (1988) Intraperitoneal mitomycin C in the treatment of peritoneal carcinomatosis following second-look laparotomy. *Semin. Oncol., 15,* 27.
177. Van Helsdingen P, De Bruyn E (1988) Toxicity, mitomycin C resorption and urinary concentrations using different instillation times in subsequent intravescial instillations for superficial bladder carcinoma. *J. Exp. Clin. Cancer Res., 7,* 49.
178. Van Helsdingen P, Rikken C, Sleeboom H et al (1988) Mitomycin C resorption following repeated intravesical instillations using different instillation times. *Urol. Int., 43,* 42.
179. Blochl-Daum B, Eichler H (1988) Escalating dose regimen of intraperitoneal mitoxantrone: Phase I study—clinical and pharmacokinetic evaluation. *Eur. J. Cancer Clin. Oncol., 24,* 1133.
180. Alberts D, Surwit E, Peng Y et al (1988) Phase I clinical and pharmacokinetic study of mitoxantrone given to patients by intraperitoneal administration. *Cancer Res., 48,* 5874.
181. Kogawa T, Togashi S, Yanagiya H et al (1988) The treatment of renal cell carcinoma with interferon. *J. Jpn. Soc. Cancer Ther., 23,* 649.
182. Nakamoto T, Usui A, Ikemoto H et al (1988) Immunotherapy of renal cell carcinoma 1. Interferon therapy (in Japanese). *Nishinihon J. Urol., 50,* 1169.
183. McLeod G (1988) Alpha-interferons in malignant melanoma. *Br. J. Clin. Pract., Suppl. 62.*
184. Aderka D, Michalevicz R, Daniel Y et al (1988) Recombinant interferon alpha C for advanced hairy cell leukemia. *Cancer, 61,* 2207.
185. Ahre A, Bjorkholm M, Osterborg A et al (1988) High doses of natural α-interferon [a-IFN] in the treatment of multiple myeloma—a pilot study from the Myeloma Group of Central Sweden (MGCS). *Eur. J. Haematol., 41,* 123.
186. Cetto G, Franceschi T, Turrina G et al (1988) Recombinant alpha-interferon and vinblastine in metastatic renal cell carcinoma: efficacy of low doses. *Semin. Surg. Oncol., 4,* 184.

187. Borden E, Hawkins M, Sielaff K et al (1988) Clinical and biological effects of recombinant interferon-β administered intravenously daily in Phase I trial. *J. Interferon Res., 8,* 357.
188. Levens W, Fischer N, Ingehag W, Rubben H (1988) Adverse reactions in long-term interferon treatment. *Semin. Surg. Oncol., 4,* 204.
189. Fentiman I, Balkwill F, Thomas B et al (1988) An autoimmune aetiology for hypothyroidism following interferon therapy for breast cancer. *Eur. J. Cancer Clin. Oncol., 24,* 1299.
190. Perez R, Lipton A, Harvey H et al (1988) A Phase I trial of recombinant human gamma interferon (IFN-γ4A) in patients with advanced malignancy. *J. Biol. Response Modif., 7,* 309.
191. Javadpour N, Lalehzarian M (1988) A Phase I–II study of high-dose recombinant human interleukin-2 in disseminated renal-cell carcinoma. *Semin. Surg. Oncol., 4,* 207.
192. Sondel P, Kohler P, Hank J et al (1988) Clinical and immunological effects of recombinant interleukin-2 given by repetitive weekly cycles to patients with cancer. *Cancer Res., 48,* 2561.
193. Webb D, Austin H, Belldegrun A et al (1988) Metabolic and renal effects of interleukin-2 immunotherapy for metastatic cancer. *Clin. Nephrol., 30,* 141.
194. Steinmetz T, Schaadt M, Gahl R et al (1988) Phase I study of 24-hour continuous intravenous infusion of recombinant human tumour necrosis factor. *J. Biol. Response Modif., 7,* 417.
195. Gonwa T, Poplawski S, Husberg B et al (1988) Cyclosporine nephrotoxicity in orthotopic liver transplantation. *Transplant. Proc., 20,* 401.
196. Dieterle A, Abeywickrama K, Graffenried B (1988) Nephrotoxicity and hypertension in patients with autoimmune disease treated with cyclosporine. *Transplant. Proc., 20,* 349.
197. Mihatsch M, Thiel G, Ryffel B (1988) Histopathology of cyclosporine nephrotoxicity. *Transplant. Proc., 20,* 759.
198. Bennett W, Porter G (1988) Cyclosporine-associated hypertension. *Am. J. Med., 85,* 131.
199. Schachter M (1988) Cyclosporine A and hypertension. *J. Hytertens., 6,* 511.
200. Tatman A, Tucker B, Amess J et al (1988) Erythraemia in renal transplant recipients treated with cyclosporin. *Lancet, 1,* 1279.
201. Teruel J, Marcen R, Pelaez E, Ortuno J (1988) Is there any relationship between azathioprine dosage and erythrocytosis after renal transplantation? *Am. J. Nephrol., 8,* 258.
202. Majer R (1988) Cyclosporine and erythraemia. *Lancet, 2,* 285.
203. Besarab A, Jarrell B, Burke J et al (1988) Erythrocytosis in renal transplantation patients treated with cyclosporine. *Transplant. Proc., 20,* 945.
204. Itami N, Akutsu Y, Yasoshima K (1988) Thrombocytosis after cyclosporin therapy in child with nephrotic syndrome. *Lancet, 2,* 1018.
205. Cadranel J, Grippon P, Mattei M et al (1988) Prevalence and causes of long-lasting hepatic dysfunction after heart transplantation: a series of 80 patients. *Artif. Organs, 12,* 234.
206. Frosch P, Ruder H, Stiefel A et al (1988) Gingivahyperpläsie und Seropapeln unter Cyclosporinbehandlung. *Hautarzt, 39,* 611.
207. Boon A, Adams D, Carey M et al (1988) Cyclosporin-associated cerebral lesions in liver transplantation. *Lancet, 1,* 1457.
208. Valbonesi M, Occhini D, Capra C et al (1988) Plasma exchange for the management of cyclosporin A-induced hypertriglyceridemia. *Int. J. Artif. Organs, 11,* 209.
209. Jerkins G, Noe H, Hill D (1987) Treatment of complications of cyclophosphamide cystitis. *J. Urol., 139,* 923.
210. Berg A, Hahlen K, Colly L (1988) Treatment of childhood acute nonlymphocytic leukemia with high-dose cytosine arabinsode, 6-thioguanine, and doxorubicin without maintenance therapy. *Pediatr. Hematol. Oncol., 5,* 93.
211. Kurrle E, Ehninger G, Freund M et al (1988) A multicentre study on intensive induction and consolidation therapy in acute myelogenous leukaemia. *Blut, 56.* 233.
212. Kantarjian H, Walters R, Keating M et al (1988) Treatment of the blastic phase of chronic myelogenous leukemia with mitoxantrone and high-dose cytosine arabinoside. *Cancer 62,* 672.
213. Walters R, Kantarjian H, Keating M et al (1988) Mitoxantrone and high-dose cytosine arabinoside in refractory acute myelogenous leukemia. *Cancer, 62,* 677.
214. Spriggs D, Robbins G, Arthur K et al (1988) Prolonged high dose ara-C infusions in acute leukemia. *Leukemia, 2,* 304.
215. Guo-cai L, Brock N, Jin-qing L et al (1988) Ifosfamide and mesna in advanced malignancies. *Chin. Med. J., 101,* 213.
216. Cavalli F (1988) Ifosfamide: an old drug recently rediscovered. *Eur. J. Cancer Clin. Oncol., 24,* 959.
217. Powell B, Craig J, Capizzi R, Richards II F (1988) Phase I–II trial of acivicin in adult acute leukemia. *Invest. New Drugs, 6,* 41.
218. Elson P, Kvols L, Vogl S et al (1988) Phase II trials of 5-day vinblastine infusion (NSC 49842), L-alanosine (NSC 153353), acivicin (NSC 163501) and aminothiadiazole (NSC 4728) in patients with recurrent or metastatic renal cell carcinoma. *Invest. New Drugs, 6,* 97.
219. Eastland G (1988) Aminothiadiazole. *Drugs Future, 13,* 711.
220. Martino S, Ratanatharathorn V, Samal BA et al (1988) Treatment of metastatic breast cancer with AZQ: a phase II trial. *Cancer Invest., 6,* 289.

221. Muramatsu T, Miyakawa K, Watanabe S et al (1988) A case of leukoencephalopathy induced by carmofur. *J. Med. Soc. Toho Univ.*, *34*, 67.
222. Hanauske A, Melink T, Harman G et al (1988) Phase I clinical trial of carbetimer. *Cancer Res.*, *48*, 5353.
223. Fromm M, Berde W, Schick H et al (1988) Phase I trial of polyelectrolyte carbetimer administered IV once every four weeks. *Invest. New Drugs*, *6*, 189.
224. Hardy J, Harvey V, Paxton J et al (1988) Phase I trial of the amsacrine analogue 9-({2-methoxy-4-[(methylsulfonyl)amino]-phenyl}amino)-*N*,5-dimethyl-4-acridinecarboxamide (CI-921). *Cancer Res.*, *48*, 6593.
225. Weiner L, Moldofsky P, Gatenby R et al (1988) Antibody delivery and effector cell activation in a Phase II trial of recombinant α-Interferon and the murine monoclonal antibody CO17-1 in advanced colorectal carcinoma. *Cancer Res.*, *48*, 2568.
226. Kris M, Kinahan J, Gralla R et al (1988) Phase I trial and clinical pharmacological evaluation of 10-ethyl-10-deazaaminopterin in adult patients with advanced cancer. *Cancer Res.*, *48*, 5573.
227. Piot G, Droz JP, Theodore C et al (1988) Phase II trial with high-dose elliptinium acetate in metastatic renal cell carcinoma. *Oncology*, *45*, 371.
228. Weiss R, Greene R, Knight R et al (1988) Phase I and clinical pharmacology study of intravenous flavone acetic acid (NSC 347512). *Cancer Res.*, *48*, 5878.
229. Leiby JM, Grever MR, Staubus AE et al (1988) Phase I clinical investigation of fludarabine phosphate by a loading-dose and continuous-infusion schedule. *J. Natl. Cancer Inst.*, *80*, 447.
230. Changliang H, Mingliang D, Renjie G et al (1988) A study on the induction of differentiation of leukemic cells by harringtonine combined with cytarabine. *Leukemia*, *2*, 518.
231. Jing-song Y, Xiao-hong W, Guang-hui F et al (1988) Small-dose harringtonine induces complete remission in patients with acute promyelocytic leukemia. *Leukemia*, *2*, 427.
232. Lippman S, Kessler J, Al-Sarraf M et al (1988) Treatment of advanced squamous cell carcinoma of the head and neck with isotretinoin: a Phase II randomized trial. *Invest. New Drugs*, *6*, 51.
233. Smith D, Lind M, Kaye S et al (1988) A negative Phase II trial of methylene dimethane sulphonate in advanced ovarian cancer (Cancer Research Campaign Phase I/II Trials Committee). *Br. J. Cancer*, *57*, 512.
234. Coleman CN, Carlson RW, Halsey J et al (1988) Enhancement of the clinical activity of melphalan by the hypoxic cell sensitizer misonidazole. *Cancer Res.*, *48*, 3528.
235. Speth PAJ, Gore ME, Pateman AJ et al (1988) Phase I and pharmacokinetic studies with the pentacylic pyrroloquinone mitoquidone. *Cancer Chemother. Pharmacol.*, *21*, 343.
236. Tsubara E, Nomura T, Niitani H et al (1988) Restorative activity of muroctasin leukopenia associated with anticancer treatment. *Arzneim.-Forsch./Drug Res.*, *38*, 1070.
237. Pazdur R, Samson MK, Baker L (1988) PCNU: Phase II evaluation in advanced colorectal carcinoma. *Invest. New Drugs*, *6*, 93.
238. Shepard K, Larson R, Le Beau M et al (1988) Acute leukemia occurring after radiotherapy and chemotherapy with a nitrosurea, PCNU. *Invest. New Drugs*, *6*, 121
239. Ohno R, Kimura K (1988) Treatment of myelodysplastic syndromes (MDS) with orally administrable N^4-palmitoyl-1-beta-D-arabinofuranosyl cytosine (PLAC). *Jpn. J. Cancer Chemother.*, *15*, 1205.
240. Pandya KJ, Kramar A, Asbury RF, Haller DG (1988) A Phase II study of spirogermanium in advanced large bowel cancer. *Am. J. Clin. Oncol.*, *11*, 496.
241. Bertino JR (1988) Trimetrexate: overall clinical results. *Semin. Oncol.*, *15*, 50.
242. Maroun JA, Natale RB, Robert F (1988) Trimetrexate combined with cisplatin or etoposide in the treatment of non small cell lung cancer: a pilot study. *Semin. Oncol.*, *2*, 38.
243. Hudes GR, Cornis RL (1988) Phase 1 and 2 studies of trimetrexate administered in combination with fluorouracil to patients with metastatic cancer. *Semin. Oncol.*, *15*, 41.
244. Stewart JA, McCormack JJ, Tong W et al (1988) Phase I clinical pharmacokinetic study of trimetrexate using a daily ×5 schedule. *Cancer Res.*, *48*, 5029.
245. Stewart JA (1988) Safety and tolerance of trimetrexate: results of a Phase II multicenter study in patients with metastatic cancer refractory to conventional therapy or for which no conventional therapy exists. *Semin. Oncol.*, *15*, 10.
246. Leiby JM (1988) Trimetrexate: a Phase 2 study in previously treated patients with metastatic breast cancer. *Semin. Oncol.*, *15*, 27.
247. Mattson K, Maasilta P, Tammilehto L et al (1988) Trimetrexate and cyclophosphamide for metastatic inoperable nonsmall cell lung cancer. *Semin. Oncol.*, *15*, 32.
248. Ota K, Taguchi T, Kimura K (1988) Report on nationwide pooled data and cohort investigation in UFT phase II study. *Can. Chemother. Pharmacol.*, *22*, 333.
249. Mukai H, Sugihara K, Kawashima K et al (1988) Effect of tegafur on oral squamous cell carcinoma (in Japanese). *Oral Ther. Pharmacol.*, *7*, 117.
250. Landys K (1988) Mitoxantrone in combination with prednimustine in treatment of unfavour-

able non-Hodgkin lymphoma. *Invest. New Drugs, 6,* 105.

251. Gale RP, Foon KA (1988) Daunorubicin or doxorubicin in acute myelogenous leukemia? *Leukemia, 2,* 209.

252. Sessa C, Gundersen S, Huinink WB, Cavalli F (1988) Phase II study of intravenous menogaril in patients with advanced breast cancer. *J. Natl. Cancer Inst, 80,* 1066.

253. Bennett W, Elzinga L, Kelley V (1988) Pathophysiology of cyclosporine nephrotoxicity: role of eicosanoids. *Transplant. Proc., 20,,* 628.

G. Ansell

48 Radiological contrast media and radiopharmaceuticals

MEDIA FOR EXAMINATION OF THE ALIMENTARY TRACT *(SED-11, 961; SEDA-12, 394; SEDA-13, 433)*

Barium sulfate *(SED-11, 961; SEDA-12, 394; SEDA-13, 433)*

Allergy It is now recognized that allergic reactions may rarely occur as a result of barium sulfate examinations (SEDA-4, 333; SEDA-6, 804; SEDA-10, 422; SEDA-12, 394). A *fatal reaction* has now been reported in a 49-year-old woman with a history of allergy who was receiving medication for asthma. During a single contrast barium enema with Sal-o-pake, the patient complained of warmth and itching. She then became intensely dyspneic and collapsed. Intravenous adrenaline was given and cardiopulmonary resuscitation performed, but this was unsuccessful. Autopsy showed severe mucous plugging of the bronchi (1^{CR}).

Barium aspiration Accidental inhalation of small quantities of barium usually causes few sequelae but several deaths have been noted in elderly patients with swallowing difficulties. Moreover, barium aspiration appears to have become more common with the high-density barium preparations used for double contrast examinations, whilst swallowing difficulties may be exacerbated by the effervescent mixtures or by anticholinergic drugs which may interfere with esophageal motility (2^{CR}). Two further cases have now been reported in debilitated elderly patients with disordered swallowing a few hours after aspirating high-density barium (E-Z HD). Autopsy showed an acute inflammatory reaction in the lungs around the aspirated barium. It is suggested that the high-density barium preparation may increase the severity of the pulmonary reaction. In patients where there might be a risk of aspiration, it is recommended that a preliminary swallow using a small quantity of a low-osmolar water-soluble medium should first be administered to ensure normal swallowing before administering high-density barium (3^{CR}).

Barium appendicitis Two additional cases of acute appendicitis have been reported following prolonged stasis of barium in the appendix (SED-11, 962; 4^{Cr}).

Perforation of colon Barium impaction in the colon is not uncommon following barium examinations (SED-11, 962). In a recent case, perforation of the sigmoid colon occurred in a 72-year-old woman at the site of an impacted barium fecolith, 10 days after a barium meal. It may be relevant that the patient was being treated with the NSAID nabumetone for osteoarthritis (5^{Cr}).

Water-soluble contrast media *(SED-11, 962; SEDA-12, 394)*

Sodium diatrizoate In a series of 7 patients with cystic fibrosis, treatment of meconium ileus equivalent with oral acetylcysteine and diatrizoate together with Gastrografin enemas resulted in acute *hypomagnesemia*, but no patient had frank tetany. It is suggested that the plasma magnesium should be monitored during treatment (6^{CR}). In rats with experimentally induced intestinal ischemia, administration of diatrizoate via a gastric tube significantly reduced the survival time of the animals. In rats given barium sulfate or the low-osmolar medium iohexol, survival time did not differ significantly from the controls. It is suggested that the effect of diatrizoate is due to the hyperos-

Side Effects of Drugs Annual 14
M.N.G. Dukes and L. Beeley, editors

molarity causing a fluid shift with distention of the bowel predisposing to a more rapid spread of bacteria through the distended bowel wall with ensuing septicemia. Dehydration may also be relevant (7[R]).

Endoscopic retrograde cholangio-pancreatography (ERCP) *(SED-11, 965; SEDA-12, 394)* Rambo et al (8[c], 9[CR]) noted higher levels of amylase and gamma-GT using meglumine ioxaglate for ERCP as compared with the lower-viscosity ionic medium meglumine ioglicate or the non-ionic medium iopromide. On the other hand, in another study, the non-ionic medium iopamidol caused significantly less hyperamylasemia and hyperlipidemia than meglumine diatrizoate despite the higher viscosity of the former medium (10[CR]).

EXCRETION UROGRAPHY AND COMPUTED TOMOGRAPHY *(SED-11, 965)*

Idiosyncratic reactions It is now generally accepted that non-ionic media produce significantly fewer mild and moderate adverse reactions than ionic media (SEDA-11, 410; SEDA-12, 411; SEDA-13, 431). Preliminary results have now been reported of a large non-randomized survey of ionic and non-ionic contrast media performed in Japan during 1987–1988 (11[C]). Ionic media were administered in 169 284 cases and non-ionic media in 168 363 cases. The combined incidence of 'severe' and 'very severe' reactions was approximately 0.25% with ionic media and 0.04% with non-ionic media, a ratio of approximately 6. It is possible that the grading of 'severe reactions' in this study may include some cases which might have been regarded as 'moderate' reactions in other studies. One *death* occurred in each group but these were considered to be non-attributable to contrast media. This appears to be an unusually low mortality rate, particularly for ionic media. Patients with asthma had a higher incidence of severe and very severe reactions viz., 1.88% with ionic media and 0.23% with non-ionic media. Other predisposing factors included atopy (0.49% and 0.11% respectively), and heart disease (0.53% and 0.1% respectively). Bolus injections and, to a lesser extent, drip infusions increased the incidence of severe and very severe reactions by a factor of approximately 1.5 with ionic media. This was less apparent with non-ionic media. In an Australian survey of 106 211 cases, non-ionic media caused a significantly lower incidence of 'moderate' and 'severe' reactions than did ionic media. This effect was evident in both 'high risk' and 'low risk' patients (12[Cr]). In a double blind trial in 1000 patients, the incidence of mild to moderate reactions was 7.7% with the non-ionic medium iohexol and 31.2% with the ionic medium metrizoate. The quality of urograms was significantly better with iohexol (13[CR]).

It is of interest that in 694 patients receiving the non-ionic medium iopamidol for urography, reports of delayed skin rashes, occurring during the following week, were received in 5.5% of patients, whereas in 687 patients receiving sodium iothalamate the figure was 2.9%. There was also a trend to a higher incidence of delayed parotid swelling with iopamidol (1.7%) as compared with sodium iothalamate (0.87%) (14[CR]).

A fatal case of *Stevens-Johnson syndrome* resulted from urography with iopamidol in a patient with systemic lupus erythematosus (SLE). At least 1 and possibly 2 reactions have previously been noted following the use of non-ionic media in SLE (SEDA-9, 411; SEDA-11, 411) and caution is advised in these cases (15[CR]). A fatal case of *toxic epidermal necrolysis* occurred following urography with diatrizoate. The patient had also had a CT scan using diatrizoate 7 weeks earlier and a possible immunological mechanism is questioned (16[Cr]).

Air embolism In 100 patients undergoing routine CT with intravenous injection of contrast media, the scan of the thorax showed evidence of venous air embolism in 23% of patients. In 20 patients, the volume of air was minimal, but in 3 patients there was a moderate amount of air. Air was visualized in the main pulmonary artery in 12 patients. There were no accompanying clinical symptoms, but caution is advised in administering intravenous fluids to patients with suspected right-to-left shunts (17[Cr]). Larger amounts of venous air embolism have been noted by CT in 5 cases over a 2-year period following pressurized injections of contrast medium (18[CR]).

ANGIOGRAPHY AND CARDIOGRAPHY (*SED-11, 970; SEDA-12,395; SEDA-13, 434*)

Pulmonary hypertension may be a serious complication of pulmonary angiography (SED-11, 970; SEDA-9, 410). In a series of 17 patients with normal pulmonary artery pressures undergoing pulmonary angiography, the effects of iohexol and diatrizoate were compared in a double-blind cross-over study. Increase in pulmonary artery pressure after iohexol was significantly less than that produced by diatrizoate and iohexol appears to be the safer medium for pulmonary angiography (19[CR]).

In a series of 82 patients with suspected coronary artery disease undergoing left ventriculography, a randomized study comparing iohexol, metrizamide and metrizoate showed that the non-ionic media iohexol and metrizamide produced markedly less hemodynamic and electrocardiographic disturbances than the ionic medium metrizoate. Subjective symptoms were also more marked with metrizoate (20[CR]).

Thromboembolic phenomena Whereas ionic contrast media have an anticoagulant action, this effect is less marked with non-ionic media and this has been suggested as a possible risk factor for thromboembolic phenomena (SEDA-10, 420, SEDA-12, 395). In a series of 1380 patients undergoing coronary angiography with iopamidol, thromboembolic complications occurred in 3 patients whereas no thromboembolic complications had been noted in some 6800 examinations performed using high-osmolality contrast media. Although the 3 patients had been heparinized, it was believed that the level of heparinization may have been suboptimal. The major factor, however, appeared to be due to withdrawal of blood into the injection syringe containing contrast medium where stasis may allow the formation of a thrombus. Withdrawal of blood should therefore be avoided and a meticulous technique is imperative combined with adequate systemic heparinization (21[CR]); risks of stasis were examined in an experimental study mimicking poor technique where 1 ml of blood was added to 9 ml of iohexol in polypropylene and styrene acrylonitrile syringes and allowed to stand for 10 minutes. Red cell aggregation occurred but was easily dispersed and was not considered to be significant. Thrombi formed in 2 cases, both being in styrene acrylonitrile syringes (22[cR]).

Transitory cortical blindness occurred in a patient following left intercostal angiography to visualize a coronary artery graft. During this procedure, contrast medium may enter the left vertebral artery. Cortical blindness is a rare complication and usually resolves spontaneously (23[CR]).

Disruption of an atheromatous plaque during angiography may cause multiple embolization of cholesterol fragments giving rise to *livedo reticularis*, multiple organ infarction hypertension and renal failure. The prognosis is poor. Palmer and Warren report 5 fatal and 2 non-fatal cases together with a review of 12 cases in the literature. They suggest that the complication may occur more frequently than the literature indicates (24[CR]).

Peripheral arteriography

In 126 patients undergoing angiography for peripheral vascular disease, the incidence of *pain* was compared in a randomized double-blind trial of 3 contrast media. Meglumine sodium diatrizoate with added lignocaine caused the most pain: Iohexol was considerably less painful but meglumine sodium ioxaglate caused the least pain (25[CR]).

Nephrotoxicity In a large series of higher-risk patients and procedures, using conventional ionic contrast media treatment with furosemide, diabetes and atopy appeared to be significant *risk factors* for nephrotoxicity. Diabetes also appeared to be a significant risk factor for moderate and severe general adverse reactions to contrast media (26[CR]).

High-dose urography in 20 patients with chronic renal failure caused worsening of renal function in 11 patients. In a subsequent series of 12 patients who received an infusion of 1 liter of normal saline in the 8 hours preceding urography and another liter in the 8 hours following urography, there was only a mild reversible deterioration of renal function in 1 patient. There was, however, temporary increase in blood pressure and weight of the patients (27[CR]). The effect of the large fluid intake on the quality of the urogram is not mentioned. In any case, urography is now less frequently used in the presence of renal failure.

The non-ionic contrast media iopamidol and iohexol are believed to be less nephrotoxic than conventional contrast media but several cases of nephrotoxicity have been described with these newer media (SEDA-13, 434). Two further cases of renal failure are reported after cardioangiography with iopamidol in patients with congestive cardiac failure (28[CR]).

Tissue toxicity A case of *priapism* occurred following cavernography with ioxaglate and diluted iothalamate. There was thrombosis of the draining veins and secondary fibrosis of the corpora cavernosa (29[C]).

MYELOGRAPHY *(SED-11, 974; SEDA-12, 396; SEDA-13, 436)*

Iofendylate

Convulsive seizures have been reported as a late complication in a 46-year-old woman 10–15 years after 4 lumbar myelograms with iofendylate. CT showed residual iofendylate in the right sylvian fissure and this corresponded to the site of focal epileptogenic abnormalities on electroencephalography (30[CR]).

Water-soluble contrast media *(SED-11, 976)*

In a double-blind randomized study of 60 patients comparing iohexol and metrizamide (180 mg I/ml) for lumbothoracic myelography, iohexol produced significantly fewer and less severe EEG changes than metrizamide. There was EEG evidence of epileptic activity in 5 patients receiving metrizamide, but no epileptic activity was detected following iohexol. There were no manifest seizures in either group. Iohexol caused significantly fewer and less severe effects than metrizamide (31[CR]).

An additional case of absence status epilepticus with confusion and disorientation has been reported after metrizamide myelography. CT showed dense accumulation of metrizamide in the cortical grey matter of the brain and EEG showed continuous high amplitude sharp and slow wave complexes. There was complete clinical recovery two minutes after intravenous injection of 10 mg diazepam with relative normalization of the EEG (32[CR]) (see also SEDA-11, 415).

In a series of 634 pediatric patients undergoing myelography with iohexol, the overall incidence of adverse reactions was 18.2%. In 6 patients with tumors (3% of tumor patients) there was an increase in focal neurological signs due to mechanical factors. Whenever possible, patients with a suspected intraspinal mass should be investigated by magnetic resonance scanning in preference to myelography (33[CR]). In a patient with multiple intraspinal neurofibromas, accidental injection of iopamidol into the spinal cord caused fatal hemorrhagic necrosis of the grey matter (34[CR]), but accidental injection of iohexol into the cervical cord in 2 patients caused no permanent sequelae (35[CR]). In 2 patients with arteriovenous fistulae of the spinal dura, myelography with metrizamide caused deterioration of the neurological findings (36[CR]).

Lymphography *(SED-11, 979)*

An additional case of cerebral lipid embolism following lymphography has recently been reported (37[Cr]).

RADIOPHARMACEUTICALS *(SED-11, 981; SEDA-12, 397) (for radioactive iodine, see Chapter 43)*

Lung scanning *(SED-11, 981)* A few cases of cardiovascular collapse and death have formerly occurred after injection of radioactive macroaggregated albumin particles (MAA) for lung perfusion scanning in patients with advanced pulmonary disease. These all occurred prior to 1975. The doses of MAA used were all in excess of current recommended doses and quality control has been improved. A recent study in 12 patients confirms that lung scanning with MAA does not significantly impair lung function as measured by carbon monoxide diffusion (38[CR]).

Cardiac imaging Intravenous thallium-201 perfusion imaging is widely used to evaluate regional coronary blood flow in patients with suspected coronary heart disease and may be combined with oral dipyridamole to produce coronary vasodilatation. During this procedure, cardiac arrest occurred in a 75-year-old patient with unstable angina. Following resuscitation there was evidence of myocardial infarction. It was suggested that vasodilatation by dipyridamole may produce a 'coronary steal' effect. Careful clinical and ECG monitoring is essential during the procedure and unstable angina should be considered as a relative contraindication (39[CR]).

Bone scanning An acute severe episode of vasculitis and erythema multiforme developed 12–24 hours after administration of labelled sodium diphosphonate in a patient with psoriatic arthritis. The condition worsened for the next 7 days. There was a slow response to topical corticosteroid, treatment being required for 4 weeks. The radiopharmaceutical contained only 0.5 mg diphosphonate as compared with doses of 15–30 mg administered by intravenous infusion for the treatment of Paget's disease. The authors suggest that skin testing for sensitivity should be considered prior to therapeutic use of disphosphonate (40[Cr]).

THORIUM DIOXIDE SOL (THOROTRAST) *(SED-11, 980; SEDA-13, 437)*

Further reports of late complications following Thorotrast administration include a Japanese clinico-pathological study of 10 patients with leukemia and 4 patients with aplastic anemia. The latent period in these cases varied from 20–44 years. Survival time after onset of hematological symptoms was short (2–8 months) (41[CR]). A case of *gliosarcoma* of the brain is reported 30–35 years after Thorotrast administration (42[CR]).

Extravasation of Thorotrast used for myelography 15 years earlier resulted in a *thorotrastoma* of the mesentery (43[Cr]). It is surprising to find that Thorotrast was still being used for myelography as late as 1973.

MISCELLANEOUS

Treatment of reactions to radiographic contrast media has recently been reviewed in depth (44[CR]).

REFERENCES

1. Feczo PF, Simms SH, Bakiri N (1989) Fatal hypersensitivity reaction during a barium enema. *Am. J. Roentgenol., 153*, 275.
2. Ansell G, Wilkins RA (1987) *Complications in Diagnostic Imaging, 2nd ed.*, p. 218. Blackwell, Oxford.
3. Gray C, Sivaloganathan S, Simkins KC (1989) Aspiration of high-density barium contrast medium causing acute pulmonary inflammation – report of two fatal cases in elderly women with disordered swallowing. *Clin. Radiol., 40*, 397.
4. Palder SB, Dalessandri KM (1988) Barium appendicitis. *West. J. Med., 148*, 462.
5. Walker AJ (1989) Case report: Perforation of the colon after barium meal examination. *Clin. Radiol., 40*, 530.
6. Godson C, Ryan MP, Brady HR et al (1988) Acute hypomagnesaemia complicating the treatment of meconium ileus equivalent in cystic fibrosis. *Scand. J. Gastroenterol., 23* (Suppl. 143), 148.
7. Stordahl A, Haider T, Laerum M (1989) Acute lethality after enteral administration of contrast media in anaesthetized rats with intestinal ischaemia. *Acta Radiol., 30, Fasc. 2*, 213.
8. Rambo A, Staritz M (1988) Contrast media for ERCP. *Endoscopy, 20*, 126.
9. Rambo A, Staritz M, Manns M et al (1988) ERCP: Welches Kontrastmittel ist geeignet? *Z. Gastroenterol., 26*, 279.
10. O'Connor HJ, Ellis WR, Manning AP et al (1988) Iopamidol as contrast medium in endoscopic retrograde pancreatography: prospective randomised comparison with diatrizoate. *Endoscopy, 20*, 244.
11. Katayama H (1988) Report of the Japanese Committee on the Safety of Contrast Media. A Scientific Poster Session presented at the Radiological Society of North America Meeting, November 1988.
12. Palmer FJ (1989) The Royal Australasian College of Radiologists (RACR) Survey of reactions of intravenous ionic and non-ionic contrast media. In: Enge I, Edgren J (Eds.), *Patient Safety and Adverse Events in Contrast Medium Examination*, p. 137. International Congress Series 816, Excerpta Medica, Amsterdam.
13. Jacobson BF, Jorulf H, Kalantar MS, Narasimhan DL (1988) Non-ionic versus ionic contrast media in intravenous urography: clinical trial in 1000 consecutive patients. *Radiology, 167*, 601.
14. McCullough M, Davies P, Richardson R (1989) A large trial of intravenous Conray 325 and Niopam 300 to assess immediate and delayed reactions. *Br. J. Radiol., 62*, 260.

15. Savill JS, Barrie R, Ghosh S et al (1988) Fatal Stevens-Johnson syndrome following urography with iopamidol in systemic lupus erythematosus. *Postgrad. Med. J., 64*, 392.
16. Kaftori JK, Abraham Z, Gilhar A (1988) Toxic epidermal necrolysis after excretory pyelography. Immunologic-mediated contrast medium reaction? *Int. J. Dermatol., 27*, 346.
17. Woodring JH, Fried AM (1988) Nonfatal venour air embolism after contrast-enhanced CT. *Radiology, 167*, 405.
18. Price DB, Nardi P, Teicher J (1987) Venous air embolism as a complication of pressure injection of contrast media: CT findings. *J. Comput. Assisted Tomography, 11*, 294.
19. Tajima H, Kumazaki T, Tajima N, Ebata K (1988) Effect of iohexol and diatrizoate on pulmonary arterial pressure following pulmonary angiography. A clinical comparison in man. *Acta Radiol., 29*, 487.
20. Vik-Mo H, Rosland GA, Følling M, Danielsen R (1988) Hemodynamic and electrocardiographic consequences of high and low osmolality contrast agents for left ventricular angiography. *Catheter. Cardiovasc. Diagn., 14*, 143.
21. Grollman JH, Liu CK, Astone RA, Lurie MD (1988) Thromboembolic complications in coronary angiography associated with the use of non-ionic contrast medium. *Catheter. Cardiovasc. Diagn., 14*, 159.
22. Dawson P, McCarthy P, Allison DJ (1988) Non-ionic contrast agents, red cell aggregation and coagulation. *Br. J. Radiol., 61*, 963.
23. Henziova MJ, Coghlan HC, Dean LS, Taylor JL (1988) Cortical blindness after left internal mammary artery to left arterial descending coronary artery graft angiography. *Catheter. Cardiovasc. Diagn., 15*, 37.
24. Palmer FJ, Warren BA (1988) Multiple cholesterol emboli syndrome complicating angiographic techniques. *Clin. Radiol., 39*, 519.
25. Murphy G, Campbell DR, Fraser DB (1988) Pain in peripheral arteriography: an assessment of conventional versus ionic and non-ionic low osmolality contrast agents. *J. Can. Assoc. Radiol., 39*, 103.
26. Moore RD, Steinberg EP, Powe NR et al (1989) Frequency and determinants of adverse reactions induced by high-osmolality contrast media. *Radiology, 170*, 727.
27. Teruel JL, Llorente MT, Herrero JA et al (1988) Presentation de la nefrotoxicidad per constrastes yodados en pacientes con insufficiencia renal. *Med. Clín. (Barc.), 91*, 281.
28. Elliot C, Reger M (1988) Acute renal failure following low osmolality radiocontract dye. *Clin. Cardiol., 11*, 420.
29. Sellam R, Economou C, Amer M et al (1988) Priapisme après cavernographie. Rapport d'un cas original. *Ann. Urol., 22*, 145.
30. Pascuzzi RM, Roos KL, Scott JA (1988) Chronic focal seizure disorders as a manifestation of intracranial iophendylate. *Epilepsia, 29*, 294.
31. Maly P, Bach-Gansmo T, Elmquist D (1988) Risk of seizures after myelography: comparison of iohexol and metrizamide. *Am. J. Neuroradiology, 9*, 879.
32. Obeid T, Yaqub B, Panayiotopoulos C et al (1988) Absence status epilepticus with computed tomographic brain changes following metrizamide myelography. *Ann. Neurol., 24*, 582.
33. Kendall B (1989) Safety aspects and tolerability of non-ionic contrast media – subarachnoid disease. In: Enge I, Edgren J (Eds.), *Patient Safety and Adverse Events in Contrast Medium Examination*, p. 47. International Congress Series 816, Excerpta Medica, Amsterdam.
34. Roos RAC, Voormolen JHC, Vielvoye GJ et al. (1988) Haemorrhagic necrosis of the grey matter of the spinal cord due to accidental injection of iopamidol in a patient with multiple neurofibromas: a clinico-pathological study. *Neuroradiology, 30*, 178.
35. Skalpe IO, Nakstad P (1988) Myelography with iohexol: a clinical report with special reference to adverse effects. *Neuroradiology, 30*, 169.
36. Roullet E, Netter JM, Chiras J et al (1988) Fistules artéroveineuses durales rachidiennes; aggravations après myélographie au métrizamide. *Rev. Neurol. (Paris), 144*, 371.
37. Marsepoil T, Levesque P, Bertaux P et al (1988) Complications neurologiques de la lymphographie. A propos d'un cas. *Rev. Méd. Interne, 9*, 191.
38. Morris TA, Thompson RT, Quinn DA et al (1988) Diffusing capacity is not measurably affected by routine lung perfusion scanning. *J. Nucl. Med., 29*, 1268.
39. Blumenthal MS, McCauley CS (1988) Cardiac arrest during dipyridamole imaging. *Chest, 93*, 1103.
40. Elliott AT, Murray T, Mackie RM, Hunter JA (1988) Severe reaction to diphosphonate: Implications for treatment of Paget's disease. *Br. Med. J., 297*, 592.
41. Kamiyama R, Ishikawa Y, Hatakeyama S et al (1988) Clinico-pathological study of hematological disorders after Thorotrast administration in Japan. *Blut, 56*, 153.
42. Wargotz ES, Sidaway MK, Jannotta FS (1988) Thorotrast-associated gliosarcoma including comments on Thorotrast use and review of sequelae with particular reference to lesions of the central nervous system. *Cancer, 62*, 58.
43. Ponzio F, Nessi F, Gaia S, De Giorgis C (1988) Su un caso di thorotrastoma del mesentere. *Minerva Chir., 43*, 1195.
44. Cohan RH, Dunnick NR, Bashore TM (1988) Treatment of reactions to radiographic contrast material. *Am. J. Roentgenol., 151*, 263.

B.C.P. Polak

49 Drugs used in ocular treatment

DIAGNOSTIC OPHTHALMIC DRUGS *(SED-11, 988)*

Phenylephrine *(SED-11, 989; SEDA-13, 439)*

Phenylephrine hydrochloride is an α-adrenergic drug which is used as mydriatic agent in 10% and 2.5% solutions; in lower concentrations it is present as a decongestant and vasoconstrictor in many ocular preparations. Local and systemic side effects from topically applied phenylephrine have been reported. They include subjective burning or stinging with lacrimation, rebound hyperemia and liberation of iris pigment into the anterior chamber. Tachycardia and elevation of systemic blood pressure were also reported.

Recently, several cases of *allergic blepharoconjunctivitis* due to phenylephrine eye drops have been reported. The reaction begins 3–4 hours after drug application, persists for 12 hours and regresses gradually within 72 hours. Conjunctival biopsy of the inflamed eyes reveals marked infiltration by lymphocytes, plasma cells and eosinophils, without predominance of any of these cells. There is clinical evidence that a sensitization mechanism is involved, but immunological studies are needed to elucidate the mechanism of this inflammation (1^C, 2^c, 3^c). The clinical picture occurs with a phenylephrine concentration as low as 0.1%; this fact is of clinical importance, since weak concentrations of phenylephrine are used in many ubiquitous ophthalmic preparations.

Side Effects of Drugs Annual 14
M.N.G. Dukes and L. Beeley, editors

THERAPEUTIC OPHTHALMIC DRUGS *(SED-11, 991)*

Timolol (Timoptol, Timoptic) *(SED-11, 992; SEDA-12, 401; SEDA-13, 440)*

Manifestations of beta-blocker-induced arthralgia range from a multisystem immunologic syndrome to less serious, isolated arthropathies (SED-11, 366). Recently a case of topical timolol-induced *arthropathy* has been reported. Because significant blood levels of beta-blockers can be achieved by topical administration, physicians should be aware of possible joint-related problems when topical beta-blocker therapy is used for the treatment of glaucoma.

A 61-year-old woman had been taking timolol 0.25% twice daily in both eyes for presumed ocular hypertension. Her systemic history included recent onset of mild arthralgias in both knees for which she took naproxen. When the optic nerve heads showed glaucomatous changes the concentration of timolol was increased to 0.5%. Several months later the patient complained of sharp, constant pains in her knees. There were no other arthritic complaints. She was taught nasolacrimal occlusion after instillation, and continued taking timolol. One month later the knee pain had decreased, but she was still uncomfortable. Her orthopedic surgeon considered bilateral knee surgery. Timolol was discontinued and the patient was treated with dipivefrine. Her intraocular pressure remained controlled. Over the next month her knee pains resolved completely, she discontinued using the knee braces and she walked without a handicap. There has been no recurrence of joint pains of any sort over the subsequent 14 months (4^c).

Preservatives used in eye drops and contact lens solutions *(SED-11, 996)*

Preservatives and local anesthetics are known to exert toxic side effects on the corneal epithelium such as disruption of cell membranes and increased permeability. The function of the corneal epithelium can be quantified by fluorophotometric determination of corneal epithelial permeability to fluorescein.

The effect of the preservatives chlorhexidine and benzalkonium chloride and the local anesthetics oxybuprocaine and tetracaine on corneal epithelial permeability was studied by fluorophotometry in normal human eyes. Five instillations of 1 drop ophthalmic solution of the compounds were administered to 1 eye at 2-minute intervals; a control solution was instilled into the fellow eye. The increase in corneal epithelial permeability expressed as the permeability ratio between the treated and the control eye was not significant after instillation of the anesthetics. The preservatives and the combination oxybuprocaine + chlorhexidine increased corneal epithelial permeability significantly. Oxybuprocaine + benzalkonium chloride and tetracaine + benzalkonium chloride increased permeability to a far greater extent (5^c).

A recent report provides a reminder of the seriousness of the problems to which benzalkonium chloride can give rise:

A 56-year-old man was seen with keratoconjunctivitis sicca and marked ocular surface disease in whom the prolonged frequent use of topical medications containing the preservative benzalkonium chloride was associated with corneal endothelial damage requiring corneal transplantation in 1 eye. The histopathological findings on examination of the excised button were consistent with toxic endothelial disease. Postoperatively the patient's symptoms continued until the preservative-containing medications were substituted with non-preserved saline eye drops (6^c).

These findings point to the potential danger of prolonged use of topical medications containing benzalkonium chloride as a preservative in the presence of extensive disruption of the corneal epithelium. The availability of non-preserved saline eye drops in unit dose dispensers should reduce the incidence of this type of complication. Caution is urged in the use of preservative-containing topical medications over an extended period in patients with extensive ocular surface disease.

REFERENCES

1. Geyer O, Yust I, Lazar M (1988) Allergic blepharoconjunctivitis due to phenylephrine. *J. Ocul. Pharmacol., 4*, 123.
2. Milpied B, Fleischmann M, Berre F et al (1988) Another case of allergic contact dermatitis from phenylephrine in eyedrops. *Contact Derm., 19*, 146.
3. Mancuso G, Errani A, Staffa M et al (1988) Dermatite allergica da contatto con fenilefrina. *Chron. Derm., 19*, 209.
4. Lustgarten JS (1988) Topical timolol-induced arthropathy. *Am. J. Ophthalmol., 105*, 687.
5. Ramselaar JAM, Boot JP, Van Haeringen NJ et al (1988) Corneal epithelial permeability after instillation of ophthalmic solutions containing local anaesthetics and preservatives. *Curr. Eye Res., 7*, 947.
6. Lemp MA, Zimmerman LE (1988) Toxic endothelial degeneration in ocular surface disease treated with topical medications containing benzalkonium chloride. *Am. J. Ophthalmol., 105*, 670.

P.A.G.M. de Smet

50 Drugs used in non-orthodox medicine

Ethnopharmacological perspectives

*A few years ago, the **Journal of Ethnopharmacology** invited scientists to respond if they were interested in the formation of an International Society for Ethnopharmacology (SEDA-12, 402). The actual creation of this Society has now been planned to take place during the First International Congress on Ethnopharmacology, which will be held in 1990 in Strasbourg, France.*

The aim of ethnopharmacology is to obtain and maintain a broad multidisciplinary perspective on the human use of crude drugs and poisons in a traditional context. It is often believed that this approach has nothing to offer but the recording and evaluation of outdated exotica, which cannot possibly have relevance for Western medicine. Admittedly, studies of traditional medicines do not often result in the addition of new valuable agents to our sophisticated drug armamentarium. This does not alter the fact, however, that ethnopharmacology can contribute to Western medicine in several ways. In one direction, it may help to provide a scientific view at the current public interest in traditional crude remedies. In another direction, it may serve as a powerful tool for drug development by leading to the discovery of pharmacologically active compounds. These principles can be useful as leads in drug design or as pharmacological tools by providing novel structures with interesting biological properties. And some of the compounds may even reach the therapeutic stage in their original non-synthetic form (1^R).

*A fascinating example of the potential relevancy of ethnopharmacology for Western medicine are the recent studies on **Phyllanthus amarus** (2^C–5^C).*

*__Phyllanthus__ species have been employed in such geographically remote areas as Asia, Africa and Latin America for the treatment of jaundice and other diseases. They have been used in traditional Indian medicine for more than 2000 years. This aroused the interest of Indian and American researchers in the therapeutic potential of **Phyllanthus amarus**, which is known in India as **Phyllanthus niruri**. In vitro experiments demonstrated that **Phyllanthus** extracts can inhibit the reaction between HBsAg (the surface antigen of HBV virus) and its corresponding antibody, and that these extracts can also inhibit the endogenous DNA polymerases, which are required for the replication of HBV virus and the woodchuck hepatitis virus. Moreover, in vivo studies in the woodchuck (**Marmota monax**) showed that carriers of the woodchuck hepatitis virus treated with **Phyllanthus** extracts were more likely to lose their carrier state than placebo-treated animals (2^C, 3^C).*

*To investigate whether such an abolishing effect could also be obtained in man, Thyagarajan et al (4^C) performed a randomized double-blind trial in 78 human subjects who had been carriers of HBV virus for at least half a year. Active treatment consisted of capsules containing 200 mg of the dried powdered whole plant (except the root) of **Phyllanthus amarus** 3 times per day for 30 days. This treatment resulted in loss of HBsAg in 22 of 37 patients without producing symptoms that could be classified as toxic side effects. Follow-up in some subjects (for up to 9 months in one subject) did not reveal reappearance of the antigen. In contrast, only 1 of 23 placebo-treated control subjects cleared the HBsAg carrier state.*

The investigators emphasized the tentative nature of these findings. They cautioned that for reasons unknown the number of drop-outs was significantly greater in the placebo group (15 of 38) than in the treated group (3 of 40). They pointed out that the response rate in HBsAg-positive carriers with HBeAg (5 of 17) was inferior to that in carriers without HBeAg (17 of 20), and that the probability of clearance was further reduced by the presence of anti-HBc IgM. They also acknowledged that no extensive laboratory studies were performed to look for subtle biochemical evidence of toxicity. However, the apparent lack of obvious side effects was consistent with results from previous acute and subchronic studies in mice, in which no clinical or histopathological evidence of toxicity had been found (3^C, 5^C).

(Biomedical Division)
Side Effects of Drugs Annual 14
M.N.G. Dukes and L. Beeley, editors

Apart from the methodological shortcomings in the trial, there is the clinical consideration that loss of HBsAg per se is not necessarily of benefit, unless it accompanies loss of HBeAg (6[r]). These preliminary findings should therefore not be taken as convincing evidence that ***Phyllanthus*** *is a valuable drug in chronic hepatitis B. The results are encouraging, however, and may serve as a guide for future studies, which will hopefully lead to the discovery of a drug that can be used in the treatment of HBV infection.*

It should be obvious that the potential relevancy of ethnopharmacology for medicine is not limited to Western society, but extends to non-Western settings. On the one hand, ethnopharmacological research may show which traditional treatments may be promoted as being clinically effective, and it may help to further the utility of native medicines by providing insight into the physicochemical and pharmacological properties of their therapeutic principles. On the other hand, it can determine which practices should be actively discouraged because they are dangerous (1[R]). The profound health hazards of certain traditionally used preparations, such as pyrrolizidine-containing herbs (7[R]), ***Gloriosa superba*** *and other toxic Liliiflorae (8[R]), surmas and similar products with high heavy metal levels (SED-10, 420) and rattlesnake meat (see below) all bear witness to the fact that ample traditional experience is not a guarantee for harmlessness.*

Proper care should be taken to avoid laying too much emphasis on the discouragement of such conspicuous poisons. In terms of health care improvement, it may be equally or more rewarding to correct the inappropriate use of less spectacular indigenous medicines. A good example is the native habit of administering herbal enemas to children with infectious diarrhea, since this practice entails the risk of life-threatening exacerbation of dehydration (9[r]). In addition, it will expose the young patient to a small but serious risk of rectal perforation (10[c]).

Aside from all medical angles, ethnopharmacology should be recognized for its cultural significance, as it pursues the basic anthropological objective of replacing ethnocentrism by cultural relativism. Scientific confirmation of the empirical rationality of certain native practices will keep us from looking down on those wandering about in ignorance (1[R]). A delightful example of aboriginal knowledge and ingenuity, which is bound to become an ethnopharmacological classic, was recently published in the ***New Scientist****.*

When Wodaabe herders in Niger were asked by a Western research team to draw maps of their region, they produced detailed maps showing the varying types of vegetation, even though they could not read or write. When questioned why they did not use certain areas of apparently good grass shown on their maps, the herders replied that their livestock would get night blindness, if allowed to graze in those areas during the dry season. This explanation fitted perfectly well with the finding of the research team that the vegetation of those regions was short of vitamin A. Surprisingly, the problem was unknown to the staff of the governmental livestock service, which was meant to improve the Wodaabe cattle. When one of the tribesmen was offered vitamin A supplementation for his animals, he was prepared to accept it, but only on the condition that half of his livestock would be treated, so that he would be able to see if the foreign remedy was really working (11[c]).

It thus appears that sophisticated methodology is not always the exclusive tool of Western trial designers.

GENERAL SOURCES OF CONCERN *(SED-11, 1002; SEDA-12, 403; SEDA-13, 443)*

During the review period, numerous publications appeared which underlined orthodox concern about the risks of alternative therapies. Most of these papers will not be discussed here, as they merely reinforce familiar arguments which have already been put forward in these volumes (SED-11, 1002; SEDA-12, 403; SEDA-13, 443). There were some reports and events, however, which gave rise to previously unnoted concerns.

Certain unorthodox medicines are capable of interference with clinical laboratory assays and may thus prevent orthodox practitioners from providing optimal health care Due to their chemical similarity to digoxin, cardiac glycosides from other natural sources than digitalis may cross-react with digoxin antibodies (12[C], 13[C]), thereby creating the false impression of high plasma digoxin levels. The practical relevance of this phenomenon became evident when Japanese investigators recently cautioned in a letter to *The Lancet* that a Chinese medicine called kyushin can interfere with digoxin immunoassays.

Fushimi et al (14[C]) found a serum digoxin level of more than 2.5 ng/ml in a patient who was taking 0.25 mg of digoxin per day and did not show any obvious sign of digoxin intoxication. They subsequently discovered that the patient had been taking kyushin, a traditional Chinese remedy, which can be purchased without prescription in Japan and contains the dried venom of the chinese toad (*Bufo bufo gargarizans*) as one of its constituents. This venom has digitalis-like cardiotonic actions due to the presence of bufalin and cinobufaginal, which are structurally related to digoxin. The digoxin-like immunoreactivity of one tablet of kyushin varied considerably from 1.5 to 72 μg of digoxin, depending on the specific immunoassay used.

Insufficient attention is still being paid to instability problems and to storage conditions of alternative medicines The Committee for Proprietary Medicinal Products (CPMP) of the European Economic Community has rightly specified in its recent note for guidance concerning the quality of herbal remedies that stability testing is one of the measures to ensure the pharmaceutical quality of botanical medicines (see the section below on Legislative developments under 'Herbal Remedies'). An eloquent example of the fact that instability of herbal remedies should not be systematically neglected is the rapid disappearance of iodine from kelp tablets.

The label of a major brand of kelp tablets in The Netherlands claims that these tablets can be used for 5 years. When the present author recently asked the responsible firm to back up this long expiry period with experimental data on the stability of the product, the firm did not have a ready answer. Yet it has been known since the early 1970s that the iodine content of kelp tablets can decline considerably with time. This came to light when Liewendahl and Turula (15[C]) observed a rare case of iodide-induced goiter and hypothyroidism in a female patient with chronic lymphocytic thyroiditis, who had taken kelp tablets made in Norway for about 3 years. Determination of the iodine content of the product revealed that tablets taken from the bottom of a fresh packet contained 1250 μg iodine a piece, whereas tablets taken from the surface layer contained only 115 μg. The tablets yielded no iodine at all, after they had been stored in the laboratory for $1\frac{1}{2}$ years. Unfortunately, the paper does not properly specify under which storage conditions this latter result was obtained.

Alternative medicines may even be promoted for use in disorders which are contraindications from the orthodox point of view As already pointed out in SEDA-13 (p. 460), it is becoming increasingly clear that fish oil products may adversely affect metabolic control in patients with non-insulin-dependent diabetes mellitus who are not being treated with a sulfonylurea derivative (16[R]). Yet a recent Dutch lay article in a free house-to-house newspaper indiscriminately tried to promote the use of fish oil in patients with non-insulin-dependent diabetes mellitus.

There is an enormous lack of reliable epidemiological data on non-orthodox medicines The information presented in these columns is all too often based on one or a few isolated case-reports, which only allow a qualitative insight into the health risks of the non-orthodox remedy in question. For obvious reasons, reliable epidemiological data on the consumption of the particular remedy and on the incidence of its side effects are usually not available. The 1989 meeting of the WHO Drug Utilization Research Group made it clear that this unsatisfactory situation will not rapidly undergo a radical change and that in-depth assessment of most alternative drug risks will remain impracticable in the foreseeable future. This does not pose a problem, of course, so long as one adheres to the conservative rule that any serious risk presented by a non-orthodox drug is an *unnecessary* threat to health and should therefore be avoided. Problems may arise, however, as soon as one starts to consider the absence of reliable evidence of risk as reliable evidence for the absence of risk.

Policy makers tend to subordinate the need of proper scientific evaluation of alternative medicines to non-scientific ideological and economic considerations The view that scientific proof of efficacy should be subordinated to the ideological benefit of therapeutic freedom has become increasingly popular in The Netherlands. Few Dutch politicians would nowadays be prepared to deny patients the basic right to choose their own treatment, even though certain treatments are known to involve the use of medicines with unproven therapeutic claims. This liberal attitude will only allow for restriction when the medicines in question have been convincingly demonstrated to represent an unacceptable threat to public health. Unfortunately, such a concept is widely open to liberal and inexpert interpretation.

In spite of repetitive warnings in the Dutch pharmaceutical press against comfrey (17[r]), which even resulted in questions being asked in parliament (18[r]), Dutch health authorities have not yet restricted in any way the free availability of this herb and preparations derived from it in health food stores and through the mail.

Recently, judgement was pronounced in a Dutch courtroom on the issue whether seized vitamin products and certain other unregistered medicines should have been submitted to official drug approval procedures. The court ruled that a serious health risk was a valid ground for making the submisssion of alternative drug products to the drug registry authorities compulsory, but at the same time overlooked the fact that toxic laetrile products were among the supplies seized (19[R]).

A political view which also seems to become increasingly influential is the hope that alternative medicine may perhaps help to cut down on the costs of the health care system. An illustrative statement was made by the Dutch Secretary for Welfare, Public Health and Culture when he announced a strategy giving lower priority to the scientific evaluation of alternative treatments in favor of other research topics, such as the effect of alternative consumption patterns on the total use of health care provisions (20[r]).

The liberal Dutch attitude towards alternative medicines has had far-reaching consequences. At the instigation of the Dutch parliament, the bill concerning health insurance reimbursement of pharmaceuticals recently underwent revision and from now onwards all homeopathic and anthroposophic drug products will be reimbursed (21[c]). Evidently, the day has come to rename alcohol and tobacco as recreational drugs, since alternative medicines have become the real social drugs of our time.

HERBAL REMEDIES *(SED-11, 1002; SEDA-12, 402; SEDA-13, 446)*

Legislative developments Drug manufacturers and license holders must apply for authorization to place medicinal products on the market. This application must be accompanied by documents which provide the results of tests and trials carried out on the product concerned. To promote the free movement of medicinal products from one member state of the European Economic Community to another, the Council of the European Communities has adopted a directive in which uniform application rules for all member states are laid down concerning the tests and trials requested, the compilation of dossiers and the examination of applications. To prevent differences between the member states in the interpretation of this general directive, the Committee for Proprietary Medicinal Products (CPMP) in Brussells regularly issues so-called notes for guidance, in which specific topics are elucidated (22[R]). Although these notes are recommendations, which are not quite as obligatory as the directive itself, they are bound to have an influence on drug registry procedures throughout the European Community.

One of the latest CPMP notes for guidance concerns the quality of herbal remedies (23[R]). This note provides rules for dealing with specific problems related to the quality assurance of medicinal products of vegetable origin and lays down standards for: (a) description of the qualitative and quantitative particulars of the constituents; (b) description of the method of preparation; (c) control of starting materials; (d) control tests carried out at an intermediate stage of the manufacturing process of the finished product; (e) control tests on the finished product; (f) stability tests.

According to section (c), a complete pharmacopeial monograph (or an equivalent monograph if a pharmacopeial one is not available) on each vegetable drug should be submitted. When constituents have known therapeutic activity, assay methods are required and a range of their contents should also be included, so as to ensure a reproducible quality of the finished product. As a general rule, vegetable drugs must be tested for microbiological contamination, residues of pesticides and fumigation agents, radioactivity, toxic metals, and adulterants, unless otherwise justified. Furthermore, if the herbal remedy does not contain the vegetable drug itself but a preparation, the monograph on the vegetable drug must be followed by a monograph on the preparation, which gives particulars on identification tests, purity tests, and quantitative determination of characteristic constituents. If the preparation is standardized on constituents with known therapeutic activity, the method of standardization should be specified.

According to section (e), control tests on the finished product should allow qualitative and quantitative determination of the vegetable ingredients and their constituents with known therapeutic activity. If constituents with therapeutic activity are unknown, control tests may be specified by using chemically defined constituents of the vegetable ingredient as markers. If ingredients of a herbal remedy cannot be quantitatively determined individually, they may be determined jointly, provided that the need for this procedure is justified.

This note for guidance touches on several orthodox concerns about the quality of herbal remedies, which have been expressed in previous annuals (SEDA-11, 424; SEDA-12, 403; SEDA-13, 442). It is somewhat disappointing, however, that the CPMP does not mention testing for the absence of certain herbal constituents as a potentially useful method of quality assurance.

The CPMP recognizes the principle that a chemically defined constituent of a herbal ingredient can be of interest for control purposes by serving as a marker: i.e., that the level of this constituent in the finished product can be taken as a measure for the quantity of herbal ingredient in the finished product (23[R]). From the point of view of drug safety, however, it may sometimes also be rewarding to ensure the absence of a particular herbal constituent. Certain medicinal plants are known to have constituents which do not contribute in any way to the established or alleged beneficial effects of the plant, but which are capable of producing adverse reactions. On the analogy of the CPMP concept of positive markers, it would be prudent to denote such superfluous and harmful compounds as 'negative markers', which should not reach unsafe levels in the finished herbal product.

Notable examples of negative markers are the carcinogenic sweet flag constituent β-asarone (SEDA-12, 408), the allergenic sesquiterpene lactone anthecotulid in chamomile (SED-11, 1007), and the hepatotoxic and carcinogenic pyrrolizidine alkaloids in comfrey and some other common medicinal herbs (SEDA-13, 450; 8[R]). In the case of sweet flag and chamomile, elimination can be readily achieved by the selection of a β-asarone-free variety (SEDA-12, 408) or an anthecotulid-free chemotype (24[CR]) respectively. In the case of pyrrolizidine alkaloids, special extraction techniques are currently being developed (25[C], 26[c]).

One's major disappointment with the CPMP note for guidance does not stem from such subtle considerations, however, but from the strict limitation of its scope to the pharmaceutical quality of herbal remedies. As a consequence, the note does not provide any guidance at all about other important aspects of herbal remedies, such as: (a) the need for adequate quality control of patient information on herbal products (see the section on this subject below); (b) the need for a rational solution of the burning issue of to what extent traditional empiricism is allowed to supplement or replace experimental data in the benefit/risk assessment of well-known medicinal plants with mild pharmacological actions.

The CPMP note for guidance does not even address the fundamental question of where and how the borderline between botanical foods and botanical medicines should be drawn. Its vague definition of herbal remedies as medicinal products which contain exclusively plant material and/or vegetable drug preparations as active ingredients leaves plenty of room for local interpretations.

Patient information As outlined in SED-11 (p. 1003), visitors to herbal drug stores can usually choose from a variety of promotional books and pamphlets which emphasize the allegedly favorable features of botanical medicines and minimize the potential dangers. It is obvious that this vast assortment of uncritical literature may lead to inappropriate practices and therefore needs to be counterbalanced by more objective patient information on herbal medicines. In other words, there is more to the quality control of herbal products than the classical monitoring of pharmaceutical quality. It is equally important to ensure that these products are provided with patient information of high quality, which adequately informs the user about acceptable uses, dosage, precautions, adverse effects and drug interactions (27[R]).

Useful examples of patient information texts on individual botanical remedies can be found in the recently updated West German handbook *Teedrogen* (28[R]). These examples are derived from the monographs of the Federal Committee for Phytotherapy in West Germany ('Kommission E') and from the so-called 'Standardzulassungen', for which another committee of the West German Federal Health Office is responsible (SEDA-12, 406).

In The Netherlands, many herbal products are not yet supplied with appropriate patient information. We have therefore developed a general patient information leaflet on the safe use of botanical remedies (20[R]), which is reproduced here below with the permission of the Royal Dutch Association for the Advancement of Pharmacy. The leaflet presents a series of cautionary notes, which are largely based on the orthodox concerns about herbal therapies expressed in these volumes (SEDA-11, 424; SEDA-12, 403; SEDA-13, 442). The leaflet is not meant to hearten those readers who already have a critical attitude towards herbal remedies. Its particular aim is to educate uninformed and credulous users of botanical medicines about the potential health risks of such products. To reach this particular audience, the leaflet deliberately speaks about phytotherapy in a sympathetic tone.

THE SAFE USE OF HERBAL REMEDIES

Back to nature A lot of our medicines today are chemically prepared, unlike in the past, when this was quite different. In the old days, all drugs originated from nature. Pills, powders, potions and ointments were prepared from medicinal plants, a variety of loose-leaf herbs were used to prepare teas. All of these botanical drugs are known as 'herbal remedies'. With the advent and advancement of chemically prepared drugs, the use of herbal remedies decreased substantially but, nowadays, botanical drugs have become 'fashionable' once again. Many people today favour natural products.

Difference with homoeopathic medicines Herbal remedies are often confused with homoeopathic medicines, yet there are major differences in use and preparation. Herbal remedies can be used in precisely the same way as chemically prepared drugs. Their action is always opposed to the disease or complaint, e.g. a laxative herb is used against constipation. In homoeopathy, however, a laxative herb is used to treat diarrhoea ('like cures like'). To give the herb a homoeopathic action, is has to be diluted first in a special way ('potentisation'). This dilution results in a homoeopathic medicine with properties different from those of the herb itself. A herbal remedy is not diluted in a homoeopathic way, and therefore retains the action (and any adverse effects) of the original herb.

There are two different kinds of herbal remedies: (1) strongly acting herbal remedies. These have strong reactions in quite small amounts. They are to be dispensed only, and exclusively, on prescription and (2) mildly acting herbal remedies. These are available without prescription from pharmacies and health food stores. Follow the safety tips given in this leaflet, and such mildly acting remedies may be used for self-medication without difficulty.

Safety tips

Buy herbal remedies from reliable and trusted sources Never bring herbal remedies from far away countries. Never order them by mail from abroad, because you will have no guarantee whatsoever that you are buying a safe product. The purity of herbal remedies is not carefully controlled everywhere in the world. Moreover, you should buy herbal remedies only from outlets where you may go back if necessary.

Purchase a herbal remedy only if the package clearly states which herb(s) it contains Do not trust herbal remedies in which the composition is kept secret. Check, before you buy anything, that the package states which herbal ingredients have been used to prepare the product. When it is a 'ready-to-use' medicine, you should also be able to see who prepared the agent (the manufacturer).

Always ask for the exact directions for use You are entitled to proper and correct directions for use, informing you of how often you may take the remedy and how much you should take per dose. In the case of a herbal tea, you should also be informed about the proper method of preparation, e.g. how much herb and (boiling) water you should use and how long the tea should be left to 'draw'. Buy your products only where this information has been given.

Do not collect herbs in the wild, unless you are well able to distinguish poisonous and innocuous herbs from one another Just as with wild mushrooms and toadstools, poisonous and nonpoisonous herbs can look very much alike. A mistake might be fatal!

Store herbal remedies with care Herbal remedies should be stored carefully, in exactly the same way as other drugs, i.e. in a cool, dry environment, which is safe from children's hands. A 'ready-to-use' product can best be stored in the package in which you have bought it. For the storage of a loose-leaf tea, a tightly closed tin is suitable. A plastic container is not suitable for the storage of herbs, particularly when they are strong-smelling herbs, because plastic may absorb the volatile oil of these herbs.

Do not use herbal remedies which you have kept for years Every herbal remedy purchased should give an indication (on its packaging) of how long it may be kept. Many loose-leaf herbs begin to loose their activity when you keep them for more than one year. 'Ready-to-use' herbal remedies are not infinitely storable either. Your pharmacist can give you advice if you are unsure whether a herbal remedy is still active after a long storage period.

Do not use herbal remedies for serious illnesses Mildly acting herbal remedies are not meant for serious diseases, such as diabetes, hypertension or epilepsy. If you suffer from such a serious condition, you should consult your physician and not try to 'play doctor' yourself, because there is a high element of risk. You should also not depend on mildly acting herbs in the case of cancer.

Stop using a herbal remedy if you start experiencing side-effects Some people have the idea that drugs from a chemical factory can be damaging, whereas natural products can not. They also think that herbal medicines cannot have adverse effects, but this is not the case. Herbal remedies can also have side-effects, such as skin eruptions or stomach ache. If such a complaint occurs, you should stop using the herbal remedy, to enable the side-effects to clear.

Do not exceed the dose range stated in the directions for use All too often, one is inclined to think that if a small amount of natural product is doing good, a larger dose would be even better. However, a herbal remedy will not be better for you if you take it upon yourself to exceed the stated dose. Quite the contrary: there are herbs which will have serious consequences if you consume too large quantities. Therefore, always take herbal remedies according to the directions for use (as with any medicine). If the remedy is not helping your ailment, it is far better to stop the treatment than to raise the dosage yourself.

Do not use herbal remedies for prolonged periods Mildly acting herbal remedies are innocuous if used in the recommended dosage, for short periods. Unfortunately, we do not yet know whether all remedies are safe to consume over a continuous period of months or years. Therefore, it is always better to err on the side of caution, and refrain from taking a herbal remedy for an extended period, unless you have previously sought the advice of your physician or pharmacist.

If you are pregnant, or breast-feeding, and want to use a herbal remedy, do this only after consulting your physician or pharmacist Certain herbal remedies should definitely not be used during pregnancy. There is also a large group of herbal remedies which cannot be entirely guaranteed to be without effect on your unborn child. Always, therefore, consult your physician or pharmacist if you are pregnant and wish to use a particular herbal remedy. Also, if you are breast-feeding, it is best to ask for expert advice first.

Your physician or pharmacist must always be informed if you are using a herbal remedy simultaneously with other medicines It is vital that this information is available, as it is a known fact that certain herbal remedies can affect (either by increasing or decreasing) the action of other medicines.

Points to remember, in brief

- Buy herbal remedies from reliable and trusted sources.
- Purchase a herbal remedy only if the package clearly states which herb(s) it contains.
- Always ask for the exact directions for use.
- Do not collect herbs in the wild, unless you are well able to distinguish poisonous and innocuous herbs from one another.
- Store herbal remedies with care.
- Do not use herbal remedies which you have kept for years.
- Do not use herbal remedies for serious illnesses.
- Stop using a herbal remedy if you start experiencing side-effects.
- Do not exceed the dose range stated in the directions for use.
- Do not use herbal remedies for prolonged periods.
- If you are pregnant, or breast-feeding, and want to use a herbal remedy, do this only after consulting your physician or pharmacist.
- Your physician or pharmacist must always be informed if you are using a herbal remedy simultaneously with other medicines.

Caffeine-containing plants

The alkaloid caffeine is widely valued because of its stimulant-like behavioral activity on mood and performance (29[C]). Its most familiar sources are coffee, tea, caffeinated soft drinks, cocoa, chocolate and certain orthodox medications (30[r]). However, caffeine may also be ingested in the more unobstrusive form of an exotic herbal remedy, such as maté tea or guarana capsules (see Table 1).

Although caffeine has been incriminated for a supposed association with various diseases, its health hazards are still considered to be relatively few. Fears of a causative role in urinary tract or pancreatic cancer, fibrocystic breast disease, and teratogenesis have largely been dispelled (36[R]). Wilcox et al (37[C], 38[c]) have now added *decreased fertility* to the long list of complications, for which a statistical association with caffeine consumption has been reported over the years. They point out that caffeine is not known to affect mammalian reproduction, but that the relevance of animal data may be limited because of wide interspecies variation in the metabolic fate of caffeine.

Wilcox et al (37[C], 38[c]) interviewed 221 healthy women who were planning to become pregnant

Table 1. *Some botanical sources rich in caffeine (other than coffee, tea and cacao) (31[R], 32[R], 33[Cr], 34[r], 35[r])*

Scientific name (family)	Vernacular name	Caffeine content (plant part)
Cola nitida (Sterculiaceae)	Cola*	1.5–3.5% (seeds)
Ilex guayusa (Aquifoliaceae)	Guayusa	1.8% (leaves)
Ilex paraguariensis (Aquifoliaceae)	Maté**	0.3–2% (leaves)
Ilex vomitoria (Aquifoliaceae)	Yaupon	0.01–1.65% (leaves)
Paullinia cupana (Sapindaceae)	Guarana	2.5–5% (seeds)
Paullinia yoco (Sapindaceae)	Yoco	2.7% (bark)

*Cola nuts may also be obtained from other *Cola* spp. containing caffeine (e.g. *C.acuminata* and *C.ballayi*).
**Several other *Ilex* spp. contain caffeine as well and are used as substitutes for Maté (e.g. *I.amara, I.conocarpa, I.theezans*).

about their consumption of alcohol, cigarettes and caffeinated beverages during the previous month. The 117 women who became pregnant within the first 3 months were not followed up. The other 104 women were interviewed at 3 months about their exposure during the preceding 3 months, and this interview was repeated at 6 months, if they still were not pregnant by that time. Analysis of the data from these 104 subjects showed that the women who had consumed more than 3.15 g of caffeine per month (approximately equivalent to 1 cup of coffee per day) showed a relative fecundability of 0.59 and 0.53 at 3 and 6 months, respectively, when compared to those with a lower caffeine intake. The association between higher caffeine consumption and impaired fertility was unaffected by adjustment for possible confounding variables, such as alcohol and smoking. When a divison was made into finer categories of caffeine exposure, a dose–response effect emerged. Women using more than 7 g per month were only one-fourth as likely to become pregnant as those taking 0.5 g or less per month (corresponding to more than 2.3 cups and less than 0.2 cups of coffee per day, respectively). The investigators examined for a subset of menstrual cycles, whether caffeine had an effect on ovulation, but the observed proportion of anovulatory cycles was too small to explain the observed association between caffeine and lower fecundability.

Wilcox and associates are commendably cautious in their interpretation of these results. They warn that their association between caffeine and decreased fertility is based on data from a special subset of women. When they analyzed the consumption data obtained from all 221 women at the start of the study, the fecundity of higher caffeine users relative to that of lower caffeine users rose to 0.8. They also acknowledge the possibility that the association could be an artifact produced by stress or some other unmeasured but correlated factor. Due to such uncertainties, it is impossible to draw firm conclusions without the benefit of additional well-designed studies. Such further research is certainly warranted, since corroboration of the findings by Wilcox and co-workers would have great practical consequences. The need for more studies is also evident from letters stimulated by their report:

Casas et al (39[c]) put forward the suggestion that caffeine may decrease fertility by lowering the plasma levels of prolactin via a dopaminergic mechanism. Christianson et al (40[c]) likewise reported a dose-related association between caffeine and decreased fertility. According to their data, women drinking less than 1 cup of coffee per day had only half a chance of difficulties in becoming pregnant compared to women who took 7 or more cups per day. This information was obtained from a much larger population of approximately 6300 women, but it was less reliable than the data of Wilcox et al, because it was entirely based on the recall of pregnant women who had been interviewed early during pregnancy.

In the period covered by this Annual, a WHO Working Group on drugs and human lactation (41[R]) concluded that caffeine-induced effects may occur in the puerperium, when infants are breast-fed by mothers who ingest this substance in large quantities. There was also the observation that caffeine can cause *fetal arrhythmias*, when excessive amounts are taken by pregnant women.

Oei et al (42[C]) described 3 cases of irregular fetal heart beat resulting from the daily intake of 1.5 liters or more of cola or coffee by the mother. In 2 of these cases, the effect was seen during labor, and heart rhythm remained irregular after delivery. Electrocardiography showed bradycardia resulting from blocking extrasystoles in one neonate and supraventricular extrasystoles in the other one. Symptoms resolved over 3 days without medical intervention.

In view of these data, it would be unwise to use excessive quantities of caffeinated products during pregnancy or breast-feeding. This advice pertains not only to coffee and other common dietary sources of caffeine, but also to some of the less conspicuous herbal remedies, which contain high levels of this alkaloid.

PLANT-DERIVED DRUGS *(SEDA-13, 455)*

Tetrahydropalmatine

It is generally recognized that oriental herbal remedies represent a particular health hazard when they are contaminated or 'fortified' with Western synthetic drugs or with high levels of heavy metals (SED-10, 894; SED-11, 1002). It seems to be less well-known, however, that such medicines may also be capable of adverse reactions by virtue of their containing a potent active principle of a traditional herb. This possibility was highlighted when we recently discovered the alkaloid *l*-tetrahydropalmatine (*l*-THP) in tablets of Chinese origin (43[C]).

The tablets were called Jin Bu Huan Anodyne, and had reached The Netherlands through a Belgian channel. The package insert claimed analgetic and hypnotic effects and recommended 2–4 tablets 1–3 times per day for pain or 1–3 tablets before sleep to treat insomnia. It suggested that 30% of an alkaloid from *Polygala chinensis* was present, but a literature search on the chemistry of this plant failed to shed light on this cryptic declaration. Only by resorting to sophisticated analytical methods were we able to demonstrate that the tablets contained approximately 25 mg of *l*-THP per piece (43[C]).

Analgesic tablets containing *l*-THP are indeed used in Chinese medicine. The alkaloid is usually extracted for this purpose from *Stephania* species. A suggested dosage regimen is 60–120 mg 1–4 times per day (44[R]).

The Chinese also value *dl*-tetrahydropalmatine (*dl*-THP) as an analgesic and hypnotic agent. This racemic form may be given to patients with insomnia in a dose of 100–200 mg at bed-time. It is the main active principle of the tubers of *Corydalis* species, which have been traditionally employed in China for relief of pain and as a blood-stimulant. Therapeutic doses of *dl*-THP may cause vertigo, fatigue and nausea (44[R]). When a single oral dose of 75 mg was tested in 64 patients, drowsiness was found as a side effect in 28% of the cases (45[c]).

Animal studies have shown that *l*-THP and *dl*-THP have analgesic and sedative activity, which is not due to affinity for opiate receptors. *l*-THP appears to be a dopamine receptor antagonist, which is more potent at presynaptic than at postsynaptic receptors. *d*-THP has no affinity for dopamine receptors, but it can lower central dopamine levels. In contrast, brain levels of dopamine are not affected by *l*-THP (44[R], 46[R], 47[C]).

As was pointed out in SEDA-13 (p. 444), Chinese pills may endanger not only the consumer himself, but also his fellow road-users, when they are adulterated with synthetic psychotropic agents, such as diazepam. The data presented here make clear, however, that the absence of Western drugs does not guarantee that a Chinese botanical medicine is safe for drivers.

HOMEOPATHIC MEDICINES *(SED-11, 1017)*

Although the risks of homeopathic medicines decrease with each dilution step in their manufacturing process, one should bear in mind that even very diluted remedies may cause *allergic reactions*. This was well illustrated by a case-report on Pentackan Sinnabaun D4 tablets. These tablets are used for rhinitis, tonsillitis and conjunctivitis. As they contain 10 μg of dichromate per piece, they are sometimes also prescribed for contact allergy to chromium, in the unproven hope that oral supplementation will lead to hyposensitization.

Van Ulsen et al (48[C]) describe a case in which such therapy did not produce relief but severe exacerbation. The patient was a 37-year-old male bricklayer, who suffered from an itchy dermatitis of the hands and forearms that worsened while working. He was found to be allergic to dichromate and cobalt. Treatment was started with 6 Pentackan Sinnabaun D4 tablets per day. This resulted in acute and severe exacerbation of eczema, with swelling and redness of the face and pemphigus of the hands. The Pentackan dose was then reduced to 2 tablets per day, and this new regimen was continued for 4 months, but his skin condition persisted.

ACUPUNCTURE *(SED-11, 1018)*

A cautionary view was advanced in SED-11 (p. 1018) in the light of reports reviewed much earlier in these volumes that acupuncture may result in serious infectious complications if insufficient care is taken to employ proper sterilization techniques. This point is now reinforced by 2 reports about acupuncture-related outbreaks of *hepatitis B virus (HBV) infection.*

Kent et al (49[Cr]) recently described one of the largest outbreaks of acupuncture-associated hepatitis B ever recorded. Suspicions as to the source arose when the health authorities of Rhode Island (United States) received 5 case-reports of jaundice due to hepatitis B infection in patients who had no apparent risk factor in common other than acupuncture treatment by the same acupuncturist. This led the authorities to close the acupuncturist's practice and to start an epidemiological investigation. The acupuncturist in question worked in a main clinic and a satellite clinic on alternate days. Of 366 persons who had undergone his treatments in the preceding period (back to one maximum incubation period before the first reported case became symptomatic), 316 subjects provided details of their treatments and symptoms of illness in a questionnaire, and submitted blood samples for hepatitis B serology. No positive serology cases were found among the 136 persons who had been treated exclusively in the main clinic. However, 18 of the 180 subjects who had received treatment in the satellite clinic were positive for HBsAg and IgM anti-HBc, and 17 other subjects in this group were negative for HBsAg but positive for IgM anti-HBc. Eleven of the 18 HBsAg-positive subjects had developed jaundice (i.e. 6% of the 180 persons treated in the satellite clinic), and 5 of these patients were hospitalized. The precise mechanism of virus transmission could not be determined, but evaluation of the acupuncturist's technique revealed potential mechanisms for contamination. He rubbed the needles with his ungloved fingers before and after use to test them for sharpness. As he repeated this procedure for subsequent patients without washing his hands, he could thus have transferred infectious material to sterile needles. He also repetitively used an instrument for applying pressure to bleeding puncture sites without resterilization. Alternatively, a lack of sterilization facilities at the satellite clinic could have led to the repetitive use of unsterilized needles. Although the acupuncturist denied this possibility, his patients reported that he replaced needles on the same tray, from which he had initially taken them, and no receptacles for used needles were found in his examination rooms. The acupuncturist denied ever having had symptoms of hepatitis. He was found to be negative for HBsAg and positive for IgM anti-HBc. As he handled hundreds of needles per day, he could very well have punctured himself with a contaminated needle. However, since no positive cases occurred among patients treated in the main clinic, it is unlikely that he was the source of the epidemic.

Slater et al (50[Cr]) reported a smaller Israelian outbreak of hepatitis B which was associated with acupuncture treatment by a physician. It involved 5 patients with clinical symptoms of hepatitis, who were all positive for HBsAg and anti-HBc, and partially positive for IgM anti-HBc, anti-HBe, and HBeAg. In addition, 6 persons who had at least one acupuncture treament date in common with the 5 hepatitis patients, were found to have anti-HBc without other HBV markers. The spread of HBV was apparently due to the use of unsterilized or improperly sterilized acupuncture needles. The most likely scenario was that transmission occurred in 2 successive steps. First the virus was transmitted from an operating room nurse, who had become infected during her work, to 2 of her acupuncture co-patients. Then it spread from one of these latter patients to a second pair of co-patients. This evidence of repeated neglect prompted the initiation of administrative measures to suspend the medical license of the physician involved.

Similar epidemics were previously reported from the United Kingdom (51[C]), Switzerland (52[C]), Belgium (53[C]) and Florida (54[C]). When the figures from Rhode Island and Israel are added to these previous data, the total number ofHBsAg-positive cases attributed to acupuncture treatment has now risen to 68 patients.

The Western experience with acupuncture-related outbreaks of hepatitis have evoked the question whether contamination of acupuncture needles may also contribute to epidemic HBV hepatitis in China.

This possibility was raised by Conn (55[r]), who pointed out that the prevalence of the HBV carrier state in the People's Republic of China is as high as 7–10%. He related that he did not notice proper sterilization techniques when he observed acupuncture practices during a visit to China. Some Chinese physicians with whom he discussed this experience acknowledged that acupuncture needles may be merely cleaned by swabbing them with alcohol and that sterile gloves are not commonly worn by acupuncturists. However, others believe that his experience was not typical and some seem sceptical of his observations.

Fortunately, acupuncture has not yet been associated with large outbreaks of *human immunodeficiency virus (HIV) infection* though it may have been responsible for individual cases.

Castro et al (56[C]) investigated 2059 AIDS patients with no previously identified risk factors, who had been reported to the U.S. Centers for Disease Control. They eliminated 921 patients because a complete risk history could not be obtained, 825 patients because risk factors were ultimately identified, and another 32 patients because they did not meet the case definition of AIDS. Of the 281 remaining patients, 178 patients or relatives received in-depth interviews with a standard questionnaire. Four of 148 persons gave a history of acupuncture, but 2 of these patients received it after the onset of symptoms.

Vittecoq et al (57[C]) described a 17-year-old boy who had received 6 acupuncture treatments once a week for his tendinitis. The week after the final treatment, a mononucleosis-like illness developed with symptoms such as diffuse lymph-node hyperplasia and a fever that lasted for 8 days. His white-cell count was normal and a Paul-Bunnell test was negative. Three months later he was found to be HIV-antibody-positive. According to the authors, the patient had never had sexual intercourse. They believe his seroconversion to be related to the acupuncture treatments, since they were unable to identify any other potential cause.

Vittecoq and associates do not explain how they were able to exclude sexual activities as a risk factor, and apparently they did not retrace the boy's infection to an HIV patient who had been treated on the same date by the same acupuncturist. As a consequence, their case can at best be classified as tentative. This should not detract from the fact, however, that AIDS is a blood-borne disease and may spread via acupuncture needles, unless adequate precautions are taken (58[r]).

As pointed out in SED-11 (p. 1018), nosocomial disease transmission can be prevented by strict adherence to aseptic skin-piercing procedures and by adequate sterilization of re-usable acupuncture needles. Overnight immersion in a solution of benzalkonium chloride or another quaternary ammonium base is not effective (54[C]), and wiping with a 70% solution of alcohol is not appropriate either (59[c]). A simple and most effective sterilization method is thorough physical cleaning followed by autoclaving at 121°C (250°F) for at least 15 minutes. The use of dry heat at 121°C for 16 hours, 161°C for 2 hours, or 171°C for 1 hour is also acceptable (49[Cr]). An alternative recommended in the *American Journal of Acupuncture* (58[r]) is the use of disposable needles.

OTHER REMEDIES *(SEDA-13, 457)*

Chondroprotective agents

The drug class of chondroprotective agents comprises the following trade products as its principal representatives (60[R], 61[R], 62[R]):

– ***Dona 200-S*** *injection and sustained-release tablet. The injection contains 400 mg of* D*-glucosamine sulfate and 10.7 mg of lidocaine hydrochloride per ampoule, while the tablet provides 250 mg of* D*-glucosamine sulfate.*

– ***Arumalon*** *injection, which may also be branded as* ***Rumalon*** *injection (63[r]). Each ampoule contains 3.5 mg of an extract of cartilage and 3.0 mg of an aqueous extract of the red bone marrow of calves. Although the product is said to be standardised to 2.5 mg/ml glycosaminoglycan peptide (64[r]), the exact chemical composition remains to be defined satisfactorily.*

– ***Arteparon*** *injection, which is prepared from bovine lung and tracheal cartilage. The content of an ampoule is declared to be 50 mg of mucopolysaccharide polysulfuric acid ester (also known as 'glycosaminoglycan polysulfate').*

These products are widely used in German-speaking parts of Europe (60[R]). In 1987, when the costs of West German prescriptions of chondroprotective agents were 92.6 million DM, they accounted for more than two-thirds of this total figure. Dona 200-S tablets alone accounted for 34 million DM, with an additional 5.6 million DM being spent on the injections. The costs of Arumalon and Arteparon injections amounted to 10 and 13 million DM, respectively (65[R]).

The drugs are all recommended for the treatment of degenerative joint disorders. The underlying hope is that the exogenous supply of substances with structural resemblance to cartilaginous components or metabolites may restore the metabolic balance in the joint, and may stop or even reverse the breakdown of the cartilage. However, there is no conclusive proof that the beneficial effects of chondroprotective agents outweigh their adverse reaction risk. This is particularly true for the parenteral preparations. Chondroprotective injections may produce a

local reaction *at the site of injection (pain, erythema, hematoma, and swelling). More rarely, they can be associated with* ***allergic symptoms****, such as exanthem, urticaria, pruritus, perspiration and dizziness. Isolated cases of anaphylactic shock and circulatory collapse have also been reported (60[R]–62[R], 66[R], 67[R]). Furthermore, there are theoretical fears that inexpert intramuscular injection might lead to* ***septicemia*** *(66[R], 67[R], 68[C]), while incorrect intra-articular administration might result in* ***septic arthritis*** *(60[R]).*

Dona 200-S

Dona 200-S injections may also cause other side effects, such as ***nausea***, ***vomiting*** *and* ***stupor****. In addition,* ***arrhythmias*** *are said to be possible, as well as isolated cases of* ***taste disturbances*** *and* ***blood disorders*** *(thrombocytopenia, pancytopenia, and leukopenia). It is likely that such reactions are partly due to the presence of lidocaine (67[R], 69[r]).*

Hunold (70[C]) treated 55 patients with Dona 200-S tablets and/or intramuscular injections. Side effects were observed in 4 patients, and consisted of skin reactions, restlessness, sleeping disturbances and stupor, and aggravation of gastric complaints. Intramuscular therapy had to be discontinued in one patient, because of an inflammatory infiltrate in the left buttock and thigh.

In 1987, the West German health authorities announced that intra-articular administration of Dona 200-S injection was no longer permitted, because painful irritation at the site of injection occurred frequently (71[r]).

Arumalon

Arumalon injections are associated only with local reactions at the site of injection and with allergic symptoms. The average incidence of immunological reactions in a total of 8540 patients was 0.2%, but this average figure was obtained by pooling studies that varied greatly in incidence of reported side effects. One research group treated more than 1700 patients without observing any adverse event, whereas another investigator reported 2 cases of immunological reactions in a series of only 62 patients (66[R]). The recent discovery of bovine serum albumin in Arumalon has resulted in a heated controversy about the clinical significance of this finding. Some argue that the formation of antibodies against this antigen should be considered as a non-pathological immune response, comparable to the formation of antibodies against bovine proteins in cow's milk and raw beef. Others classify it as a hazardous contaminant, and suggest that it may be responsible for suspected cases of serious allergic reactions to Arumalon treatment (72[r], 73[r]).

According to an undetailed statement in ***Arznei-Telegramm*** *(74[r]), polymyositis and fatal dermatomyositis have been recorded as potential side effects of Arumalon injections in the so-called 'Network of Mutual Information'. This Network is used by West German doctors and pharmacists to inform each other about suspected cases of drug toxicity. Unfortunately, insufficient details were provided to allow an independent assessment of these cases.*

A West German group (75[C], 76[C]) reported allergic reactions to Arumalon in 2 other patients. One patient reacted with fever, malaise and symptoms of pronounced inflammation after she had received a total of 5 intramuscular injections. Her lymphocytes showed a positive response in a lymphocyte transformation test for the diagnosis of drug allergy (75[C]). The other patient had been treated for several years with series of Arumalon injections twice a year, and developed a nephrotic syndrome 6 weeks after her last injection. In a lymphocyte transformation test, her lymphocytes gave a borderline positive response when incubated with heterologous serum (76[C]).

As was to be expected, these reports were immediately challenged by the Swiss manufacturer, Robapharm (64[c], 77[c]). With respect to the nephrotic syndrome following the use of Arumalon, spokesmen of the company pointed out that the patient had also received bezafibrate and that this nephrotoxic drug was not examined in the lymphocyte transformation test. They emphasized that the response in this test was borderline positive and that it reflected long-term treatment rather than an immunopathological reaction, as the patient had tolerated many Arumalon injections over the years without apparent side effects (64[r]).

This reply did not properly acknowledge, however, that short-term use of Arumalon has also been associated with a positive lymphocyte transformation test (75[C]). It did not acknowledge either that progressive proteinuria had already been diagnosed 2 weeks before bezafibrate had been prescribed and that the lymphocyte transformation test was positive, in spite of the fact that the patient had been taking 100 mg of the immunosuppressive drug prednisolone daily for 4 weeks (76[C]). Furthermore, the manufacturer's spokesmen did not present experimental evidence to back up their claim that long-term treatment with Arumalon produces a positive response in the lymphocyte transformation test.

Arteparon

The Arteparon principle, glycosaminoglycan polysulfate, resembles heparin in its molecular structure (78[C], 79[CR]). It is well established that heparin may cause increased platelet aggregation resulting in thrombocytopenia through induction of antibodies that can bind to platelets (80[C], 81[R], 82[C]). Arteparon may have a similar adverse effect on platelet aggregation and one should be aware that cross-reactivity between ***heparin*** *and Arteparon is possible.*

Wolf et al (78[C]) studied the plasma or serum of 6 patients with Arteparon-induced thrombocytopenia and of 17 patients with heparin-associated thrombocytopenia. The majority of samples agglutinated Arteparon-coated thrombocytes as well as heparin-coated thrombocytes. Indirect immunofluorescence tests revealed involvement of IgG antibodies (with one exception in which IgM antibodies were also involved) and complement binding.

Dettmer et al (79[CR]) described 2 women with increased platelet aggregation following intramuscular administration of Arteparon forte 125 mg 3 times per week. One patient complained of headaches, pain and twitching of the hands, and paresthesias, while the other patient suffered from headaches, coldness, shivers, and stupor, as well as pain in the hip and left leg. The immunological basis of the Arteparon effects was suggested by the identification of an IgG antibody acting as aggregating factor in the plasma of one of the patients.

In the 2 cases recorded by Dettmer and associates, symptoms receded after discontinuation of the Arteparon therapy. It is well documented, however, that heparin-induced increased platelet aggregation may be complicated by thromboembolic events, such as recurrent or multiple pulmonary embolus, myocardial infarction, and death (80[C]). Similar grave effects have been observed following the parenteral use of pentosane polysulfate. This substance, which is also known as xylan polyhydrogen sulfate or SP 54, belongs to the group of low-molecular-weight heparinoids (83[c], 84[R]). It is therefore not surprising that Arteparon has also been associated with life-threatening ***thromboembolic manifestations****.*

Arteparon forte 125 mg injections were withdrawn from the market in 1982, after their use had been associated with isolated cases of myocardial infarction, pulmonary embolus, hemiplegic apoplexia, and 4 deaths (60[r], 85[r]).

Arteparon 50 mg injections remained available until 1988, when a female patient in Switzerland reportedly died from cerebral hemorrhage after receiving 3 injections. Although an evaluation was still needed to refute or confirm a causal relationship, the incident prompted the manufacturer to suspend sales temporarily (83[r], 86[r]).

Other reported side effects of Arteparon injections include ***arthropathy***, ***subcutaneous fat necrosis****, and reversible* ***alopecia*** *(60[R], 87[R], 88[R]).*

Concluding remarks

There is no conclusive evidence that the negative effects of chondroprotective agents are outweighed by a beneficial influence. Advocates of this controversial drug class point to positive results in in-vitro experiments, animal studies and human investigations. However, there are no well-designed and well-documented clinical trials which provide objective and unequivocal proof of their therapeutic efficacy, and the recommended dosage regimens for Dona 200-S and Arumalon lack the rational basis of pharmacokinetic data and dose-finding studies in man (60[R], 61[R], 66[R], 67[R]).

Because chondroprotective drugs have such a poor benefit/risk ratio, the West German Health Office announced in 1987 its intention to withdraw the license for the Dona 200-S injection (67[R]) and the Arumalon injection (66[R]). At the time when this review was written, the jury for Arumalon was still out (89[r]), but the license for Dona 200-S injections has been withdrawn permanently (69[r]). Also, the marketing license for the Arteparon 50 mg injection was suspended for 5 years (unless additional studies would provide such convincing proof of efficacy that premature annulment of this suspension would be justified) (90[r]).

Remarkably, the measures of the West German Health Office have not affected the availability of the biggest chondroprotective seller, Dona 200-S tablets, even though the usefulness of this oral dosage form is as poorly documented as that of the injection. The reason is that the West German Drug Law does not permit the Health Office to ban a drug product only because there is insufficient proof of efficacy (89[r]).

Rattlesnake meat

Dried rattlesnake meat is a well-known Mexican folk remedy. It is used for the treatment of various ailments, such as systemic lupus erythematosus (SLE), diabetes, skin disorders, cancer, and AIDS. It can be purchased without prescription in Mexico, El Salvador, and the southwestern part of the United States. It is available as such and in the form of powder, capsules or pills, which may be labeled in Hispanic as *víbora de cascabel*, *pulvo de víbora*, or *carne de víbora* (91[CR], 92[CR], 93[C]). These products represent a serious health threat, since the rattlesnake is a well-established reservoir for *Salmonella arizona*. This pathogenic Gram-negative bacillus was formerly denominated as *Arizona hinshawii* and has how been reclassified as *Salmonella enterica* subspecies *arizonae*. It causes clinical syndromes similar to those seen with other *Salmonella*: gastroenteritis, enteric fever, septicemia, and localized infections of the urinary tract or the joint.

Eleven cases have now been reported, in which rattlesnake meat was incriminated as the proven or most likely cause of a severe extragastrointestinal infection with *S. arizona*. Eight of these cases have been described in detail (91[CR], 92[CR], 93[C]–96[C]). Typically, victims were Hispanic patients with an underlying medical illness that undermined their immunological integrity, such as SLE or AIDS. In most cases *S. arizona* was isolated from the blood. Additional isolation sites were lymph nodes, pleural fluid, peritoneal fluid, urine, joint fluid, bone marrow, stool, urine, sputum, and cerebrospinal fluid. In several cases, *S. arizona* was also recovered from the patient's rattlesnake preparation, and it was sometimes even shown to be of the same serotype as the organism isolated from the patient (91[CR]). Although most patients responded well to intravenous therapy with ampicillin or co-trimoxazole, 2 cases had a fatal outcome.

Bhatt et al (92[CR]) described a 27-year-old Hispanic woman who was taking prednisone and hydroxychloroquine for systemic lupus erythematosus. She presented with weakness, fever and chills, and arthralgias. After her blood cultures had grown *S. arizona*, she admitted that she had used raw dried rattlesnake meat purchased in a Mexican herb shop. She received a course of intravenous ampicillin, but restarted her intake of the rattlesnake meat at home. She returned 2 weeks later with a relapse, which required 4 weeks of intravenous therapy with co-trimoxazole. She did well until 4 months after her discharge, when a second relapse occurred. She was found to have developed gastroenteritis, bacteremia, peritonitis, and meningitis. The *S. arizona*, isolated after this readmission was of the same serotype as the previous one. This time she had been using a fluid Mexican folk medicine, but cultures of this potion were only positive for *Enterobacter* and *Citrobacter*. The patient seemed to respond well to intravenous ampicillin and repeated lumbar punctures, but her condition deteriorated after 1 month, and she finally died with renal failure, *Pseudomonas* pneumonia, and gastrointestinal bleeding. Rattlesnake capsules bought in the same Mexican neighborhood where the patient had obtained her rattlesnake meat were positive for *S. arizona* of a different serotype.

Fainstein et al (95[C]) reported the death of a 66-year-old male cancer patient who developed recurrent overwhelming infection and septicemia due to *S. arizona* after taking rattlesnake capsules for lymphoma.

An additional point of concern is that rattlesnake products may also be infested with *Escherichia coli*, *Klebsiella* species, and *Pseudomonas aeruginosa* (91[CR]).

Adverse esophageal effects of non-orthodox medicines

There were two direct reasons for preparing a special review on this subject. One reason was that several products and substances which are commonly used in non-orthodox medicine were incriminated as causative agents in recent case-reports on drug-induced esophageal injury (97[C]–100[C]). The other reason was that slimming aids containing guar gum have recently been banned in the United Kingdom because of the fact that guar gum and related bulk-producing substances have been repeatedly associated with esophageal obstruction (101[R], 102[r], 103[r]).

Indirect effects

Drug-induced esophageal disease may be caused by local effects or by indirect mechanisms. Although the latter type of injury will not be fully reviewed here, it should be noted that there are at least two ways in which drugs of natural origin may damage the esophagus indirectly. One mechanism is a reduction in the lower esophageal sphincter pressure, which will predispose the patient to reflux esophagitis (104[R], 105[R]). Medications capable of this side effect include the anticholinergic alkaloid, atropine (106[C]). Another possibility is that induction of violent vomiting by a natural drug results in laceration of the esophago-gastric junction. The serious nature of this complication is highlighted by rare cases of Mallory-Weiss syndrome secondary to ipecac-induced emesis (107[C], 108[C]).

Direct injury

In addition to producing indirect esophageal damage, drugs may also injure the esophagus by direct contact with the esophageal mucosa. This effect may occur when a tablet or capsule does not advance into the stomach following ingestion, but sticks in the esophagus. This will be especially hazardous, of course, when the drug has considerable caustic potential, e.g. if it can rapidly dissolve to produce an acidic or hyperosmotic solution. Factors predisposing to the lodgment of solid dosage forms in the eosphagus include large size and strong adhesiveness of the drug product, swallowing with insufficient liquid or in a supine position, and anatomical or motility disorders of the esophagus. Characteristic symptoms are retrosternal pain, odynophagia, and dysphagia, which may occasionally be severe enough to require hospitalization. Serious sequelae, including death, have been linked to slow-release preparations of potassium chloride, but serious complications with other medications have been rare. The effects usually reside within 7–10 days of symptomatic therapy (105[R], 109[R]–113[R]).

A handful of orthodox agents (notably doxycycline hyclate and emepronium bromide) account for the majority of cases reported so far (111[R], 112[R]). In some cases, however, the offending agent is either a non-orthodox medicine or an orthodox drug, which could be taken for non-orthodox reasons.

Vitamin products *Ascorbic acid (vitamin C) produces a distinctly acidic solution, when dissolved. Although it would not ordinarily be regarded as a non-orthodox remedy it merits this classification when used in mega-doses, and it is precisely these doses which are likely to give rise to risk. The drug has been associated with esophageal injury on 3 separate occasions.*

Walta et al (114[C]) described a 24-year-old woman with an esophageal motor disorder, who developed localized proximal esophagitis following ingestion of a 500-mg ascorbic acid tablet. The caustic effect of the tablet was confirmed in an animal model.

Kikendall et al (97[Cr]) observed drug-induced esophageal ulceration and stricture in a 61-year-old woman who was at special risk for tablet retention because of cardiomegaly and recent mitral valve surgery. Although the offending agent could not be identified with absolute certainty, the patient specifically related the onset of her symptoms to the ingestion of an ascorbic acid tablet.

Bonavina et al (110[CR]) reported an association between ascorbic acid intake and the development of esophageal ulceration and stricture in a 58-year-old woman who apparently did not have a pre-existing esophageal abnormality. Dilatation of her esophagus resulted in a perforation, which required resection and colon interposition.

In addition to the reports on ascorbic acid, two publications have associated esophagitis with the use of a multivitamin.

Kobler et al (115[C]) attributed a case of esophageal ulceration to Pantogar, a multivitamin preparation with thiamine HCl, calcium pantothenate, para-aminobenzoic acid, cystin, faex and keratin. Bova et al (116[c]) ascribed another case of esophagitis to an unidentified multivitamin product.

Herbal cough remedies *Most reports about esophageal side effects of herbal drug products relate to obstruction by bulk-producing laxatives or slimming aids (see below). Only a single case-report has been recovered from the literature which incriminated a herbal tablet as the cause of focal esophagitis.*

Fiedorek and Casteel (98[C]) examined a 9-year-old boy who was referred to hospital after suffering for 1 week from retrosternal pain that was exacerbated by swallowing. Radiography and esophagoscopy showed 2 opposing circumscribed erythematous mucosal abrasions at the level of the aortic notch. The patient had swallowed a eucalyptus oil/menthol cough tablet (Halls Mentho-Lyptus) without water. The symptoms abated within 1 week.

Tryptophan *This amino acid is advocated in non-orthodox medicine for the treatment of depression and insomnia. Its use in the form of a tablet was recently associated with a case of intramural esophageal hematoma.*

Piccione et al (99[C]) reported an 81-year-old woman with diuretic-treated hypertension, who presented to hospital because of chest pain, nausea and blood vomiting. The evening before her admission she had taken 2 tryptophan tablets before retiring, and she had felt that the second one stuck in her midchest. Endoscopy demonstrated partial occlusion of the esophageal lumen by a hemorrhagic mass arsing from the posterior wall and extending for about 15 cm. Biopsy specimens contained talc, a common filler in pharmaceutical dosage forms. Radiographic examination showed an intramural esophageal mass. The barium stream became eccentric just below the cricopharyngeal muscle and remained thin for the entire length of the esophagus. At the level of the aortic arch, a 3-cm mucosal tear could be observed. Computed tomography revealed eccentric compression of the lumen by a para-esophageal mass of a density consistent with a hematoma. Symptoms resolved over 4-5 days.

The exact mechanism by which the tryptophan tablet induced the esophageal hematoma in this case remains to be clarified.

Papain *This proteolytic enzyme is obtained from the fruit juice of* ***Carica papaya****. It is included in health food tablets and capsules because of its digestive properties. There are no actual case-reports associating such papain products with esophageal injury. However, in view of adverse experiences with the use of a papain solution to treat esophageal meat impaction, it is difficult to exclude the possibility that a papain-rich health food might cause topical damage, once it remains stuck in the esophagus.*

Davis et al (100[C]) treated a 54-year-old man with a papain solution because of food lodging in his esophagus. The impaction resolved within 90 min without pain or discomfort, but radiographic and endoscopic examination showed numerous tiny ulcerations at the level of the previous obstruction. A second examination on the 5th hospital day revealed minimal residual ulceration and inflammation.

Andersen et al (117[C]) described a 27-year-old woman who died from esophageal perforation after the use of papain for meat impaction. Approximately half a day after the ingestion of the proteolytic enzyme, the patient experienced rapidly progressive mediastinitis, which terminated in perforation of the common carotid artery and sudden massive hemorrhage. Although actual perforation of the esophagus could not be reproduced in dog experiments, these experiments showed that papain is capable of damaging the esophageal wall.

A similar case of fatal esophageal perforation following papain ingestion to soften and dislodge impacted meat was reported by Holsinger et al (118[C]).

Another potentially lethal complication of the use of papain to relieve esphageal meat impaction was recently described by Hall and Huseby (119[C]) who observed hemorrhagic pulmonary edema due to inadvertent aspiration of the papain solution.

Fumaric acid derivatives *These compounds are currently used in certain European countries as therapeutic agents for psoriasis. Although there are no well-documented cases in which esophagitis following the use of these agents was confirmed by esophagoscopy, dimethylfumarate was reported to cause esophageal pain (113[c], 120[c]). In view of the potential of fumaric acid derivatives to produce gastrointestinal problems (SEDA-13, p. 458), it would be far from surprising if they proved capable of exerting a caustic effect on the esophagus.*

Esophageal obstruction

In addition to being caused by systemic effects or local injury, esophageal adverse reactions may also be induced by bulk-forming medications. Such drugs may swell up before having passed the esophagus and may thus result in esophageal obstruction. There are two distinct classes of botanical medicines which have actually been associated with esophageal blockade because of their ability to swell up in contact with fluids. One is the well-known group of herbal bulk laxatives, such as ispaghula, psyllium, and sterculia gum. The other group consists of natural vegetable fibers, such as glucomannan and guar, which quickly form a non-absorbable viscous gum with water. While these fibers are under investigation for their potential usefulness in regular medicine (121[C], 122[R], 123[C]), they are also heavily promoted outside the orthodox circuit as weight-control agents.

Herbal laxatives *Bulk-forming herbal laxatives have an excellent safety record. However, this does not alter the fact that at least 17 cases of esophageal obstruction due to these agents have been published over the past 50 years (124[C]–137[C]).*

The offending drugs were bassorin, which is the major insoluble constituent of tragacanth

(2×), sterculia gum (4×), ispaghula (10×), and psyllium (1×). In 5 cases, these bulk-forming substances were combined with a natural anthranoid laxative. The patients were 8 males and 9 females with a mean age of 70.8 years (range 47–87 years). Typical symptoms were a sudden onset, progressive substernal pain and inability to swallow food or water, sometimes accompanied by pseudohypersialorrhea. Radiography and esophagoscopy usually revealed complete obstruction of the lower third of the esophagus by a gelatinous mass. Inflammation of the esophagal mucosa (130[C], 131[C], 133[C]) or a shallow esophageal ulcer (134[C]) were reported in some cases. The obstructing mass was mostly removed by mechanical means and was taken out by esophagotomy in one patient (129[C]). One patient did not recover uneventfully:

A sterculia-induced esophageal obstruction in an 80-year-old woman was complicated by consolidation in the pulmonary lobes, which was attributed to aspiration. On her 20th hospital day, she developed fever and X-raying revealed an abscess cavity in the apex of the right lower lobe posteriorly. Sputum culture yielded ***Pseudomonas aeruginosa***. The patient did not respond to antibiotics and died 10 days later (133[C]).

Some patients had no disorder of the esophagus to explain the obstruction (131[C], 134[C]), whereas others had esophageal or gastric abnormalities, such as hiatal hernia (129[C], 133[C], 137[C]), a small epibronchic diverticulum (130[C]) or subtotal gastric resection (128[C]). It usually remained uncertain, however, whether this pathology had played a contributory role. The majority of patients took an overdose or swallowed the drug without sufficient water.

Bulk-producing slimming aids Certain types of slimming tablets, capsules and granules contain a dehydrated vegetable fiber with considerable capacity to absorb water. When swallowed, these products may swell up rapidly inside the stomach to several times their original volume. This is claimed to produce a sensation of satiety, which will help overweight patients to lose weight. Concern has arisen, however, that such products may put users at the risk of esophageal obstruction and even rupture of the esophagus, because they may also swell up rapidly, when they accidentally stick in the esophagus. Recent Australian experiences with glucomannan tablets have shown that this is not an imaginary health hazard.

Glucomannan is a hygroscopic fiber obtained from ***Amorphophallus knojac***. It is considerably hygroscopic and on contact with water swells and becomes a viscous gel. After tablets containing dry non-expanded glucomannan had been introduced in Australia as an over-the-counter appetite suppressant, the Australian Adverse Drug Reaction Advisory Committee received 8 reports of partial or complete esophageal obstruction (138[CR], 139[r]).

Most patients were non-elderly women without esophageal disease, who were taking the tablets for weight reduction. Two cases resolved spontaneously after 5 and 17 hours, but the other 6 patients required removal by rigid esophagoscopy. In at least 4 of these latter cases the obstruction was in the upper third of the esophagus. In one patient, esophagoscopy was complicated by esophageal perforation leading to mediastinitis, which necessitated a 2 months' stay in hospital. When the tablets were placed in water or diluted hydrochloric acid solution, they rapidly expanded from <1 ml to 12–16 ml after 10 min immersion. Their viscosity increased to the extent that they became rubbery and would bounce when thrown on the floor.

These reports led to a ban of glucomannan tablets in Australia, which did not affect the availability of encapsulated and powdered forms (138[R]). In the United Kingdom, the sale of slimming aids containing glucomannan or the related galactomannan had already been prohibited for years. This ban was recently expanded to include slimming products containing more than 15% of guar gum or the related locust bean gum (101[R], 102[r], 103[r]).

Guar gum comes from the endosperm of the seeds of the cluster bean (***Cyanopsis tetragonoloba***). Although it is reported to produce a smaller gel volume and lower gel viscosity than glucomannan (140[c]), its use has likewise been associated with esophageal obstruction.

A Danish guar gum granulate called Lej-guar was incriminated in 3 cases. According to the directions for use, this granulate has to be taken by sprinkling 5–10 g on 50 ml of water and by ingesting the stirred mixture immediately. Two of the cases concerned patients in their 50s who developed total obstruction without serious complications (141[C], 142[C]). In the 3rd case, the obstruction in a 60-year-old woman was complicated by respiratory problems and esophageal rupture (143[C]). The latter case as well as one of the other 2 cases were observed in Sweden and prompted a prohibition of Lej-guar as a health food product by the Swedish National Board of Health and Welfare (144[r]). Even though this decision was challenged, inter alia with the argument that there was no causal relationship between the esophageal rupture and the Lej-guar obstruction (145[r]), the Board upheld its decision (146[r]).

The German antidiabetic medicine Glucotard, which is also a guar gum granulate, was responsible for a case of complete obstruction of the distal esophagus in a 63-year-old man. This patient ingested 5 g with 250 ml of water as usual and experienced a feeling of retrosternal pressure, which made him drink 20 ml of liquor. This did not bring relief, however, and symptoms deteriorated rapidly. Esophagoscopy revealed an obstructive bolus, which had to removed with the aid of pincers. In vitro testing of the granulate suggested a contributing effect of the liquor intake: the addition of 20 ml of water to 5 g of granulate resulted in a viscous fluid, whereas mixing of the same amount with 10 ml of water and 10 ml of 40% alcohol produced a solid mass within 1 min (147[C]).

On basis of these case-reports, the British Ministry of Agriculture, Fisheries and Foods decided that it would be illegal in the United Kingdom to sell slimming products containing more than 15% of guar gum or locust bean from June 1989 (103[r]). One might wonder whether this ban is overshooting the mark a little, because it does not take into account the fact that the viscosity of guar gum products may vary considerably (148[c]), depending on factors such as the exact method of processing (149[C]). It might also be added that we were unable to reproduce the reported solidifying effect of alcohol on the German medicine Glucotard, when we tested Lej-guar granulate in our laboratory (150[c]).

However, even if the British ban were too indiscriminate, this should no be regarded as any serious injustice, because there is no substantial proof that guar gum helps obese users to loose weight (151[r], 152[R]). Promotional sources would like us to belief that guar gum reduces the desire to eat by swelling up inside the stomach and producing a sense of satiety. Radiographic experiments have shown, however, that tablets containing 0.5 or 1.0 g of the bulk-producer methylcellulose rapidly advance from the stomach into the small bowel, when they are taken on an empty stomach (153[c]). There is no evidence that tablets or capsules providing a similar dose of guar gum will behave differently.

Concluding remarks

It should be borne in mind that the cases which have been reviewed here may not reflect the true prevalence of non-orthodox drug-induced esophageal problems. Many cases probably go unrecognized, because patients with mild symptoms often do not consult a physician (105[R]), and when patients present with an esophageal complaint following the use of a herbal product or other alternative medicine, the chances seem low that this will actually result in a published case-report.

When Noble and Grannis (137[Cr]) brought their observation of acute esophageal obstruction by a psyllium-based bulk laxative to the attention of the manufacturer, the manufacturer replied that 21 reports about esophageal blockage by the product (apparently unpublished) had been received in the previous 3 years.

The Australian experience with glucomannan-containing slimming tablets shows that a non-orthodox product can present such a substantial risk of esophageal problems that an irreversible ban is warranted. This regulatory step would be unrealistic, however, for most of the alternative products which have been associated here with esophageal injury or obstruction. Nevertheless, prescribers and users should be made aware that even commonly used non-orthodox medicines, such as vitamin C tablets, tryptophan tablets and herbal laxatives, can result in a painful and frightening experience, which may be complicated by potentially serious sequelae, if such products are not administered in the appropriate way. Users should be clearly instructed to take a bulk-forming product without exceeding the recommended dose and to take sufficient water simultaneously with the preparation. Users of unorthodox capsules and tablets should be advised to swallow these products in an upright position with a liberal amount of water. Caution should be exercised by elderly and bed-ridden people and by other groups at special risk (113[R]), such as patients who have undergone valvular heart surgery (97[R]).

It is almost needless to say that these recommendations demonstrate the need for adequate patient information on alternative medicines, as has already been emphasized in the section on herbal remedies.

REFERENCES

1. De Smet PAGM, Rivier L (1989) A general outlook on ethnopharmacology. *J. Ethnopharmacol.*, *25*, 127.
2. Thyagarajan SP, Thiruneelakantan K, Subramanian S, Sundaravelu T (1982) In vitro inactivation of HBsAg by *Elipta alba* Hassk and *Phyllanthus niruri* Linn. *Indian J. Med. Res.*, *76*, 124.
3. Venkateswaran PS, Millman I, Blumberg BS (1987) Effects of an extract from *Phyllanthus niruri* on hepatitis B and woodchuck hepatitis viruses: in vitro and in vivo studies. *Proc. Natl. Acad. Sci. USA*, *84*, 274.
4. Thyagarajan SP, Subramanian S, Thirunalasundari T et al (1988) Effect of *Phyllanthus amarus* on chronic arriers of hepatitis B virus. *Lancet*, *2*, 764.
5. Jayaram S, Thyagarajan SP, Panchanadam M, Subramanian S (1987) Anti-hepatitis B properties of *Phyllanthus niruri* Linn. and *Elipta alba* hassk: in vitro and in vivo safety studies. *Biomedicine*, *7*, 9.
6. Brook MG (1988) Effect of *Phyllanthus amarus* on chronic carriers of hepatitis B virus. *Lancet 2*, 1017.
7. Anonymous (1988) *Pyrrolizidine Alkaloids*. Environmental Health Criteria 80, World Health Organization, Geneva.
8. Hutchings A, Terblanche SE (1989) Observations on the use of some known and suspected toxic Liliiflorae in Zulu and Xhosa medicine. *South Afr. Med. J.*, *75*, 62.
9. Green EC (1988) Can collaborative programs between biomedical and African indigenous health practitioners succeed? *Soc. Sci. Med.*, *27*, 1125.
10. Walker HC, Nivatvongs S, Gedgaudas E (1983) Rectal injury during barium enema examination. *J. Am. Med. Assoc.*, *249*, 2780.
11. Anonymous (1988) Developers need to keep their ears open. *New Sci.*, *119*, 62.
12. Radford DJ, Gillies AD, Hinds JA, Duffy P (1986) Naturally occurring cardiac glycosides. *Med. J. Aust.*, *144*, 540.
13. Cheung K, Hinds JA, Duffy P (1989) Detection of poisoning by plant-origin cardiac glycoside with the Abbott TDx Analyzer. *Clin. Chem.*, *35*, 295.
14. Fushimi R, Tachi J, Amino N, Miyai K (1989) Chinese medicine interfering with digoxin immunoassays. *Lancet*, *1*, 339.
15. Liewendahl K, Turula M (1972) Iodide-induced goitre and hypothyroidism in a patient with chronic lymphocytic thyroiditis. *Acta Endocrinol.*, *71*, 289.
16. Sorisky A, Robbins DC (1989) Fish oil and diabetes. The net effect. *Diabetes Care*, *12*, 302.
17. De Smet PAGM (1988) Vrij verkrijgbare kruidenmiddelen met fatale leverbeschadiging in verband gebracht. *Pharm. Weekbl.*, *123*, 804.
18. Anonymous (1988) Vragen. Tweede Kamer der Staten-Generaal, Vergaderjaar 1988–1989, 29 september 1988, 1.
19. De Smet PAGM (1988) Laetrile tussen wal en schip. *Med. Contact*, *43*, 976.
20. De Smet PAGM (1989) Dutch patient information on the safe use of herbal remedies. *Int. Pharm. J.*, *3*, 98.
21. Anonymous (1989) Wijziging Besluit farmaceutische hulp ziekenfondsverzekering. *Staatscourant, 6 februari*, 8.
22. Battaglino G (1987) *EEC Directives and Recommendations in the Pharmaceutical Field.* Organizzazione Editoriale Medico Farmaceutica, Milan.
23. Anonymous (undated) *Quality of Herbal Remedies*. Committee for Proprietary Medicinal Products, Brussels.
24. Hausen B, Busker E, Carle R (1984) Über das Sensibilierungsvermögen von Compositenarten. VII. Experimentelle Untersuchungen mit Auszügen und Inhaltstoffen von *Chamomilla recutita* (L.) Rauschert und *Anthemis cotula* L. *Planta Med.*, *50*, 229.
25. Mauz Ch, Candrian U, Lüthy J et al (1985) Methode zur Entfernung von Pyrrolizidin-Alkaloiden aus Arzneipflanzenextrakten. *Pharm. Acta Helv.*, *60*, 256.
26. Van de Dungen FM, Vermeulen NPE, Fischer FC et al (1987) Removal of pyrrolizidine alkaloids from *Symphytum* tinctures – their toxicity towards isolated hepatocytes. *Pharm. Weekbl. Sci. Ed.*, *9*, 222.
27. De Smet PAGM (1987) Kruidenmiddelen en volksgezondheid. *Pharm. Weekbl.*, *122*, 1069.
28. Wichtl M (1989) *Teedrogen. Ein Handbuch für die Praxis auf wissenschaftlicher Grundlage, 2. Aufl.* Wissenschaftliche Verlagsgesellschaft mbH, Stuttgart.
29. Lieberman HR, Wurtman RJ, Emde GG et al (1987) The effects of low doses of caffeine on human performance and mood. *Psychopharmacology*, *92*, 308.
30. Gallant CJ, Macaulay T, Chandler RF (1981) Caffeine: a hazardous drug? *Can. Pharm. J.*, *114*, 212.
31. Hegnauer R (1964–1973) *Chemotaxonomie der Pflanzen, Band 3–Band 6*. Birkhäuser Verlag, Basel.
32. List PH, Hörhammer L (1973–1977) *Hagers Handbuch der Pharmazeutischen Praxis, Vierte Neuausgabe, Band 4–Band 6*. Springer-Verlag, Berlin.
33. Holmstedt B, Lindgren JE (1972) Alkaloid analyses of botanical material more than a thousand years old. *Etnol. Stud.*, *32*, 139.
34. Hoppe HA (1975) *Drogenkunde, Band 1: Angiospermen, 8. Aufl.* Walter de Gruyter, Berlin.
35. Lewis WH, Elvin-Lewis PF (1977) *Medical Botany – Plants Affecting Man's Health*, p. 386. John Wiley and Sons, New York.
36. Ashton CH (1987) Caffeine and health. *Br. Med. J.*, *295*, 1293.

37. Wilcox A, Weinberg C, Baird D (1988) Caffeinated beverages and decreased fertility. *Lancet, 2*, 1453.
38. Wilcox AJ (1989) Caffeinated beverages and decreased fertility. *Lancet, 1*, 840.
39. Casas M, Ferrer S, Calaf J et al (1989) Dopaminergic mechanism for caffeine-induced decrease in fertility? *Lancet, 1*, 731.
40. Christianson RE, Oechsli FW, Van den Berg BJ (1989) Caffeinated beverages and decreased fertility. *Lancet, 1*, 378.
41. Bennett PN (1988) *Drugs and Human Lactation*. Elsevier, Amsterdam.
42. Oei SG, Vosters RPL, Van der Hagen NLJ (1989) Fetal arrhythmia caused by excessive intake of caffeine by pregnant women. *Br. Med. J., 298*, 568.
43. De Smet PAGM, Elferink F, Verpoorte R (1989) Linksdraaiend tetrahydropalmatine in Chinese tablet. *Ned. Tijdschr. Geneeskd., 133*, 308.
44. Quansheng C (1986) Yanhusuo. In: Chang H-M, But PP-H (Eds) *Pharmacology and Applications of Chinese Materia Medica, Vol. I*, p. 515. World Scientific Publishing Co., Singapore.
45. Yang YC (1959) Clinical observations on the analgesic action of Corydalis B. *Acta Acad. Med. Primae Shanghai, 6*, 581.
46. Jin G-Z (1987) (−)-Tetrahydropalmatine and its analogs as new dopamine receptor antagonists. *Trends Pharmacol. Sci., 8*, 81.
47. Xu S-X, Jin G-Z, Yu L-P et al (1987) Brain dopamine depleted by *d*-tetrahydropalmatine. *Acta Pharmacol. Sin., 8*, 212.
48. Van Ulsen J, Stolz E, Joost T (1988) Chromate dermatitis from a homeopathic drug. *Contact Derm., 18*, 56.
49. Slater PE, Ben-Ishai P, Leventhal A et al (1988) An acupuncture associated outbreak of hepatitis B in Jerusalem. *Eur. J. Epidemiol., 4*, 322.
50. Kent GP, Brondum J, Keenylside RA et al (1988) A large outbreak of acupuncture-associated hepatitis B. *Am. J. Epidemiol., 127*, 591.
51. Boxall EH (1978) Acupuncture-associated hepatitis in the West Midlands, 1977. *J. Med. Virol., 2*, 377.
52. Kobler E, Schmuziger P, Hartmann G (1979) Hepatitis nach Akupunctur. *Schweiz. Med. Wochenschr., 109*, 1828.
53. De Galocsy C, Geubel AP, Gulbis A, Dive C (1982) Hépatite sur acupuncture: rapport de sept cas. *Acta Gastro-Enterol. Belg., 45*, 224.
54. Stryker WS, Gunn RA, Francis DP (1986) Outbreak of hepatitis B associated with acupuncture. *J. Fam. Pract., 22*, 155.
55. Conn H (1988) Acupuncture in epidemic HBV hepatitis: in China too? *Hepatology, 8*, 1176.
56. Castro KG, Lifson AR, White CR et al (1988) Investigations of AIDS patients with no previously identified risk factors. *J. Am. Med. Assoc., 259*, 1338.
57. Vittecoq D, Mettetal JF, Rouzioux C et al (1989) Acute HIV infection after acupuncture treatments. *N. Engl. J. Med., 320*, 250.
58. Denzin M (1987) Acupuncture and AIDS: some guidelines for the prevention of nosocomial disease transmission. *Am. J. Acupunct., 15*, 355.
59. Sisco V, Winters LL, Zange LL, Brennan PC (1988) Efficacy of various methods of sterilization of acupuncture needles. *J. Manipulative Physiol. Ther., 11*, 94.
60. Anonymous (1986) 'Knorpelschutzstoffe' – gibt es eine 'Basistherapie der Arthrose'? *Arznei-Telegr., 1*, 3.
61. Loosen W, Morck H (1988) Chondroprotektiva – eine Wirkstofgruppe noch ohne Profil. *Pharm. Ztg., 133/8*, 9.
62. Anonymous (undated) *Novitätenkartei*. Werbe- und Vertriebsgesellschaft Deutscher Apotheker mbH, Frankfurt am Main.
63. Anonymous (1989) *Codex Galenica 1989*. Documentation Galenica, Bern.
64. Schacht E, Roetz R (1989) Nephrotic syndrome after injections of bovine cartilage and marrow extract. *Lancet, 1*, 963.
65. Schmidt G (1988) Antirheumatika und Antiphlogistika. In: Schwabe U, Paffrath D (Eds), *Arzneiverordnungs-Report '88. Aktuelle Daten, Kosten, Trends und Kommentare*, p. 90. Gustav Fischer Verlag, Stuttgart.
66. Anonymous (1987) Vorinformation Arumalon Injektionslösung. *Pharm. Ztg., 132*, 2838.
67. Anonymous (1981) Vorinformation Dona 200 S Injektionslösung. *Pharm. Ztg., 132*, 3007.
68. Zuber M, Mall T (1987) Staphylokokkensepsis nach intramuskulärer Injektion. *Schweiz. Med. Wochenschr., 117*, 328.
69. BGA Pressedienst (1989) *Widerruf der Zulassung für Dona 200-S, Injektionslösung*. Pressebericht nr. 17, April 26, 1989, Bundesgesundheitsamt, Berlin.
70. Hunold W (1981) Fingergelenkarthrose. Ergebnisse einer Kurzzeittherapie mit Dona 200 S. *Z. Allg. Med., 57*, 1686.
71. BGA Pressedienst (1987) *Dona 200 S Injektionslösung*. Pressebericht nr. 2, January 6, 1987, Bundesgesundheitsamt, Berlin.
72. Anonymous (1988) Soll Arumalon die Zulassung entzogen werden? *Dtsch. Apoth. Ztg., 128*, 2322.
73. Anonymous (1988) Arumalon enthält nicht deklariertes Rinderserumalbumin. *Arznei-Telegr., 11*, 100.
74. Anonymous (1987) Dermatomyositis/Polyserositis nach Arumalon-Injektionskuren. *Arznei-Telegr., 10*, 92.
75. Glogner P, Berg PA, Becker W (1989) Nebenwirkungen eines Knorpelextrakts. *Dtsch. Med. Wochenschr., 114*, 319.

76. Dürk H, Haase K, Saal J et al (1989) Nephrotic syndrome after injections of bovine cartilage and marrow extract. *Lancet, 1*, 614.
77. Roetz R, Schacht E (1989) Nebenwirkungen eines Knorpelextrakts. *Dtsch. Med. Wochenschr., 114*, 809.
78. Wolf H, Nowack H, Wick G (1983) Detection of antibodies interacting with glycosaminoglycan polysulfate in patients treated with heparin or other polysulfated glycosaminoglycans. *Int. Arch. Allergy Appl. Immunol., 70*, 157.
79. Dettmer N, Nowack H, Raake W (1983) Thrombozyten-Aggregation nach Heparin und Arteparon. Klinische Bedeutung. *Münch. Med. Wochenschr., 125*, 540.
80. Chong BH, Pitney WR, Castaldi PA (1982) Heparin-induced thrombocytopenia: association of thrombotic complications with heparin-dependent IgG antibody that induces thromboxane synthesis and platelet aggregation. *Lancet, 2*, 1246.
81. Böttiger LE (1985) Heparin-induced thrombocytopenia. *Acta Med. Scand., 218*, 257.
82. Wolf H, Wick G (1986) Antibodies interacting with, and corresponding binding site for, heparin on human thrombocytes. *Lancet, 2*, 222.
83. Anonymous (1988) 'Chondroprotektiva' in der Diskussion. *Arznei-Telegr., 6*, 49.
84. Anonymous (1988) Xylan-polyhydrogensulfat: Thrombocytopenien und Thromboembolien. *Pharm. Ztg., 133/21*, 6.
85. Anonymous (1988) Nachwirkungen. *Arznei-Telegr., 5*, 47.
86. Anonymous (1988) Nutzen-Risiko-Bewertung von Chondroprotektiva. *Dtsch. Apoth. Ztg., 128*, 1007.
87. Anonymous (1987) 'Knorpelschutzstoffe' im Spiegel der Nachzulassung. *Arznei-Telegr., 1*, 2.
88. BGA Pressedienst (1987) *'Bundesgesundheitsamt beabsichtigt Zulassungswiderruf für 'Arteparon'. Ein Ergebnis der Aufbereitung des Marktes von Alt-Arzneimitteln durch unabhängige Sachverständigenkommission.* Pressebericht nr. 36, July 15, 1987, Bundesgesundheitsamt, Berlin.
89. Anonymous (1989) 'Aus' für DONA-S Injektionslösung. *Arznei-Telegr., 5*, 51.
90. Anonymous (1988) Ruhen der Zulassung – Arteparon Injektionslösung. *Pharm. Ztg., 133/40*, 122.
91. Riley KB, Antoniskis D, Maris R, Leedom JM (1988) Rattlesnake capsule-associated *Salmonella arizona* infections. *Arch. Intern. Med., 148*, 1207.
92. Bhatt BD, Zuckerman MJ, Foland JA et al (1989) Disseminated *Salmonella arizona* infection associated with rattlesnake meat ingestion. *Am. J. Gastroenterol., 84*, 433.
93. Fleischman S, Haake DA, Lovett MA (1989) *Salmonella arizona* infections associated with ingestion of rattlesnake capsules. *Arch. Intern. Med., 149*, 701.
94. Anonymous (1983) *Arizona hinshawii* septicemia associated with rattlesnake powder – California. *Morbid. Mortal. Wkly Rep., 32*, 464.
95. Fainstein V, Yancey R, Trier O, Bodey GP (1982) Overwhelming infection in a cancer patient caused by *Arizona hinshawii*: its relation to snake pill ingestion. *Am. J. Infect. Control, 10*, 147.
96. McIntyre Jr KE, Malone JM, Richards E, Axline SG (1982) Mycotic aortic pseudoaneurysm with aortoenteric fistula caused by *Arizona hinshawii. Surgery, 91*, 173.
97. Kikendall JW, Schmidt Jr M, Graeber GM et al (1986) Pill induced esophageal ulceration and stricture following cardiac surgery. *Mil. Med., 151*, 539.
98. Fiedorek SC, Casteel HB (1988) Pediatric medication-induced focal esophagitis. *Clin Pediatr., 27*, 455.
99. Piccione PR, Winkler WP, Baer JW, Kotler DP (1987) Pill-induced intramural esophageal hematoma. *J. Am. Med. Assoc., 257*, 929.
100. Davis M, Thomas LC, Guice KS (1987) Esophagitis after papain. *J. Clin. Gastroenterol., 9*, 127.
101. Anonymous (1988) *Minister Proposes Ban on Certain Slimming Products.* News Release 3 October, 1988, Ministry of Agriculture, Fisheries and Food, London.
102. Anonymous (1989) Guar gum safety questioned. *Pharm. J., 242*, 70.
103. Anonymous (1989) Guar slimming tablets ban. *Pharm. J., 242*, 611.
104. Bramble MG, Record CO (1978) Drug-induced gastrointestinal disease. *Drugs, 15*, 451.
105. Bott S, McCallum RW (1986) Medication-induced esophageal injury: survey of the literature. *Med. Toxicol., 1*, 449.
106. Bettarello A, Tuttle SG, Grossman MI (1960) Effect of autonomic drugs on gastroesophageal reflux. *Gastroenterology, 39*, 340.
107. Tanberg D, Liechty EJ, Fisbein D et al (1981) Mallory-Weiss syndrome: an unusual complication of ipecac induced emesis. *Ann. Emerg. Med., 10*, 521.
108. Timberlake GA (1984) Ipecac as a cause of the Mallory-Weiss syndrome. *South. Med. J., 77*, 804.
109. Kikendall JW, Friedman AC, Oyewole MA et al (1983) Pill-induced esophageal injury. Case reports and review of the medical literature. *Dig. Dis. Sci., 28*, 174.
110. Bonavina L, DeMeester TR, McChesney L et al (1987) Drug-induced esophageal strictures. *Ann. Surg., 206*, 173.
111. Bott S, Prakash C, McCallum RW (1987) Medication-induced esophageal injury: survey of the literature. *Am. J. Gastroenterol., 82*, 758.
112. Wienbeck M, Berges W, Lübke HJ (1988) Drug-induced oesophageal lesions. *Baillière's Clin. Gastroenterol., 2*, 263.

113. Stricker BHCh, De Smet PAGM (1989) Slokdarmbeschadiging door geneesmiddelen. In: De Smet PAGM, Van Loenen AC, Van der Does E, Offerhaus L (Eds.) *Medicatiebegeleiding, Medisch-Farmaceutische Achtergronden van een Veranderend Geneesmiddelgebruik,* p. 398. Bohn Staflen Van Loghum, Houten-Deurne.

114. Walta DC, Giddens JD, Johnson LF et al (1976) Localized proximal esophagitis secondary to ascorbic acid ingestion and esophageal motor disorder. *Gastroenterology, 70*, 766.

115. Kobler E, Bühler H, Nüesch HJ, Deyhle P (1978) Medikamentös induzierte Ösophagusulzera. *Dtsch. Med. Wochenschr., 103*, 1038.

116. Bova JG, Dutton NE, Goldstein HM, Hoberman LJ (1987) Medication-induced esophagitis: diagnosis by double-contrast esophagography. *Am. J. Radiol., 148*, 731.

117. Andersen HA, Bernatz PE, Grindlay JH (1959) Perforation of the oesophagus after use of a digestant. Report of a case and experimental study. *Ann. Otol. Rhinol. Laryngol., 68*, 890.

118. Holsinger Jr JW, Fuson RL, Sealy WC (1968) Esophageal perforation following meat impaction and papain ingestion. *J. Am. Med. Assoc., 204*, 188.

119. Hall ML, Huseby JS (1988) Hemorrhagic pulmonary edema associated with meat tenderizer treatment for esophageal meat impaction. *Chest, 94*, 640.

120. Nieboer C, De Hoop D, Van Loenen AC, Van Dijk E (1987) De therapie van fumaarzuurderivaten bij psoriasis. *Ned. Tijdschr. Geneeskd., 131*, 1885.

121. Hopman WPM, Huiben PGMP, Speth PAJ, Lamers CBHW (1988) Glucomannan prevents postprandial hypoglycaemia in patients with previous gastric surgery. *Gut, 29*, 930.

122. Peterson DB, Mann JI (1985): Guar: pharmacological fibre or food fibre? *Diabetic Med., 2*, 345.

123. Superko HR, Haskell WL, Sawrey-Kubicek L, Farquhar JW (1988) Effects of solid and liquid guar gum on plasma cholesterol and triglyceride concentrations in moderate hypercholesterolemia. *Am. J. Cardiol., 62*, 51.

124. Goldman JL (1937) Esophageal obstruction from a hygroscopic gum laxative (Saraka). *J. Am. Med. Assoc., 108*, 1408.

125. Waltz MR (1939) Esophageal obstruction resulting form an injudicious method of ingesting a hygroscopic gum laxative (Saraka). *J. Am. Med. Assoc., 112*, 229.

126. Hinkel CL (1951) Complete obstruction of the esophagus following Serutan ingestion. *J. Am. Med. Assoc., 146*, 1129.

127. Roden V (1951) Esophageal obstruction due to Serutan. *J. Am. Med. Assoc., 147*, 777.

128. Melamed A, Marck A (1953) Esophageal obstruction due to Serutan. *J. Am. Med. Assoc., 152*, 318.

129. Gautier-Benoit C (1971) Bézoard de l'oesophage. *Sem. Hôp. Paris, 47*, 1474.

130. Voinchet O, Mouchet A (1974) Obstruction de l'oesophage par mucilage. *Nouv. Presse Méd., 3*, 1223.

131. Laroche C, Caquet R, Remy R, Duflo B (1975) Obstruction aiguë de l'oesophage par mucilage. *Sem. Hôp. Paris, 51*, 2531.

132. Bléry M, Bismuth V, Loiseau B, Chagnon S (1979) Les obstructions oesophagiennes aiguës d'origine alimentaire ou par mucilage. A propos de 15 observations. *J. Radiol., 60*, 395.

133. Sandeman DR, Clements MR, Perrins EJ (1980) Oesophageal obstruction due to hygroscopic gum laxative. *Lancet, 1*, 364.

134. Sauerbruch T, Kuntzen O, Unger W (1980) Agiolax® bolus in the esophagus. Report of two cases. *Endoscopy, 12*, 83.

135. Lyden E, Spandow O (1981) Totalstopp i esofagus efter intag av bulklaxativ. *Läkartidningen, 78*, 4456.

136. Roux E, Nicole A, Capitaine Y (1984) Complication aiguë d'un traitement par laxatif mucilagineux. *Schweiz. Med. Wochenschr., 114*, 1470.

137. Noble JA, Grannis Jr FW (1984) Acute esophageal obstruction by a psyllium-based bulk laxative. *Chest, 86*, 800.

138. Henry DA, Mitchell AS, Aylward J et al (1986) Glucomannan and risk of oesophageal obstruction. *Br. Med. J., 292*, 91.

139. Henry DA, McEwen J (1987) Monitoring the safety of over the counter drugs. *Br. Med. J., 295*, 1414.

140. Garcia MJ, Charlez M, Fauli C et al (1988) Physicochemical comparison of the dietary fibers glucomannan, galactomannan, carboxymethylcellulose, pectin, and wheat bran. *Curr. Ther. Res., 43*, 1010.

141. Ahlman H (1982) Totalstopp i esofagus efter intag av hälsekostmedel. *Läkartidningen, 79*, 1479.

142. Sørensen J, Rasmussen OR (1983) Synkestop efter indtagelse af fiberholdig helsekostprodukt Lej-Guar. *Ugeskr. Laeg., 145*, 171.

143. Edström S, Pettersson G (1982) Esophagusruptur efter intag av naturmedel. *Läkartidningen, 79*, 1478.

144. Anonymous (1982) Socialstyrelsen förbjuder Lej-Guar. *Läkartidningen, 79*, 1478.

145. Tibbling L (1982) Bulkaxativ – är reglerna hardare mot naturmedel än mot läkemedel? *Läkartidningen, 79*, 2621.

146. Mandahl H, Sjöholm I (1982) Ett naturmedel till skall stoppas. *Läkartidningen, 79*, 2622.

147. Ranft K, Imhof W (1983) Bolusobstruktion des distalen Ösophagus durch pflanzliche Quellstoffe (Guarmehl). *Dtsch. Med. Wochenschr., 108*, 1968.

148. Leeds AR, Bolster NR, Andrews R, Truswell AS (1979) Meal viscosity, gastric empyting and glucose absorption in the rat. *Proc. Nutr. Soc., 38*, 44A.

149. Bolliger R (1960) Der Einfluss der Herstellungsmethode und der Wasserstoffionen-Konzentration auf die Viskosität von Guar-Gummi-Schleimen. *Pharm. Acta Helv.*, *35*, 316.
150. De Smet PAGM, Elferink F (1989) Unpublished data.
151. Temme D (1984) Guarmehl als Schlankheitsmittel? *Dtsch. Apoth.-Ztg.*, *124*, 816.
152. Anonymous (1987) Guar gum: of help to diabetics? *Drug Ther. Bull.*, *25*, 65.
153. Drenick EJ (1975) Bulk producers. *J. Am. Med. Assoc.*, *234*, 271.

N.H. Choulis

51 Miscellaneous drugs and agents

Activated charcoal *(SED-11, 790; SEDA-12, 319; SEDA-13, 339)*

Fifteen patients who presented with acute poisoning due to various compounds, such as barbiturates, organophosphates and antihistamines were treated with repeated doses of activated charcoal in order to promote so-called gastrointestinal dialysis (1[R]). During the treatment, 3 patients developed *pulmonary aspiration* and died, despite prior administration of parenteral metoclopramide and ranitidine. To overcome this problem, in the next 6 patients a cuffed endotracheal tube was passed before starting charcoal treatment. The tube was retained for 48 hours, and thereafter no problems with aspiration were encountered.

In another study by Danel (2[R]), dealing with about 800 patients a year, *nausea* and *vomiting* were not uncommon complications. In the opinion of the author, these side effects may be due, apart from the charcoal, also to the far from negligible water load that goes with it. At this center too, all patients who are unrousable on admission and respond poorly to stimulation are intubated before gastric lavage and the charcoal is administered through an orogastric tube.

Contact lenses and fluids *(SED-11, 966, 1035)*

The FDA has sent a safety alert letter to approximately 50 000 ophthalmologists, optometrists and opticians asking them to warn patients about the hazards of improper use of homemade saline solutions in caring for contact lenses. Such use can result in serious infections that could cause *blindness* (3[C]).

Side Effects of Drugs Annual 14
M.N.G. Dukes and L. Beeley, editors

The solutions, generally prepared by dissolving salt tablets or capsules in distilled water, are non-sterile and may be contaminated with such pathogenic micro-organisms as bacteria and Acanthamoeba. Although Acanthamoeba infections are relatively rare, they are very painful and difficult to treat, and can cause blindness.

It must be stressed that homemade saline solutions can be safely used in the heat disinfection of contact lenses since the high temperatures are sufficient to kill the organisms. If they are however used as a rinse or eye drop after disinfection, or in chemical disinfection of the lenses, serious infection can result.

Cyclamate *(SED-11, 1038)*

Despite the onward march of aspartame, cyclamate is still a widely used artificial sweetening agent and has been the subject of numerous studies seeking to clarify the safety margin and possible carcinogenic potential of this substance. One case-report (4[r]) describes a patient with long-standing high-dose cyclamate abuse associated with histological and radiological abnormalities of the small intestine and moderate malabsorption:

The patient had taken excessive amounts of a cyclamate-based candy (Kandisin) up to 400 pieces (14.72 g cyclamate)/d. He developed rapid weight loss for which he received repeated psychiatric treatment; Kandisin abuse could only be stopped by administration of neuroleptic drugs for 3 months.

After discharge, the patient started using the sweetener once more, increasing the intake up to 600 pieces (22.08 g cyclamate)/d. He developed *diarrhea* with up to 10 watery stools per day, and weight loss. Because of hallucinations the patient required neuroleptic drugs and cyclamate abuse could then be reduced to 100 pieces/d. He was admitted to hospital.

Three months after stopping cyclamate intake he required no further dietary restrictions or medical treatment. Diarrhea disappeared resulting in increasing body weight.

The histological and radiological abnormalities of the small intestine and the malabsorption were completely reversible within 3 months after discontinuation of cyclamate.

Dacron arterial prostheses *(SED-11, 1034)*

Cases have been reported in the literature of non-anastomotic rupture of Dacron prostheses and investigations have been carried out into the late degeneration of Dacron fiber.

Recently, Magee and Teague (5[r]) reported 3 cases in which *rupture* of a Dacron prosthesis with false *aneurysm formation* had occurred.

In Case 1, a 61-year-old man had had an aortobifemoral graft carried out in 1972 for claudication due to aortoiliac stenotic disease. In 1986 false aneurysms were noted in both groins and the aortogram showed an unusual appearance of an aneurysm related to the right limb of the Dacron graft, as well as a small shadow near the left limb. A false aneurysm due to rupture of the Dacron prosthesis was found. It was replaced with a new knitted Dacron graft.

In Case 2, a 74-year-old female had an aortobifemoral bypass graft for aneurysmal disease inserted in 1978. She was referred in 1987 because of large false aneurysms in each groin. An aortogram suggested that there was a false aneurysm, very similar in appearance to that in the first case.

The last case was that of a 60-year-old man who had a Cooley double velour knited Dacron graft, inserted in 1976 for claudication. In 1987 he presented with a large pulsative swelling above the left knee. At operation there was a large pulsative hematoma, due to a split near the lower end of the Dacron graft. The graft was excised and replaced with another one.

Finally, Gossetti et al (6[c]) describe 389 surgical procedures employing autologous saphenous vein, polytetrafluoroethylene, Dacron (12 cases) and homologous saphenous vein. The results showed that Dacron prostheses had the highest incidence of *thrombosis*.

Disulfiram *(SED-11, 1039; SEDA-12, 417; SEDA-13, 475)*

Administration of disulfiram can produce *peripheral neuropathy* and the incidence may be higher than previously supposed if subclinical cases are taken into consideration. Pilliyath and Schwartz (7[R]) report a neurological study of 15 alcoholics, 32–61 years of age with no clinical evidence of peripheral neuropathy, on 250 mg/d treatment. The findings nevertheless indicated that a therapeutic dosage of disulfiram over 3 months produces electrophysiological changes in the peripheral nerves which are detectable if function is specifically tested.

In another study (8[r]) a 45-year-old man was hospitalized with a 6-month history of progressive leg weakness, associated with dysesthesias in the feet. Neurological examination revealed distal weakness in all 4 limbs. He had abused alcohol for 25 years and he was on disulfiram therapy at 500 mg/d, 18 months prior to admission. Disulfiram administration was discontinued and he was placed on folic acid therapy. Three months later, examination showed marked improvement in strength and sensation. The electrophysiological findings in the legs slightly improved.

Acheson and Howard (9[r]) report disulfiram *optic neuropathy* in a 54-year-old man who had progressive bilateral visual loss. He gave a 5-year history of medical treatment for alcohol dependency on 250 mg disulfiram/d, 5 times weekly but had taken no other medication. He was unable to read any of the Ishihara color test plates with either eye, and visual field analysis showed bilateral centrocecal scotomata, but all other ocular examinations were normal. He discontinued the treatment. Two months later a detailed examination showed no immunological, biochemical and hematological abnormalities. On examination the right and left visual acuities were again both 6/6 without correction, and he could read the Ishihara color test plates correctly.

Ethanol embolization

A case of infarction of the left testis secondary to transcatheter embolization of a malignant left renal tumor with absolute alcohol is reported by Siniluoto et al (10[C]).

A 53-year-old male was sent for urological examination because of intermittent gross hematuria. Multiple pulmonary metastases were seen on chest radiography. Intravenous urography showed a nonfunctioning left kidney, and ultrasonography and computed tomography showed a central left renal tumor with enlarged left para-aortic lymph nodes.

Palliative transcatheter embolization using the balloon occlusion technique was performed to control the hematuria. The smaller left renal artery was embolized with 6 ml of ethanol, and the larger artery with 12 ml of ethanol. The patient complained of slight flank pain during the embolization. The following night the left testis became painful and then tender and swollen. During follow-up the testis became smaller and at 4 months it was clearly atrophic. The patient died of progressive *pulmonary disease* 1 month later.

This is the first reported case of *testicular infarction* following ethanol embolization of a renal tumor, although colonic infarction following ethanol embolization of a renal tumor has been attributed primarily to a reflux of ethanol from the renal artery into the aorta (11[r]).

Intrauterine contraceptive devices (IUDs) *(SED-11, 1035; SEDA-13, 476)*

Experience in 600 IUD users is outlined by Calzolari et al (12[R]). The investigators indicate that in 21.8% of the cases this contraception technique had to be abandoned, and that the most common reason for IUD removal was *bleeding*. In this group, there were 18 pregnancies, 3 of them ectopic, as well as 4 cases of pelvic inflammatory disease. The failure rate was higher among the nulliparous women. Progesterone-containing IUDs were effective and well-tolerated, though it must be borne in mind that these were mostly used by multiparous women over 30 years of age.

In another case-report (13[r]) the tissue effects of IUDs containing copper were evaluated. Abnormal cells were observed on the surface of the device as well as in the endometrium. It is suggested that the copper ions escaping to the surface of the device may be responsible for the local endometrial damage.

Nicotine *(SED-11, 1042; SEDA-12, 418)*

Cigarette smoking is the principal source of nicotine intake, and the latter is a known cause of *tremor*, yet in the past the phenomenon has been poorly quantified. In a number of case-reports, the relation of nicotine to tremor has been examined in otherwise normal individuals. Lippold et al (14[c]) found that 30 of 35 normal subjects had a twofold increase in tremor when smoking one cigarette as compared with sham smoking (mimic smoking of an unlit cigarette). In another paper, Stiffman et al (15[r]) assessed tremor in 12 chronic smokers by measuring the current induced in a coil by a magnet attached to the finger. In uncontrolled observations, both smoking a cigarette and chewing 4 mg of nicotine gum increased 'tremometer' scores.

Marshall and Schneider (16[r]) studied the effect of intravenous nicotine in an uncontrolled manner in parkinsonian and essential tremor. They reported tremor increase in 5 parkinsonian patients within minutes after receiving 2 mg of nicotine. Four patients with essential tremor showed an increase after nicotine, but in a fifth the tremor was reduced.

Rautokorpi (17[r]) concluded from data taken from a questionnaire that smoking may exacerbate tremor in some cases of essential tremor and attenuate it in others. However, Zdonczyk et al (18[r]) indicate that nicotine, when investigated in a controlled study with patients receiving nicotine or chewing gum, does not lead to subjective changes in tremor sensitivity, either physiological or pathological.

Propylene glycol *(SED-11, 1042; SEDA-12, 103, 112; SEDA-13, 119)*

Propylene glycol-induced side effects have frequently been reported. More recently, Lolin et al (19[r]) described a case of propylene glycol poisoning in a 39-year-old woman which resulted in her admission to hospital in *status epilepticus*. The diagnosis of the poisoning resulted directly from the finding of a high plasma osmolal gap on admission. During the year following her discharge from the hospital, the patient had no further seizures. Plasma osmolality and the osmolal gap should clearly be considered as first-line investigations in patients presenting with metabolic acidosis and cerebral signs and symptoms.

In another study (20[r]) 28 patients (16 male, 12 female) aged 36–72 years, were administered intravenous nitroglycerin therapy containing propylene glycol as stock solution. Three of 28 patients developed *acute hemolysis* with elevated lactic dehydrogenase, bilirubin and free plasma hemoglobin; hemoglobinuria was present in 1/28 cases. In addition 6/28 patients had elevated lactate levels. Five of them had serious underlying conditions with hemodynamic instability and tissue hypoxia.

Sorbitol *(SED-11, 1038; SEDA-12, 307; SEDA-13, 339)*

A 55-year-old white male with mild mental retardation was admitted to hospital because of renal failure. He had previously been in good health and was taking no medication. On examination the urinary bladder was markedly distended and the prostate was markedly enlarged (21[r]). Since, after the diagnosis, continuous urinary catheter drainage was required, transurethral resection of the prostate (TURP) was performed under general anesthesia on the 13th hospital day. Large volumes of 3% sorbitol solution were used for urethral irrigation. Following the procedure, he developed symptomatic *hyponatremia*, but had only mild hypo-osmolality. The 'osmolal gap' was 47 mosmol/kg, probably from sorbitol absorbed systemically during TURP.

The presence of severe hyponatremia with only modest hypo-osmolality may occur in patients with renal failure following systemic absorption of hypotonic fluids containing solutes such as sorbitol mannitol. Hemodialysis offers the advantages of correcting the hyponatremia while removing the unmeasured solute, thus preventing rapid increases in serum osmolality.

Synthetic food coloring

In a study of 220 children referred for suspected '*hyperactivity*', 55 were subjected to a 6-week trial of the Feingold diet, which is free of artificial colorants. Forty demonstrated improved behavior and 26 remained improved following liberalization of the diet. However, the parents of the children claimed that a particular cluster of behavior was associated with the ingestion of foods containing synthetic colorants. A double-blind cross-over study using 8 of these children was therefore carried out. Subjects were maintained on a diet free from synthetic additives and were challenged daily for 18 weeks with either placebo or 50 mg of either tartrazine or carmoisine, each for 2 separate weeks. Two significant factors were identified whose behavioral pattern featured extreme *irritability, restlessness* and *sleep disturbance*. One of the reactors did not have inattention as a feature (22[CR]).

The findings raise the issue of whether the strict criteria for inclusion in studies concerned with hyperactivity based on 'attention deficit disorders' may miss children who indicate behavioral changes associated with the ingestion of food colorants.

Talc *(SED-11, 1036; SEDA-12, 33)*

Lange et al (23[r]) assessed as part of a still ongoing study the long-term effects on lung function of treatment of idiopathic spontaneous pneumothorax by talc poudrage or simple chest drainage. 114 patients were studied, 22–35 years of age, after their first pneumothorax with measurement of static and dynamic lung volumes. Of these 114 subjects, 80 had been treated with talc pleurodesis, and the rest with simple pleural drainage. 75 participated fully in the study.

The group treated with talc poudrage showed a mild *restrictive impairment of lung function* with a mean total lung capacity (TLC) of 89% of that predicted. In subjects treated with simple drainage mean TLC was 96% of that predicted. One patient treated with talc poudrage had extensive *pleural calcification* and a substantial reduction in lung function (TLC 58% predicted) with some evidence of lung fibrosis. None of the subjects had developed a mesothelioma. The authors conclude that talc poudrage may cause a mild restrictive impairment of lung function and pleural thickening on the chest radiograph.

Teflon(politef)-Proplast implants *(SED-11, 1034)*

Internal derangements of the temporomandibular joint (TMJ) are quite common and among recent popular surgical treatments is interposition of Teflon-Proplast implants.

In a recent case study, Kaplan et al (24[r]) report on 6 patients who had *osseous destructive changes* of the TMJ after placement of Teflon-Proplast implants for the treatment of internal derangements. The implants were surgically removed from all 6 joints, and foreign-body reactions were found to account for the radiographic appearance. The plain film radiographic features included simple or multiple osseous erosions of the mandibular condyle in all cases and of the temporal bone on the glenoid fossa in 2 cases. Some erosions were poorly defined, whereas other were well defined, either with or without sclerotic margins.

Table 1. *Miscellaneous reports*

Drug/Product	Complication	Ref. no.
Cyanamide	diffuse edematous and erythematous eruptions	25[c]
Ciclosporin A	serum creatinine increase (21 cases)	26[c]
Dialyzer membranes	leukopenia, hypoxemia	27[r]
Fluoride	reticuloendothelial malignancy (3 cases)	28[c]
Food allergies	respiration and cutaneous contamination	29[r]
Intraventricular catheters	leukoencephalopathy (10 cases)	30[r]
Mechanical aortic prosthesis	thrombosis (1 case)	31[c]
Mechanical valves	thromboembolic complications	32[c]
Medium-chain triglyceride diet	fatty infiltration (1 case)	33[c]
Resin restorations	lichenoid lesions (17 cases)	34[r]
Silicone breast prosthesis	hardening, discomfort, pain	35[c]
Sodium morrhuate sclerosant solution	fever, pneumonia (18 cases)	36[c]

Radiologists must be aware of this possible complication of alloplastic TMJ implants in order to suggest the diagnosis in the appropriate clinical setting.

MISCELLANEOUS

Other reports on miscellaneous drugs and their effects are listed in Table 1.

REFERENCES

1. Rau NR, Nagavaj MV, Prakash PS et al (1988) Fatal pulmonary aspiration of oral activated charcoal, *Br. Med. J., 297*, 918.
2. Danel V (1988) Fatal pulmonary aspiration of oral activated charcoal. *Br. Med. J., 297*, 684.
3. Anonymous (1989) Safety alert on homemade solutions for contact lens care. *FDA Drug Bull., 19*, 5.
4. Derfler K, Siegfried M, Herold C et al (1988) Reversible malabsorption caused by high doses of cyclamate. *Am. J. Med., 85*, 446.
5. Magee HR, Teague CA (1988) Late rupture of knitted velour Dacron arterial prosthesis. *Aust. NZ J. Surg., 58*, 549.
6. Gossetti B, Irase L, Intrieri F et al (1988) The salvage of the lower limbs: choice of the prosthetic material in femorodistal and axillofemoral bypass. *Ital. J. Surg. Sci., 18*, 69.
7. Pilliyath S, Schwartz BD (1988) Disulfiram neuropathy: electrophysiological study. *Electromyogr. Clin. Neurophysiol., 28*, 245.
8. Bergouignan FX, Vital C, Henry P et al (1988) Disulfiram neuropathy. *J. Neurol., 235*, 382.
9. Acheson JF, Howard RS (1988) Reversible optic neuropathy associated with disulfiram. *Neuroophthalmology, 8*, 175.
10. Siniluoto TMJ, Hellstrom PA, Paivansalo MJ et al (1988) Testicular infarction following ethanol embolization of a renal neoplasm. *Cardiovasc. Intervent. Cardiol., 11*, 162.
11. Cox GG, Lee KR, Price HI et al (1982) Colonic infarction following ethanol embolization of renal cell carcinoma. *Radiology, 145*, 343.
12. Calzolari E, Girolametti C, Parisi C et al (1988) Esperienze di contraccezione intrauterina. Rilievi su 600 utenti di IUD presso l'ospedale universitario S. Anna in Roma. *Minerva Ginecol., 40*, 317.
13. Patai K, Balogh I (1988) Clinicopathological problems of tissue effects caused by IUDs containing copper. *Mag. Noorv. Lapja, 51*, 240.
14. Lippold OC, Williams EJ, Wilson CG (1980) Finger tremor and cigarette smoking. *Br. J. Clin. Pharmacol., 10*, 83.

15. Stiffman SM, Gritz ER, Maltese J et al (1983) Effects of cigarette smoking and oral nicotine on hand tremor. *Clin. Pharmacol. Ther., 33*, 800.
16. Marshall J, Schneider H (1966) Effects of adrenaline, noradrenaline, atropine and nicotine on some types of human tremor. *J. Neurol. Neurosurg. Psychiatry, 29*, 214.
17. Rautokorpi I (1958) Essential tremor. An epidemiological clinical and genetic study. *Res. Rep. Dept. Neurol. Univ. Turku, Finland.*
18. Zdonczyk D, Royce V, Coller WC (1988) Nicotine and tremor. *Clin. J. Neuropharmacol., 11*, 282.
19. Lolin Y, Francis DA, Flanagan RJ et al (1988) Cerebral depression due to propylene glycol in a patient with chronic epilepsy. The value of the plasma osmolal gap in diagnosis. *Clin. Toxicol., 64*, 610.
20. Demey HE, Dealamans RA, Verpooten GA et al (1988) Propylene glycol-induced side effects during intravenous nitroglycerin therapy. *Intens. Care Med., 14*, 221.
21. Campell HT, Fincher ME, Sklar AH (1988) Severe hyponatremia without severe hypoosmolality following transurethral resection of the prostate (TURP) in end-stage renal disease. *Am. J. Kidney Dis., 12*, 152.
22. Rowe KS (1988) Synthetic food colouring and hyperactivity: a double-blind cross-over study. *Aust. Paediatr. J., 24*, 143.
23. Lange P, Mortensen J, Groth S (1988) Lung function 22 to 35 years after treatment of idiopathic spontaneous pneumothorax with talc poudrage or simple drainage. *Thorax, 43*, 559.
24. Kaplan PA, Ruskin JD, Tu HK et al (1988) Erosive arthritis of the temporomandibular joint caused by Teflon-Proplast implants. Plain film features. *Am. J. Radiol., 151*, 337.
25. Iwasa M, Matsumura T, Higashi N (1988) A case of drug eruption from cyanamide. *Skin Res., 30*, 348.
26. Deray G, Hoang Le P, Cacoub et al (1988) Renal function and blood pressure in patients treated with cyclosporin A for uveitis. *Eur. J. Clin. Pharmacol., 34*, 601.
27. Wiegmann TB, MacDougall ML, Diederich DA (1988) Dialysis leukopenia, hypoxemia and anaphylatoxin formation: effect of membrane, bath and citrate anticoagulation. *Am. J. Kidney Dis., 11*, 418.
28. Smith G (1988) Genotoxic effects of fluoride and implications for its use in the treatment of osteoporosis. *NZ J. Med., 101*, 213.
29. Gervais P, Gervais A (1988) Respiratory and cutaneous contaminants and food allergies. Consequences for prevention and treatment. *Sem. Hôp., 64*, 2482.
30. Lemann W, Wiley R, Posner JB (1988) Leukoencephalopathy complicating intraventricular catheters: clinical, radiographic and pathologic study of 10 cases. *J. Neuro-Oncol., 6*, 67.
31. Sadoun N, Komajda M, Drobinski G et al (1988) Early postoperative thrombosis of an aortic Saint-Jude prosthesis. Success of fibrinolitic therapy. *Ann. Cardiol. Angeiol., 37*, 365.
32. Perier P, Deloche A, Chauvaud S et al (1988) Clinical comparison of mitral valve replacement using porcine, Starr, and Björk valves. *J. Cardiac Surg., 3*, 359.
33. Beverley D, Arthur R (1988) Fatty liver and medium chain trygliceride (MCT) diet. *Arch. Dis. Child., 63*, 840.
34. Lind P (1988) Oral lichenoid reactions related to composite restorations. *Acta Odontol. Scand., 46*, 64.
35. Anonymous (1989) Safety of silicone breast prostheses. *FDA Drug Bull., 19(1)*, 2.
36. De Puey EG, Richards WO, Millikan WJ et al (1988) Scintigraphic detection of pulmonary embolization of esophageal variceal sclerosant. *Endoscopy, 20*, 91.

International drug monitoring*

For two decades an international collaboration in monitoring adverse drug reactions, under the auspices of the World Health Organization, has been in operation. The program started in 1968 as a pilot project with the participation of 10 countries. The intent was to render it easier through international collaboration to detect adverse drug reactions not revealed during clinical trials. Some years later, the Swedish government assumed operational and financial responsiblity for the program and a WHO Collaborating Centre for International Drug Monitoring was created in Uppsala.

The system is today based on the interchange of adverse reaction information between national drug monitoring centres in 28 countries (listed on pp. 461–465). Collectively these centres annually provide 60000–70000 individual reports of reactions suspected of being drug-induced. The cumulative database that has been constructed from these reports now comprises over 660000 records (Fig. 1).

In each country it is the national centre which processes and evaluates adverse reaction reports, sent to them either from medical professionals or in some countries from pharmaceutical manufacturers. Information obtained from these reports is passed back to the medical profession on a national basis, but also contributes to drug experience at the international level.

The collected material in the WHO database is screened 4 times a year for new and serious reactions and the reporting frequencies of associations of particular interest chosen by national centres or by WHO Collaborating Centre staff. In addition, the national centres receive an annual reference document containing summary data on all suspected reactions reported to the WHO program.

The main aim of the international program, i.e. the early identification of new adverse reactions, has been re-emphasized during the last few years. At the start of the program it was hoped that by applying carefully designed statistical analysis to the large amount of data available, it would be possible to identify new, unexpected reactions of medical significance. However, a purely statistical approach does not identify important clinical problems; a combination of automatic signalling devices and scanning of the data by experienced medical personnel is crucial to successful interpretation. The review of adverse reaction signals has been intensified during the last few years by the appointment of reviewers in national centres to analyze reactions pertaining to particular body systems. Short summaries of their findings are circulated to participating national centres. The succes of the signalling function is also dependent on a speedy input of reports from national centres to the WHO Collaborating Centre. One of the main objectives at the moment is to reduce delay in this input as much as possible.

The increased communication between national centres during the past few years has resulted in a number of publications in medical journals. The focal point of the analyses behind many of these publications is the WHO database. There are plans to intensify research activities on the basis of the WHO register. The intention is that interested researchers would stay at the WHO Collaborating Centre for short periods to study specific drug-related problems.

An important part of the Centre's activities is also to act in other ways as a communication centre – a clearing house for information on drug safety at the service of drug regulatory agencies.

---

* Contributed by Prof. Kjell Strandberg, on behalf of the WHO Collaborating Centre for International Drug Monitoring, Uppsala, Sweden. Director of the Centre: Prof. I.R. Edwards.

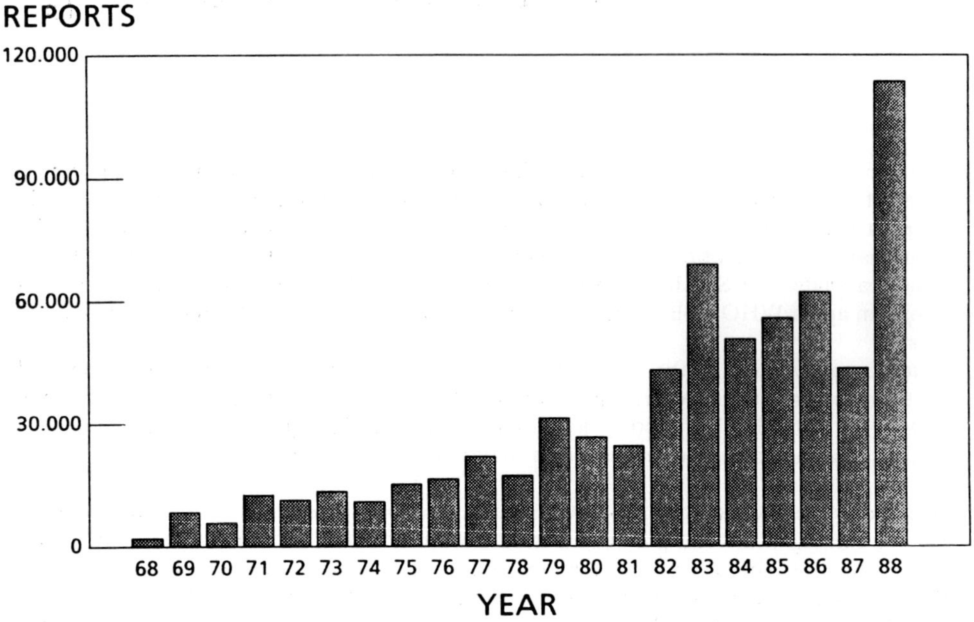

Fig. 1. Number of reports processed at the WHO Collaborating Centre for International Drug Monitoring, Uppsala, Sweden.

Requests for special database searches and investigations are also accepted by the Centre from participating national centres. Through searches in the WHO register, direct communication can be established between centres with a similar drug problem. The fastest way for a national centre to gain access to international experience is through an on-line connection to the WHO Centre computer.

Since 1982, the WHO Collaborating Centre has been distributing an *Adverse Reactions Newsletter* to participating centres, with reviews of national adverse reaction bulletins and news of drug problems being investigated in the various countries, supplemented with figures from the WHO register.

Finally, the WHO program has assumed responsibility for developing a standardized adverse reaction terminology and a comprehensive index of reported drugs, both of which have a utility beyond their importance to the monitoring system.

Address list of national centres participating in the WHO drug monitoring scheme

Australia	
Dr J. McEwen Secretary Tel. +61 62 897605 Telex 71 62149 Telefax +61 62 816946	Drug Evaluation Support Branch Department of Community Services and Health P.O. Box 9848 CANBERRA ACT 2601 Australia
Belgium	
Mr J. Allard General Inspector Tel. +32 2 2104909 Telex 46 25768	Centre National de Pharmacovigilance Ministère-de la Santé Publique et de la Famille Inspection Générale de la Pharmacie Cité Administrative de l'Etat Quartier Vésale 1010 BRUSSELS Belgium
Bulgaria	
Prof. P. Zikolov Director Tel. +359 2 446566 Telex 67 22430	Committee on Adverse Reactions to Drugs Institute for State Control of Drugs 26 Buld 'VI Zaimov' 1040 SOFIA Bulgaria
Canada	
Dr E. Napke Chief Tel. +1 613 9570337 Telex 21 0533679 Telefax +1 613 9527767	Product Related Desease Division Bureau of Pharmaceutical Evaluation Health Protection Branch Health and Welfare Finance Annex Building Tunney's Pasture OTTAWA Ontario K1A OL2 Canada
Czechoslovakia	
Dr H. Fouskova Tel. +42 2 722751 Telex 66 122662	Committee on Adverse Drug Reactions State Institute for Drug Control Srobarova 48 100 41 PRAGUE Czechoslovakia

Denmark	
Prof. J. Schou Ms I. Kovacs, M.Sc. Tel. +45 2 943773 Telex 55 35333 Telefax +45 2 847077	Pharmaceutical Laboratories National Board of Health Frederikssundsvej 378 DK-2700 BRØNSHØJ Denmark
Finland	
Dr E. Alhava Medical Officer Tel. +358 0 7723254	National Board of Health Siltasaarenkatu 18 A SF-00530 HELSINKI Finland
France	
Prof. P. Ambroise-Thomas Tel. +33 1 40566000 +33 1 40565359 Telex 42 250001359	Direction de la Pharmacie et du Médicament Ministère de la Solidarité, de la Santé et de la Protection 1 Place de Fontenoy F-75 700 PARIS France
Prof. R.J. Royer Tel. +33 83 576161 Ext. 1758 Ext. 1759 Telex 42 960561 SANTSEC 250011 F	Commission Nationale de Pharmacovigilance Centre Hospitalier Universitaire 29 ave de Lattre de Tassigny P.O. Box CO 34 F-54037 NANCY France
Federal Republic of Germany	
Dr G. Kreutz Head Tel. +49 30 4502311 Telex 004117 308062 Telex +49 30 4502207	Division of Drug Experience Institute für Arzneimittel des Bundesgesundheitsamtes P.O. Box 33 00 13 D-1000 BERLIN Federal Republik of Germany
Dr K. Kimbel Secretary-General Tel. +49 221 4004350 Telex 41 8882161 Telefax +49 221 4004266	Drug Commission of the German Medical Profession P.O. Box 41 01 25 D-5000 KÖLN Federal Republic of Germany
Iceland	
Dr O. Olafsson Director Tel. +354 91 27555 Telex 501 2050 or 2225	Directorate-General of Public Health Laugavegur 116 IS-105 REYKJAVIK Iceland

Indonesia

Dr Andajaningsih
Chairman
Tel. +62 21 415459
Telex 73 46142

National Centre for Monitoring of Adverse Drug Reactions
Directorate General of FDA
Ministry of Health
Jalan Percetakan Negara 23
JAKARTA
Indonesia

Ireland

Ms N. Arthur
Tel. +353 1 7649717
Telex 500 90542

Adverse Reaction Section
National Drugs Advisory Board
63-64 Adelaide Road
DUBLIN 2
Ireland

Israel

Dr D. Hemo, M.Sc. Pharm.
Tel. +972 2 782508
or 692344
Telex 606 25206

Department of Clinical Pharmacology
Drug Monitoring Centre (MOH)
2 Ben Tabai St.
P.O.B. 1176
JERUSALEM 91010
Israel

Italy

Prof. D. Poggiolini
General Director
Tel. +39 65 925863
Telex 43 625205
Telefax +39 65 924774

Pharmaceutical Division
Ministry of Health
Viale della Civiltà Romana, 7
I-00144 ROMA
Italy

Prof. L. Rossini
Tel. +39 71 5893636
Telex 43 561838
Telefax +39 71 5893324

WHO-ITA
University of Ancona Medical School
Via Ranieri Monte d'Ago
I-60100 ANCONA
Italy

Japan

Dr T. Ebihara
Director
Tel. +81 3 5014507
Telex 72 02225132
Telefax +81 3 5084364

Pharmaceuticals and Chemicals Safety Division
Ministry of Health and Welfare
2-2, 1-Chome, Kasumigaseki
Chiyoda-Ku
TOKYO
Japan

Netherlands

Dr R.H.B. Meyboom
Head
Tel. +31 70 406793
Telex 44 31680
Telefax +31 70 405048

Netherlands Centre for Monitoring of Adverse Reactions
to Drugs
P.O. Box 5406
2280 HK RIJSWIJK
Netherlands

New Zealand

Director	National Toxicology Group
Tel. +64 24 740999	University of Otago Medical School
ext. 8345	P.O. Box 913
Telex 74 5706	DUNEDIN
Telefax +64 24 770509	New Zealand

Norway

Ms K. Myhr	Adverse Drug Reaction Section
Tel. +47 2 257550	Norwegian Medicines Control Authority
Telex 56 72400	Sven Oftedals vei 6
Telefax +47 2 257454	N-0950 OSLO 9
	Norway

Poland

Dr A. Czarnecki	Centre for Monitoring of Adverse Effects of Drugs
Head	Institute for Drug Research and Control
Tel. +48 22 416742	30/34 Chelmska Street
	00-725 WARSZAWA
	Poland

Romania

Prof. C. Baloescu	Institute for State Control of Drugs and Pharmaceutical
Director	Research
Tel. +40 0 666070	Str. Aviator Sanatescu 48, Sector 1
Telex 65 11595	850510 BUCHAREST
	Romania

Spain

Prof. J.R. Laporte	Secció de Farmacologia Clinica
Tel. +34 3 3582852	Universitat Autònoma de Barcelona
Telex 52 97341	Ciutat Sanitària de la Vall d'Hebron
Telefax (man.):	P. Vall d'Hebron, s.n
34 3 3582711	08035 BARCELONA
	Spain

Sweden

Dr B.E. Wiholm	Adverse Drug Reaction Section
Tel. +46 18 174600	Division of Drug Epidemiology and Information
Telex 76059	Department of Drugs
Telefax +46 18 148566	National Board of Health and Welfare
	P.O. Box 607
	S-751 25 UPPSALA
	Sweden

Thailand

Dr P. Pothisiri	Drug Information Center and NADRM
Director	Food and Drug Administration
Tel. +66 282 9967	Ministry of Public Health
Telex 86 82573	Devaves Palace
	BANGKOK 10200
	Thailand

Turkey

Ms S. Öksüz
Chemist
Tel. +90 41 1314829
Telex 42770
Telefax +90 41 1314829

Adverse Drug Reactions Monitoring Centre
Directorate of Pharmaceuticals
Ministry of Health and Social Ass.
Sihhiye, ANKARA
Turkey

United Kingdom

Dr S.M. Wood
Principal Medical Officer
Tel. +44 1 7202188
Telex 51 883669
Telefax +44 1 7205647

Committee on Safety of Medicines
Market Towers
1 Nine Elms Lane
LONDON SW8 5NQ
United Kingdom

United States of America

Dr G. Faich
Director
Tel. +1 301 4434227
Telex 23 898488
Telefax +1 301 4432763

Office of Epidemiology and Biostatics (HFD-700)
Food and Drug Administration
5600 Fishers Lane
ROCKVILLE
Maryland 20857
U.S.A.

Yugoslavia

Prof B. Vrhovac
Tel. +38 41 213861
Telex 62 21252

Section of Clinical Pharmacology
Department of Medicine
University Hospital Rebro, Medical School
12, Kispatićeva
41000 ZAGREB
Yugoslavia

WHO-HQ

Dr John F. Dunne
Tel. +41 22 7912111
Telex 45 27821
Telefax +41 22 910746

World Health Organization Pharmaceuticals
CH-1211 GENEVA 27
Switzerland

Index of drugs

Page numbers in **bold** type indicate where a given drug is discussed in detail.

Index of side effects

The index is divided according to the system or phenomenon involved into the following principal classes:

Abuse/Dependence/Intoxication
Allergic/Immunologic disturbances
Blood disturbances
Cardiovascular disturbances
Ear/Nose/Throat disorders
Endocrinopathy
Eye disorders
Gastrointestinal disorders
Liver/Gallbladder disorders
Metabolic/Nutritional disorders
Miscellaneous
Muscle/Bone diseases
Nervous system disorders
Pharmacogenetics/Pharmacokinetics
Psychic disturbances
Reproductive system/Breast disorders
Respiratory tract disorders
Second-generation effects
Skin disorders
Tumor induction
Urinary tract disorders

The following is a list of the primary (**bold**) entries with the principal class headings under which they can be found:

abdominal pain – gastrointestinal disorders
abortion – reproductive system/breast disorders
abscess – miscellaneous
abuse – abuse/dependence/intoxication
acute kidney failure – urinary tract disorders
adrenal dysfunction – endocrinopathy
adrenal insufficiency – endocrinopathy
aggression – psychic disturbances
agitation – psychic disturbances
agranulocytosis – blood disturbances
air embolism – miscellaneous
airway resistance – respiratory tract disorders
akathisia – nervous system disorders
alopecia – skin disorders
amnesia – nervous system disorders
anaphylactic reaction – allergic/immunologic disturbances
anaphylactic shock – allergic/immunologic disturbances
anemia – blood disturbances
angina pectoris – cardiovascular disturbances
angioedema – allergic/immunologic disturbances
anorexia – gastrointestinal disorders
antibody formation – allergic/immunologic disturbances
antinuclear antibody/SLE – allergic/immunologic disturbances
anxiety – psychic disturbances
aplastic anemia – blood disturbances
apnea – respiratory tract disorders
arthralgia – muscle/bone diseases
arthritis – muscle/bone diseases
arthropathy – muscle/bone diseases

ABUSE/DEPENDENCE/INTOXICATION

ALLERGIC/IMMUNOLOGIC DISTURBANCES

BLOOD DISTURBANCES

CARDIOVASCULAR DISTURBANCES

EAR/NOSE/THROAT DISORDERS

ENDOCRINOPATHY

EYE DISORDERS

GASTROINTESTINAL DISORDERS

LIVER/GALLBLADDER DISORDERS

METABOLIC/NUTRITIONAL DISORDERS

MISCELLANEOUS

MUSCLE/BONE DISEASES

NERVOUS SYSTEM DISORDERS

PHARMACOGENETICS/PHARMACOKINETICS

PSYCHIC DISTURBANCES

REPRODUCTIVE SYSTEM/BREAST DISORDERS

RESPIRATORY TRACT DISORDERS

SECOND-GENERATION EFFECTS

SKIN DISORDERS

TUMOR INDUCTION

URINARY TRACT DISORDERS